16.99

KT-464-369

Jim Stoppani's
ENCYCLOPEDIA OF MUSCLE & STRENGTH

SECOND EDITION

JIM STOPPANI, PHD

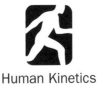

Human Kinetics

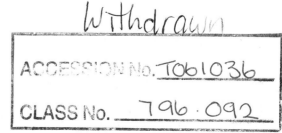

Withdrawn

ACCESSION No. TO61036

CLASS No. 796.092

16.99

Library of Congress Cataloging-in-Publication Data

Stoppani, James, 1968-
  [Encyclopedia of muscle & strength]
  Jim Stoppani's encyclopedia of muscle & strength / Jim Stoppani. -- Second Edition.
     pages cm.
  Includes bibliographical references and index.
  1. Weight training. 2. Bodybuilding. 3. Muscle strength. I. Title. II. Title: Jim Stoppani's encyclopedia of muscle and strength.
  GV546.S74 2014
  613.7'13--dc23

                         2014024299

ISBN: 978-1-4504-5974-7 (print)

Copyright © 2015, 2006 by Jim Stoppani

All rights reserved. Except for use in a review, the reproduction or utilization of this work in any form or by any electronic, mechanical, or other means, now known or hereafter invented, including xerography, photocopying, and recording, and in any information storage and retrieval system, is forbidden without the written permission of the publisher.

This publication is written and published to provide accurate and authoritative information relevant to the subject matter presented. It is published and sold with the understanding that the author and publisher are not engaged in rendering legal, medical, or other professional services by reason of their authorship or publication of this work. If medical or other expert assistance is required, the services of a competent professional person should be sought.

The web addresses cited in this text were current as of June 2014, unless otherwise noted.

Acquisitions Editor: Justin Klug; **Senior Managing Editor:** Amy Stahl; **Associate Managing Editor:** Anne Mrozek; **Copyeditor:** Jan Feeney; **Indexer:** Michael Ferreira; **Permissions Manager:** Martha Gullo; **Graphic Designer:** Nancy Rasmus; **Cover Designer:** Keith Blomberg; **Photograph (cover):** Pavel Ythjall; **Photographs (interior):** Neil Bernstein, unless otherwise noted; figures 4.1, 4.7, 4.9, 4.14, 4.15, 4.32, and 4.37 courtesy of Jim Stoppani; figure 4.35 courtesy of Power Plate North America, Inc.; figure 4.36 courtesy of Robert Q. Riley Enterprises; **Visual Production Assistant:** Joyce Brumfield; **Photo Production Manager:** Jason Allen; **Art Manager:** Kelly Hendren; **Associate Art Manager:** Alan L. Wilborn; **Illustrations:** © Human Kinetics, unless otherwise noted; **Printer:** Sheridan Books

We thank Metroflex Gym in Long Beach, California, for assistance in providing the location for the photo shoot for this book.

Human Kinetics books are available at special discounts for bulk purchase. Special editions or book excerpts can also be created to specification. For details, contact the Special Sales Manager at Human Kinetics.

Printed in the United States of America   10 9 8 7 6 5 4 3 2 1

The paper in this book is certified under a sustainable forestry program.

Human Kinetics
Website: www.HumanKinetics.com

United States: Human Kinetics
P.O. Box 5076
Champaign, IL 61825-5076
800-747-4457
e-mail: humank@hkusa.com

Canada: Human Kinetics
475 Devonshire Road Unit 100
Windsor, ON N8Y 2L5
800-465-7301 (in Canada only)
e-mail: info@hkcanada.com

Europe: Human Kinetics
107 Bradford Road
Stanningley
Leeds LS28 6AT, United Kingdom
+44 (0) 113 255 5665
e-mail: hk@hkeurope.com

Australia: Human Kinetics
57A Price Avenue
Lower Mitcham, South Australia 5062
08 8372 0999
e-mail: info@hkaustralia.com

New Zealand: Human Kinetics
P.O. Box 80
Torrens Park, South Australia 5062
0800 222 062
e-mail: info@hknewzealand.com

E6002

Jim Stoppani's

ENCYCLOPEDIA OF MUSCLE & STRENGTH

SECOND EDITION

CONTENTS

PART I

TRAINING ESSENTIALS

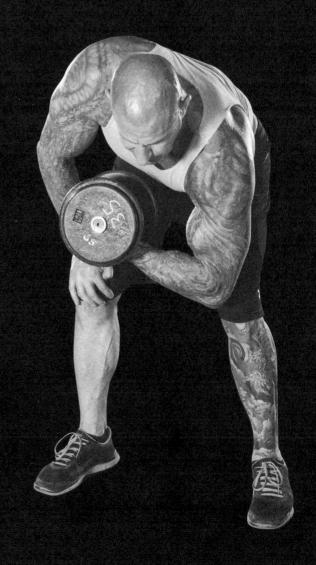

Strength training can be traced back to the beginning of recorded time. As early as 2000 b.c.e., the ancient Egyptians lifted sacks of sand to strength-train for hunting and military duty. According to military records, the Chinese also used strength training for their military personnel as early as 700 b.c.e. But the historical association that most people are familiar with is the ancient Greeks. Many of the athletes who competed in the ancient Olympics lifted heavy stones to develop strength and boost their athletic performance. Besides those functional results, strength training provided the development of a muscular physique. This masculine physique was honored in classic Greek art and writing. In fact, it may be the ancient Greek culture's celebration of muscle that is responsible for spawning the modern sport of bodybuilding. Several famous athletes during that period, such as Milo and Heracles, often performed feats of strength and displayed their muscularity to spectators. In the 19th century, the appreciation by the masses for heavily muscled physiques made celebrities out of many performing strongmen of that time. The most famous was Eugen Sandow, who is considered the father of bodybuilding.

Despite the fact that humans have a longstanding fascination with strength and muscularity, the concept of strength training is one that few have familiarized themselves with. Even during the fitness boom of the 1970s in the United States, most Americans participated in some form of aerobic exercise but neglected the strength component of physical fitness. Over the years, with help from pioneers of strength training (such as Bob Hoffman, Joe Weider, and Charles Atlas) and through advances in research on the developing science of resistance training, strength became viewed as a necessary component of physical fitness and athletic performance. And participation in strength training grew faster than participation in any other physical activity.

As the popularity of strength training grew, so did awareness that this practice was a complicated science that participants must fully understand in order to reap the true benefits. That is why part I of this book is so important for anyone interested in strength training at any level. Unless you clearly understand the principles of strength training, you will never fully comprehend how to implement an effective strength training program.

So before you skip ahead to one of the strength training programs in parts II, III, and IV, be sure you have a decent grasp of the fundamentals presented in these first four chapters. Armed with this background, you will have a much fuller understanding of the exercises, techniques, and programs presented in the other chapters. You also will be more capable of individualizing these techniques to create specialized programs for yourself and for others.

CHAPTER 1

Core Concepts

Strength training is performed by a wide range of people for a variety of reasons. Most are interested in gaining muscle strength and muscle mass with a concomitant loss of body fat. In addition, many people expect these physical adaptations to carry over into improvements in performance of athletic endeavors and daily life activities. Strength training can provide these adaptations as long as you follow certain principles, which are discussed here to help you realize your strength training goals. These principles are integral to understanding how strength training works, how to individualize it to meet your needs and goals, and how to change it to continue making adaptations as you progress.

In addition to understanding the concepts of strength training, you must be familiar with the terminology that is often used in discussions of strength training. Having the ability to understand and use this lexicon will help you to learn the fundamentals of strength training and to communicate with others who participate in strength training. To familiarize yourself with this vocabulary, refer to the glossary at the end of this book.

Before we can discuss the principles of strength training, we must define the major terms that will be discussed throughout this book. First and foremost is the actual term *strength training*. If you've done a fair share of reading on the topic of strength training—be it on the Internet, in magazines, or in other books—you've probably discovered that the terms *strength training, weight training,* and *resistance training* are often used interchangeably. While there are definite similarities in the three terms, a more precise interpretation of the definitions points out the differences. *Resistance training* is the broadest of the three terms. It describes any type of training in which the body must move in some direction against some type of force that resists that movement. This could include lifting free weights, pushing against a hydraulic apparatus, or running up a set of stairs. *Strength training* is a type of resistance training (although not all types of resistance training are strength training). Specifically, strength training refers to any type of training that involves the body moving in some direction against a force that specifically induces changes in muscle strength or hypertrophy (muscle growth). This could include lifting free weights or moving against a hydraulic apparatus, but not running up a set of stairs. *Weight training* is also a type of resistance training and can be a type of strength training. By strict terms of its definition, it refers to any type of training in which the body moves in some direction against a force that resists that movement and is supplied by some type of weight. This could include free weights and weight machines but not training with a hydraulic apparatus or running up a set of stairs. See table 1.1 for a list of training methods that are categorized under each of these types of training.

This book covers strength training (most of it will be weight training), because it best describes the types of training that we are interested in—exercise that involves the body moving against a force in an effort to induce changes in muscle strength or hypertrophy.

TABLE 1.1   Categories and Methods of Training

Type of training	Sample training methods
Resistance training	Free weights (including common objects) Weight machines (linear guided, cable or pulley system, cam based) Hydraulic machines Pneumatic machines Isokinetic machines Body-weight training Sled dragging Parachute running
Strength training	Free weights (including common objects) Weight machines (linear guided, cable or pulley system, cam based) Hydraulic machines Pneumatic machines Body-weight training
Weight training	Free weights (including common objects) Weight machines (linear guided, cable or pulley system, cam based)

DEFINITIONS OF STRENGTH

The basic definition of *strength* is the maximal amount of force a muscle or muscle group can generate in a specified movement pattern at a specified velocity (speed) of movement (Knuttgen and Kraemer 1987). But defining strength is not that simple. That's because strength has many manifestations. The following definitions are all forms of strength.

absolute strength—The maximal amount of force a muscle can produce when all inhibitory and protective mechanisms are removed. Because of this, it is rare that a person could ever demonstrate his or her **absolute** strength. This can take place only under extreme measures such as during an emergency, under hypnosis, or with certain ergogenic aids.

maximal strength—The maximal amount of force a muscle or muscle groups can produce in a specific exercise for one repetition. This is also referred to as *one-repetition maximum,* or *1RM.* Some estimate that the 1RM usually amounts to only about 80 percent of absolute strength. This type of strength is important for powerlifters.

relative strength—The ratio between a person's maximal strength and his or her body weight. This is important when comparing the strength of athletes who are much different in body size. Relative strength is determined by dividing the 1RM by the body weight of the person. For

example, a 200-pound (91-kilogram) athlete who can bench-press 400 pounds (400 ÷ 200 = 2) has the same relative strength as a 100-pound (45-kilogram) athlete who can bench-press 200 pounds (200 ÷ 100 = 2). This type of strength is important for powerlifters as well as for football players and other strength athletes who are often compared with other teammates as a means of predicting performance on the field.

speed strength—The ability to move the body or an object quickly. This term is more commonly known as *power*. This type of strength is important for most sports but is most critical in track and field events such as the shot put, javelin, and long jump.

starting strength—The ability to generate a sharp rise in power during the initial phase of the movement. This type of strength is important in Olympic weightlifting, deadlifts, boxing, martial arts, and offensive line positions in football, where strength must be generated immediately.

acceleration strength—The ability to continue the sharp rise in power throughout most of the movement of the exercise. This type of strength takes over after starting strength and is important for sports such as judo, wrestling, and sprinting.

endurance strength—The ability to maintain force production for a longer time or through multiple repetitions of an exercise. This type of strength is important in wrestling, cycling, swimming, and training for bodybuilding.

Considering these numerous types of strength that a person can train for specifically, it's easy to understand that the term *strength training* encompasses many types of training approaches. Regardless of whether you are training for maximal strength, power, or endurance strength, you are following some form of strength training. Each of these types of strength is developed with the use of resistance of some type, be it free weights, machines, or body weight. Although this book focuses on strength training for muscle mass and strength, as well as fat loss, other muscle adaptations can take place with the use of strength training.

TYPES OF MUSCLE ACTION

During a typical strength training session, muscles may contract from tens to hundreds of times to move the body or the implement they are training with. Neural stimulation of the muscle causes the contractile units of the muscle to attempt to shorten. But contraction does not always involve shortening of the muscle fibers. Depending on the load and the amount of force supplied by the muscle, three different muscle actions may occur during a muscle contraction (see figure 1.1):

1. *Concentric muscle action.* This type of muscle action occurs when the muscle force exceeds the external resistance, resulting in joint movement as the muscle shortens. In other words, concentric contractions are those in which the muscle fibers shorten while contracting to lift the weight. This is demonstrated by the upward phase of a biceps curl and is often referred to as the *positive phase of the repetition.*

2. *Eccentric muscle action.* This type of muscle action occurs when the external resistance exceeds the force supplied by the muscle, resulting in joint movement as the muscle lengthens. Eccentric muscle actions are demonstrated by the downward phase of the biceps curl. This is often referred to as the *negative portion of the repetition.* Even though the fibers are lengthening, they're also in a state of contraction, permitting the weight to return to the starting position in a controlled manner.

3. *Isometric muscle action.* This type of muscle action occurs when the muscle

contracts without moving, generating force while its length remains static. Isometric muscle actions are demonstrated in an attempt to lift an immovable object or an object that is too heavy to move. The muscle fibers contract in an attempt to move the weight, but the muscle does not shorten in overall length because the object is too heavy to move.

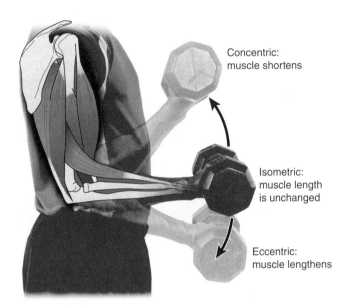

Concentric:
muscle shortens

Isometric:
muscle length
is unchanged

Eccentric:
muscle lengthens

FIGURE 1.1 Major types of muscle actions: concentric, isometric, *and* eccentric.

Among strength training scientists there is much debate about the importance of each of these types of muscle actions regarding increases in strength and muscle mass. Studies have been conducted in an effort to determine whether one type of muscle action is most important for enhancing muscle strength and mass. Because it is possible to produce greater force during eccentric and isometric muscle actions as compared to concentric muscle actions, it has been hypothesized that these muscle actions may be more important than concentric muscle actions for inducing changes in muscle strength and size.

Researchers have found that training with isometric muscle actions can increase muscle strength and size (Fleck and Schutt 1985). However, the strength gains from isometric training are realized only during the specific joint angles at which the muscles were trained. In other words, if someone trains isometrically on the bench press at the point halfway between the start and finish, that person will gain muscle strength only at that specific point in the exercise. This would not equate to greater overall strength in the bench press unless a variety of joint angles between the start and finish were also trained isometrically. Therefore, while isometric training can be beneficial, concentric and eccentric muscle actions should also be included for better overall muscle adaptations. For a sample training program that uses isometric muscle actions, see Static Strength Training in chapter 9.

Because it is possible to overload a muscle more during eccentric muscle contractions, these contractions cause more muscle damage. It has been hypothesized that this greater overload can induce greater gains in strength. Indeed, research has shown that eccentric-only training does induce significant strength gains; however, this training appears to offer no greater strength benefit than concentric-only training. Therefore, to maximize muscle adaptations, strength training programs need to incorporate both concentric and eccentric muscle actions. For sample training programs that incorporate eccentric training, see Negative Repetitions in chapter 6 and Negative-Rep Strength Training in chapter 9.

The use of concentric, eccentric, and isometric muscle actions in strength training will yield somewhat different adaptations. Although isometric muscle actions can improve strength and muscle size to some degree, they provide mainly static strength. This does not necessarily carry over to dynamic strength used for most sports. Therefore, most strength training programs should focus on concentric and eccentric muscle actions. Greater improvements in strength and muscle mass can be achieved when repetitions include both concentric and eccentric muscle actions.

Another type of muscle action that should be considered here is called *voluntary maximal muscle action*. This type of muscle action does not refer to the actual movement of the muscle but to the intensity of the resistance. When a muscle undergoes a voluntary maximal muscle action, it is moving against as much resistance as its current fatigue level will allow. Regardless of how many repetitions are performed in a set— whether it be 1 or 10—it is the last repetition, when momentary concentric muscle failure is reached, that is considered the voluntary maximal muscle action. In other words, not another single repetition can be performed. This is also referred

to as the *repetition maximum (RM)* and is usually represented with a number preceding the RM. For example, 1RM would represent the amount of weight that induces a voluntary maximal muscle action with one repetition. A 10RM is the amount of weight that induces a voluntary maximal muscle action on the 10th repetition.

PRINCIPLES OF STRENGTH TRAINING

Countless principles of strength training are being employed today. But the validity of many of these principles is questionable, because few strength training professionals agree on the majority of them. However, there are a few principles that are revered by all strength training professionals: the principle of specificity, the principle of progressive overload, the principle of individuality, the principle of variation, the principle of maintenance, and the principle of reversibility. So important are these principles that few would argue against their being considered laws of strength training.

principle of specificity—One of the seminal principles in designing strength training programs. It is often referred to as SAID, which stands for "specific adaptation to imposed demands." In its most basic definition, it means to train in a specific manner to produce a specific outcome. For instance, if the immediate goal is to increase 1RM strength, then training with the appropriate range of repetition, proper rest periods, and apposite frequency to optimize strength gains is a necessity. Or if the goal is to increase athletic performance in a specific sport, the exercises should mimic the types of movements performed in the sport, and they should be performed at a similar speed as those movements. This principle is one of the most important in strength training because if it is not being met, all other principles are negated.

principle of progressive overload—The practice of continually increasing the intensity of the workout as the muscle becomes accustomed to that intensity level. This can be done by increasing the weight lifted, the number of repetitions performed, or the total number of sets; or it can be done by decreasing the rest between sets. Continually increasing the stress placed on the muscle allows the muscle to increase its strength and prevents stagnation. This is one of the most critical principles of strength training as well as one of the earliest developed. This principle was established just after World War II by the research of DeLorme (1945) and DeLorme and Watkins (1948). Without providing the muscles with progressive overload, continual adaptations in muscle strength and size would cease. For example, at the start of a strength training program, performing three sets of 10 reps on the bench press with 135 pounds may be a challenge. After several weeks of training, performing three sets of 10 reps on the bench press with 135 pounds will become easy. At this stage, training adaptations will cease unless the weight is increased above 135 pounds, the reps are increased above 10 reps, the sets are increased to more than three, or the rest between sets is decreased.

principle of individuality—The theory that any training program must consider the specific needs or goals and abilities of the person for whom it is designed. For example, a beginning bodybuilder with the goal of adding muscle mass would have a much different training program than an advanced bodybuilder with the same goal. The difference in their training programs is based not on their desired training outcomes but on their training experiences. The advanced trainer would require more volume and high-intensity training techniques to reach the same goal as the beginner. On the other hand, an advanced lifter who has the goal of gaining muscle mass would train much differently than an advanced lifter with the goal of gaining muscle strength. Here the difference in their training programs is based on their different goals. In general, the advanced lifter with the goal of gaining more muscle strength would train with fewer reps, heavier weight, and lower volume than the advanced lifter with the muscle mass goal.

principle of variation—The simple fact that no matter how effective a program is, it will be effective only for a short period. Once a person has experienced the specific adaptations that a particular training program is designed to provide, a new stimulus must be imposed on the muscles or continued progress will be stagnated. This is the foundation of periodization (discussed in chapter 3) and is the reason that training cycles must be employed.

principle of maintenance—As a person reaches his or her goals, it takes less work to maintain that level of strength or muscle mass. If he or she is happy with that level, the frequency of training can be reduced. This is typically a good time to involve more cross-training so that other fitness components can be developed.

principle of reversibility—The fact that once the strength training program is discontinued or not maintained at the minimal level of frequency and intensity, the strength or hypertrophy adaptations that were made with that program will not only stop forward progression but will also revert back to the starting level.

WARMING UP, STRETCHING, AND COOLING DOWN

You might have trouble finding the time to sneak in a workout, let alone worry about properly warming up before and stretching after the workout. However, how you prepare and end your strength training sessions can have a big impact on your results as well as your quality of life, especially as you get older. Try your best to warm up properly before each workout and do some stretching to cool down after the workout.

A general warm-up of 5 to 10 minutes on a treadmill or stationary bike, some calisthenics, or, better yet, dynamic stretches such as high kicks and arm circles will raise your body temperature sufficiently. A study by Taylor and colleagues (2011) found that just a 0.3 °F increase in body temperature allowed athletes to jump 6 percent higher and have 10 percent more power. In other words, a short warm-up allows you to be stronger and perform better in the gym. Doing dynamic stretches as a warm-up further increases muscle power and strength during the warm-up. On the other hand, static stretching before strength training may impair muscle power and strength during the workout.

Your best bet is to save static stretching for the cool-down and as a way to increase your flexibility. This form of stretching is particularly effective for maximizing flexibility when done after workouts when the body is warmer and the muscles are more fatigued. This book does not focus on stretching exercises, so for a good resource, pick up the book *Full-Body Flexibility, Second Edition*, by Jay Blahnik (Human Kinetics 2011).

SUMMARY

To properly apply any discipline, you must first familiarize yourself with the principles of the discipline. Without a clear understanding of the foundation of strength training, the application of it will be lacking. Just as an athlete who doesn't understand the basics of his sport will do poorly in that sport, not understanding the basics of strength training will severely limit your potential. Regardless of whether your goal is to increase muscle mass or muscle strength, having this knowledge will have a positive effect on your ability to reach your goal.

First you must understand the different types of strength that you can train for: absolute, maximal, relative, speed, starting, acceleration, and endurance. Being familiar with the different muscle actions is essential to understanding the components of any repetition you perform. You will learn the concepts to follow in order for adaptations to take place. This basic information is just the starting point. This knowledge base will continue to grow with information contained in the following chapters of part I. Once you are armed with this seminal information, applying the training techniques and programs in the later sections will be easier and the results will be more substantial.

CHAPTER 2

Training Variables

The average strength training program will last several weeks to several months before a new training phase is implemented. Considering this time frame, a single workout may seem inconsequential to the overall program. Yet the design of each single workout is just as important as the overall program. This is because each workout adds up sequentially to create the long-term training program that will provide the adaptations that the program imparts. This chapter discusses the principles involved in designing a single strength training workout.

Every workout is composed of at least five specific program variables that you can manipulate in order to alter the workout: choice of exercises, order of exercises, number of sets, resistance, and rest taken between sets. You must carefully choose these variables to get a workout that is appropriate for your level of fitness and that initiates the desired adaptations.

Although strength athletes such as Olympic weightlifters, powerlifters, and bodybuilders have manipulated these variables for many years, William J. Kraemer, PhD, is credited with scientifically determining and recording what he has termed the five specific clusters of acute program variables (see table 2.1). The systematic alteration of these acute variables results in the periodized training program.

CHOICE OF EXERCISES

While all acute variables of a program are critical to a person's progress, choice of exercise is arguably one of the most critical. The reasoning behind this is that if you are not training the appropriate muscle groups, then all other variables are somewhat meaningless. Simply put, muscles that are not trained will not benefit from the program. Therefore, choosing the proper exercises for each workout is the first step in creating an effective strength program.

TABLE 2.1 Program Design Details

Variable	Specifics
Choice of exercises	Primary exercises Assistance exercises Multijoint exercises Single-joint exercises Exercise equipment
Order of exercises	Primary exercises followed by assistance exercises Larger muscle groups followed by smaller muscle groups Lagging muscle groups trained first Straight sets for each exercise Supersets
Number of sets	Volume effects Single sets Multiple sets Number of sets performed per exercise Number of sets performed per muscle group Number of sets performed per workout
Resistance (intensity)	Percentage of 1RM RM target zone OMNI-resistance exercise scale
Rest period between sets	Dependent on resistance used Dependent on muscle adaptation desired Dependent on metabolic pathway being trained Dependent on training technique

Adapted from S.J. Fleck and W.J. Kraemer, *Designing resistance training programs,* 3rd ed. (Champaign, IL: Human Kinetics), 158-73.

For those interested in gaining muscle strength, all exercises in a workout can be categorized as either a primary exercise or an assistance exercise. Refer to table 2.2 for a list of common primary and assistance exercises. Primary exercises are those that are most specific to the goals of the individual. These exercises must involve the

TABLE 2.2   Primary and Assistance Exercises

Primary exercises	Assistance exercises
Power clean	Knee extension
Deadlift	Leg curl
Squat	Chest fly
Leg press	Deltoid lateral raise
Bench press	Biceps curl
Military press	Triceps extension
Barbell row	Wrist curl
Pull-up	Calf raise
	Abdominal crunch

muscle groups in which the person is most interested in gaining strength. For competitive athletes, the primary exercises not only should target the same muscle groups that are used in competition but should also include some exercises that mimic the movements performed in their sports. For example, the primary exercises for an Olympic weightlifter are the clean and jerk and the snatch; for a powerlifter they are the bench press, squat, and deadlift; for an offensive lineman they are the squat and incline bench press.

Primary exercises usually are multijoint movements such as the bench press, squat, and deadlift. These exercises require the coordinated use of multiple muscle groups. Because several large muscle groups are used in performing these exercises, they tend to be the ones in which the most weight can be lifted. For instance, the world records in the deadlift and the squat are well over 900 and 1,100 pounds (408 and 499 kilograms), respectively. The world record in the barbell biceps curl (although this is not a lift that is sanctioned by any powerlifting federation), a single-joint exercise (typically referred to as an assistance exercise), is not much more than 400 pounds (181 kilograms). Because the primary exercises call for great strength and coordination, they should be performed early in the workout when the muscle groups are the least fatigued.

Assistance exercises typically are single-joint exercises such as the biceps curl, triceps extension, and deltoid lateral raise. These exercises often involve only a single muscle group. Because only one muscle group is working to lift the weight, these exercises usually involve much lighter weight than primary exercises do. For powerlifters and other strength athletes, assistance exercises are usually done toward the end of the

workout after the major muscle groups are fairly fatigued from performing the primary exercises. An exception to the rule that most assistance exercises are single-joint exercises is core training. Training the core (the deep muscles in the abdominal cavity and lower back) involves complicated movement patterns that involve multiple joints and force the core musculature to work at stabilizing the body.

For those interested in building muscle size, all exercises also can be divided into multijoint and single-joint exercises. However, the terms used in bodybuilding circles are *multijoint* and *isolation* exercises. *Isolation* implies that the single-joint movement is isolating the major muscle group and forcing it to perform all the work in that exercise without the help from other muscle groups. An example of this is the leg extension. While most major muscle groups have both multijoint and isolation exercises that target them, the biceps, forearms, calves, and abdominals are muscle groups that are trained usually with just isolation exercises. For a list of multijoint and isolation exercises for most major muscle groups, refer to table 2.3.

TABLE 2.3   Multijoint and Isolation Exercises

Muscle group	Multijoint exercises	Isolation exercises
Chest	Bench press Dumbbell bench press	Dumbbell fly Cable crossover
Shoulders	Barbell overhead press Upright row	Lateral raise Front raise
Triceps	Close-grip bench press Dips	Triceps pressdown Lying triceps extension
Biceps		Barbell curl Seated incline curl
Forearms		Wrist curl Reverse wrist curl
Quadriceps	Squat Leg press	Leg extension
Hamstrings	Squat Deadlift	Leg curl Romanian deadlift
Calves		Standing calf raise Seated calf raise
Abdominals		Crunch Reverse crunch

Exercise equipment is another factor to consider when choosing exercises for an individual workout. While free weights are used in the majority of the primary exercises, other equipment has its benefits depending on the overall goals of the person. For example, to mimic movements that occur in a more horizontal plane while an athlete is in an upright position (such as swinging a baseball bat), free weights are a poor choice because they offer resistance only in a vertical plane. Here, the use of a cable apparatus or resistance tubing would be a better exercise choice. Choosing appropriate strength training equipment is discussed in more detail in chapter 4.

ORDER OF EXERCISES

How the specific exercises that make up a single workout are ordered will determine not only the effectiveness of the workout but also the particular adaptations that the program imparts. Therefore, the order in which exercises are performed must correspond with the specific training goals.

In training for strength, the primary exercises are performed first in the workout relative to assistance exercises. The logic behind this is the fact that primary exercises typically involve numerous large muscle groups working together to lift relatively heavy weight. Therefore, these exercises must be done early enough in the program that fatigue is not an issue. Performing single-joint exercises first will compromise the amount of weight a person can lift on the primary exercises and may even make the person more susceptible to injury, because form tends to suffer when muscles are fatigued.

If building muscle size is the primary goal, then multijoint exercises should be performed first with isolation exercises performed later in the workout. The multijoint exercises help to build muscle size because it is possible to train with heavier weight on them. An exception to this rule involves a common bodybuilding technique known as preexhaust. This technique involves the use of single-joint exercises before multijoint exercises in an effort to exhaust a particular muscle group so that it becomes the weak link in the multijoint exercise. This concept is discussed in detail in chapter 6.

If multiple muscle groups are trained in a workout, such as in whole-body workouts, and only one exercise per major muscle group is performed, then ordering exercises involves determining the most critical muscle groups based on the goals of the person. Typically, larger-sized muscle groups (such as the legs and back) are trained before smaller muscle groups (such as the shoulders and biceps) for the same reason mentioned previously: Larger muscle groups need to be trained before fatigue is an issue.

NUMBER OF SETS

A set is a grouping of repetitions that is followed by a rest interval. The number of sets performed in a workout is one of the factors affecting the total volume (sets × repetitions × resistance) of exercise. Therefore, it must be consistent not only with the individual's strength goals but also with his or her current level of fitness.

Generally speaking, it is accepted that multiple sets are more beneficial for developing strength and muscle mass. In fact, this stance is supported in guidelines set by the National Strength and Conditioning Association (Pearson et al. 2000) and the American College of Sports Medicine (Kraemer et al. 2002). Single sets are effective for building strength for beginning weightlifters or for maintaining strength during periods when it is necessary or desired to reduce the volume performed. Beginners starting with a single-set program should progressively increase the number of sets to make continued adaptations in strength.

When designing a workout, one should consider the number of sets performed per exercise, the number of sets per muscle group, and the total number of sets for the workout. The number of sets per exercise typically varies depending on the strength training program. Most programs designed for the intermediate to advanced weight trainer incorporate between three and six sets per exercise. This set range is considered optimal for increasing strength. How many sets one should perform per muscle group is a question that is most applicable to bodybuilding-type training, in which numerous exercises are performed for each muscle group. This is in opposition to strength training programs for conditioning athletes, which may typically involve only one exercise per major muscle group. The number of sets per muscle group may range from 3 to 24 but ultimately depends on the number of exercises performed for that muscle group, the number of muscle groups trained in that workout, the intensity used, and where the person is in his or her training cycle. The total number of sets performed for a workout may vary from about 10 to 40, depending on the type of training and the number of sets per exercise. Care must be taken so that not too many total sets are performed, particularly when intensity is high, since these variables greatly influence total work. Performing too much total work over time stresses the body and can lead to overtraining in the long run. Although defining how much work is too much is a difficult task because many factors are involved, such as the person's training experience and genetics, general recommendations can be made. Typically doing more than 20 sets per muscle group for an extended period can lead to overtraining. In addition, doing more than 40 sets per workout, even when multiple muscle groups are trained in that workout, can lead to overtraining if done too frequently or if proper nutrition is not being followed.

As for any other acute variables of training, the number of sets should be manipulated to prevent stagnation of training adaptations. The most important variable of training that influences the number of sets that should be performed is intensity (the amount of weight lifted). The greater the intensity, the greater the stress placed on the muscle, and thus the lower the number of sets that should be performed. Therefore, the total number of sets in a training cycle should vary inversely with training intensity. In fact, training with too many total sets can be detrimental to the adaptations of strength training and lead to overtraining.

RESISTANCE

The term *intensity* refers to the amount of weight lifted (or resistance used) on a particular set. Alternatively, many bodybuilders use *intensity* to refer to the difficulty of a set or a workout, regardless of the amount of weight used. For example, a bodybuilder may perform a high-intensity set involving very light weight at extremely high repetitions until muscle failure is reached. The intensity of that set would be even higher if the spotter helped the bodybuilder get three extra forced reps at the end of that set. However, according to the formal definition of *intensity,* that set would be categorized as low intensity. Therefore, to avoid confusion, the term *resistance* will be used when referring to the amount of weight used.

The resistance used is one of the most important variables in a training program, ranking second only to exercise choice. The amount of resistance

used for a set is inversely related to the number of repetitions performed. That is, the heavier the weight, the fewer the repetitions that can be performed. One of the most common ways that resistance is measured is through the use of a percentage of the repetition maximum (RM). For example, an exercise can be prescribed at 80 percent of the individual's 1RM.

If, for instance, the person's 1RM on the bench press is 300 pounds (136 kilograms), then

$$300 \text{ pounds} \times .80 = 240 \text{ pounds}$$

Using this method does require frequent 1RM testing to ensure that accurate training resistance is used. This method may be desirable for certain strength athletes because recurrent testing is a commonly used measure of an athlete's progress and a predictor of preparedness for competition. Olympic weightlifters should use this method regularly because of the skill component required for that type of lifting. Competitive weightlifters must use precisely measured resistance for their training phases. Powerlifters also commonly use this method because the defining moment in their sport is the amount of weight they can perform at 1RM on the bench press, squat, and deadlift. However, many top powerlifters train with percentages that are based on the 1RM they are predicting to lift in competition. The down side to prescribing exercise intensity with RM percentages is the fact that the amount of reps you can perform at a certain percentage of 1RM can vary depending on experience, the muscle group being trained, and the exercise equipment used.

For bodybuilders and other fitness enthusiasts, frequent testing of 1RM is not convenient or often feasible. It would be too time consuming because of the larger number of exercises they typically use. In addition, many of the exercises they perform are not conducive to 1RM testing. Although charts are devised for estimating 1RM based on the number of reps that can be completed at a certain weight, these are far from accurate. For serious weight trainers, an RM target zone is the easiest way to monitor training resistance. This is depicted as 10RM or 5RM and refers to a resistance that limits them to that number of repetitions. As their strength increases, they simply move to a heavier weight but shoot for the same RM goal. This allows them to continually stay in the repetition range they are shooting for without the need to test their 1RM. Worth mentioning here is that many strength coaches and strength training scientists suggest that repetitions (resistance) should be kept in a fairly small range for any given workout. They believe that muscle can be trained for only one goal in any acute situation. Yet bodybuilders often train with a wide range of repetitions in a single workout. For example, they may do one set of an exercise with a very heavy weight for 5 to 7 reps and follow it with another set with light weight for reps in the 15 to 20 range.

A more recently developed method of prescribing and monitoring resistance involves the use of the OMNI-resistance exercise scale (Robertson et al. 2003; Robertson 2004). This is a 10-point subjective scale (see figure 2.1) that is a modified version of the rating of perceived exertion (RPE) scale that was originally described by Borg (1982) and used mostly for monitoring aerobic exercise. Each value from 1 to 10 on the OMNI represents approximately a 10 percent increase in repetition maximum. For example, the use of 100 percent of a person's 1RM elicits a rating of 10 on the OMNI-resistance exercise scale, while the use of 50 percent of the person's 1RM corresponds to a rating of 5 on the scale. The OMNI-resistance exercise scale is not a precise quantitative scale but more a qualitative scale that determines how hard the weight feels to the lifter. For this reason, it is

best used by trainers who are prescribing strength training to inexperienced lifters.

Today, thanks to the many years of trial and error by athletes and the numerous research studies to confirm the original inclinations, it is now well established that using certain resistance intensities provides corresponding results. This information can be used in designing a repetition maximum continuum as seen in figure 2.2. This figure is a modification of the continuum devised by Fleck and Kraemer (2004) that is recognized as the most acceptable by exercise scientists and strength coaches. The continuum in figure 2.2 ranges in maximal repetitions from 1 to 25, as does the original, but adds the adaptation of muscle hypertrophy. On the lower end of the continuum, strength gains are more pronounced, particularly when using maximal repetitions in the range of 1 to 6, or about 80 to 100 percent of 1RM (O'Shea 1966; Weiss, Coney, and Clark 1999). Enhanced muscle hypertrophy is most notable when training with repetition maximums in the 8 to 12 range, which corresponds to about 70 to 80 percent 1RM (Kraemer, Fleck, and Evans 1996). And muscular endurance benefits occur when repetition maximums of 12 and above, or 70 percent of 1RM and below, are used (Stone and Coulter 1994). New evidence also suggests that these

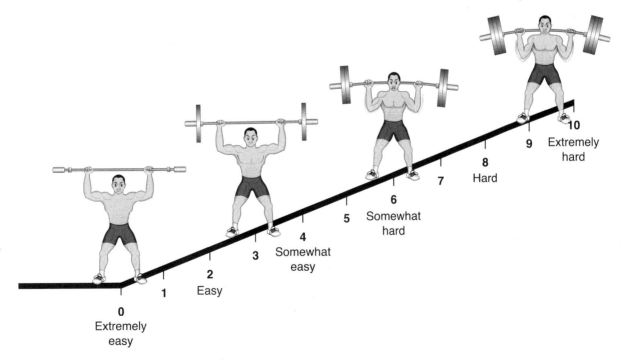

FIGURE 2.1 OMNI-resistance exercise scale.

Reprinted from R.J. Robertson, 2004, *Perceived exertion for practitioners: Rating effort with the OMNI picture system* (Champaign, IL: Human Kinetics), 49, with permission of the author.

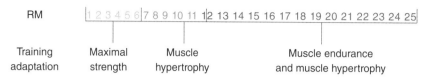

FIGURE 2.2 Continuum of repetition maximums.

Modified from S.J. Fleck and W.J. Kraemer, *Designing resistance training programs*, 3rd ed. (Champaign, IL: Human Kinetics), 167.

higher rep ranges are also effective for muscle hypertrophy as long as sets are taken to muscle failure (Burd 2010; Burd 2011; Mitchell 2012). These varied muscle adaptations underscore the importance of periodization for producing the most desirable changes in a muscle, whether the person's goal is increasing muscle endurance or increasing maximal strength. This is because each adaptation is related to the others. For example, increasing both maximal strength and muscle endurance beneficially affects muscle hypertrophy. So while the person should spend the majority of training time using the repetition range that best fits his or her major goals, the periodic cycling of other intensities will enhance this goal.

One major assumption that the continuum of repetition maximums makes is that all repetitions are performed at a moderate speed. Yet the speed of a rep can be increased or decreased, particularly at light to moderate loads. And this change in speed will dramatically alter the muscle adaptations. In general, fast repetition speeds with very light weight are best for building speed strength, or power, when few repetitions are performed. In contrast, slow to moderate repetitions with a submaximal weight are better for producing adaptations in muscle endurance and hypertrophy as the time the muscle is under tension is increased. As an example, using a weight that is about 30 to 45 percent of 1RM to do three reps as fast as possible builds speed strength (power) and has little effect if any on muscle hypertrophy or endurance.

REST PERIOD BETWEEN SETS

How long a weightlifter should rest between sets is dependent on numerous factors. These include the resistance being used, the goals of the lifter, and the metabolic pathways that need to be trained. The general consensus is that the lower the reps being performed (that is, the higher the resistance intensity), the longer the rest periods that should be taken. And so as the periodized routine alters resistance intensity, so too do the rest periods change accordingly.

If a person is training for maximal strength or power, he or she should take long rest periods between sets. This is because lifting heavy weight for low reps requires energy derived from anaerobic metabolism, called the ATP-PC (adenosine triphosphate-phosphocreatine) system. This metabolic pathway provides the immediate energy required for lifting heavy weight or performing explosive movements for a short period. This system requires more than 3 minutes of rest for the majority of recovery to occur. Therefore, the recommendation is to rest at least 3 to more than 5 minutes when training for maximal strength or power. The general guidelines are as follows: resistance at less than 5RM requires over 5 minutes of rest, 5-7RM requires 3-5 minutes, 8-10RM requires 2-3 minutes, 11-13RM requires 1-2 minutes, and over 13RM requires about 1 minute (Kraemer 2003). This level of rest ensures that fatigue will be minimal at the start of a new set, and in turn, strength can be near maximal. Similarly, if a strength athlete or other athlete performs short bouts of high-intensity exercise with long rest periods between, the athlete should rest at least three minutes between sets.

When training for muscle hypertrophy (which is best attained with reps in the range of 8 to 12), shorter rest periods appear to be the most beneficial. Resting less than three minutes between sets stresses the anaerobic energy systems, and this is often recommended for bodybuilding training. This is because fatigue is believed to play some role in the pathways leading to muscle growth. One possibility involves lactate, which dramatically increases as reps increase and rest between sets decreases.

For athletes interested in improving muscle endurance, low intensity (less than 60 percent 1RM), high repetitions of 15 and beyond, and short rest periods (under one minute) seem to be the best plan. This plan allows them to train to the point of fatigue and beyond, which enhances the body's ability to use lactate as an energy source and even improves aerobic capacity to some degree. Because fatigue is associated with muscle hypertrophy, many bodybuilders also frequently use this style of training.

Some styles of training use such minute rest periods between sets that they are classified in gym circles as using "no rest" between sets. This means that you would take no deliberate rest but instead immediately move to the next exercise. Such training methods include circuit training and the various forms of superset training, which includes compound sets, triple sets, and giant sets (see chapter 6 for more detailed explanations of these methods). With each of these methods, a certain number of sets of different exercises are done back to back with no rest between exercise sets. Only after you complete the prescribed number of exercises (which can vary from 2 to as many as 12) would you take a rest period. Then you would repeat the cycle anywhere from one to five times depending on the program.

ADDITIONAL FACTORS

The five original acute training variables discussed earlier were classified and organized decades ago. As with any science, progress has been made to further our understanding of resistance training. Besides determining the best exercises to use, the correct order of those exercises, the proper resistance to use, the optimal number of sets to do, and the right amount of rest to take between sets, other factors are to be considered.

Another acute training variable that can be added to the list is repetition speed, or rep tempo. Generally speaking, typical rep speed in strength training lasts about two to three seconds to complete the positive (concentric) and negative (eccentric) portions of each rep. This is considered a controlled pace and is the pace taught by most strength coaches and personal trainers. However, some programs rely on the manipulation of rep speed. Speeding up the time it takes to complete a rep—in the range of one second or less—has been shown to be an effective way to increase muscle power. See Ballistic Strength Training in chapter 9 for an explanation of how to train with fast, explosive reps. Some strength training

experts also believe that slowing down a rep—in the range of 10 to 20 seconds—can enhance muscle endurance as well as size. Research in this area is limited, but anecdotal reports are positive. See Slow-Repetition Training in chapter 6 for an explanation of how to train using very slow reps, and see Speed-Set Training in chapter 6 as well.

Another factor you should also be concerned about is how frequently you train. The frequency at which muscle groups are trained can be more critical than any of the acute variables of training discussed previously. The reason has to do with recovery. It is generally accepted that you should wait until a muscle has recovered from a previous workout before training the muscle again. Muscle recovery, however, is an individual thing that is influenced by factors such as lifting experience, intensity of the workout, and total volume. In most instances it is best to get 2 to 7 days of rest for each muscle group. This will be determined by how you split your training. *Training splits* refer to how you break down training days. For example, do you train your whole body during every workout, or do you train only one or two muscle groups each workout? For obvious reasons, the more workouts it takes you to train all the major muscle groups of the body, the more rest you will take between workouts for the same muscle group. Training splits and training frequency are discussed in more detail in chapters 5 and 8.

SUMMARY

The design of every workout is a critical component of the design of the strength training program. Regardless of your goal, you must carefully select appropriate acute variables to optimize the adaptations that occur in every workout. In designing the most effective training programs to reach your goals, you must carefully consider the choice of exercises and the order, intensity used, number of sets performed, and rest periods between sets. In addition to these variables, you may want to consider the speed at which you perform your reps. Last but not least is the frequency at which you train muscle groups. This basic information in this chapter will make more sense after you read about training details in parts II, III, and IV.

CHAPTER 3

Training Cycles

The term *periodization* refers to the systematic manipulation of the acute variables of training (as discussed in chapter 2) over a period that may range from days to years. The original concept was developed in the former Eastern Bloc countries in the late 1950s to optimize athletes' adaptations to resistance training. More important, periodization revolves around the athlete's competitive calendar so that he or she is at a competitive peak for competition.

The basis of periodization is general adaptation syndrome (GAS), which describes three stages that an organism—such as an athlete—goes through when exposed to a novel stress (Selye 1936). As a new stress is placed on the body (for example, heavy training in the range of three to five reps), the muscle first goes through an alarm reaction. During this stage the athlete momentarily gets weaker. But with continued exposure to the stress (successive workouts), the body enters the stage of adaptation. In this stage the body supercompensates for the stress—such as increasing muscle strength—to better deal with the stress. If the body is continually exposed to the same stress for too long, it may enter the stage of exhaustion, where its adaptation to the stress may actually decline. This may mean that the strength gains the athlete made during the adaptation stage will cease, and stagnation may set in. It may even lead to an actual decline in strength. Although this theory is now considered a simplistic take on the body's response to stress, it does hold true and explains the reason periodization is so important for proper adaptation to strength training.

You must expose the muscle to any one training style for just long enough to reap the benefits but avoid a nosedive of those positive adaptations. At this stage a new training style should be introduced, and the cycle continues. A simplistic take on periodization is the maxim of "everything works, but nothing works forever." This is a major theme of this book and is the reason it offers so many training methods. Having a large arsenal of training methods (as provided in chapters 6 and 9) to use for short periods and continually cycling them in a systematic order will prevent stagnation and maximize training adaptations.

The three periodization schemes most commonly used by strength coaches, which are the three most extensively researched, are classic strength and power periodization, reverse linear periodization, and undulating periodization. Although there are many other more obscure periodization schemes out there, a discussion including these three will cover the premise behind periodization. Regardless of the exact plan, periodized strength training programs have been shown through research to be significantly more effective than nonperiodized programs for increasing strength, power, and athletic performance in both men and women (Kraemer et al. 2003; Marx et al. 2001; Rhea and Alderman 2004; Willoughby 1993).

CLASSIC PERIODIZATION

The name implies that this system is the hallmark periodization scheme most associated with the term *periodization*. In its most general form, classic periodization divides a long-term training period called the *macrocycle* (which typically involves six months to one year but may be up to four years, such as with Olympic athletes) into smaller phases called *mesocycles* (usually lasting several weeks to months), which are also subdivided into weekly *microcycles.* The strength training progresses over the macrocycle from low resistance (intensity) to high intensity with total volume following the opposite progression, from high to low. A schematic overview of the classic strength and power periodization scheme can be seen in figure 3.1 and table 3.1.

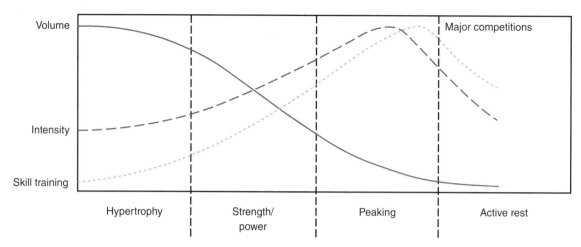

FIGURE 3.1 Classic strength and power periodization scheme.

Adapted, by permission, from S.J. Fleck and W.J. Kraemer, *Designing resistance training programs*, 3rd ed. (Champaign, IL: Human Kinetics), 213.

TABLE 3.1 Classic Strength and Power Periodization Model

Training phase	Hyper-trophy	Strength	Power	Peak-ing	Active rest
Sets	3-5	3-5	3-5	1-3	Light physical activity
Reps per set	8-12	2-6	2-3	1-3	
Intensity	Low	Moderate	High	Very high	
Volume	Very high	High	Moderate	Low	

Adapted from M.H. Stone, H. O'Bryant, and J. Garhammer, 1981, "A hypothetical model for strength training," *Journal of Sports Medicine and Physical Fitness* 21(4): 342-351.

Figure 3.1 represents the most common periodization format used for increasing strength and power. The first phase, or mesocycle, is classified as the hypertrophy phase and is categorized as being low intensity. Reps are around 8 to 12 and sometimes as high as 20. It is considered very high in volume because sets are usually in the range of 4 to 5 for each exercise. The goal of this phase is typically to prepare the athlete for the high-intensity training that is to follow. The muscle hypertrophy experienced in this phase will enhance the gains in strength and power an athlete will make in the later stages. Although this is termed the *hypertrophy phase,* it should not be confused with a periodized program a bodybuilder would use. Hypertrophy is the main

goal in a bodybuilding program, not something an athlete may do only for several months. In some periodized programs designed for athletes, the hypertrophy phase may be preceded by what is known as a *general preparedness (GP) phase.* This is especially true if the person being trained is a rank beginner or an athlete who is returning after an off-season where little, if any, training took place. This would provide a means of preparing an athlete for the hypertrophy phase with very low intensity and moderate- to high-volume training.

The next mesocycle is usually the strength phase. As the name implies, the major goal during this phase is to maximize muscle strength. This phase is typically moderate to high in intensity with reps in the range of two to six and the goal to build up muscle strength. It's somewhat high in volume, with three or four sets performed per exercise and fewer total exercises performed per muscle group than during the hypertrophy phase. Following the strength phase is the power phase. It is similar to the strength phase in that the intensity is high (reps are in the range of two to three). The volume is a bit lower; sets usually are about three per exercise. The point of this phase is to start transferring the strength gains made during the first two phases into more explosive power that serves well for competition.

The final two mesocycles prepare the athlete for competition. The peaking phase follows the power phase. It is categorized by low volume (only one to three sets per exercise are formed) and very high intensity (reps as low as one per set). This phase gets the athlete ready for competition by maximizing strength and power. After this phase, the athlete drops the strength training and undergoes a period of active rest just before competition. The active rest phase is categorized by activity other than strength training such as swimming, hiking, or sport activities like basketball and tennis. This phase usually lasts for only about one to two weeks before a competition to allow the body to recover from all the strenuous training so that it can perform at its best. After competition, this phase may actually continue for several weeks before the periodized training scheme starts again. For this reason, the active rest phase is often referred to as the *transition phase*. Most strength experts using the classic strength and power periodization program will continue the mesocycle phases for anywhere from three weeks to three months. However, a compressed version of this program would involve changing the phases (hence the intensity and volume) every week. Then the cycle repeats itself.

Although classic strength periodization schemes can allow for adaptations in strength training, some issues need to be considered with these models. The first consideration is the fact that the higher-volume training phase may lead to fatigue if followed consecutively for too long. This could be a problem for athletes who must compete at various times throughout the year. The second consideration is the fact that the muscle hypertrophy gained during the hypertrophy phase may not be maintained very well during the later stages, where volume gets considerably low. This could be a problem for bodybuilders and other athletes who are concerned about muscle mass. Therefore, other periodized schemes have been developed and tested in the gym as well as in the lab.

REVERSE LINEAR PERIODIZATION

Reverse linear periodization takes the classic strength and power periodization scheme and runs it backward. Whereas the goal of the classic periodization model is to maximize an athlete's strength and power, the goal of the reverse linear model is to maximize muscle hypertrophy or endurance strength, depending on the rep range that the program concludes with (8 to 12 for hypertrophy and 20 to 30 for endurance strength). Research supports the concept that the reverse

linear periodization scheme is more effective for increasing endurance strength than the classic model (Rhea et al. 2003).

In essence, the reverse linear model starts with the power phase, where intensity is very high (two or three reps per set) and volume is low (three sets per exercise). The peaking phase is usually skipped because the athlete is not preparing for a competition in which power and strength matter. After the athlete follows the power phase for several weeks, the strength phase starts. Again, the strength phase uses moderate to high intensity (two to six reps per set) and slightly higher volume than the power phase (three or four sets per exercise). The goal of these first two phases is to build the strength and power to optimize gains in mass or endurance strength.

Being able to lift heavier weight for the desired number of reps during the hypertrophy phase can result in significant gains in muscle mass as well as muscle endurance. The hypertrophy stage comes last in the program and involves lower intensity (8 to 12 reps per set) and high volume, which is the best prescription for building muscle mass. This stage is a good systematic approach to gaining muscle mass, which makes it a smart periodized plan for bodybuilders. See figure 3.2 for a sample reverse linear periodization scheme for muscle hypertrophy.

To make the reverse linear model a better fit for optimizing endurance strength, the power phase can be eliminated. That means it would start with the strength phase, then move to the hypertrophy phase, then move to an endurance phase (where the reps are in the range of 20 to 30), and finally move to an active rest phase if the athlete is training for a competition. A diagram of this model is shown in figure 3.3. As with any periodization scheme, the acute variables can be manipulated within each stage to improve the result of the program. For instance, a reverse linear model can start with reps in the 8 to 10 range, then progress to the range of 12 to 15, and end in the range of 20 to 30.

UNDULATING PERIODIZATION

As the name implies, undulating periodization follows a less linear scheme than does the classic strength (power) scheme or the reverse linear periodization scheme. Undulating models are gaining

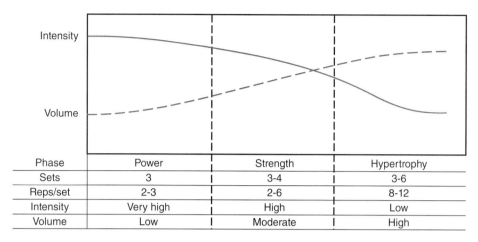

Phase	Power	Strength	Hypertrophy
Sets	3	3-4	3-6
Reps/set	2-3	2-6	8-12
Intensity	Very high	High	Low
Volume	Low	Moderate	High

FIGURE 3.2 Reverse linear periodization scheme for hypertrophy.

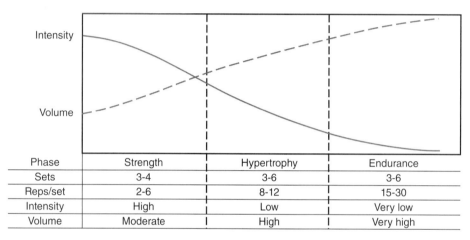

Phase	Strength	Hypertrophy	Endurance
Sets	3-4	3-6	3-6
Reps/set	2-6	8-12	15-30
Intensity	High	Low	Very low
Volume	Moderate	High	Very high

FIGURE 3.3 Reverse linear periodization scheme for endurance strength.

in popularity in strength rooms because of their convenience and effectiveness.

Undulating periodization schemes typically follow a 14-day mesocycle with three or four different workouts to stagger (see table 3.2). This way, instead of sticking with one training phase for several weeks or more, the lifter can change intensity and volume from one workout to another. For example, if the lifter were following a whole-body training split, he or she might perform the strength workout on Monday, the endurance strength workout on Wednesday, and the hypertrophy workout on Friday. The following week the lifter may train the endurance strength workout on Monday, the hypertrophy workout on Wednesday, and the strength workout on Friday. If the lifter trained the upper body on Mondays and Thursdays and the lower body on Tuesdays and Fridays, he or she might then do hypertrophy workouts on Monday and Tuesday and strength workouts on Thursday and Friday. The following week the lifter might train with endurance workouts on Monday and Tuesday and strength workouts on Thursday and Friday. After the two-week mesocycle the lifter could

TABLE 3.2 Undulating Workouts

Type of workout	Sets	Reps	Rest between sets
Strength workout	3-5	2-4	4-5 min
Hypertrophy workout	3-4	8-12	2-3 min
Endurance strength workout	3-4	15-30	1-2 min

switch back to a different workout and perform the mesocycle over again, or the lifter can take a week off (especially if a competition is scheduled) and then return to the 14-day mesocycle.

One of the great things about undulating periodization is that it requires less organization and planning than linear periodized programs require. For instance, if a person felt tired or sick (or conversely, the person felt exceptionally motivated and strong one day), the workout could be changed for that day to better suit mood and physical health. Or if scheduling was a problem and the lifter was short on time one day, he or she could switch to a workout with lower volume. Although it seems that such a training system that requires little planning would be less effective than a program that is scheduled months in advance, research has found that undulating periodized programs are just as effective as linear periodized models for the development of strength, power, and muscle mass (Marx et al. 2001; Kraemer et al. 2000) and are more effective than nonperiodized programs. One study by Rhea, Ball, Phillips, and Burkett (2002) found that undulating periodized training was more effective for developing strength compared to a linear periodized plan.

In actuality, the sporadic nature of the undulating program works as a default for building muscle, strength, and power. That's because periodization is based on the fact that a physiological system makes adaptations to a stress that it is exposed to. Yet if the system is exposed to the stress for too long, the adaptations will plateau and even reverse to some degree. Given that, the undulating periodized scheme allows the stress (strength training) to be encountered for very short periods before it is changed and then cycled back in. In this model, the different types of strength training (heavy, light, fast, or whatever) are cycled repeatedly from day to day. So it helps to keep the muscle from getting used to the stimulus, yet it exposes it frequently enough to cause progressive adaptations.

MICROCYCLES

With the classic linear periodization model and the reverse linear periodization model, sticking with the same rep range for a full mesocycle,

which can last many weeks, can have some drawbacks. Some athletes get bored using the same rep ranges for several weeks. Another issue discussed earlier is the fact that some of the adaptations made in a previous mesocycle may be lost in a later mesocycle. For example, gains in muscle size made during the hypertrophy phase may be lost during the strength and power phases where repetitions performed each set rarely exceed 6.

Undulating periodization is one way to remedy the issues of the mesocycles. However, using a linear model, whether it is the classic linear scheme or the reverse linear scheme, has merit. Microcycles may be an even more effective way of using linearly periodized training schemes.

The term *microcycle* refers to weekly changes in the weight used and reps performed. For example, if following the classic linear model, week 1 might be a muscle endurance microcycle with reps of 12 to 15. Week 2 might be the hypertrophy microcycle with reps of 8 to 12. Week 3 continues increasing the weight and decreasing the reps for the strength microcycle with reps of 4 to 6. Then in week 4, which could be the power microcycle, reps drop again to just 2 or 3 per set. After week 4, the cycle repeats itself with week 5 returning to the muscle endurance microcycle. These microcycles can keep repeating in this order until the athlete is ready for competition, or for a noncompetitive strength trainer, the program is over after 12 weeks or so. See table 3.3 for a sample linear scheme that uses microcycles. This is very similar to the Shortcut to Size (Micromuscle) program that has gained great popularity online due to the extraordinary gains in muscle size and strength that are possible with this 12-week program. For more details on this program, see chapter 7.

TABLE 3.3 Microcycle Scheme*

Week/Microcycle	Weight	Rep range
1: Muscle Endurance	Light	12-15
2: Hypertrophy	Moderate	8-12
3: Strength	Moderate-heavy	4-6
4: Power	Heavy	2-3

* This table shows the weight and rep range changes that occur each week/microcycle when using a linear scheme with microcycles.

COMBINING PERIODIZED SCHEMES

There is no rule that states that you have to pick one and only one form of periodization and follow it until the end of the program. A great way to increase muscle size and strength is to use programs that combine periodization models.

A good example of this is pendulum training. In pendulum training, you start off using a classic linear periodization model usually with microcycles. Therefore, you might start with reps in the range of 8 to 12 in week 1. Then in week 2, reps drop to 6 to 8. In week 3, reps drop again to 3 to 5. In week 4, the order switches to a reverse linear periodization model with reps going back up to the 6-to-8 range and then in week 5 to the 8-to-12 range. Then in week 6 it is back to a linear progression with reps dropping to 6 to 8 reps. The program would continue swinging back and forth like this similar to a pendulum—hence the name. See table 3.4 for a sample pendulum scheme.

Another way to combine periodization models is to use both linear and reverse linear models simultaneously. This works well with a program that trains each muscle group twice per week. For example, with a program that uses a two-day split with chest, back, and shoulders trained in workouts 1 and 3 and legs and arms trained in workouts 2

TABLE 3.4 Pendulum Scheme*

Week/Microcycle	Weight	Rep range
1: Hypertrophy	Moderate	8-12
2: Strength	Moderate-heavy	6-8
3: Power	Heavy	3-5
4: Strength	Moderate-heavy	6-8
5: Hypertrophy	Moderate	8-12
6: Strength	Moderate-heavy	6-8
7: Power	Heavy	3-5

* This table shows the weight and rep range changes that occur each week/microcycle when using a pendulum scheme.

and 4, workouts 1 and 2 could follow a linear order using a microcycle system of increasing weight and decreasing reps with each week. Weeks 3 and 4 could follow a reverse linear order using a microcycle system in which the weight decreases and the reps increase each week. See table 3.5 for an example of this scheme. What's interesting when you consider the order of the rep ranges with two separate rep ranges being used each week is that the scheme is similar to an undulating periodization model. Here workouts 1 and 2 progress from 9 to 11 reps in week 1, to 6 to 8 reps in week 2, and to 3 to 5 reps in week 3. Workouts 3 and 4 start at 12 to 15 reps in week 1, then jump to 16 to 20 reps in week 2, and finally go to 21 to 30 reps in week 3. But when you consider the order

TABLE 3.5 Combined Linear and Reverse Linear Scheme

Multijoint Linear periodization Increase weight/decrease reps				Single joint Reverse linear periodization Increase reps/decrease weights			
Microcycle 1/4	Monday: Chest Triceps Abs	Tuesday: Shoulders Legs Abs	Wednesday: Back Traps Biceps	Thursday: Chest Triceps Abs	Friday: Shoulders Legs Abs	Saturday: Back Traps Biceps	Sunday: Off
9 to 11 reps per set				**12 to 15 reps per set**			
Microcycle 2/5	Monday: Chest Triceps Abs	Tuesday: Shoulders Legs Abs	Wednesday: Back Traps Biceps	Thursday: Chest Triceps Abs	Friday: Shoulders Legs Abs	Saturday: Back Traps Biceps	Sunday: Off
6 to 8 reps per set				**16 to 20 reps per set**			
Microcycle 3/6	Monday: Chest Triceps Abs	Tuesday: Shoulders Legs Abs	Wednesday: Back Traps Biceps	Thursday: Chest Triceps Abs	Friday: Shoulders Legs Abs	Saturday: Back Traps Biceps	Sunday: Off
3 to 5 reps per set				**21 to 30 reps per set**			

Adapted from J. Stoppani, 2013, Jim Stoppani's six-week shortcut to shred. [Online]. Available: www.bodybuilding.com/fun/jim-stoppani-six-week-shortcut-to-shred.html [September 4, 2014].

from workouts 1 and 2 to workouts 3 and 4 each week, the reps actually go in this order: 9 to 11, 12 to 15, 6 to 8, 16 to 20, 3 to 5, 21 to 30. It is actually an undulating order. This is very similar to my Shortcut to Shred (1-2-3 Lean) program that has gained a lot of popularity online because it allows trainees to build significant strength and size despite the fact that they are drastically reducing body fat. See chapter 13 for more details on this program.

TYPES OF TRAINING CYCLES

Periodization is a term used by strength coaches, experts, and athletes who have been educated on the matter. Rarely will you hear the term used in the gym by bodybuilders or powerlifters. These athletes refer to the concept of periodization as *cycling*. It may sound cooler, but cycling is just a simpler term for periodization. Although the minor details of cycling for powerlifters and bodybuilders are slightly different from the three periodized schemes discussed previously, they rely on the same premise: Change is good.

Powerlifters use several types of cycles to prepare for a competition. A multitude of these are presented in chapters 9 and 10. The most common cycle uses a gradual increase in the amount of weight used over time. Usually this starts out as low as 50 percent of the lifter's 1RM and progresses up to 100 percent of the 1RM weight for that lift over a 6- to 12-week period. See table 3.6 for a sample 11-week powerlifting cycle.

Bodybuilders also use numerous cycling strategies. In fact, an unlimited number of bodybuilding cycles could be used. These are covered in chapters 6 and 7. The most common ones used are similar to the reverse linear periodization scheme (table 3.7) and the undulating periodization scheme (table 3.8). Although these athletes mix up their training frequently, the focus tends to stay on reps in the moderate to high range (8 to 20). Occasionally, these athletes train with heavy weight and low reps, but these phases are short and infrequent.

TABLE 3.6 Strong Cycle

Week	% 1RM	Reps	Sets
1	55%	5	5
2	60%	5	5
3	65%	5	5
4	70%	5	5
5	75%	5	5
6	85%	3	3
7	90%	3	3
8	95%	3	3
9	95%	2	2
10	100%*	2	2
11**	–	–	–

*Based on previous max.

**Active rest.

TABLE 3.7 Linear Muscle

Weeks	Reps	Sets (per exercise)	Rest between sets
1-2	6-8	3	3-4 min
3-4	8-10	3	2-3 min
5-6	10-12	3	1-2 min
7-8	12-15	3	<1 min

TABLE 3.8 Undulating Muscle

WEEK 1			
Day and muscle groups	Reps	Sets (per exercise)	Rest between sets
Monday (chest, shoulders, triceps)	8-10	3	2-3 min
Tuesday (back, biceps)	12-15	3	<1 min
Wednesday (legs)	6-8	3	3-4 min
Thursday (chest, shoulders, triceps)	12-15	3	<1 min
Friday (back, biceps)	6-8	3	3-4 min
Saturday (legs)	10-12	3	1-2 min

WEEK 2			
Day and muscle groups	Reps	Sets (per exercise)	Rest between sets
Monday (chest, shoulders, triceps)	6-8	3	3-4 min
Tuesday (back, biceps)	10-12	3	1-2 min
Wednesday (legs)	8-10	3	3 min
Thursday (chest, shoulders, triceps)	10-12	3	1-2 min
Friday (back, biceps)	8-10	3	3 min
Saturday (legs)	12-15	3	<1 min

SUMMARY

Regardless of whether the goal is to increase power and strength or muscle growth, periodization (or cycling) is a necessary method for making continual progress. Only by cycling the training phases is it possible to keep the muscles adapting and prevent them from stagnating. Fortunately, numerous periodization methods can be employed. These include classic linear periodized schemes, reverse linear schemes, and undulating schemes.

So while any one periodization scheme will provide sufficient variability in the training program, using different periodization schemes promotes training variability and progress. Over time you should try them all to decide what scheme works best for you. From there, you can choose to use that cycle as your primary scheme or frequently change up your cycles as you should for acute variables of training. You can even combine periodized schemes into one training program, such as with pendulum training.

CHAPTER 4

Strength Training Equipment

There is an abundance of equipment that you can use for the purpose of strength training. Although some of these pieces of equipment are more complicated or sophisticated than others, all have their advantages and disadvantages. Regardless of how simple or innovative, most strength training devices fall into one of three categories: those that provide constant resistance throughout the range of motion, those that provide variable resistance (whether controlled or not) throughout the range of motion, and those that provide a constant speed throughout the entire range of motion. In addition, some novel pieces of strength training equipment do not fit into the standard categories, such as vibration. This chapter covers the more common forms of strength training equipment as well as some that are not so common.

SIMPLE RESISTANCE

The first category of strength training equipment provides constant resistance throughout the entire range of motion. This is the simplest form of resistance and is composed of little more than objects that provide weight. The mass of the object, whether it be a dumbbell or a weight stack, provides resistance through gravity. Any time you attempt to pick up a free object, you are fighting the force of gravity, which pulls the object to the ground. The type of contraction that the muscle goes through when lifting a free object is termed *isotonic*. It literally means same tone or tension, because the weight stays the same while you lift it. If the object is too heavy to move, the type of contraction the muscle goes through is *isometric*. Because the mass of any object can be used in this manner, this category of strength training equipment is the largest and is composed of the widest range of equipment.

Free Weights

The term *free weights* refers to equipment moved in the performance of an exercise, which is simply raised and lowered as a complete unit. It is called *free weight* because the weight is free to move in any direction and in any manner. Technically, any object can be considered free weight; however, the term usually refers to the weight plates and barbell or dumbbell systems and related items found in home and commercial gyms.

barbell—The bar that weight plates are loaded onto for purposes of strength training. Barbells normally measure between five and seven feet in length, depending on the type of barbell. There are several different types of barbells:

Olympic barbell—A special type of barbell used in Olympic weightlifting and in powerlifting competitions as well as in gyms (see figure 4.1). These bars weigh 20 kilograms (just under 45 pounds) and are seven feet in length. The ends of the bar are two inches (five centimeters) in diameter to fit Olympic weight plates, and the handle section where you grab the bar is one inch (two and a half centimeters) in diameter. Parts of the handle section are knurled for better gripping. Some gyms have shorter versions of these bars.

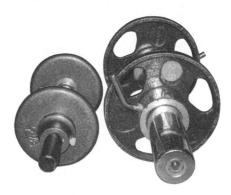

FIGURE 4.1 Standard bar and plates (left) contrasted with Olympic bar and plates (right).

standard barbell—Similar to Olympic barbells in that the gripping portion is usually one inch in diameter and knurled in sections. However, these barbells have ends that are one inch in diameter to fit standard weight plates.

fixed barbell—A barbell with a predetermined weight (see figure 4.2).

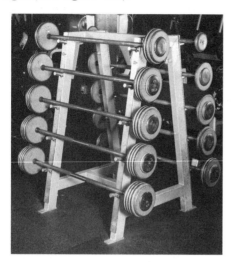

FIGURE 4.2   Fixed barbells on a rack.

EZ curl bar—A special type of barbell that is bent at several points so that it looks like a stretched-out W (see figure 4.3). This allows the user to have a grip that is somewhere between a fully supinated grip (underhand grip) and a neutral grip. The purpose of this is to take stress off the wrists as well as place more stress on the long head of the biceps (outer biceps). An EZ curl bar is occasionally called a cambered curling bar.

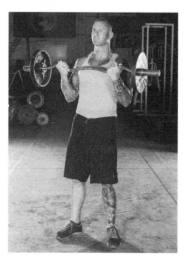

FIGURE 4.3   Curls with an EZ curl bar.

fat bar—A special barbell or dumbbell that is larger in diameter on the gripping portion of the bar than the conventional bars that are one inch in diameter. Fat bars usually come in two-inch and sometimes three-inch (five- or eight-centimeter) diameters. Training with fat bars allows users to develop greater grip strength than they would by using a standard one-inch bar. However, research has shown that using fat bars on pulling exercises, such as deadlifts, rows and curls can limit the weight used on those exercises, which could interfere with strength and muscle hypertrophy gains of the target muscle.

safety squat bar—A bar that resembles a barbell with two short padded bars (about 12 inches, or 30 centimeters) that run perpendicular to the bar from the middle. These padded bars rest on the shoulders and allow the user to grab them as a handle while squatting (see figure 4.4).

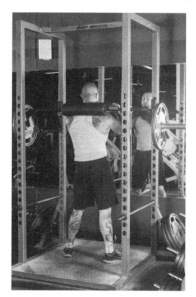

FIGURE 4.4   Squatting with a safety squat bar.

trap bar—A weight bar with a diamond-shaped or hexagon section in the middle. During the exercise, the lifter stands inside the diamond and grips the transverse handholds on either side of the diamond. This type of bar is sometimes called a hex bar, due to its shape, and is typically used for shrugs and deadlifts (see figure 4.5).

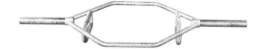

FIGURE 4.5   Trap bar.

weight plates—The round steel plates that add weight to barbells and plate-loaded weight machines. There are generally two types of weight plates, but regardless of the type of weight plate, these are commonly available in weights of 1.25, 2.5, 5, 10, 25, 35, 45, and even 100 pounds:

Olympic weight plates—These plates have center holes that are 2-1/8 inches (about 5.4 centimeters) in diameter to fit on Olympic barbells.

standard weight plates—These plates have center holes that are about 1-1/8 inches (about 3 centimeters) in diameter to fit on a 1-inch standard bar.

bumper plates—An Olympic weight plate with a rubber outer rim and/or coating to reduce damage to the floor and the weight plate in the event that it is dropped. These are most commonly used in Olympic weightlifting where very heavy weights are lifted overhead and then dropped.

collar—The clamp used to hold plates securely in place on a barbell or adjustable dumbbell. The collars used in powerlifting and Olympic weightlifting weigh 5.5 pounds (2.5 kilograms).

dumbbell—A short-handled barbell intended primarily for use with one hand. It is usually about 8 to 12 inches (20 to 30 centimeters) in total length; the knurled gripping portion is about 6 inches (15 centimeters) on most dumbbells. Some dumbbells are solid steel with round or hexagon ends, while others use weight plates and can be adjusted to different weights.

Specialty Free-Weight Objects

Some free-weight objects don't fall under the typical category of dumbbell or barbell. These unique objects provide weight for many conventional and unconventional exercises.

medicine ball—A weighted leather or rubber ball that varies in size from that of a volleyball to a basketball, depending on the weight (2 to 30 pounds, or 0.9 to 14 kilograms). Medicine balls can be used for throwing exercises or to simulate most typical exercises done with barbells or dumbbells (see figure 4.6).

kettlebell—This cast-iron free weight resembles a cannonball with a solid handle welded to it. Kettlebells come in weights as low as 15 pounds to as high as 50 (about 7 to 23 kilograms), usually

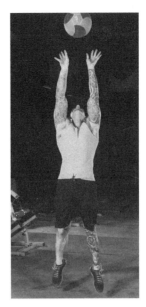

FIGURE 4.6 Throwing a medicine ball.

in 5- or 10-pound increments. They can be used for a variety of exercises but are mainly used for performing swings, snatches, and cleans.

head harness—A leather or nylon head strap that has a chain attached from one side to the other. Weight plates are added to the chain and the device is worn on the head to provide resistance for neck-strengthening exercises (see figure 4.7).

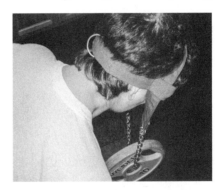

FIGURE 4.7 Neck extensions with a head harness.

weighted belt—This equipment resembles a short weight belt that fits around the small of the back along with a long chain that runs from one side of the belt to the other. Weight plates are added to the chain and supported around the waist for adding resistance during bodyweight exercises such as dips and pull-ups.

weight vest—This device is simply a nylon vest with pockets that hold 1- to 2-pound weights. Total weight usually adjusts between 2 and 40 pounds (0.9 to 18 kilograms), although a few extreme vests go up to 80 pounds or more. This is often used to increase the weight on body-weight exercises such as push-ups as well as bounding and running exercises.

sand bags—These devices are typically made of canvas, leather or neoprene and are filled with sand or steel bee bees. This creates a weighted device that changes the distribution of the weight depending on how you hold it and move it.

wrist roller—This device is simply composed of a short steel or wooden handle with a three- to four-foot (91- to 122-centimeter) rope attached to it (see figure 4.8). On the other end of the rope weights are attached. To train the forearm flexors, a lifter would roll the handle with a forward motion to lift the weight from the floor until the rope is completely wrapped around the handle. To train the forearm extensors, the lifter would roll the handle in a reverse motion.

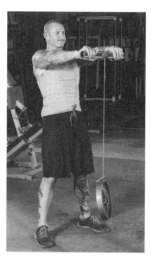

FIGURE 4.8 Wrist curls with a wrist roller.

arm blaster—This aluminum device is used to prevent movement of the upper arms when doing biceps curls. It has straps that suspend it from the shoulders so that it sits firmly against the waist allowing the backs of the arms to press against the arm blaster while the lifter performs curls (see figure 4.9).

land mine—This device is a weighted plate (many look like home plate on a baseball diamond) that holds a sleeve that fits the end of a barbell. The sleeve is connected to the base with a number of free moving joints that allow the barbell to be rotated from the free end to work the core muscles, as well as the lower body and upper body muscles (see figure 4.10).

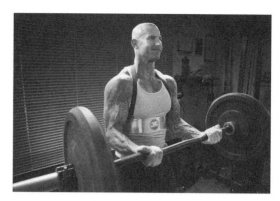

FIGURE 4.9 Barbell curls with an arm blaster.

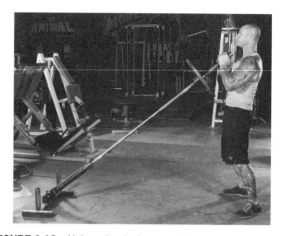

FIGURE 4.10 Using a land mine to perform a dead land mine.

Free-Weight Accessories

Besides the resistance component of strength training with free-weight objects, many exercises require the use of various benches and racks to support the lifter and the free weight.

weight benches—Various benches are used along with free weights and are specifically designed for certain barbell exercises. These weight benches have supports for barbells to allow the lifter to easily rack the barbell at the end of the set. Following are some types of benches:

bench-press bench—A horizontal bench with vertical barbell supports.

incline bench-press bench—A bench that is angled up at about 35 to 45 degrees from the floor so that when a lifter sits on it the head is higher than the hips. The bench is welded to a steel structure that has vertical barbell supports and a step platform for a spotter to watch over the lifter performing the incline bench press exercise.

decline bench-press bench—A bench that angles down about 30 to 40 degrees so that the head is lower than the feet. There are barbell supports for doing decline barbell bench presses.

shoulder press bench—A bench that has a padded seat and vertical seat back so that when the lifter sits on it the torso is vertical, as it should be when doing the barbell shoulder press exercise. The bench is welded to a steel structure that has vertical barbell supports that sit behind the lifter's head so that he or she can easily grab the bar at the start of the set and can rack it without stressing the shoulder joint at the end of the set.

preacher bench—A bench that has a seat and a padded armrest that is angled at about 45 degrees to the floor and set in front of the lifter. In front of the armrest is a barbell support. The lifter sits on the seat with the upper arms supported on the armrest and performs biceps curls.

free-standing benches—Some benches do not have barbell supports because they are used mainly with dumbbells. These benches consist of just the padded bench and leg supports and include the following:

flat bench—A fixed horizontal bench that is used for seated or lying exercises that are performed prone or supine.

adjustable-incline bench—A bench that allows the angle of the surface to be adjusted from horizontal to vertical with various points in between.

adjustable-decline bench—A bench that angles down at varying degrees so that the head is lower than the feet. This is often used for chest and abdominal exercises.

low-back bench—A bench that has a short horizontal seat and a low vertical back pad to support the back during exercises such as overhead presses and triceps extensions.

weight rack—A rack that supports a barbell to allow the lifter to grab it from a variety of positions. The following are some types of weight racks:

power rack—The most versatile rack is this safety apparatus that is made of four vertical steel beams to create a cage that is usually about five feet (one and a half meters) long, five feet wide, and seven feet (two meters) tall. The vertical beams have holes drilled into them every one to two inches from top to bottom. The holes allow the barbell hooks to be adjusted to different heights. The holes also fit safety bars that can be used to catch the barbell if the lifter fails to lift the weight. Power racks are typically used for squats, shrugs, and presses (see figure 4.11a).

squat rack—A steel structure that has barbell-support hooks at different heights so that lifters of various statures can easily unrack the barbell to perform the squat or other standing exercises. Some squat racks have two horizontal beams that are about three feet (91 centimeters) high and run parallel to each other off the front of the squat rack. These beams act as a safety rack so that if a lifter fails to complete a squat, he or she can rack the weight on the safety beam (see figure 4.11b).

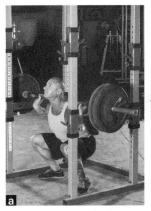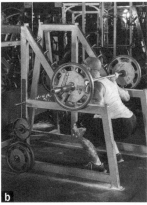

FIGURE 4.11 *(a)* Squatting in a power rack contrasted with *(b)* squatting in a squat rack.

stability objects—A multitude of objects can provide unstable support. Unlike a bench, which has a stable foundation to support the lifter's body weight, stability objects are unstable objects that make an exercise more difficult to perform. This helps to develop the strength of the core and stabilizer muscles.

exercise ball—Also known as a stability ball. These inflatable balls come in several sizes (30 to 85 centimeters in diameter). They offer a platform that rolls and gives when a person sits or lies on it, making seated or lying exercises with dumbbells or barbells much more difficult to perform (see figure 4.12). These can also be used with body-weight exercises such as crunches and push-ups.

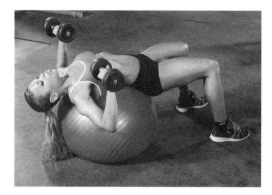

FIGURE 4.12   Dumbbell presses on an exercise ball.

BOSU balance trainer—This object resembles the top half of a large exercise ball with a solid and stable base. It offers most of the benefits of an exercise ball without the rolling, which makes it ideal for building core strength with standing exercises (see figure 4.13).

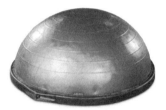

FIGURE 4.13   BOSU balance trainer.

stability disc—Small (about 12 to 14 inches in diameter and 2 to 3 inches in height) pancake-like disc made of pliable plastic that a person can stand on or sit on while doing strength exercises (see figure 4.14).

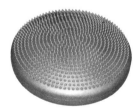

FIGURE 4.14   Stability disc.

balance board—A wooden base that has a rounded bottom to provide wobbling when stood on. These are sometimes used for performing standing strength exercises (see figure 4.15).

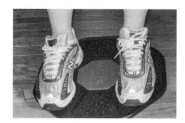

FIGURE 4.15   Balance board.

Common Objects

Long before dumbbells and barbells were available, athletes and others needing to enhance their strength and fitness used a variety of common objects that served as free weight, such as stones and sacks of sand. Today, although balanced barbells and dumbbells are available, some people use common objects (such as food cans or gallon milk jugs) when they don't have access to standard free-weight implements or choose to lift awkward and unbalanced objects (such as stones and beer kegs) to develop more functional strength. Obviously, any object with mass can be used as a strength training tool—a can of soup, a bucket of water, or a cement cylinder block. Rocks, logs, and tires are common implements to be lifted in strongman competitions. The disadvantage to lifting common objects is the awkwardness. Without a clear handle to grab and without an even balance of weight, lifting common objects requires more functional ability than free weights require. But lifting such awkward implements helps to develop core strength and functional strength.

strongman implements—Strongmen are required to lift a number of awkward objects during competition. Most events combine strength and muscle endurance by requiring the competitors to outdo each other by lifting such objects for the most repetitions or carrying them the most quickly over a certain distance. Some common strongmen implements include the following:

Atlas stone—Atlas stones are large, heavy balls made of granite or concrete that strongmen must lift and carry in competition. Sizes range from 14 inches to more than 60 inches (36 to 152 centimeters) in diameter and weights range from about 140 pounds to well over 300 pounds (64 to 136 kilograms). Competitors typically must lift progressively heavier Atlas stones from the ground and load them onto progressively higher pedestals (up to 60 inches). The competitor who completes the task in the least amount of time wins.

logs—These awkward objects are common to strongman competitions. The modified ones found in competitions have handles carved into them for easier gripping when lifting. These can range in weight from about 200 to well over 300 pounds (91 to 136 kilograms). The winner is the competitor who lifts the heaviest log from the ground to overhead. Aluminum logs are available that have Olympic barbell ends to allow Olympic weight plates to be added for training with different weights.

tractor tires—These can range in weight from about 500 pounds to more than 900 pounds (227 to 408 kilograms), depending on the size. In strongman competitions the competitor who flips the tire the fastest over a predetermined distance is the winner.

training adjuncts—Some common objects are used for enhancing strength in the gym or on the playing field. The unique mass characteristics of the object (unbalanced weight or progressive weight) offer benefits that free weights don't. Such implements include the following:

chains—Steel chains can be attached to an Olympic bar to provide progressive resistance during barbell exercises such as the bench press or squat. The unique thing about chains is that as each link lifts off the ground, the weight being lifted increases, offering linear variable resistance throughout the range of motion. This type of resistance provides greater resistance the further you move through the range of motion of an exercise.

beer keg—An empty beer keg weighs approximately 30 pounds (14 kilograms). The handles on a beer keg make it easy to grip, but the rotund shape makes it awkward to lift and control. Some strength coaches have their football, basketball, baseball, and hockey players as well as other athletes lift kegs as a way to develop more functional strength.

everyday objects—Objects that are found in most homes can be used in place of free weights when free weights are unavailable for standard strength training exercises. Some objects commonly used include the following:

soup cans—These can range in weight from 10 ounces to a little over 1 pound (.28 to .45 kilogram). Similar to dumbbells, soup cans can be held in the hands for almost any exercise that would normally be performed with dumbbells. Because of the limit in weight available, cans are best suited for people with poor strength or for those performing workouts that have very high reps.

gallon jugs—Plastic gallon jugs weigh about 8 pounds (4 kilograms) when filled with fluid or 14 pounds (6 kilograms) when filled with sand. The handles allow them to be gripped in a fashion similar to that of dumbbells (although they're more awkward to lift). The weight can be adjusted by altering the amount of fluid or sand in the jugs.

Human Body

Your own body weight or that of a training partner can be used as a form of resistance.

own body weight—Exercises such as push-ups, chin-ups, dips, body-weight squats, and crunches use pure body weight, nothing else, to get the job done (see figure 4.16).

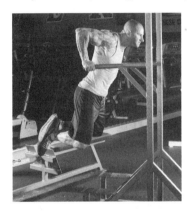

FIGURE 4.16 Dips.

partner body weight—When training with a partner, you can do a variety of exercises that use the partner's body weight as resistance. For example, rows, bench presses, and squats can all be done with the weight of a training partner (see figure 4.17).

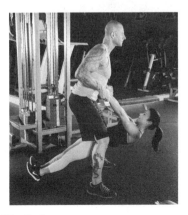

FIGURE 4.17 Body rows.

body-weight exercise accessories—Certain equipment has been designed for use with exercises that primarily rely on one's body weight:

chin-up bar—A chin-up bar is simply a horizontal bar that is mounted to its own stand, wall, ceiling, doorway, or other exercise apparatus (such as a power rack or cable crossover).

dip bars—Parallel bars set high enough above the floor to allow dips to be performed between them. They can also be used for leg raises for the abdominals and for a variety of other exercises. Some dipping bars are angled inward at one end so that the distance between the two bars is different. This allows you to perform dips with varying grip width.

vertical bench—This device is composed of a long, vertical, padded bench that is attached to a metal platform that has handles and armrests. The lifter suspends the body by supporting the weight with the forearms and pressing the back against the pad. This bench is used for leg raises (see figure 4.18) and is sometimes referred to as a captain's chair. Some vertical benches have dip bars extended off the front.

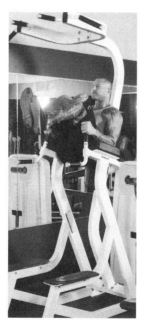

FIGURE 4.18   Knee raises on a vertical bench.

back extension bench—A high, short, padded bench that has leg pads set at the same height as the bench. This allows the lifter to lie prone with the pelvis resting on the padded bench and the feet secured under the leg pads while doing back extensions.

Suspension trainer—The TRX is responsible for making suspension training popular. But long before TRX, chains or ropes with handles were used. Today there are numerous other suspension trainer brands that have followed in the footsteps of TRX. Suspension training involves straps, often made of canvas or nylon that suspend part of the body (usually from the arms or feet) to allow the person's own body to provide resistance. For example, you can do inverted rows using a suspension trainer to work the lats (see figure 4.19).

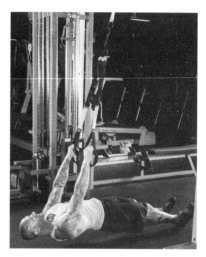

FIGURE 4.19   Inverted rows on a TRX.

Simple Weight Machines

Simple weight machines are those machines and apparatuses that provide a constant level of resistance throughout the entire range of motion. These devices include linear guided machines and cable pulley machines. They contain a weight that must be moved. The lifter directly moves the weight along its guide rods or through a cable pulley system.

Linear Guided Machines

Linear guided machines consist of an apparatus that rides on two guide rods. This limits the movement to a linear, or straight, movement. These types of machines usually require the addition of weight plates for added resistance.

Smith machine—A type of machine that consists of a barbell that rides along two vertical rods that serve as guides. The bars permit the barbell to move only in a vertical direction, but they have safety catches at several points from the bottom of the machine to the top to allow the user to start or stop the exercise at any point. This machine is typically used just for exercises that require vertical pushing or pulling, such as the squat, bench press, and row (see figure 4.20).

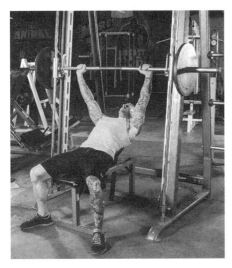

FIGURE 4.20   Incline bench press on a Smith machine.

leg press—This machine consists of a sled that rides along two rods that are angled at approximately 45 degrees. There is a seat for a lifter to sit in while placing the feet on the sled (see figure 4.21). After the lifter disengages the safety bar, the sled is free to move up and down the linear guide rod. However, the natural arc of motion of the legs in that position is curvilinear (a combination of a curve and a straight line). This has prompted some manufacturers of weight machines to design leg press machines that follow a curvilinear path. This more natural motion places less stress on the knees.

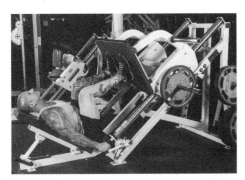

FIGURE 4.21   The leg press.

hack squat—This machine for leg exercises is similar to the leg press except that the lifter stands rather than sits. A padded sled rides along two guide rods that are angled at about

50 to 80 degrees. The lifter stands in the hack squat with the back against the padded sled and the shoulders under the shoulder pads. After disengaging the safety bars, the lifter squats down and back up, allowing the sled to follow.

Cable Pulley Machines

Cable pulley machines refer to exercise machines that are based on a simple system of cables and pulleys. In their most basic form they consist of a cable that routes through a pulley (or several pulleys) and connects to a weight stack. A pulley is a freely rotating wheel used to change the direction of force applied by a cable. This allows for force to be applied to a muscle in a variety of directions, such as horizontal. A weight stack is a stack of specialized weight plates (usually rectangular in shape and weighing 5 to 20 pounds each) that are fixed so that they can slide vertically on the guide rods of a weight machine. Each weight plate is drilled with a horizontal hole that allows a pin to be placed through the plate. This weight and all those above it may then be lifted by the moveable rod, which is typically attached to a cable or lever arm. When tension is placed on the cable (that is, the cable is pulled), the weight stack is lifted along its guide rods, thereby supplying resistance. Some home machines, such as Bowflex, use flexible rods for resistance instead of a weight stack. Cables offer a number of benefits to weightlifters. Because the cable can be pulled in a number of directions, it offers constant tension on the muscle throughout the entire range of motion (see figure 4.22).

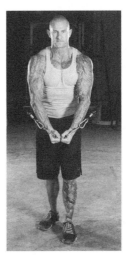

FIGURE 4.22   The cable crossover.

cable attachments—A handle must be attached to the end of the cable in order for a cable machine to be used. A variety of cable attachments are used for a variety of exercises:

carabiner—This clip mechanism allows for easy attachment of bars to the cable (see figure 4.23).

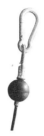

FIGURE 4.23   A carabiner that can be attached to a cable.

lat bar—Primarily used when training the latissimus dorsi and other back muscles on the pulldown machine. The most common lat bar is a long shaft that bends down on both sides (see figure 4.24).

parallel-arm lat bar—This bar has handles on the end that are perpendicular to the bar and allow a neutral grip to be maintained during pulldowns and cable rows (see figure 4.24).

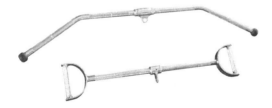

FIGURE 4.24   Lat bar (top) and parallel-arm lat bar (bottom).

EZ bar—The EZ bar attachment is shaped similar to the EZ curl bar: a stretched-out W (see figure 4.25). Most have a rotating sleeve that allows the bar to swivel to reduce the stress placed on the wrists. This bar is typically used for cable biceps curls and triceps pressdowns.

short straight bar—This bar attachment is similar to an Olympic bar in shape but is much shorter in length (about 20 inches or 51 centimeters). Most have a rotating sleeve. This bar can be used for a variety of exercises, including triceps pressdowns, curls, reverse curls, and upright rows (see figure 4.25).

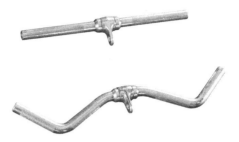

FIGURE 4.25   Short straight bar (top) and EZ bar (bottom) attachments.

low row bar—This attachment has two short parallel handles connected to two triangle-shaped bars (see figure 4.26). It is used primarily for cable rows and close-grip pulldowns.

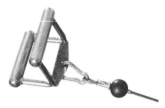

FIGURE 4.26   Low row bar.

long multiple-use V-bar—This bar looks like an upside-down V, with long handles for gripping projecting out to the sides. Because of its design, this bar may relieve some of the load on the wrists during heavy triceps pressdowns. Rows and pulldowns are other exercises that can be performed with the V-bar.

single-handle D-grip—This handle looks like a stirrup with a swiveling handle to grasp (see figure 4.27). It is designed for unilateral cable exercises such as lateral raises, rows, curls, and triceps pressdowns.

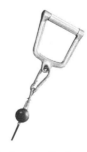

FIGURE 4.27   Single-handle D-grip.

pressdown bar—This bar looks like an inverted V or U and is used primarily for triceps pressdowns.

rope—As the name implies, this attachment is literally a thick rope with a metal sleeve where it attaches to the cable (see figure 4.28). This attachment can be used for performing various cable exercises such as triceps pressdowns, hammer curls, and cable crunches.

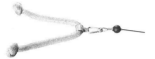

FIGURE 4.28   Rope attachment.

ankle collar—A wide ankle bracelet that clips to pulleys to allow leg exercises to be performed with cables, such as leg lifts and leg curls (see figure 4.29).

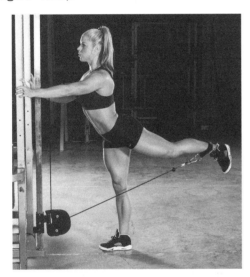

FIGURE 4.29   Leg raises with an ankle collar attachment.

VARIABLE RESISTANCE

This category of strength training equipment provides variable resistance, whether controlled or not. It includes machines that purposely vary the resistance throughout the range of motion and equipment that varies the resistance throughout the range of motion in an uncontrolled fashion.

Cam-Based Resistance Machines

Cam-based resistance machines are the type of weight machines found in most gyms. They are often called *selectorized machines* because of the weight stack that is on most of these machines. However, some cam-based machines are plate loaded. The most popular brands are Cybex, Life Fitness, Nautilus, PreCor, Hoist, and Paramount.

The cam is an ellipse connected to the movement arm of the machine on which the cable or belt travels. The purpose of the cam is to provide variable resistance, which changes how heavy the weight feels (but the actual weight never changes) as the lifter moves through the range of motion of the exercise. The reason the perception of the weight needs to change is that each joint movement has an associated strength curve. That is, at different angles of the joint the strength of the agonist muscle varies. For example, during a biceps curl, the strength of the agonist muscles (mainly the biceps) progressively gets stronger up to about 90 degrees of bend at the elbow. After that, the strength progressively decreases as the curl continues. This is known as an ascending and descending strength curve.

There are three types of strength curves and, therefore, three basic cam shapes that correspond to each strength curve:

ascending and descending curve—This type of strength curve was described previously with the biceps curl as an example. In this type of curve the strength increases up to about the halfway point of the movement and then decreases through the rest of the movement. For this reason it is often referred to as bell shaped. The shape of the ascending and descending cam is similar to a bell or an inverted U with the largest radius in the middle (see figure 4.30a).

ascending curve—In the ascending curve the strength progressively increases through the entire range of motion. An example of this is the bench press. The farther the weight moves away from the chest, the stronger the agonist muscles are. The shape of the ascending cam is oblong with the largest radius at the distal end (see figure 4.30b).

descending curve—In the descending curve the strength progressively decreases through the entire range of motion. This type of strength curve can be experienced during the row exercise. As the handles are pulled closer to the body, the strength of the agonist muscles decreases. The shape of the descending cam is oblong with the largest radius at the proximal end (see figure 4.30c).

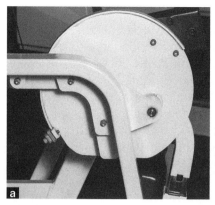
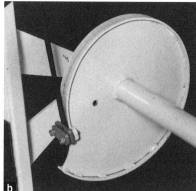
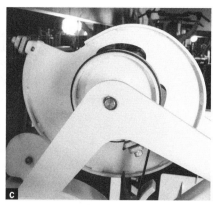

FIGURE 4.30 Types of cam machines: *(a)* ascending and descending cam, *(b)* ascending cam, and *(c)* descending cam.

Lever-Arm Resistance Machines

Lever-arm resistance machines use counterbalanced lever arms to mimic the strength curves of the muscles being trained. Therefore, much like cam-based machines, the counterbalanced lever arms vary the resistance throughout the range of motion by altering the amount of weight that counterbalances the weight being moved. These are usually plate-loaded machines; however, some of them use a weight stack system. The most popular line of lever-arm resistance machines is Hammer Strength by Life Fitness (see figure 4.31).

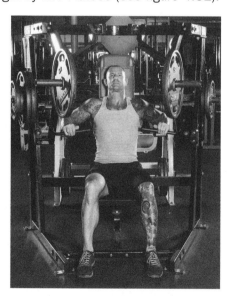

FIGURE 4.31 A Hammer Strength chest press.

Resistance With Pull

Some exercise devices don't rely on mass for resistance but on the energy their material supplies. Springs, bands, and other material that resist being pulled are such devices. These devices provide only ascending resistance, because the resistance progressively increases over the range of motion.

Springs

The force generated by a spring is a restoring force, which attempts to move the two attachment points back to their original resting positions when they are either pulled farther apart or pushed closer together. The force a spring supplies depends on its material and the diameter of its coils. The distance the spring is pulled or compressed also changes the force, because the farther the ends are moved away from their original position, the more force they will supply. This is known as the *spring rate*—the rate at which tension increases as the ends move. This characteristic makes it impossible to maintain a particular resistance level over the movement of the exercise.

As the spring is deflected, resistance goes up; as it is relaxed, resistance goes down. Because of spring rate, users are forced to select a resistance that will be within their strength capability at maximum deflection, or they won't be able to do the exercise movement at all. As a result, during the first 50 percent or more of the movement, resistance is often too low to produce much benefit. Spring-resistance exercise devices come in a variety of setups. These include simple handheld devices that were popular in the 1950s, such as the Bull Worker, Chest Expander, and Grip Master (see figure 4.32). Although strength training has progressed far beyond spring resistance, some spring devices are still being used in certain products such as hand grippers (see figure 4.33), Pilates exercise machines, and the Stamina Gyrotonics spring-resistance exercise machine.

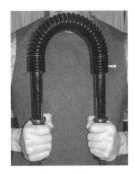

FIGURE 4.32   Bull Worker.

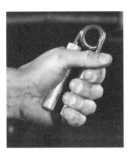

FIGURE 4.33   Hand gripper.

Elastic Bands and Tubing

Elastic bands and tubing supply a restoring force similar to that of springs. However, the force is applied only when the ends of the material are being pulled away from one another. Like springs, elastic bands and tubing have a spring rate. That is, as they are lengthened, the resistance they provide increases (see figure 4.34). This type of resistance is known as linear variable resistance and provides numerous benefits that free weights cannot. Because the resistance gets harder as you pull the bands, it is great for targeting the fast-twitch muscle fibers and developing greater muscle power. Because they are lightweight and portable, bands and tubing allow exercisers to work out at home or while away from home. They can also be added to free weights to provide both isotonic

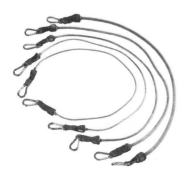

FIGURE 4.34   Elastic bands.

resistance from the free weights and the linear variable resistance from the bands. Research shows that this method can produce superior gains in muscle strength and power than using free weights alone. Bands and tubes are color coded to represent a certain resistance level. See table 4.1 for color and resistance codes.

TABLE 4.1   Tube and Band Resistance

Band or tube color	Resistance level
Yellow	Extra light
Green	Light
Red	Medium
Blue	Heavy
Black	Extra heavy
Orange	Extra, extra heavy

Resistance levels are measured at 100 percent elongation and twice the unstretched length. They should not be stretched beyond this point.

SPEED MACHINES

This category of strength training equipment deals with machines that control the rate of speed of movement. The type of muscle contraction where the speed remains constant is considered isokinetic. Equipment that controls the speed of movement provides resistance simply by moving through a range of motion at a particular set speed while the lifter applies as much force as possible to the lever arm without altering the speed at which the lever arm moves. Because the lever arm must be moved at a controlled, constant rate, the machines that provide this type of resistance—known as isokinetic dynamometers—are controlled by a computer.

> **isokinetic dynamometer**—This computerized resistance machine can be programmed to move at a variety of set speeds. These are commonly found only in laboratory settings or sports medicine clinics as a tool for measuring the amount of force that an athlete can apply. This type of equipment is usually interfaced with a computer to not only control the rate of speed of the movement but to measure force applied as well. There are several disadvantages of isokinetic dynamometers. The first is the fact that the only motion they permit is angular. In other words, they permit only flexion or extension at the elbow, wrist, knee, or ankle. They cannot be used for pressing

exercises, such as the bench press, shoulder press, or squat. The other disadvantage of isokinetic dynamometers is that no isokinetic muscle actions actually occur in real-life movements.

NONTRADITIONAL AND NEW APPARATUS

The last category of strength training equipment covers equipment that is typically not categorized among the other more common forms of strength training equipment. These devices include vibration machines, electronic and computerized resistance machines, pneumatic resistance machines, hydraulic resistance machines, and the Bodyblade. Common to them all is the fact that the way they provide resistance is novel.

Vibration Machines

Whole-body vibration machines usually consist of a device that the user can stand, lie, sit, or place the hands or any other part of the body on to transmit vibration to the body tissues the user wishes to stimulate (see figure 4.35). Most of these vibration machines are about the size of a typical stair stepper, and the vibration platform is about 32 inches by 20 inches (81 by 51 centimeters). The control panel allows the user to change the speed (or frequency) and the magnitude of the vibration.

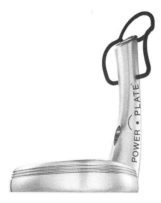

FIGURE 4.35 Vibration machine.

Most machines have vibration plates that move up and down and side to side, while others work as a high-speed wobble board. The energy from the mechanical vibration (of the plate) is transferred through the body, causing the muscle fibers to contract and relax at an extremely rapid rate and with very high force. Research shows that performing vibration training for several weeks can increase muscle strength and power (Issurin and Tenenbaum 1999) as well as increase the release of growth hormone and testosterone, which are anabolic hormones (Bosco et al. 2000). Although most people cannot understand how vibration can be considered a method of strength training, it is slowly being recognized for its ability to increase strength, power, and possibly muscle growth.

Electronic and Computerized Resistance Machines

Electronic and computerized machines provide resistance through gears and belts connected to a motor. These are programmed to provide variable resistance throughout the range of motion to follow the strength curve of the muscle being trained. Resistance can be increased in increments as small as one pound through a touch screen, button, or foot pedal. Some machines can be programmed to provide greater resistance during the eccentric portion of the exercise.

Pneumatic Resistance Machines

Pneumatic resistance machines use a compressor to supply air pressure for resistance. This allows the lifter to adjust the resistance on his or her own throughout the range of motion (see figure 4.36). The benefit of this is that as the muscles fatigue during a set, the resistance can be reduced to allow more reps to be completed.

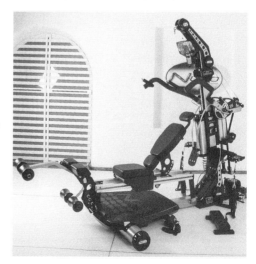

FIGURE 4.36 Pneumatic machine.

Both electronic and pneumatic machines work in one plane, so the user's motion is predefined. Electronic and pneumatic machines can be less intimidating and safer for beginning exercisers because weight stacks aren't visible and plates do not have to be loaded. Some exercisers do not like electronic or pneumatic equipment, however, because they don't provide the feel of lifting an actual weight stack, dumbbell, or barbell. These modalities also can be more expensive than other strength training equipment, and they require special wiring for electricity or a layout to accommodate an air compressor and hoses.

Because of their uniqueness and ability to suit any population, electronic and pneumatic machines can be an excellent investment and provide variety in strength training for all exercisers.

Hydraulic Resistance Machines

Hydraulic resistance machines provide resistance through hydraulics. The lever arm on these machines is connected to a hydraulic piston that provides resistance against the oil-filled chamber it resides in. The problem with hydraulic resistance machines is that they allow for concentric contractions only. Therefore, most hydraulic machines train dual muscles but only through the concentric portion. For instance, the hydraulic biceps machine is a biceps–triceps machine because after the user curls the weight up, he or she must press it back down using the triceps muscles.

Bodyblade

Bodyblade, shown in figure 4.37, is a five-foot-long fiberglass beam that resembles a snow ski and works by the laws of inertia (an object set in motion remains in motion until another force acts on it to stop or change its direction). The user holds the middle of it and pushes and pulls on the apparatus to start it oscillating. During use, it oscillates at an average rate of about 270 times per minute. These oscillations in the ends of the blade create a force that the holder must resist to literally keep it from flying out of the hands. With each oscillation the muscles of the arms and core must resist the movement by contracting. The greater the amplitude of the blade ends (the farther they flex up and down), the more force the user must apply to resist the movement. By varying the positions of the body or direction of the flexing blade, the user can target specific muscle groups throughout the body. Since the blade can be used at any angle and position, a major benefit to this piece of equipment is that it can mimic the movements in a particular sport and provide the required specificity of training. The disadvantage of the Bodyblade is the fact that it is limited mainly to upper-body and core exercises with little application for the lower-body muscles.

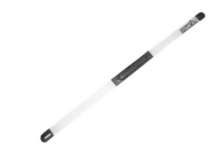

FIGURE 4.37 Bodyblade.

SUMMARY

Strength training equipment has developed over the decades from simple free weights to complex machinery that provide resistance through novel mechanisms. This, however, is not to say that the more modern equipment is better than the simplest form of free weights. In fact, free weights have many advantages and very few disadvantages. Modern resistance machines, on the other hand, tend to have many more disadvantages than free weight equipment. Because all forms of strength training equipment offer different advantages and are limited by different disadvantages, it is best to use a variety of training equipment in your strength training program.

PART II

TRAINING FOR MUSCLE MASS

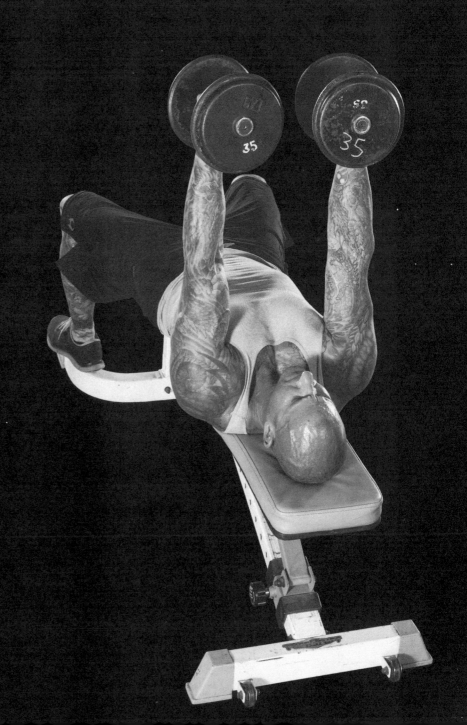

Muscle growth—known scientifically as muscle hypertrophy—involves a complex integration of multiple factors. Strength training initiates many of these factors through both the mechanical stress and the metabolic stress that it places on the muscle fibers. The mechanical stress is the actual physical weight the muscle fibers must resist by contracting. This damages muscle fibers and initiates a biochemical cascade that leads to growth of muscle fibers. The metabolic stress comes from the energy demands placed on the muscle to fuel muscle contractions. This type of stress initiates biochemical cascades that influence growth of muscle fiber through various mechanisms that mainly result in an increase in muscle protein synthesis. Although the details of many of these biochemical cascades are well defined, it is currently unknown exactly how all these factors work together to result in muscle growth. Yet, through both trial and error and scientific investigation, we do know what training techniques and programs work best to influence the factors that are responsible for causing muscle growth. These techniques and programs are presented in part II.

Chapter 5 covers the basics of creating strength training programs for maximizing muscle growth.

This chapter teaches you how to organize your workouts for the week based on your training experience and schedule. It presents guidelines for designing workouts that are effective at producing gains in muscle mass. In addition, it breaks down training into exercises for each major muscle group to allow maximal growth of each.

Chapter 6 introduces you to more advanced training strategies that you can add to the training foundations in chapter 5. These techniques are designed to exaggerate the mechanical stresses and metabolic stresses that are placed on the muscle fibers to encourage muscle growth. These are strategies that are critical to the advanced lifter because the advanced lifter's muscle fibers are better able to handle the stress of strength training.

Chapter 7 concludes this section with long-term training cycles that are designed for beginning, intermediate, and advanced lifters. In addition, training cycles are designed for specific overall goals as well as for emphasizing the growth of specific muscle groups. Whether you're a beginner or an advanced weightlifter, if your current goal is to build more muscle, in part II you will discover all you need to know to realize that goal.

Tactics for Building Muscle Mass

Regardless of whether your goal is to maximize muscle mass or strength gains, knowing how to develop an individualized training program that delivers results is critical to your pursuit. While advanced training techniques—like those described in chapter 6—can help you rapidly advance muscle gains, you must first understand how to organize a basic training program. This chapter demonstrates how to put together a basic yet highly effective program that you can build on later with more advanced training methods as you progress.

If your primary goal is to build muscle mass, then you must consider several things when structuring your strength training program. You will need to consider the variables discussed in chapter 2. These include the choice of exercises you will perform, the order of those exercises, how many sets of each exercise you will do, how heavy a weight you will use on those exercises, how much rest you will allow between sets, and even how fast or slow your reps are. You will also need to consider how often you will train each muscle group, how you will split up your training, and how you will periodize (or cycle) your training for optimal results.

WEEKLY SPLITS

Most weightlifters break their training down into a weekly period. While this isn't a necessity, it seems to be the simplest approach to split up training days because our calendar revolves around a weekly schedule. All other activities in our lives—school, work, television programs, and leisure activities—all follow a weekly schedule. It's only logical to break your strength training down into a similar period. How you split your training will influence how often you train each muscle group

per week. Choosing a training split that is the most advantageous for you depends on several factors, such as your training experience, your overall goals, your schedule, and even convenience.

The following seven training splits are the most common and effective for the majority of bodybuilders. These splits start with the easiest (whole-body training) split for beginners (those with less than six months of consistent strength training) and progressively become more intense as they advance through push–pull training splits and two-day training splits, which are ideal for intermediate lifters (those with less than one year of consistent strength training) and end with five-day training splits and twice-a-day training splits, which are geared for the advanced lifter (those with over a year of consistent strength training). Choosing the right split will depend primarily on your training experience, but you should also take into consideration your schedule.

Whole-Body Training

Whole-body training refers to single workouts that stress every major muscle group. In other words, the entire body is trained in every workout. Because you will need to train up to 11 major muscle groups (chest, shoulders, back, quadriceps, hamstrings, biceps, triceps, forearms, trapezius, calves, and abdominals) in each workout, the number of exercises and sets you can do per muscle group is minimal. This allows you to train each muscle group more frequently because it receives a limited amount of stress at each workout. Typically, most whole-body training workouts use one or two exercises per muscle group, and total sets per muscle group rarely exceed six. Compare this to the four-day and five-day training splits, which allow the weightlifter to hit three to six exercises and a total of 12 to 30 sets per muscle group. The fewer total sets a muscle group receives, the less recuperation it usually needs before being trained again.

Whole-body training splits allow you to train each muscle group about three times per week. This type of training split is best for beginning weightlifters (those with up to six months of training experience), those who want to train each muscle group more frequently, and those who are interested in cutting down on body fat. The reason whole-body training is the best choice for beginners is that the initial adaptations made in a strength training program involve the nervous system. That is, in the first few months of strength training, the primary improvements are seen in the motor units (the nerve fibers that serve the muscle cells). These improvements allow the muscles to contract more efficiently and are best trained by repetition. This means that the best way for beginners to train is with high repetitions and more frequent training to program the nervous system. They should use the same exercises in each workout to maximize the learning effect that will have the greatest benefit on the nervous system.

Whole-body training is effective for building muscle mass for two reasons. The first benefit is known as the staircase effect. Training each muscle group every other day (or about three days per week) allows you to build onto the effects of the previous workout. If you wait too long between workouts, you're back to square one—almost as if you are starting over from the original point. Some experts believe that the staircase effect is critical to muscle adaptation. The second benefit to whole-body training is that it stimulates a large portion of the body's muscle mass. This leads to higher production of growth hormone and testosterone (important for stimulating muscle growth) than workouts that train fewer muscle groups. If you are an advanced weightlifter, the best way to use whole-body training is to mix up the exercises at every workout. This allows you to hit each muscle group from a variety of angles for better stimulation of the majority of muscle fibers within each muscle group.

When it comes to shedding body fat, no workout split is more conducive to that goal than whole-body training. Training all the major muscle groups revs up cellular processes in all the muscle cells, which increases the metabolic rate for up to 48 hours after the workout is over. This means you will burn more calories while sitting around doing nothing. See tables 5.1 and 5.2 for beginner and advanced whole-body training splits.

TABLE 5.1   Beginner Whole-Body Training Split

Exercise	Sets	Reps
Incline barbell bench press	3	8-10
Dumbbell row	3	8-10
Barbell shoulder press	3	10-12
Leg press	3	8-10
Triceps pressdown	3	8-10
Standing dumbbell curl	3	10-12
Standing calf raise	3	12-15
Crunch	3	15-20

TABLE 5.2   Advanced Whole-Body Training Split

MONDAY		
Exercise	**Sets**	**Reps**
Bench press	4	8-10
Pulldown	4	8-10
Lateral raise	4	10-12
Squat	4	8-10
Barbell curl	4	8-10
Triceps extension	4	10-12
Seated calf raise	4	12-15
Crunch	4	15-20
WEDNESDAY		
Barbell row	4	8-10
Barbell shoulder press	4	8-10
Incline fly	4	10-12
Leg extension	3	10-12
Lying leg curl	3	10-12
Lying triceps extension	4	8-10
Incline dumbbell curl	4	10-12
Standing calf raise	4	10-12
Reverse crunch	4	12-15
FRIDAY		
Incline dumbbell press	4	8-10
Dumbbell row	4	8-10
Upright row	4	10-12
Leg press	4	8-10
Preacher curl	4	8-10
Close-grip bench press	4	8-10
Leg press calf raise	4	15-20
Hanging leg raise	4	10-12

Upper- and Lower-Body Training

Upper- and lower-body training is a training split that simply breaks the body down into upper-body (chest, back, shoulders, trapezius, biceps, triceps) and lower-body (quadriceps, hamstrings, calves, and often abdominals to limit the volume of work done in upper-body workouts). This allows you to train each muscle group two or three times per week depending on whether your schedule allows for four or six days of training each week. The four-day-per-week schedule is a good advancement for the beginner who is progressing from whole-body training. The advantage of upper- and lower-body training over whole-body training is that you can do more volume for each muscle group with upper- and lower-body training. Because you train fewer muscle groups each workout, you have the time to do more exercises and total sets for each muscle group. This means you can train each muscle group more intensely than with whole-body training. However, this means the muscles will require more rest on an upper- and lower-body training split. For this reason most bodybuilders using this split train four days per week, as shown in table 5.3. This allows for two or three days of rest for each muscle group between workouts and allows for different exercises to be done for each muscle group on the separate workouts.

TABLE 5.3   Upper- and Lower-Body Training Split

UPPER BODY (MONDAY)			
Muscle group	**Exercise**	**Sets**	**Reps**
Chest	Incline bench press	3	6-8
	Dumbbell fly	3	8-10
Back	Pull-up	3	6-8
	Dumbbell row	3	8-10
Shoulders	Dumbbell shoulder press	3	6-8
	Lateral raise	3	10-12
Trapezius	Smith machine shrug	3	6-10
Biceps	Barbell curl	3	8-10
	Preacher curl	2	10-12
Triceps	Close-grip bench press	3	8-10
	Triceps pressdown	2	10-12
LOWER BODY (TUESDAY)			
Quadriceps	Leg press	3	6-8
	Leg extension	3	10-12
Hamstrings	Seated leg curl	3	10-12
Calves	Leg press calf raise	3	15-20
	Seated calf raise	3	15-20
Abdominals	Hanging leg raise	3	10-12
	Crunch	3	15-20

UPPER BODY (THURSDAY)			
Muscle group	**Exercise**	**Sets**	**Reps**
Chest	Dumbbell bench press	3	8-10
	Incline dumbbell fly	3	8-10
Back	Barbell row	3	6-8
	Reverse-grip pulldown	3	8-10
Shoulders	Barbell shoulder press	3	6-8
	Upright row	3	10-12
Trapezius	Dumbbell shrug	3	8-10
Biceps	Incline dumbbell curl	3	8-10
	Cable curl	2	10-12
Triceps	Lying triceps extension	3	8-10
	Triceps dip	2	8-10
LOWER BODY (FRIDAY)			
Quadriceps	Squat	3	6-8
	Dumbbell lunge	3	10-12
Hamstrings	Romanian deadlift	3	8-10
Calves	Seated calf raise	3	15-20
	Standing calf raise	3	15-20
Abdominals	Cable crunch	3	10-12
	Reverse crunch	3	15-20

Two-Day Training Split

The two-day training split is very similar to the upper- and lower-body training split. The minor difference is that some upper-body muscle groups are trained with the legs (see table 5.4). This is because the upper body is composed of more muscle groups than the lower body. Many weightlifters use a scheme similar to the upper- and lower-body training split, but they train biceps and triceps with legs. This splits the two workouts into a workout for the chest, back, shoulder, trapezius, and abdominals and a workout for the quadriceps, hamstrings, calves, biceps, and triceps. The benefits of the two-day training split are the same as for the upper- and lower-body training split. However, the advantage to the two-day training split is that it better balances the number of muscle groups trained for each workout. You can use the two-day training split to train each muscle group either twice a week or three times per week, depending on your schedule and the amount of time you want to allow muscle groups to recover.

TABLE 5.4　Two-Day Training Split

MONDAY

Muscle group	Exercise	Sets	Reps
Chest	Decline bench press	3	6-8
	Incline cable fly	3	8-10
Back	Close-grip pulldown	3	8-10
	Smith machine row	3	8-10
Shoulders	Smith machine shoulder press	3	6-8
	Cable lateral raise	3	10-12
Trapezius	Barbell shrug	3	6-8
Abdominals	Hanging leg raise	3	10-12
	Oblique crunch	3	15-20

TUESDAY

Muscle group	Exercise	Sets	Reps
Quadriceps	Smith machine squat	3	6-10
	One-leg leg extension	3	12-15
Hamstrings	Dumbbell Romanian deadlift	3	8-10
Calves	Donkey calf raise	3	15-20
	Seated calf raise	3	15-20
Biceps	Barbell curl	3	8-10
	Cable concentration curl	2	10-12
Triceps	Seated triceps extension	3	8-10
	Triceps pressdown	2	10-12

THURSDAY

Muscle group	Exercise	Sets	Reps
Chest	Incline dumbbell press	3	8-10
	Machine fly	3	10-12
Back	Seated cable row	3	8-10
	Wide-grip pulldown	3	8-10
Shoulders	Dumbbell shoulder press	3	8-10
	Barbell front raise	3	10-12
Trapezius	Behind-the-back barbell shrug	3	8-10
Abdominals	Hip thrust	3	15-20
	Exercise-ball crunch	3	15-20

FRIDAY

Muscle group	Exercise	Sets	Reps
Quadriceps	Leg press	3	6-8
	Dumbbell lunge	3	10-12
Hamstrings	Lying leg curl	3	10-12
Calves	Seated calf raise	3	15-20
	Leg press calf raise	3	15-20
Biceps	Alternating dumbbell curl	3	8-10
	Preacher curl	2	10-12
Triceps	Triceps dip	3	6-10
	Lying triceps extension	2	8-10

Three-Day Training Split

The three-day training split is a common training split used by many bodybuilders to break the major muscle groups into three separate workouts. Although it is not critical how you pair muscle groups, a very common way to break up muscle groups with a three-day split is to separate workouts into a leg day (quadriceps, hamstrings, calves), a push day that trains the muscle groups involved in pushing movements (chest, shoulders, and triceps), and a pull day that trains muscle groups that perform pulling movements (back and biceps). Muscle groups such as abs can be trained on the first and third workout (if training each muscle group once per week) or on the second workout (if training each muscle group twice per week). Dividing the body into three separate workouts allows you to further increase the volume that is typically used in whole-body training, upper- and lower-body training, and two-day training splits. This type of split allows

you to give each muscle group three to seven days of rest between workouts. Most bodybuilders using this system train each muscle group either once or twice per week. When training muscle groups just once per week, the typical three-day training split is done on Monday, Wednesday, and Friday, as shown in table 5.5. Although the training doesn't have to take place on these precise three days, it is best to provide one day of rest between workouts. However, if your schedule does not allow for this, it is perfectly fine to train two or even all three of the workouts on consecutive days. This three-day training split is convenient for bodybuilders who train with high intensity or high volume because of the amount of rest allowed. For those interested in training each muscle group twice per week, the three-day training split can be done on Monday, Tuesday, and Wednesday and then repeated Thursday, Friday, and Saturday with a rest day on Sunday. Lower volume should be used for most muscle groups when training this frequently.

TABLE 5.5 Three-Day Training Split

MONDAY

Muscle group	Exercise	Sets	Reps
Chest	Bench press	3	8-10
	Incline dumbbell press	3	8-10
	Cable crossover	3	10-12
Shoulders	Dumbbell shoulder press	3	8-10
	Upright row	3	8-10
	Bent-over lateral raise	3	10-12
Trapezius	Dumbbell shrug	3	6-8
Triceps	Seated triceps extension	3	8-10
	Triceps pressdown (rope)	3	10-12
Abdominals	Hanging leg raise	3	10-12

WEDNESDAY

Muscle group	Exercise	Sets	Reps
Quadriceps	Squat	3	8-10
	Leg press	3	6-8
	Leg extension	3	10-12
Hamstrings	Lying leg curl	3	10-12
Calves	Standing calf raise	3	10-12
	Seated calf raise	3	12-15

FRIDAY

Muscle group	Exercise	Sets	Reps
Back	Pull-up	3	6-10
	Barbell row	3	6-8
	Seated cable row (wide grip)	3	8-10
	Straight-arm pressdown	3	10-12
Biceps	Barbell curl	3	8-10
	Preacher curl	3	8-10
Forearms	Wrist curl	3	10-12
Abdominals	Standing cable crunch	3	10-12
	Reverse crunch	3	12-15

Four-Day Training Split

The four-day training split divides all the major muscle groups of the body into four separate training days. This allows you to train fewer muscle groups each workout. By training fewer muscle groups per workout, you can increase the volume and intensity of your workouts. Both of these factors are important for continued progress as your training experience grows. Most four-day training splits are done on a Monday, Tuesday, Thursday, and Friday schedule, and rest days are taken on Wednesday, Saturday, and Sunday. A common way to break up the body's muscle groups is by training chest, triceps, and abdominals on Mondays; quadriceps, hamstrings, and calves on Tuesdays; shoulders, trapezius, and abdominals on Thursdays; and back, biceps, and forearms on Friday, as covered in table 5.6.

The four-day training split pairs larger muscle groups with smaller ones that assist the larger muscle groups, such as chest with triceps. The triceps assist the chest muscles (pectorals) in all pressing exercises such as the bench press. The logic behind this technique is that the chest workout also works the triceps muscles. With this in mind, it makes sense to continue with exercises that further target the triceps. This is the same with pairing back, biceps, and forearms as well as quadriceps, hamstrings, and calves. Along this line of reasoning, you could also pair chest with shoulders and trapezius because the shoulder (deltoid) muscles assist the chest during all exercises that target the chest. The most important rule here is that larger muscle groups are trained before the smaller muscle groups that assist them, because if you train the smaller muscle groups first, they will be fatigued when you are training the larger muscle group and will limit strength on the exercises for the larger muscle group.

TABLE 5.6 Four-Day Training Split for Pairing Like Muscle Groups

MONDAY

Muscle group	Exercise	Sets	Reps
Chest	Incline bench press	3	8-10
	Dumbbell bench press	3	8-10
	Incline dumbbell fly	3	10-12
	Cable crossover	3	10-12
Triceps	Triceps dip	3	6-10
	Lying triceps extension	3	8-10
	Overhead rope extension	3	10-12
Abdominals	Hanging leg raise	3	10-12
	Crunch	3	15-20

TUESDAY

Quadriceps	Smith machine squat	4	8-10
	Lunge	3	8-10
	Leg extension	3	10-12
Hamstrings	Lying leg curl	3	10-12
	Romanian deadlift	3	8-10
Calves	Standing calf raise	3	10-12
	Seated calf raise	3	12-15

THURSDAY

Muscle group	Exercise	Sets	Reps
Shoulders	Barbell shoulder press	3	8-10
	Lateral raise	3	10-12
	Front raise	2	10-12
	Standing cable reverse fly	2	10-12
Trapezius	Barbell behind-the-back shrug	4	8-10
Abdominals	Hip thrust	3	12-15
	Cable crunch	3	12-15

FRIDAY

Back	Wide-grip pulldown to front	3	8-10
	One-arm dumbbell row	3	8-10
	T-bar row	3	8-10
	Reverse-grip pulldown	3	10-12
Biceps	EZ bar curl	3	8-10
	Dumbbell concentration curl	3	10-12
	Alternating hammer curl	3	8-10
Forearms	Dumbbell wrist curl	3	10-12
	Reverse wrist curl	3	10-12

Of course, this isn't your only option for pairing muscle groups. On the flip side of pairing muscle groups that work together is the concept of separating muscle groups that work together. The reasoning for this is that the smaller muscle group is often fatigued after training the larger muscle group. This will limit the strength of the smaller muscle group and cause it to fatigue earlier when doing exercises that target it. This in turn can limit growth of that muscle. The option here would be to split up the muscle groups into those that perform opposite actions. For example, on Monday train chest and back; Tuesday train shoulders, trapezius, and abdominals; Thursday train quadriceps,

hamstrings, and calves; and Friday train biceps, triceps, forearms, and abdominals, as shown in table 5.7. The Monday and Friday workouts best exemplify this training strategy. Training chest and back allows you to train two muscle groups that don't fatigue each other. The same can be said for training biceps and triceps together. Each muscle group performs an opposite motion of its training pair. The biceps flex the elbow while the triceps extend it. Not only does this help to prevent fatigue of the second muscle group trained, but it can also enhance muscle strength, as explained in chapter 9, with the technique known as *front-to-back training*.

TABLE 5.7 Four-Day Training Split for Pairing Opposite Muscle Groups

MONDAY

Muscle group	Exercise	Sets	Reps
Chest	Smith machine bench press	3	8-10
	Incline dumbbell press		8-10
	Dumbbell fly	3	10-12
	Pec deck	3	10-12
Back	Pull-up	3	6-10
	Reverse-grip barbell row	3	6-8
	Seated cable row	3	8-10
	Wide-grip pulldown	3	10-12

TUESDAY

Muscle group	Exercise	Sets	Reps
Shoulders	Dumbbell shoulder press	3	8-10
	Smith machine upright row	3	8-10
	One-arm cable lateral raise	3	10-12
	Bent-over lateral raise	3	10-12
Trapezius	Barbell shrug	4	6-8
Abdominals	Incline sit-up	3	12-15
	Oblique crunch	3	12-15

THURSDAY

Muscle group	Exercise	Sets	Reps
Quadriceps	Squat	3	6-8
	Leg press	3	8-10
	Step-up	3	8-10
	Leg extension	3	10-12
Hamstrings	Standing leg curl	3	10-12
Calves	Smith machine calf raise	3	10-12
	Seated calf raise	3	12-15

FRIDAY

Muscle group	Exercise	Sets	Reps
Biceps	Alternating dumbbell curl	3	8-10
	Lying cable curl	3	8-10
	Dumbbell preacher curl	3	8-10
Forearms	Reverse-grip curl	3	10-12
	Behind-the-back wrist curl	3	10-12
Triceps	Close-grip bench press	3	6-10
	Triceps pressdown	3	8-10
	One-arm overhead dumbbell extension	3	10-12
Abdominals	Exercise-ball crunch	3	10-12
	Reverse crunch	3	12-15

BISHOP BURTON COLLEGE

Five-Day Training Split

The five-day split lets you train most muscle groups solo. This means that each workout you can focus on one major muscle group. Training this way lets you radically increase the intensity factor of training and the total volume you perform. This is because each major muscle group is trained when it is rested and at its strongest. A sample five-day training program might be chest on Monday, legs (quadriceps, hamstrings, and calves) on Tuesday, back on Wednesday, shoulders and trapezius on Thursday, and arms (triceps, biceps, and forearms) on Friday. Abdominals can be thrown in on any day such as Monday and Thursday, as shown in table 5.8. This lets you have the weekends off for rest. When you take the rest days is not critical because you could essentially take any two days off during the week. Rest days with this split are more a matter of your schedule. If training on the weekends is not a problem, then train Saturday and Sunday, but take two weekdays off for rest.

TABLE 5.8 Five-Day Training Split

MONDAY

Muscle group	Exercise	Sets	Reps
Chest	Smith machine incline press	4	6-10
	Dumbbell bench press	3	8-10
	Decline dumbbell press	3	8-10
	Incline dumbbell fly	3	10-12
	Cable fly	3	10-12
Abdominals	Hanging leg raise	3	12-15
	Oblique crunch	3	12-15
	Cable crunch	3	10-12

TUESDAY

Muscle group	Exercise	Sets	Reps
Quadriceps	Squat	4	6-10
	Hack squat	3	8-10
	Lunge	3	8-10
	Leg extension	3	10-12
Hamstrings	Romanian deadlift	3	8-10
	Lying leg curl	3	10-12
Calves	Standing calf raise	3	10-12
	Donkey calf raise	3	12-15
	Seated calf raise	3	15-20

WEDNESDAY

Muscle group	Exercise	Sets	Reps
Back	Pull-up	3	6-10
	Barbell row	3	6-8
	One-arm dumbbell row	3	8-10
	Reverse-grip pulldown	3	10-12
	Straight-arm pressdown	3	10-12

THURSDAY

Muscle group	Exercise	Sets	Reps
Shoulders	Barbell shoulder press	3	6-8
	Dumbbell shoulder press	3	8-10
	Cable upright row	3	8-10
	Seated dumbbell lateral raise	3	10-12
	Reverse pec deck	3	10-12
Trapezius	Smith machine shrug	3	6-8
	Dumbbell shrug	3	8-10
Abdominals	Reverse crunch	3	12-15
	Standing cable crunch	3	10-12
	V-up	3	12-15

FRIDAY

Muscle group	Exercise	Sets	Reps
Triceps	Lying triceps extension	3	8-10
	Reverse-grip cable pressdown	3	8-10
	Overhead dumbbell extension	3	8-10
	Dumbbell kickback	2	12-15
Biceps	Barbell curl	3	8-10
	EZ bar preacher curl	3	8-10
	Prone incline dumbbell curl	3	8-10
	Seated hammer curl	2	10-12
Forearms	Dumbbell wrist curl	3	10-12
	Dumbbell reverse wrist curl	3	10-12

Twice-a-Day Training Split

This is a demanding split that offers several advantages for only the most advanced bodybuilders. As the name implies, the twice-a-day training split involves training at two separate times a day. Typically, most bodybuilders who train twice a day train one muscle group earlier in the day and one muscle group later in the day (see table 5.9). The break between the two training sessions usually is at least six hours. Depending on your goal, this allows you to either train more frequently or get more complete rest days. With twice-a-day training you can train all the major muscle groups of the body in three or four days. This means you can get either three or four days of rest each week if you train the muscle groups once per week. However, this method also allows you to train each muscle group up to twice per week. Another way to use twice-a-day training is to follow a typical five-day training split that incorporates a not-so-typical twist: train the same muscle group twice per day. According to research, this may be a beneficial way to train muscles. See chapter 6 for more details on this training method.

TABLE 5.9 Twice-a-Day Training Split

MONDAY (8:00 A.M.)			
Muscle group	**Exercise**	**Sets**	**Reps**
Chest	Bench press	3	8-10
	Incline dumbbell bench press	3	8-10
	Incline dumbbell fly	3	10-12
	Cable crossover	3	10-12
MONDAY (6:00 P.M.)			
Triceps	Triceps dip	3	6-10
	Dumbbell lying triceps extension	3	8-10
	Triceps pressdown	2	10-12
	Overhead dumbbell triceps extension	2	10-12
Abdominals	Hanging leg raise	3	10-12
	Cable crunch	3	10-12
TUESDAY (8:00 A.M.)			
Quadriceps	Leg press	4	6-8
	Smith machine squat	4	8-10
	Step-up	3	8-10
	One-leg leg extension	4	12-15
TUESDAY (6:00 P.M.)			
Hamstrings	Romanian deadlift	3	8-10
	Lying leg curl	3	10-12
	Back extension	2	12-15
Calves	Standing calf raise	4	10-12
	Seated calf raise	4	12-15

THURSDAY (8:00 A.M.)			
Muscle group	**Exercise**	**Sets**	**Reps**
Shoulders	Barbell shoulder press	4	8-10
	Dumbbell upright row	3	8-10
	Dumbbell lateral raise	3	10-12
	Bent-over lateral raise	3	10-12
THURSDAY (6:00 P.M.)			
Trapezius	Smith machine barbell shrug	3	6-8
	Seated dumbbell shrug	3	8-10
Abdominals	Hip thrust	3	12-15
	Exercise-ball crunch	3	12-15
FRIDAY (8:00 A.M.)			
Back	Wide-grip pulldown to front	4	8-10
	Barbell row	4	8-10
	Close-grip pulldown	3	10-12
	Seated cable row	3	8-10
FRIDAY (6:00 P.M.)			
Biceps	Barbell curl	3	8-10
	Incline dumbbell curl	3	10-12
	Cable concentration curl	2	10-12
	Dumbbell hammer curl	2	8-10
Forearms	Dumbbell wrist curl	3	10-12
	Reverse wrist curl	3	10-12

BODY-PART TRAINING

Regardless of what type of split you choose, you need to be informed about the best ways to train each muscle group according to your training split of choice. The training split you use will influence factors such as the number of exercises you perform and the total number of sets you do per muscle group. But generally speaking, your training split does not have to influence the type of exercises you choose, the amount of weight used, the number of reps performed, or the amount of rest you allow between sets. Therefore, there are general rules to consider when designing a strength training program, regardless of the spilt you are employing.

If your goal is to maximize muscle mass, then your most important rule has to deal with taking all sets to muscle failure. Although the sweet spot for muscle growth is said to be in the range of 8 to 12 reps, newer research from McMaster University in Canada suggests that the amount of weight and rep range used may not matter as much as once proposed as long as sets are taken to muscle failure. One of their studies reported that participants training for 10 weeks using weights that allowed them to complete 20 to 30 reps and taking each set to muscle failure gained as much muscle mass as those training with weights that limited them to 8 to 12 reps per set and taking each set to muscle failure (Burd et al. 2010). Other studies done by this group demonstrate that the higher rep ranges (20-30) with light weight taken to muscle failure increase muscle protein synthesis to an equivalent amount or even better than lower rep ranges (4-5 reps) taken to muscle failure (Burd et al. 2011). So the smartest plan of attack is to cycle through a variety of rep ranges from very low (3-5 per set) with heavy weight to very high (20-30+ per set) with light weight, and a multitude of rep ranges in between, such as 6 to 8 per set, 9 to 11 per set, and 12 to 15 per set. This way you get the benefit that each rep range imparts, aside from the direct influence on muscle protein synthesis. For example, heavier-weight workouts have been shown to increase testosterone levels higher than workouts with lighter weight. Testosterone is an anabolic hormone that initiates the process of muscle growth. However, higher reps, such as 15 or more, are associated with a higher rate of release of growth hormone compared to workouts involving heavier weight. Because growth hormone is involved in muscle growth, maximizing its release after a workout can be critical. Higher reps also enhance the capillarization of muscle fibers. That is, the amount of blood vessels that supply the muscles increases with higher-repetition training. By increasing the number of blood vessels that supply a muscle fiber, there is an accompanying increase in the delivery of blood to the muscle fibers. Enhancing blood flow to the muscle fibers increases the supply of critical nutrients for energy and growth such as carbohydrate, amino acids from protein, and fat. There also is greater provision of oxygen. Oxygen not only is essential for muscle energy for recovery between sets but is also critical for lessening the indirect muscle damage that follows a weightlifting workout. Another benefit of increased blood flow to muscle fibers is the greater supply of anabolic hormones, such as testosterone and growth hormone, to the muscles.

The order in which you cycle the rep ranges may not be critical. Periodized models using linear schemes, reverse linear schemes, and undulating schemes have all been effective in producing muscle growth. So a variety of periodized programs that cycle a variety of rep ranges but take each working set to failure appear to be the best tactic for focusing on muscle growth.

Another important consideration for building muscle mass is the rest time allowed between sets. Most bodybuilders use shorter rest periods of around one to two minutes. Shorter rest periods—those that are two minutes or less—have also been shown to increase the surge of growth hormone that follows a weightlifting workout. Shorter rest periods also increase the capillarization of the muscles as well as enhance the activity of enzymes that are involved in energy supply to the muscle. One study reported that participants following an eight-week strength-training program who decreased the rest period between sets by 15 seconds every week had greater gains in muscle mass than those keeping rest periods steady at 2 minutes (Souza-Junior et al. 2011). See chapter 6 for programs that decrease rest period between sets over time.

Exercise selection and order of those exercises are other important things to consider for building muscle mass. For larger muscle groups that employ several multijoint exercises, such as the chest, back, shoulders, and legs, you should primarily do those multijoint exercises early in the workout when the muscle is strongest. Then follow those exercises with isolation exercises that involve movement at one single joint and best isolate the targeted muscle group. The reason for this is that multijoint exercises recruit the help of other muscle groups to perform the exercise. The targeted muscle group of that exercise is considered the primary mover, while the muscle groups that help the primary mover perform the exercise are considered assistance muscles. An example of this is the bench press, a multijoint exercise for the chest. In the bench press, the chest is considered the primary mover while the shoulders, triceps, and even the lats are considered the assistance muscles. Because multijoint exercises involve synergy of several muscle groups, you can lift more weight with multijoint exercises. It is a good idea to do the exercises that you can lift the most weight with first. This is when all the muscles used in that exercise are freshest and therefore can all help to lift the greatest amount of weight they are capable of lifting. Using more weight places more overload on the target muscles, which can lead to increased muscle hypertrophy over time. All that said, on occasion it's a good idea to flip this rule on its head and use the training technique known as preexhaust. With this technique you do the single-joint exercises for a muscle group first in the workout and the multijoint exercises last. For more on preexhaust

and why it works and to see a program that uses it, go to chapter 6.

For gains in strength, the general consensus among experts is that fewer sets tend to be best. But there is some debate over the ideal volume—or total sets—to use for optimizing gains in muscle mass. One reason may be that there is no ideal number of sets for increasing muscle mass. In general, beginners should start out with fewer sets and gradually increase them as their training experience progresses. But when you consider experienced bodybuilders, there are few generalizations that can be made in regard to volume. Some bodybuilders train with very low volume (6 to 10 total sets per muscle group), while others use extremely high volume (20 to 30 total sets per muscle group), as did the most famous bodybuilder of all time, Arnold Schwarzenegger. One bit of advice for advanced lifters is to cycle training volume from periods of low volume to high volume. This will depend on the training intensity as well as the training frequency.

Just remember that these are general guidelines for building a solid foundation for your training program. Many of the methods you will read about in chapter 6 contradict these guidelines. The reason is that the techniques presented in chapter 6 are techniques for those with moderate to extensive training experience. For experienced lifters, changing the convention from time to time better enables muscle growth because of the radical change in the training program.

Changing Your Split

No matter the training split that currently is your best fit, you should consider changing your split to offer your body some variety in the way you train it. Just as it is important to change your weight and reps or rest time between sets, altering how you split up your training is another way to maintain continual progress in training adaptations and avoid stagnation. For beginners, starting on a whole-body training split and then slowly progressing to splits that allow more volume to be done for each muscle group is a necessity. See the table for a suggested succession of training splits based on training experience. Start with the split that corresponds to your level of training experience and progress to the next split as you reach a new level of training experience.

Training experience (months)	Optimal training split
1 to 3	Whole-body training split
4 to 9	Upper- and lower-body training split or two-day training split
10 to 18	Three-day training split
19+	Four- or five-day training split

Chest

The chest refers to the muscle group known as the pectoralis major. This consists of the upper pectoralis major and lower pectoralis major (see figure 5.1). The pectoralis muscles perform movements such as horizontal adduction of the upper arms, as in the dumbbell fly. For detailed descriptions of chest exercises, refer to chapter 14. Basic, multijoint exercises for the chest involve pressing movements, such as the bench press, incline dumbbell press, and push-up. Isolation exercises for the chest are flylike exercises that involve movement of the arms without any change occurring at the elbow joint. Examples of isolation exercises for the chest include the dumbbell fly, cable crossover, and pec deck. The upper and lower sections of the chest are hit differently by the various chest exercises. Therefore, the first order of importance when it comes to chest training is to ensure that you include exercises that target the upper, middle, and lower pectoralis. Refer to table 5.10 for basic guidelines in designing a chest workout based on the current training split used.

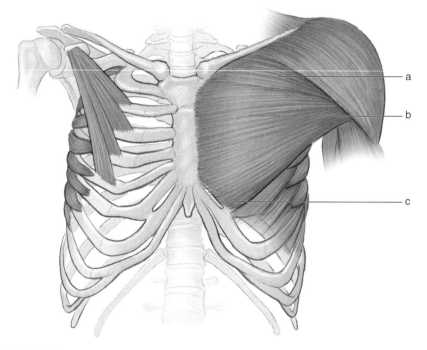

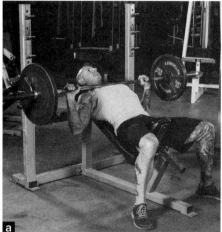
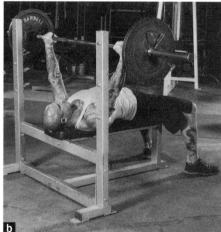
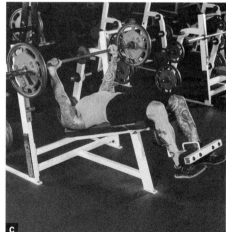

FIGURE 5.1 Pectoralis muscle: *(a)* the upper pectoralis is targeted by the incline bench press; *(b)* the middle pectoralis is targeted by the flat bench press; and *(c)* the lower pectoralis is targeted by the decline bench press.

TABLE 5.10 Chest Training Guidelines Based on Training Split

Training split	Number of exercises	Exercise order	Total sets
Whole-body training split	1	Swap pressing exercises and fly-type exercises every other workout. Swap incline- and flat-bench exercises every other workout.	3-6
Upper- and lower-body training split or two-day training split	2	Choose one incline- and one flat-bench exercise every workout. First: A pressing exercise* Second: A fly-type exercise Swap the incline movement from the pressing exercise to the fly-type exercise every other workout. Perform one decline exercise or the cable crossover at least once every other week.	6-8
Three-day training split	3	First: A barbell exercise* Second: A dumbbell press Third: A fly-type exercise Alternate incline and flat benches for the first two exercises every other workout. The third exercise should match the type of incline used for the first. Perform one decline exercise or the cable crossover at least once every other week.	6-12
Four-day training split	4	First: A barbell exercise* Second: A dumbbell press Third: A dumbbell fly exercise Fourth: A machine or cable fly-type exercise Alternate incline and flat benches for the first two exercises every other workout. The third exercise should match the type of incline used for the first. Perform one decline exercise or the cable crossover at least once every other week.	8-16
Five-day training split	4-5	First: A barbell exercise* Second: A barbell or a dumbbell press Third: A dumbbell press exercise if doing five exercises total; if doing only four exercises total, the third should be a dumbbell fly exercise Fourth: A dumbbell, machine, or cable fly-type exercise Fifth: A machine or cable fly-type exercise Alternate incline, flat, and decline benches for the first three exercises every other workout. The fourth exercise should match the type of incline used for the first.	10-20
Twice-a-day training split	4	First: A barbell exercise* Second: A dumbbell press Third: A dumbbell fly exercise Fourth: A machine or cable fly-type exercise Alternate incline and flat benches for the first two exercises every other workout. The third exercise should match the type of incline used for the first. Perform one decline exercise or the cable crossover at least once every other week.	8-16

*Can supplement Smith machine version here.

Shoulders

The shoulders refer to the deltoid muscles found on top of the upper arm. The deltoid is composed of three heads that originate on different points of the shoulder girdle but all converge on one common tendon that inserts on the humerus (upper arm bone). The three heads are the anterior deltoid (front head), the middle deltoid, and the posterior deltoid (rear head). Although these three heads work together to lift the upper arm at the shoulder joint, such as during the lateral raise, each head is stressed differently by different exercises (see figure 5.2). That is why it is important to structure shoulder workouts around basic multijoint movements (such as the shoulder press) that hit all three heads as well as isolation exercises (such as front raise for the anterior head, lateral raise or upright row for the middle head, and rear deltoid raise for the posterior head). Refer to chapter 15 for detailed descriptions of all shoulder exercises. See table 5.11 for guidelines for designing a shoulder workout based on the current training split being used.

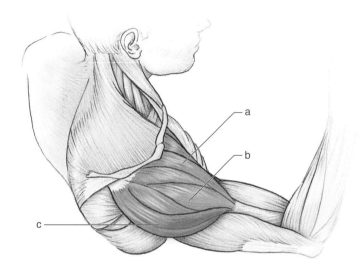

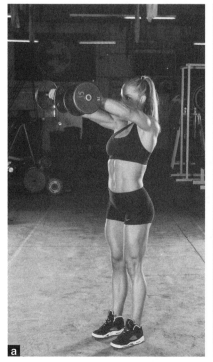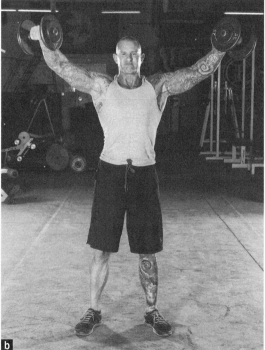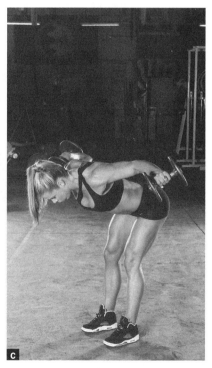

FIGURE 5.2 Deltoid muscle: *(a)* the anterior head is targeted by the front raise; *(b)* the middle head is targeted by the lateral raise; and *(c)* the posterior head is targeted by the bent-over lateral raise.

TABLE 5.11 Shoulder Training Guidelines Based on Training Split

Training split	Number of exercises	Exercise order	Total sets
Whole-body training split	1	Swap pressing exercises and isolation exercises every other workout. Frequently swap between barbell* and dumbbell pressing exercises. Periodically swap upright rows for lateral raises. Try to perform a rear deltoid exercise for the isolation exercise at least once a month.	3-6
Upper- and lower-body training split or two-day training split	2	Choose one pressing exercise and one isolation exercise every workout. First: A pressing exercise Second: An isolation exercise Swap barbell pressing* exercises with dumbbell pressing exercises every other workout. Frequently alternate isolation exercises by switching up on lateral raises, front raises, upright rows, and rear deltoid exercises.	6-8
Three-day training split	3	First: A pressing exercise* Second: A lateral raise or upright row exercise Third: A front raise or a rear deltoid exercise Alternate barbell* and dumbbell presses for the first exercises every other workout. Alternate upright row and lateral raise exercises every other workout. Alternate front raise and rear deltoid exercises every other workout.	6-12
Four-day training split	4	First: A pressing exercise* Second: A lateral raise or upright row exercise Third: A front raise exercise Fourth: A rear deltoid exercise Alternate barbell* and dumbbell presses for the first exercises every other workout. Alternate upright row and lateral raise exercises every other workout.	8-16
Five-day training split	4	First: A pressing exercise* Second: A lateral raise or upright row exercise Third: A front raise exercise Fourth: A rear deltoid exercise Alternate barbell* and dumbbell presses for the first exercises every other workout. Alternate upright row and lateral raise exercises every other workout.	8-16
Twice-a-day training split	4	First: A pressing exercise* Second: A lateral raise or upright row exercise Third: A front raise exercise Fourth: A rear deltoid exercise Alternate barbell* and dumbbell presses for the first exercises every other workout. Alternate upright row and lateral raise exercises every other workout.	8-16

*Can supplement Smith machine version here.

Back

Back refers to the muscles that make up the backside of the torso. Although the term *back* refers mostly to the large latissimus dorsi muscles, or lats, that run from the upper arms all the way down to the buttocks (see figure 5.3), it can also include the teres major, the rhomboids, and even the middle and lower portions of the trapezius, because these muscles are often involved in performing exercises that are considered back exercises. The two major types of lat exercises are the pulling exercises (which include pull-ups and pulldowns) and rowing exercises (which include bent-over barbell rows, T-bar rows, and seated cable rows). Pull-up and pulldown exercises tend to concentrate more on the upper and outer lats as well as the teres major. Rowing exercises tend to concentrate more on the middle and lower lats as well as the rhomboids and middle trapezius muscles. Other types of lat exercises are the pullover and straight-arm pulldown. For detailed descriptions of all back exercises, refer to chapter 16. See table 5.12 for basic guidelines for designing a back workout based on the current training split used.

The term *back* also refers to the musculature of the low back. The muscles in the lower back are those that support the spinal column and allow it to extend back, such as when you recline in a chair. These are deeper muscle fibers such as the spinal erectors, which include the longissimus thoracis, iliocostalis lumborum, and spinalis thoracis. Exercises that train the low back are back extension exercises and good mornings.

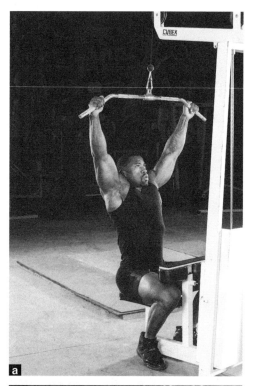

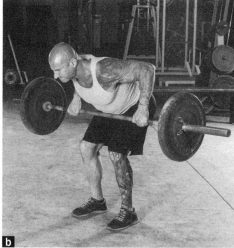

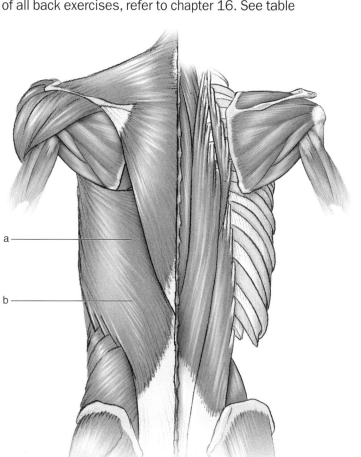

FIGURE 5.3 Back musculature: *(a)* the upper and outer lats are worked by the lat pulldown, and *(b)* the lower and middle lats are worked by the barbell row.

TABLE 5.12 Back Training Guidelines Based on Training Split

Training split	Number of exercises	Exercise order	Total sets
Whole-body training split	1	Swap pulling exercises and rowing exercises every other workout. At least once a month include a pullover or straight-arm pulldown exercise. It's also wise to include one low-back exercise once a week.	3-6
Upper- and lower-body training split or two-day training split	2	Choose one pulling and one rowing exercise every workout (swap the order every week). Occasionally replace the pulling exercise with a straight-arm pulldown or pullover exercise. It's also wise to include one low-back exercise once a week.	6-8
Three-day training split	3	Choose one pulling and one rowing exercise as the first two exercises every other workout (swap the order every week). The third exercise should be a straight-arm pulldown or pullover exercise. It's also wise to include one low-back exercise once a week.	6-12
Four-day training split	4	Choose one pulling and one rowing exercise as the first two exercises every other workout (swap the order every week). Third: A pulling or rowing exercise (swap the exercise choice every other week) Fourth: A straight-arm pulldown or pullover exercise It's also wise to include one low-back exercise once a week.	8-16
Five-day training split	4-5	Choose one pulling and one rowing exercise as the first two exercises every other workout (swap the order every week). Third: A pulling or rowing exercise (swap the exercise choice every other week) Fourth: A straight-arm pulldown or pullover exercise Fifth: A low-back exercise	10-20
Twice-a-day training split	4	Choose one pulling and one rowing exercise as the first two exercises every other workout (swap the order every week). Third: A pulling or rowing exercise (swap the exercise choice every other week) Fourth: A straight-arm pulldown or pullover exercise It's also wise to include one low-back exercise once a week.	8-16

Trapezius

The trapezius is the large diamond-shaped muscle on the upper back, often referred to as traps. This muscle has upper, middle, and lower portions that all perform different movements (see figure 5.4). The upper trapezius primarily lifts and rotates the shoulder blades upward as when shrugging the shoulders (such as during dumbbell shrugs). The middle trapezius primarily pulls the shoulder blades together (such as during face pulls). The lower trapezius rotates the shoulder blades downward (such as when lifting a barbell overhead with straight arms like during the snatch). Trapezius training can be paired with shoulders or back. Most bodybuilders train the traps after shoulders because their primary interest is in developing the upper portion of the traps. The upper traps are involved in most deltoid exercises. Therefore, they are sufficiently warmed up after training shoulders. However, because it is technically a back muscle and assists during many back exercises, upper traps are often trained with back. Most lifters typically pick one or two exercises for trap workouts and perform three to eight sets. If both a barbell and a dumbbell trap exercise are done in the same workout, the barbell exercise is typically done first. For detailed descriptions of trapezius exercises, see chapter 17.

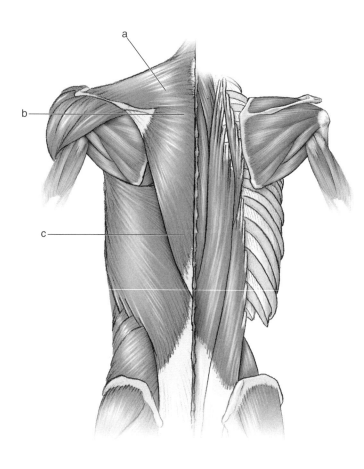

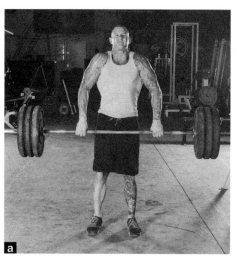 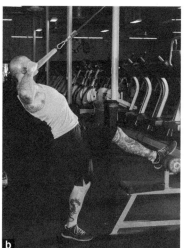 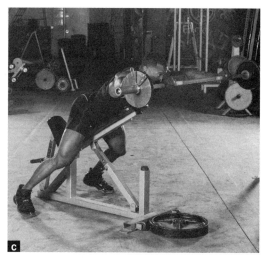

FIGURE 5.4 Trapezius muscle: *(a)* the upper traps are worked by the barbell shrug; *(b)* the middle traps are worked by the facepull; and *(c)* the lower traps are worked by the prone front raise.

Triceps

The triceps consist of three muscle heads that are on the back of the upper arm. The three heads of the triceps are the lateral head, long head, and medial head (see figure 5.5). Each head has a distinct attachment on the upper end, but they all meet at one common tendon that crosses the elbow and attaches on the ulna. Contracting the triceps results in extension at the elbow such as the motion the arm makes when hammering.

The two types of triceps exercises are compound movements and isolation movements. Compound triceps exercises involve extension at the elbow and movement at the shoulder. These include close-grip bench presses and dips. Isolation triceps exercises involve just extension at the elbow with no other joint movement, such as dumbbell kickbacks. When choosing triceps exercises, you should include some compound exercises, which are beneficial for adding on overall triceps mass, as well as a good variety of isolation exercises. The isolation exercises you choose should hit the three different triceps heads. While you may not be able to do this in every workout, depending on your split, you should try to rotate your exercise selection from workout to workout to hit the different heads.

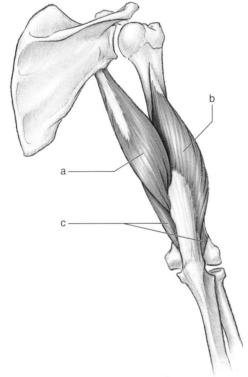

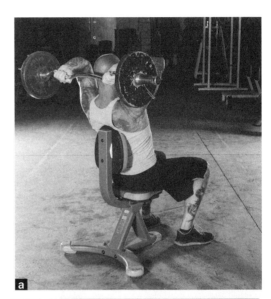

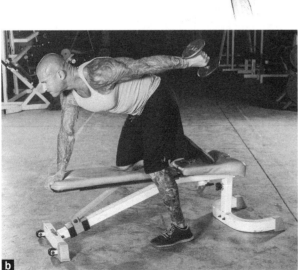

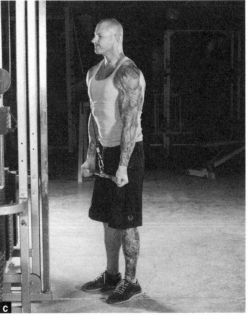

FIGURE 5.5 Triceps: *(a)* the long head is targeted by the overhead triceps extension; *(b)* the lateral head is targeted by the dumbbell kickback; and *(c)* the medial head is targeted by the reverse-grip cable pressdown.

Although every triceps exercise hits all three heads to some degree, certain ones are better than others at stressing the different heads because of the biomechanics involved. Because the long head of the triceps attaches to the scapula (shoulder blade), it is more strongly contracted during exercises where the arms are brought overhead or in front of the body. This is because that action stretches the long head. Muscles contract the strongest when they are stretched to their longest length. Therefore, exercises that are done overhead such as overhead extensions (with dumbbells, barbells, or cables) best stress the long head of the triceps. Exercises that place the arms in front of the body, such as lying triceps extensions (with barbells, dumbbells, or cables) also hit the long head to some degree. Extensions that are done with the arms at the sides of the torso while holding a neutral or overhand grip—such as triceps pressdowns and dumbbell kickbacks—best target the lateral triceps head. The same exercises done with an underhand grip seem to stress the medial head. For detailed descriptions of all triceps exercises, go to chapter 18. Refer to table 5.13 for basic guidelines for designing a triceps workout based on the current training split used.

TABLE 5.13   Triceps Training Guidelines Based on Training Split

Training split	Number of exercises	Exercise order	Total sets
Whole-body training split	1	Swap compound and isolation exercises every other workout. Rotate isolation exercises to target all three triceps heads.	2-4
Upper- and lower-body training split or two-day training split	2	Choose one compound and one isolation exercise every workout. First: A compound exercise (alternate between pressing and dipping exercises every other workout) Second: An isolation exercise (rotate isolation exercises to target all three triceps heads)	4-8
Three-day training split	3	Choose one compound and two isolation exercises every workout. First: A compound exercise (alternate between pressing and dipping exercises every other workout) Second: An overhead or lying extension (alternate between the two every other workout) Third: An extension done with the arms held at the sides (alternate between overhand, neutral, and underhand grips on different workouts)	6-12
Four-day training split	3-4	Choose one compound and two or three isolation exercises every workout. First: A compound exercise (alternate between pressing and dipping exercises every other workout) Second: An overhead or lying extension (alternate between the two every other workout if doing only three exercises) Third: If doing four exercises total, an overhead or lying extension (if the second exercise is an overhead extension the third should be a lying extension, and vice versa); if doing only three exercises total, the third should be an extension with the arms held at the sides Fourth: An extension with the arms held at the sides (alternate between overhand, neutral, and underhand grips on different workouts)	6-16

Training split	Number of exercises	Exercise order	Total sets
Five-day training split	3-4	Choose one compound and two or three isolation exercises every workout. First: A compound exercise (alternate between pressing and dipping exercises every other workout) Second: An overhead or lying extension (alternate between the two every other workout if doing only three exercises) Third: If doing four exercises total, an overhead or lying extension (if the second exercise is an overhead extension the third should be a lying extension and vice versa); if doing only three exercises total, the third should be an extension with the arms held at the sides Fourth: An extension with the arms held at the sides (alternate between overhand, neutral, and underhand grips on different workouts)	6-16
Twice-a-day training split	3-4	Choose one compound and two or three isolation exercises every workout. First: A compound exercise (alternate between pressing and dipping exercises every other workout) Second: An overhead or lying extension (alternate between the two every other workout if doing only three exercises) Third: If doing four exercises total, an overhead or lying extension (if the second exercise is an overhead extension, the third should be a lying extension, and vice versa); if doing only three exercises total, the third should be an extension with the arms held at the sides Fourth: An extension with the arms held at the sides (alternate between overhand, neutral, and underhand grips on different workouts)	6-16

Biceps

Biceps refers to two muscle heads that run down the front of the upper arm that are called the biceps brachii (see figure 5.6). The two heads are the long head (or outer head) and the short head (or inner head). The major difference between them is where each muscle attaches on the scapula (shoulder blade). The tendon of the long head attaches farther back on the scapula than the short head. This is why they are referred to as *long head* and *short head.* Both biceps heads converge into one tendon near the elbow, and this attaches to the radius to cause flexion of the elbow when the muscles contract, such as when curling a dumbbell.

To flex the elbow, the biceps brachii receives help from the assistance muscle called the brachialis. This muscle lies underneath the biceps muscles and starts at the humerus (upper arm bone) and attaches to the ulna. The bulk of this muscle is lower than the bulk of the biceps muscle, which allows it to offer the most help during the first 30 degrees of elbow flexion. The brachialis is also strongly involved in elbow flexion when the hands maintain an overhand grip on the bar. The brachioradialis, although considered a forearm muscle, also helps at the initiation of elbow flexion. It is strongly involved in elbow flexion when the hand is in a neutral position, such as during hammer curls.

With the exception of underhand chin-ups, there are no compound exercises for biceps. Even the underhand chin-up is considered a back exercise. Therefore, almost all true biceps exercises are single-joint or isolation exercises. However, the exercises you choose should stress the different biceps heads as well as the brachialis, which helps to make the biceps appear larger (particularly the lower portion) when it is properly developed. For detailed descriptions of all biceps exercises, refer to chapter 19. For basic guidelines for designing biceps workouts based on the current training split used, see table 5.14. Most exercise choices for the biceps workout should be underhand (supinated) grip curls, such as barbell curls, dumbbell curls, and preacher curls. With barbell curls you should frequently change your grip to stress the heads differently. Doing curls with a closer grip

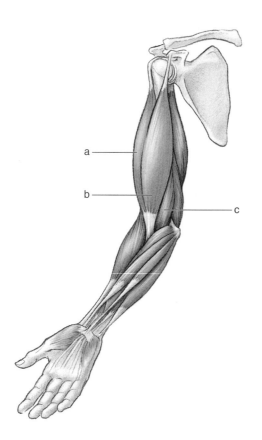

(hip width or closer) puts more stress on the long head of the biceps—the part of the biceps that is responsible for the peak that is seen when a bodybuilder flexes the biceps. Also consider alternating between using a straight barbell and an EZ curl bar. The EZ curl bar places the hands halfway between an underhand and a neutral grip. This places greater emphasis on the long head of the biceps. Therefore, doing hammer curls (using a neutral grip) with dumbbells or a rope attachment emphasizes the long head of the biceps in addition to the brachialis and brachioradialis (forearm muscle on the thumb side of the forearm) muscles. Another exercise that hits the brachialis and brachioradialis and, to a lesser extent, the biceps is reverse-grip curls with a pronated grip. One other way to place greater emphasis on the long head is by doing dumbbell curls while sitting back on an incline between 30 and 60 degrees. This position stretches the long head of the biceps to put it in its strongest position for contraction.

To emphasize the short head, you can do the opposite of the incline curl and do curls on a preacher bench. This places the arms in front of the body, which shortens the long head and reduces its

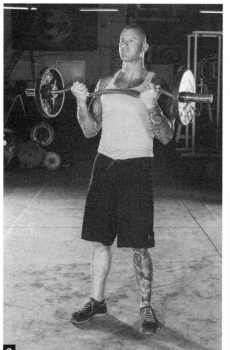

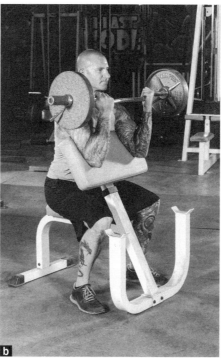

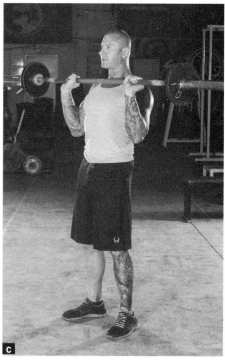

FIGURE 5.6 Biceps: *(a)* the long head is targeted by the EZ bar curl; *(b)* the short head is targeted by the preacher curl; and *(c)* the brachialis, located beneath the biceps, is targeted by the reverse curl.

TABLE 5.14 Biceps Training Guidelines Based on Training Split

Training split	Number of exercises	Exercise order	Total sets
Whole-body training split	1	The majority of exercise choices should be basic underhand curls. Frequently alter the type of curl from workout to workout to hit each biceps head differently as well as the brachialis.	2-4
Upper- and lower-body training split or two-day training split	2	First: A basic underhand curl (alternate every workout for variety) Second: Should target the long head or the short head (alternate between long-head and short-head exercises) Periodically swap the second exercise with a brachialis exercise.	4-8
Three-day training split	3	First: A basic underhand curl (alternate every workout for variety) Second: Should target the long head or the short head (alternate every workout between long-head and short-head exercises) Third: A brachialis exercise	6-12
Four-day training split	3-4	First: A basic underhand curl (alternate every workout for variety) Second: Should target the long head or the short head (if doing only three exercises total, alternate every workout between long-head and short-head exercises) Third: If doing four exercises total, an exercise that stresses the long head or short head (opposite of what the second exercise stressed); if doing three exercises total, the third should target the brachialis Fourth: A brachialis exercise	6-16
Five-day training split	3-4	First: A basic underhand curl (alternate every workout for variety) Second: Should target the long head or the short head (if doing only three exercises total, alternate every workout between long-head and short-head exercises) Third: If doing four exercises total, an exercise that stresses the long head or short head (opposite of what the second exercise stressed); if doing three exercises total, the third should target the brachialis Fourth: A brachialis exercise	6-16
Twice-a-day training split	3-4	First: A basic underhand curl (alternate every workout for variety) Second: Should target the long head or the short head (if doing only three exercises total, alternate every workout between long-head and short-head exercises) Third: If doing four exercises total, an exercise that stresses the long head or short head (opposite of what the second exercise stressed); if doing three exercises total, the third should target the brachialis Fourth: A brachialis exercise	6-16

contraction strength. Other ways to stress the short head are to do curls with a wider grip (shoulder width and wider) or to perform supination during dumbbell curls. Supination requires the movement of the hand from a neutral position to an underhand position while curling. The order in which you stagger your biceps exercises is not as critical as involving a variety of movements that emphasize both biceps heads as well as the brachialis.

Since the brachioradialis and other forearm muscles are involved in assisting most biceps exercises, it is wise to train the forearms after the biceps. Doing hammer curls and reverse-grip curls at the end of your biceps workout is a smart way to segue from a biceps workout into a forearm workout. These exercises involve the brachialis and biceps as well as the brachioradialis muscle.

Forearms

The forearms are the muscles that make up the entire lower arm. Though you do not need to familiarize yourself with all the different forearm muscles shown in figure 5.7, you should recognize the difference in those referred to as the wrist flexor group and those referred to as the wrist extensor group. The wrist flexor group is composed of forearm muscles that perform wrist flexion—the movement of the palms toward the inner forearm, such as during a wrist curl. The wrist extensors, on the other hand, are involved in performing wrist extension—moving the back of the hand toward the back of the forearm, such as when you twist the throttle on a motorcycle. It is wise to train the forearms after the biceps because they are used so strongly during all biceps exercises. Typically, choosing one wrist curl (flexion) exercise and one reverse wrist curl (extension) exercise is sufficient for working the forearm muscles after biceps, especially if reverse-grip or hammer-grip curls were performed. If grip strength is a limiting factor on back and biceps exercises, including a specific grip exercise may be warranted. The grip exercise should be done before the wrist curl and reverse wrist curl exercises. For a complete listing and detailed descriptions of all forearm exercises, see chapter 20. If training with a whole-body, upper- and lower-body, or two-day split, you may consider skipping specific forearm work and relying on the fact that the forearm muscles are used during back and biceps exercises. For basic guidelines for designing forearm workouts based on the current training split used, see table 5.15.

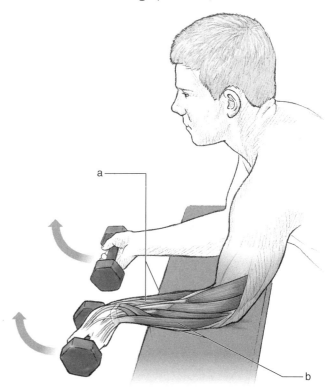

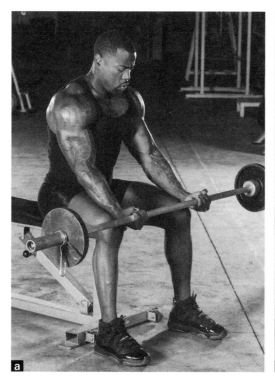
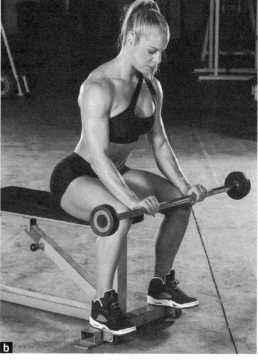

FIGURE 5.7 Forearm muscles: *(a)* the flexor muscles are worked by the wrist curl, and *(b)* the extensor muscles are worked by the reverse wrist curl.

TABLE 5.15 Forearm Training Guidelines Based on Training Split

Training split	Number of exercises	Exercise order	Total sets
Whole-body training split	1	Alternate wrist curl exercises and reverse wrist curl exercises every other workout.	2-4
Upper- and lower-body training split or two-day training split	1	Alternate wrist curl exercises and reverse wrist curl exercises every other workout.	2-4
Three-day training split	2	Choose one wrist curl and one reverse wrist curl exercise every workout; alternate the order every other workout. Frequently change the type of wrist curl and reverse wrist curl exercises.	4-8
Four-day training split	2	Choose one wrist curl and one reverse wrist curl exercise every workout; alternate the order every other workout. Frequently change the type of wrist curl and reverse wrist curl exercises.	4-8
Five-day training split	2	Choose one wrist curl and one reverse wrist curl exercise every workout; alternate the order every other workout. Frequently change the type of wrist curl and reverse wrist curl exercises.	4-8
Twice-a-day training split	2	Choose one wrist curl and one reverse wrist curl exercise every workout; alternate the order every other workout. Frequently change the type of wrist curl and reverse wrist curl exercises.	4-8

Quadriceps

The quadriceps are the four muscles that make up the front of the thigh. The vastus lateralis, vastus medialis, vastus intermedius, and rectus femoris all originate from different attachment points on the thigh and hip bone, but they all converge on one common tendon to perform knee extension, such as when you kick a ball (see figure 5.8). Because the rectus femoris originates on the hipbone, not the femur (thigh bone) as with the other three quadriceps muscles, it also is involved in hip flexion, such as when you lift your knee up. Although all four muscles work together to straighten the knee, certain exercises are better for targeting specific parts of the quad. For instance, the leg extension best targets the rectus femoris muscle. However, doing leg extensions with the toes turned in places more stress on the outer quad (vastus lateralis), and doing leg extensions with the toes pointed out better targets the inner quads (vastus medialis). The leg press hits all four quad muscles, but research shows that the emphasis is on the medialis muscle. Conversely, the hack squat tends to place more emphasis on the outer quads (vastus lateralis). Squats and lunges, however, hit the four quadriceps muscles fairly evenly, along with the leg adductors, hamstrings, gluteus maximus, and other muscles. For detailed descriptions of all quadriceps exercises, see chapter 21.

For maximizing leg size, you should start your quadriceps workout with one or two squat exercises (with barbells, Smith machine, or dumbbells) or leg press exercises, depending on the type of split you are training with. These exercises are compound exercises that involve extension at the knees and hips. Therefore, they use not only the quadriceps muscles but also the hamstring and gluteus maximus muscles (powerful hip extensors). Because these large muscle groups work together to perform the exercise, they provide great strength. This is the reason that these exercises should be at the beginning of your leg workout. You should train these muscles when they are at their strongest so that the greatest amount of weight can be used for stimulating the most muscle growth.

With the squat and leg press exercises you should routinely alter your foot position to slightly change the specific muscle fibers that are used during the exercise. Although squats hit all four quadriceps muscles pretty equally, slightly greater emphasis can be directed to certain muscles by changing the distance the feet are spaced apart. It is generally agreed that squats done with the feet close together place slightly more emphasis on the outer quads than squats done with the feet shoulder-width apart. Conversely, when squats are done with the feet spaced much wider than shoulder width, greater emphasis is placed on the inner quad and adductor muscles. However, one study suggested that little difference in the use of the medialis or lateralis was observed with a wide or narrow stance (Paoli, A., et al. 2009). Squats done on a Smith machine or on a squat machine allow you to change not only the width of your feet but also the distance they are out in front of your hips.

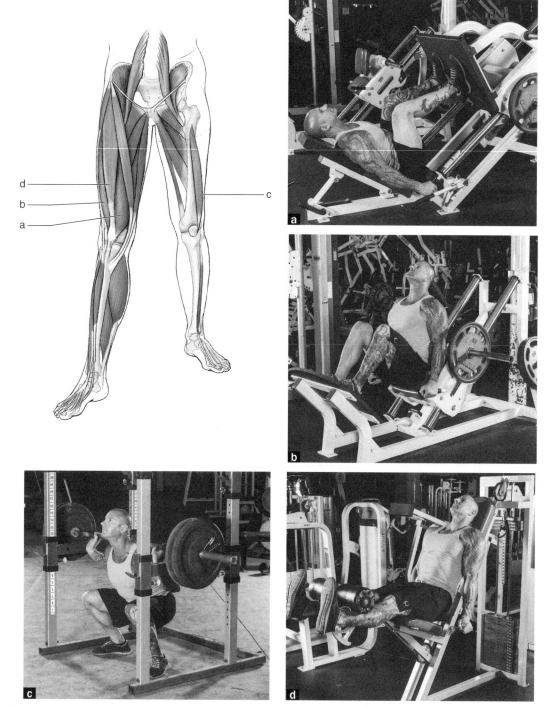

FIGURE 5.8   Quadriceps muscle: *(a)* the vastus medialis is worked by the leg press; *(b)* the vastus lateralis is worked by the hack squat; *(c)* the vastus intermedius, located underneath the rectus femoris, is worked by the squat; and *(d)* the rectus femoris is worked by the leg extension.

For these exercises the same rules apply in regard to how wide the feet are spaced apart. It also is possible to reduce the emphasis on the quadriceps and increase the emphasis on the hamstrings and gluteus maximus by moving the feet farther forward from the hips. The farther the feet are placed in front of the hips, the greater the stress placed on the hamstrings and gluteus maximus and the less stress the quadriceps receive.

The leg press, on the other hand, reduces the amount of stress placed on the hamstrings and gluteus maximus and maximizes the stress placed on the quadriceps; the majority of stress hits the vastus medialis muscle. This is due to the seated position of the angled leg press. The seated position keeps the hips flexed at about 90 degrees when the legs are fully extended. Since the hamstrings and gluteus maximus are involved in extension of the hips during compound leg movements, their involvement is minimized on the leg press.

It's optimal to include some form of lunging or stepping exercises to train the legs unilaterally. Because these exercises are compound movements done one leg at a time, they require a lot of stabilization from small and large muscle groups. That means they use most of the leg muscles including the quads, hamstrings, glutes, and adductor and abductor muscles. Not only do these types of exercises help develop overall size of the thigh muscles, but they also build functional strength, which transfers to more strength on other exercises, such as squats.

The only type of isolation exercise for quadriceps is leg extension exercises, where the only movement that occurs is extension at the knee. This focuses a good deal of the stress on the rectus femoris muscle, although you can encourage more involvement from the vastus lateralis or vastus medialis by altering the position of the feet, as described previously. You should perform leg extension exercises at the end of the quadriceps workout after you perform the more demanding compound exercises. However, some bodybuilders prefer to warm up their quads before heavy compound exercises by doing several light sets of leg extensions. For basic guidelines for designing quadriceps workouts based on the current training split used, see table 5.16.

TABLE 5.16 Quadriceps Training Guidelines Based on Training Split

Training split	Number of exercises	Exercise order	Total sets
Whole-body training split	1	Swap squat exercises, leg press or machine squat exercises, lunge or step exercises, and leg extension exercises each workout.	3-6
Upper- and lower-body training split or two-day training split	2	Choose one compound exercise (such as squat, leg press or machine squat, or lunge or step exercise) and one leg extension exercise every workout. First: A compound exercise (alternate different ones every other workout) Second: An isolation exercise	6-8
Three-day training split	3	Choose two compound exercises and one leg extension exercise every workout. First: A squat exercise Second: A leg press or machine squat or lunge or step exercise Third: A leg extension exercise	9-12
Four-day training split	4	Choose three compound exercises and one leg extension exercise every workout. First: A squat exercise Second: A leg press or machine squat exercise Third: A lunge or step exercise Fourth: A leg extension exercise	12-16

> *continued*

TABLE 5.16 Quadriceps Training Guidelines Based on Training Split *(continued)*

Training split	Number of exercises	Exercise order	Total sets
Five-day training split	4-5	Choose three or four compound exercises and one leg extension exercise every workout. First: A squat exercise Second: If doing four exercises total, do a leg press or machine squat exercise; if doing five exercises total, the second can be another squat or a leg press Third: If doing only four exercises total, do a lunge or step exercise; if doing five exercises and the second is a squat, the third could be a leg press exercise; if doing five exercises and the second is a leg press, the third could be a squat machine exercise or a lunge exercise Fourth: If doing only four exercises total, do a leg extension exercise; if doing five exercises and the third is a leg press or squat machine exercise, the fourth could be a lunge or step exercise; if doing five exercises and the third is a lunge, the fourth should be a step exercise Fifth: A leg extension exercise	12-20
Twice-a-day training split	4	Choose three compound exercises and one leg extension exercise every workout. First: A squat exercise Second: A leg press or machine squat exercise Third: A lunge or step exercise Fourth: A leg extension exercise	12-16

Hamstrings and Gluteus Maximus

The hamstrings are the muscles on the back of the thigh. The gluteus maximus, also referred to as the *glutes,* are the large buttock muscles. The glutes are involved in extending the legs back (as when standing up from a seated position) and kicking the legs back behind the body. The hamstrings are composed of the biceps femoris, the semitendinosus, and the semimembranosus. Collectively the hamstring muscles not only flex the knee, as when you bend your knee, but they also work in conjunction with the glutes to extend the legs at the hips (see figure 5.9).

Although compound quadriceps exercises like the squat, hack squat, lunge, and step-up are traditionally considered quadriceps exercises, they also largely involve the glutes and the hamstring muscles. For this reason, most bodybuilders perform fewer hamstring exercises than quadriceps exercises.

Even though the hamstrings involve three different muscles that work together to perform leg flexion and hip extension, specific exercises better target each muscle. The Romanian deadlift hits the entire hamstring fairly evenly along with the glutes because of the hip extension involved in this exercise. The biceps femoris is better targeted with lying and standing leg curls. The semitendinosus and semimembranosus, on the other hand, are better targeted with seated leg curls. Therefore, a thorough hamstring workout should include one exercise that involves hip extension (such as the Romanian deadlift) and knee flexion (such as the leg curl). For a complete listing and detailed descriptions of all hamstring exercises, see chapter 22. If following a whole-body training split, you may forfeit specific hamstring exercises since the compound quadriceps exercises also use the hamstrings and glutes very strongly. For basic guidelines for designing hamstring and glute workouts based on the current training split used, see table 5.17.

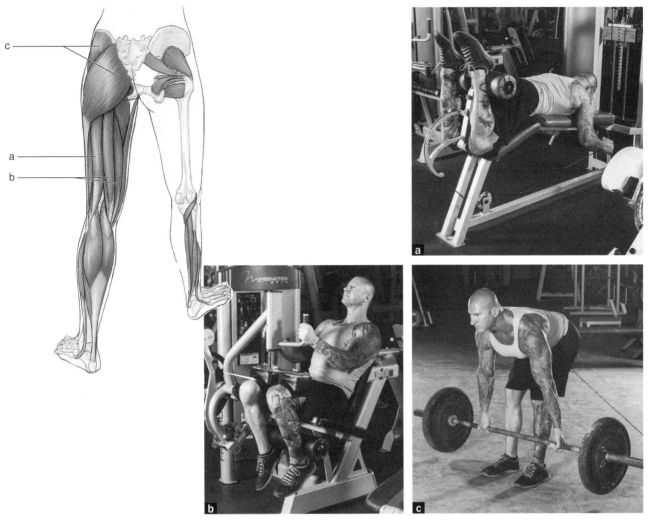

FIGURE 5.9 Hamstrings and gluteus muscles: *(a)* the biceps femoris is targeted by the lying leg curl; *(b)* the semitendinosus and semimembranosus are targeted by the seated leg curl; and *(c)* the glutes are targeted by the Romanian deadlift.

TABLE 5.17 Hamstrings and Glutes Training Guidelines Based on Training Split

Training split	Number of exercises	Exercise order	Total sets
Whole-body training split	1	Alternate hip extension exercises and leg curl exercises every other workout.	2-4
Upper- and lower-body training split or two-day training split	2	First: A hip extension exercise Second: A leg curl exercise Frequently change the type of hip extension and leg curl exercises used.	4-8
Three-day training split	2	First: A hip extension exercise Second: A leg curl exercise Frequently change the type of hip extension and leg curl exercises used.	4-8

> continued

TABLE 5.17 Hamstrings and Glutes Training Guidelines Based on Training Split *(continued)*

Training split	Number of exercises	Exercise order	Total sets
Four-day training split	2-3	First: A hip extension exercise Second: A leg curl exercise (whether doing two or three total exercises) Third: Another leg curl exercise Frequently change the type of hip extension and leg curl exercises used.	4-12
Five-day training split	2-3	First: A hip extension exercise Second: A leg curl exercise (whether doing two or three total exercises) Third: Another leg curl exercise Frequently change the type of hip extension and leg curl exercises used.	4-12
Twice-a-day training split	2-3	First: A hip extension exercise Second: A leg curl exercise (whether doing two or three total exercises) Third: Another leg curl exercise Frequently change the type of hip extension and leg curl exercises used.	4-12

Calves

Calves refer to two separate muscles on the lower leg. These muscles are the gastrocnemius (a muscle shaped like an upside-down heart) and the soleus (a muscle that lies underneath the gastrocnemius), as shown in figure 5.10. Both muscles perform extension at the ankle, such as when you stand up on your toes.

Certain exercises are better than others at targeting the two calf muscles. For detailed descriptions of all calf exercises, refer to chapter 23. Standing calf raises, or any calf raise that involves a fairly straight knee, is better at focusing the stress to the gastrocnemius. The soleus, on the other hand, is better targeted with seated calf raises or any calf raise that is performed with the knee bent to about 90 degrees.

The best way to train calves is to include one or two exercises that target the gastrocnemius muscle and one exercise that targets the soleus muscle. Most bodybuilders train their calves after thighs. Some also include a second or third workout of the calves if they do not train legs twice a week. The reason for this is that the calves, particularly the soleus, are made up of a slightly higher percentage of slow-twitch muscle fibers. These muscle fibers have a high-endurance capacity and recover more quickly than fast-twitch muscle fibers. This is also the reason that many bodybuilders train their calves with very high reps (20 to 30 reps per set). However, the best way to train calves is with the use of a periodized program that cycles the number of reps performed. For basic guidelines for designing calf workouts based on the current training split used, see table 5.18.

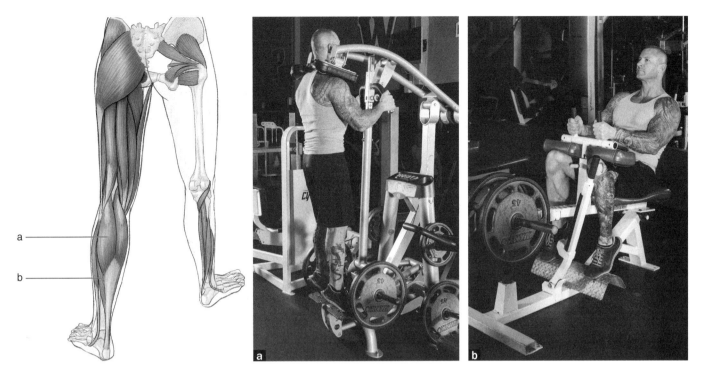

FIGURE 5.10 Calf muscles: *(a)* the gastrocnemius is targeted by the standing calf raise, and *(b)* the soleus is targeted by the seated calf raise.

TABLE 5.18 Calf Training Guidelines Based on Training Split

Training split	Number of exercises	Exercise order	Total sets
Whole-body training split	1	Alternate gastrocnemius exercises and soleus exercises every other workout.	3-6
Upper- and lower-body training split or two-day training split	2	First: A gastrocnemius exercise (frequently change the type) Second: A soleus exercise (on occasion perform the soleus exercise first)	6-10
Three-day training split	2	First: A gastrocnemius exercise (frequently change the type) Second: A soleus exercise (on occasion perform the soleus exercise first)	6-10
Four-day training split	2-3	First: A gastrocnemius exercise (frequently change the type) Second: If doing only two exercises, do a soleus exercise (on occasion perform the soleus exercise first); if doing three exercises, the second should be a gastrocnemius exercise Third: A soleus exercise (on occasion perform it first or second)	6-12
Five-day training split	2-3	First: A gastrocnemius exercise (frequently change the type) Second: If doing only two exercises, do a soleus exercise (on occasion perform the soleus exercise first); if doing three exercises, the second should be a gastrocnemius exercise Third: A soleus exercise (on occasion perform it first or second)	6-12
Twice-a-day training split	2-3	First: A gastrocnemius exercise (frequently change the type) Second: If doing only two exercises, do a soleus exercise (on occasion perform the soleus exercise first); if doing three exercises, the second should be a gastrocnemius exercise Third: A soleus exercise (on occasion perform it first or second)	6-12

Abdominals

Abdominals refer to four muscles that are on the midsection, informally called abs by most body-builders. These include the rectus abdominis, the external obliques, the internal obliques, and the transverse abdominis (see figure 5.11). The best abdominal program uses exercises that target all four areas of the abdominal region—upper abs, lower abs, internal and external obliques, and the transverse abdominis.

The upper abs are best targeted with crunch exercises that involve flexing the upper spine forward by bringing the shoulders toward the hips, such as the standard crunch. The lower abdominals are best trained with exercises that involve flexing the lower spine forward by bringing the knees toward the chest, such as hanging knee raises. Both the internal and external obliques are best targeted by exercises that flex the spine later-ally to the left and right, such as oblique crunches. They also are targeted with exercises that involve flexing the spine forward and rotating it to the left or right, such as with crossover crunches. The deep transverse abdominis is best trained with core exercises that force the flexing of the transverse abdominis (pulling the navel in toward the spine) to stabilize the spine and pelvis. For a complete listing and detailed descriptions of all abdominal exercises, see chapter 24.

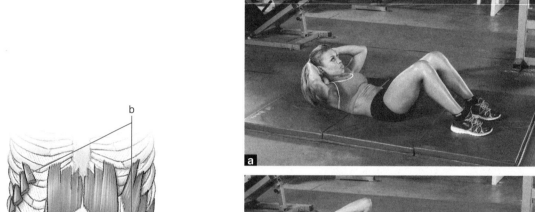

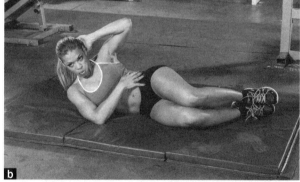

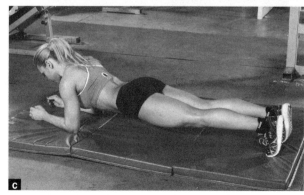

FIGURE 5.11   Abdominal muscles: *(a)* the rectus abdominis is worked by the crunch; *(b)* the external and internal obliques are worked by the oblique crunch; and *(c)* the transverse abdominis, located deep beneath the rectus abdominis and the obliques, is worked by the plank.

Most bodybuilders train the abdominals more frequently and with higher reps than they use with most other major muscle groups. This is because the abdominals are postural muscles that stay flexed for long periods to support the spine. Therefore, they tend to be slightly higher in slow-twitch muscle fibers than the other muscle groups. Most bodybuilders train the abdominals a minimum of three times per week and some train them every day. For most people, training abdominals on two or three nonconsecutive days per week will suffice. Because the abdominals are often trained with no more resistance than the person's body weight, they are frequently trained with reps in the range of 15 to 30. However, even abdominal training should be periodized to cycle the rep range and resistance used. Although many people fear that using heavy resistance on ab exercises will make the waist too big and blocky, it is essential to train the abdominal muscles like any other muscle group. Increasing the development of the abdominal muscles improves definition, when body fat is low. It also helps to increase core strength, which can cross over to help increase overall strength.

The best way to train the abdominals is by choosing four exercises that each target a different area of the abdominals for each workout. However, if you train with a whole-body, upper- and lower-body, or two-day training split, you won't have the time to do four separate abdominal exercises. In this case, you should choose one or two exercises that target one area of the abdominals and rotate the abdominal region trained for every workout. For basic guidelines for designing abdominal workouts based on the current training split used, see table 5.19.

TABLE 5.19 Abdominal Training Guidelines Based on Training Split

Training split	Number of exercises	Exercise order	Total sets
Whole-body training split	1	Alternate upper abdominal exercises, lower abdominal exercises, oblique exercises, and core exercises every other workout.	3-4
Upper- and lower-body training split or two-day training split	2	Choose two exercises that target one area of the abdominals and alternate upper-abdominal exercises, lower-abdominal exercises, oblique exercises, and core exercises every other workout.	6-8
Three-day training split	3	First: A lower-ab exercise (frequently change the type) Second: An upper-ab exercise (frequently change the type) Third: An oblique exercise Every other ab workout, do a core exercise as the first exercise and skip the oblique exercise.	6-10
Four-day training split	3-4	If doing only three exercises total: First: A lower-ab exercise Second: An upper-ab exercise Third: An oblique exercise Every other ab workout, do a core exercise as the first exercise and skip the oblique exercise. If doing four exercises total: First: A core exercise Second: A lower-ab exercise Third: An upper-ab exercise Fourth: An oblique exercise	6-16
Five-day training split	4	First: A core exercise Second: A lower-ab exercise Third: An upper-ab exercise Fourth: An oblique exercise	8-16
Twice-a-day training split	4	First: A core exercise Second: A lower-ab exercise Third: An upper-ab exercise Fourth: An oblique exercise	8-16

CHAPTER 6

Programs for Building Muscle Mass

Building muscle mass takes considerable time and consistency in the gym. But one problem that arises from consistency is that the muscles quickly adapt to a workout when it is used for too long. To prevent muscle adaptation from turning into stagnation, you need to frequently expose your muscles to different training techniques. Having numerous techniques to draw from allows you to continually provide new training stimuli to your muscles for optimal growth. This chapter presents training methods that are effective for maximizing muscle mass.

The techniques are categorized by the type of acute variable of training that is being manipulated in each workout. Each technique is rated on a scale of 1 to 5 for four critical areas:

1. **Time**—the amount of time that a specific workout typically takes to complete. This helps you immediately determine whether this training technique will fit your training schedule. The higher the number, the longer the workouts for that specific technique will take to complete.

2. **Length**—the amount of time required for following the program consistently before appreciable results are noticeable. This helps you determine whether you have the patience required in order for a certain program to demonstrate results. The higher the number, the longer you must follow this technique in order to realize results.

3. **Difficulty**—the amount of weightlifting experience required for using the program effectively. This helps you decide whether you have enough training experience to take on specific training techniques. The higher the number, the more training experience you should have before attempting that particular technique.

4. **Results**—how effective the program seems to be for mass gains in most people. This helps you estimate how much muscle mass you can expect to gain with each program. The higher the number, the greater gains in muscle mass you can expect from a particular program.

Each training technique provides a sample workout to give you an indication of how the particular technique can be used. Some provide details on exercise selection, rep ranges, total sets, and training frequency that you need to follow closely. However, others offer just a snapshot for one particular workout or one workout cycle. These are just templates, and you are encouraged to substitute your own exercises where warranted to maintain variety.

Although you need not use every method listed in this chapter, if you have more than a year of training experience, you should eventually try a majority of the methods to determine those that work best for you. Then you can cycle these techniques, along with the basic programs covered in chapter 5, to create a periodized program that delivers the desired results and prevents the muscles from stagnating. Chapter 7 covers periodized schedules for building muscle mass using the programs and techniques covered in chapters 5 and 6. In the programs, weights are given in pounds; please see appendix for metric conversions.

PROGRAMS THAT MANIPULATE SETS

The following training techniques alter the sets performed during a workout. This can be done by increasing the number of exercises performed that make up one set, by limiting the number of sets performed per muscle group, or by increasing the number of sets performed for an exercise in a given time. They all are effective ways to increase your training intensity.

Superset Training

Superset training is a method that pairs exercises for agonist and antagonist muscle groups, such as biceps and triceps, and involves performing a set for each muscle group back to back with no scheduled rest between exercises. See table 6.1 for sample exercise pairs that work well for supersets. Superset workouts typically consist of two or three exercise pairs for each muscle group. See table 6.2 for a sample triceps and biceps superset workout. Superset training offers several advantages over straight-set training. The most obvious advantage is time. Because of the limited rest between exercises, superset workouts are generally quicker to perform than other training methods that allow rest periods between sets and exercises. Another advantage of supersets is that you'll actually be stronger in the second exercise. Research has found that a muscle will be stronger if preceded immediately by a contraction of its antagonist, or opposing muscle group. For example, when you do a superset of barbell curls and triceps extensions, in that order, you'll be stronger on the triceps extension and vice versa. This happens because normally the muscle you're training is somewhat limited by its antagonist. When bench-pressing using straight sets, for instance, the back muscles inhibit the contraction of your pecs to a certain extent. Doing a set of rows shortly before benching, however, lessens this inhibitory effect, allowing your pecs to contract more forcefully. As a result, you'll be able to train with more weight and get stronger and bigger. Another benefit to superset training is enhanced recovery. When you alternate every set of triceps with a set of biceps, you increase blood flow to those muscles because when you're doing curls, your triceps are still contracting, which increases blood flow to them and aids in recovery. This helps your body remove waste products and damaged muscle tissue as a result of exercise. Keep rest periods short between supersets (1 to 2 minutes).

RATING

Time	1	2	3	4	5
Length	1	2	3	4	5
Difficulty	1	2	3	4	5
Results	1	2	3	4	5

TABLE 6.1   Superset Training Pairs

Muscle pair	Exercises
Chest and back	Bench press and barbell row
Shoulders and back	Shoulder press and pull-up
Biceps and triceps	Barbell curl and triceps pressdown
Quadriceps and hamstrings	Leg extension and leg curl

TABLE 6.2   Supersets for Biceps and Triceps

Exercise	Sets	Reps
Barbell curl	3	8-10
Superset with triceps pressdown	3	8-10
Preacher curl	3	8-12
Superset with lying triceps extension	3	8-10
Seated dumbbell curl	3	8-12
Superset with triceps bench dip	3	8-12

Compound-Set Training

Compound-set training is similar to superset training except that the two exercises that are done back to back are performed for the same muscle group. As an example for shoulders, a lifter would perform a set of shoulder presses and immediately follow that set with a set of lateral raises with no break. That equals one compound set. After the set of lateral raises is finished, the lifter would rest for a couple of minutes and then start back with shoulder presses. This might be performed for two or three compound sets. The compound can then be followed with other shoulder exercises that are performed either in straight sets or as another compound set. While the exercise choices are not that critical, there are two strategies that are usually used with compound sets. Exercise choices can be made either to target a different section of the desired muscle group (such as the dumbbell shoulder press and the bent-over lateral raise) or to target a similar part of the muscle group (such as the dumbbell shoulder press and the machine shoulder press). The major benefits of compound-set training are intensity and time. Training two exercises for one muscle group without any rest between exercises significantly increases the intensity of the workout and places greater demands on the muscle fibers being trained as well as on your entire body. It also dramatically reduces the amount of time required to train a muscle group. This makes it a great workout technique when you want to push a particular muscle group beyond its comfort zone or when you are short on time. Because compound-set training is a very high-intensity technique, you should use it infrequently or for short periods, because overtraining is possible if done for too long. See table 6.3 for a sample compound-set shoulder workout.

RATING

	1	2	3	4	5
Time	1	2	3	4	5
Length	1	2	3	4	5
Difficulty	1	2	3	4	5
Results	1	2	3	4	5

TABLE 6.3   Shoulder Compound Set

Exercise	Sets	Reps
Dumbbell shoulder press	3	6-8
Compound set with lateral raise	3	10-12
Front raise	3	10-12
Compound set with upright row	3	8-10

Tri-Set Training

Tri-set training is an extended compound set. It uses three exercises for the same muscle group back to back with no rest between sets, as opposed to just two exercises. For smaller muscle groups like biceps, triceps, and deltoids, one group of tri-sets performed for two to four sets is typically enough to train the muscle group effectively. When smart exercise choices are selected, one tri-set can properly target all areas of most major muscle groups. As with compound-set training, the major benefits of tri-set training are higher-intensity training and less training time required. Of course, it also means that the technique should be used infrequently and for short periods to prevent overtraining. See table 6.4 for an example of a triceps tri-set workout.

RATING

	1	2	3	4	5
Time	1	2	3	4	5
Length	1	2	3	4	5
Difficulty	1	2	3	4	5
Results	1	2	3	4	5

TABLE 6.4   Triceps Tri-Set

Exercise	Sets	Reps
Triceps pressdown	3	8-10
Seated overhead triceps extension	3	6-8
Bench dip	3	8-12

Giant-Set Training

Giant-set training is similar to compound-set and tri-set training in that multiple exercises are done for a single muscle group back to back with no rest between sets. The difference is in the number of exercises performed. Giant sets incorporate four or more exercises. Giant sets or tri-sets are a great way to quickly hit any muscle group from a variety of angles. The benefits are similar to those of compound and tri-sets. See table 6.5 for a sample giant-set routine for abs.

Without taking a rest, perform one set of each exercise listed. Then rest for a few minutes and follow the exercise order again.

RATING

Time	1	2	3	4	5
Length	1	2	3	4	5
Difficulty	1	2	3	4	5
Results	1	2	3	4	5

TABLE 6.5 Giant Set for Abdominals

Exercise	Sets	Reps
Hanging knee raise	3	15
Crossover crunch	3	20
Reverse crunch	3	15
Cable crunch	3	12

High-Intensity Training

High-intensity training (HIT) is a method based on the one-set training concept that was popularized by Arthur Jones (founder of Nautilus) and professional bodybuilder Mike Mentzer. The foundation of this training method involves very low volume and very high intensity. Most followers do as few as one set per exercise and only one to three exercises per muscle group (see table 6.6). Intensity for this technique is not so much about the weight used but about training beyond the point of muscle failure. Every set must be taken beyond failure with the use of forced reps, negative-rep training, and even partial-rep training (where as much of the range of motion of the exercise is performed until the weight cannot be budged). The theory behind HIT is that if multiple sets of an exercise are performed, every set cannot be trained with maximal intensity. By doing one and only one set of an exercise, you have a better chance of training with maximal intensity.

Volume is also kept low with HIT to minimize the time spent in the gym. Because volume is low with HIT, it allows the lifter to follow a whole-body training split or a two-day training split, depending on whether the lifter wants to train each muscle group two or three times per week.

There is no research to specifically support the theory of HIT, and anecdotal reports are varied.

Some lifters experience considerable gains in strength and muscle mass. But for most, the progress soon comes to a halt. The problem may lie in the fact that volume is an acute variable that does not get manipulated in this program. Therefore, following HIT for only four to six weeks would be a smart way to use it. After training with HIT you should switch to a training program that uses fairly high volume. The sample HIT program in table 6.6 is a two-day split done twice a week. In this program, each set should be preceded with one short warm-up set before each exercise with approximately 50 percent of the weight you will use for the main working set. Do only about four to six reps with this lighter weight. Perform each set to muscle failure and have a spotter help you perform three or four forced reps after reaching muscle failure. Resist the negative portion of the forced reps for added intensity and consider attempting a few partial reps at the very end of the set.

RATING

Time	1	2	3	4	5
Length	1	2	3	4	5
Difficulty	1	2	3	4	5
Results	1	2	3	4	5

TABLE 6.6   Big HIT Workout

MONDAY AND THURSDAY			TUESDAY AND FRIDAY		
Exercise	Sets	Reps	Exercise	Sets	Reps
Barbell incline bench press	1	8-10	Squat	1	8-10
Dumbbell pullover	1	8-10	Leg extension	1	8-10
Dumbbell fly	1	8-10	Leg curl	1	8-10
Barbell shoulder press	1	8-10	Standing calf raise	1	8-12
Dumbbell lateral raise	1	8-10	Barbell biceps curl	1	8-10
Dumbbell shrug	1	8-10	Seated incline curl	1	8-10
Barbell row	1	8-10	Triceps dip	1	8-10
			Triceps pressdown	1	8-10
			Hanging knee raise	1	10-15

Nubret Pro-Set Method

This method, named after International Federation of Bodybuilding and fitness professional bodybuilder Serge Nubret of France, incorporates a progression method that increases the number of sets done on an exercise with each workout. It also requires that you do that in the same amount of time as for the previous workout. For example, if you do three sets of barbell curls for 10 reps in five minutes in one workout, you must try to get four sets of 10 reps in five minutes in the following workouts until you reach that goal. The only way to do more sets in the same amount of time is to reduce your rest period between sets. Therefore, this method increases strength and muscle mass by enhancing the ability of the muscles to recover between sets. The best way to use this technique is to do it first in your workout using one exercise for each muscle group. See table 6.7 for a sample progression of the Nubret pro-set workout in which the lifter required four weeks to increase his total work from three sets of 10 in five minutes to four sets of 10 in five minutes.

RATING

Time	1	2	3	4	5
Length	1	2	3	4	5
Difficulty	1	2	3	4	5
Results	1	2	3	4	5

TABLE 6.7   Nubret Pro-Set Method

Week	Sets	Reps	Total time
1	3	10	5 min
2	2	10	5 min
	1	8	
	1	6	
3	3	10	5 min
	1	8	
4	4	10	5 min

PROGRAMS THAT MANIPULATE REPETITIONS

Although the rep is the smallest part of the workout, manipulating it can lead to big gains in muscle mass. The following training techniques alter the reps performed in each workout. This can be done by using specific rep ranges, using extremely high-rep training, dividing the reps up throughout the day, altering the range of motion of specific reps, performing reps with additional help after muscles have fatigued, changing the speed at which reps are performed, or emphasizing a certain part of the rep. These all work to boost muscle growth one rep at a time.

5–10–20 Training

This program is actually an advanced version of tri-sets (see Tri-Set Training earlier in this chapter). With most tri-set programs you perform equal reps on all three exercises, but this one uses very specific repetition ranges for each exercise. The first exercise in the tri-set is done for just 5 reps. This is a good rep range for boosting muscle strength. The second exercise is done for 10 reps. This is the ideal rep range for building muscle mass. The last exercise in the tri-set is done for 20 reps. This rep range enhances muscle endurance but also further promotes muscle hypertrophy. Combining all three of these rep ranges gives you a program that trains the muscles in every respect necessary to get them big, lean, and strong.

Exercise selection plays an important role in the 5–10–20 program because of the imposed rep ranges. The first exercise should be a basic exercise, preferably using a barbell. Because the reps on this exercise are so low for building strength, basic multijoint exercises with a barbell are best (see table 6.8 for sample exercise choices for each exercise). The second exercise is done with a moderate number of reps for putting on muscle size; therefore, it should be another basic exercise (similar to the first) but performed with either dumbbells or a machine. The third exercise is the high-rep set, so the best exercise choices are single-joint isolation moves. These can be done with dumbbells, but cables or machines are your preferred method to give your muscles continuous tension throughout the entire range of motion.

Because this program is so demanding on the muscles and on your entire body, you'll need to get plenty of rest for optimal recovery. Allow each muscle group trained with the 5–10–20 program at least five days of rest before training them again. I suggest you plan on working each muscle group just once per week, as shown in table 6.9. Remember that you can substitute these exercises for any of the appropriate ones in table 6.8. Perform one set of each exercise, resting just long enough to get set up on the next exercise. After the last exercise is completed, rest two minutes before repeating in the same order. Repeat for a total of two to four tri-sets. Follow the program for no longer than 6 weeks. This is a fairly grueling regimen to maintain for any longer. But don't think that you have to train every body part with 5–10–20. You can choose to train just one or a few of your troublesome body parts with the 5–10–20 program to bring them up to par with the rest of you.

RATING

Time	1	2	3	4	5
Length	1	2	3	4	5
Difficulty	1	2	3	4	5
Results	1	2	3	4	5

TABLE 6.8 Choosing 5s, 10s, 20s

FIRST EXERCISE	
Muscle group	**Exercise choices**
Chest	Barbell bench press, incline barbell bench press, decline barbell bench press
Deltoids	Barbell shoulder press (seated or standing)
Back	Barbell row, pull-up
Thighs	Squat
Triceps	Close-grip bench press, triceps dip
Biceps	Barbell curl
SECOND EXERCISE	
Chest	Dumbbell bench press, machine chest press (flat, incline, or decline versions)
Deltoids	Overhead dumbbell press, machine overhead press
Back	Dumbbell row, cable row, machine row, pulldown (various grips)
Thighs	Leg press, lunge, dumbbell step-up
Triceps	Lying or seated triceps extension
Biceps	Dumbbell curls (standing, seated, or incline)
THIRD EXERCISE	
Chest	Dumbbell fly or cable fly (incline, flat, or decline), cable crossover, pec deck
Deltoids	Dumbbell, cable, or machine lateral raise; bent-over lateral raise; front raise
Back	Straight-arm pulldown
Thighs	Leg extension, leg curl (lying, seated, or standing)
Triceps	Triceps pressdown, machine triceps extension
Biceps	Cable concentration curl or machine curl

TABLE 6.9 5–10–20 Blocks

THIGHS				CHEST		
Exercise	**Sets**	**Reps**		**Exercise**	**Sets**	**Reps**
Barbell squat	4	5		Incline bench press	3	5
Dumbbell lunge	4	10		Flat dumbbell press	3	10
Leg curl	4	20		Cable crossover	3	20
BACK				**TRICEPS**		
Bent-over barbell row	3	5		Triceps dip	2	5
Pulldown	3	10		Lying triceps extension	2	10
Straight-arm pulldown	3	20		Triceps pressdown	2	20
BICEPS						
Barbell curl	2	5				
Incline dumbbell curl	2	10				
Machine preacher curl	2	20				

Finish Pump Method

This method involves training with basic exercises and heavy weight in the beginning of the workout. For example, a chest workout would start with an exercise such as the bench press for sets of 6 to 8 reps, and then continue with the dumbbell press for sets of 8 to 10 reps, and then finish with dumbbell flys for sets of 12 to 15 reps and cable crossovers for sets of 15 to 20. This concept takes advantage of the enhanced blood flow from the higher-rep training to deliver more water (which enters the muscle to create the pump), oxygen, nutrients, and anabolic hormones to the muscles and help flush the waste products away from the muscle at the end of the workout. This helps to enhance recovery and stimulate muscle growth. See table 6.10 for a sample finish pump workout.

RATING

Time	1	2	3	4	5
Length	1	2	3	4	5
Difficulty	1	2	3	4	5
Results	1	2	3	4	5

TABLE 6.10   Finish Pump for Quadriceps

Exercise	Sets	Reps
Squat	3	6-8
Leg press	3	8-10
Lunge	3	12-15
Leg extension	3	15-20

Hundreds Training

Hundreds training is an extremely hard-core method that incorporates very high repetitions—100 reps per set, to be exact. The weight you will use to complete 100 reps is around 20 to 30 percent of a weight you can use for 10 strict reps. For example, if you use 50-pound dumbbells for 10 reps on dumbbell curls, you will use 10- to 15-pound dumbbells when you do hundreds training. Try the 10-pound dumbbells to start, because you always want to start lighter than heavier. Your goal is to perform at least 70 reps before you stop for a quick breather. That is, you should fail before you reach 100 reps. If you can do all 100 reps with a given weight, without stopping, then the weight is too light and you will need to increase it for the next workout. You need to find a weight that allows you to complete 60 to 70 reps without stopping. Your mark for increasing the weight is when you can get 70 reps or more with a weight.

Let's walk through a sample set of standing dumbbell curls using the hundreds training approach. Grab your appropriately weighted dumbbells and perform dumbbell curls as you normally would with a heavier weight. Keep your form on the dumbbell curls strict as described in chapter 19 and keep your reps moderately paced and under control at all times. If you chose the correct weight, you will reach momentary muscle

failure somewhere between rep 60 and rep 70. Here's where you get a rest but only for as many seconds as the number of reps you have left to complete. In other words, rest 1 second for every remaining rep you have left. If you completed 65 reps, then you rest 35 seconds, and then attempt to do the remaining 35 reps. If you fail to complete those final 35, use the same method—rest 1 second for every rep you have left until you reach the 100-rep mark. Sounds simple . . . until you actually try it. This method is only for those with at least one full year of consistent strength training experience.

The benefit of hundreds training is how it incorporates the muscle fibers in the muscle. Because the weight is so light and the reps are so high, it thoroughly trains the slow-twitch muscle fibers in the beginning of the set. All muscles are composed of two major types of muscle fibers—slow-twitch and fast-twitch muscle fibers. Slow-twitch muscle fibers tend to be used for endurance-type activities—therefore, higher reps tend to train them best. Fast-twitch muscle fibers are used for more powerful activities—therefore, they are better trained with heavy weight and low reps, or with fast, explosive-type movements. Most muscles are close to 50 percent slow-twitch and 50 percent fast-twitch muscle fibers. This means it's a good idea to use techniques that train both types of muscle fibers. With hundreds training you will hit the slow-twitch muscle fibers during the first 60 reps or so. After that, your muscles will have to call on the fast-twitch muscle fibers to help out the fatigued slow-twitch fibers. Doing this many repetitions causes biochemical changes in the muscle, which aid in muscle growth. It also leads to greater growth of blood vessels that feed the muscle fibers to enhance the delivery of blood, oxygen, nutrients, and hormones to the muscle cells. This environment increases the growth potential of the muscle fibers.

The best way to use hundreds training is to train each muscle group twice per week. Therefore, following an upper- and lower-body training split or a two-day is ideal with this style of training. The only difference is that you can do up to three exercises for larger muscle groups (chest, back, and quadriceps) because you perform only one set per exercise with hundreds training. Try hundreds training for about two to four weeks; it is very intense and will be difficult to follow for any longer. Then follow it with a standard mass training that uses heavy weight and low reps. Another way to use hundreds training is to sporadically train one muscle group or your entire body with hundreds training for just one or two workouts to change your training style and shock the muscles for added growth. See table 6.11 for a sample training regimen using the hundreds training technique. Each of the workouts in this program is to be done twice weekly. For instance, you can do workout 1 on Monday and Thursday and workout 2 on Tuesday and Friday. Or you can allow a day of rest between every workout and do workout 1 on Monday and Friday and workout 2 on Wednesday and Sunday.

RATING

	1	2	3	4	5
Time	**1**	2	3	4	5
Length	1	2	**3**	4	5
Difficulty	1	2	3	4	**5**
Results	1	2	3	**4**	5

TABLE 6.11 Hundreds Workouts

WORKOUT 1

Muscle group	Exercise	Sets	Reps
Chest	Bench press	1	100
	Incline dumbbell fly	1	100
	Cable crossover	1	100
Back	Wide-grip pulldown	1	100
	Seated cable row	1	100
	Straight-arm pulldown	1	100
Shoulders	Smith machine shoulder press	1	100
	Dumbbell lateral raise	1	100
Trapezius	Dumbbell shrug	1	100
Abdominals	Cable crunch	1	100

WORKOUT 2

Muscle group	Exercise	Sets	Reps
Quadriceps	Smith machine squat	1	100
	Leg press	1	100
	Leg extension	1	100
Hamstrings	Lying leg curl	1	100
Calves	Standing calf raise	1	100
	Seated calf raise	1	100
Biceps	Barbell curl	1	100
	Preacher curl	1	100
Triceps	Lying triceps extension	1	100
	Triceps pressdown	1	100

50–50 Method

This program helps to bring up the development of lagging muscle groups. Simply stated, this program involves the completion of 100 reps per day on one exercise for any body part that you deem is behind in growth. It is different from hundreds training in that you don't perform all 100 reps at one time, plus you do this for one muscle group every day for eight weeks. By doing so many reps every day, you enhance the endurance capacity of the muscle. Enhanced endurance is facilitated by an increase in the capillary density of the muscle. Capillary density refers to the number of capillaries (small blood vessels where nutrient and gas exchange take place between the blood and the muscle cells) a muscle is supplied with. Muscle hypertrophy tends to lower the capillary density because of the greater amount of muscle present. This also happens with low-rep, heavy-weight training, because this style of training forces the muscle to rely more on the energy it can derive within the muscle cell, not from the blood. By doing the 50–50 method, you can boost the capillary density of a muscle and therefore enhance the delivery of nutrients, anabolic hormones, and oxygen to the muscle. In addition, you enhance the removal of biochemical waste products from the muscle. This results in bigger muscle pumps, more rapid recovery of the muscle, and ultimately greater potential for muscle growth.

To follow the 50–50 method, choose the muscle group you want to bring up to par with the others. Then choose one exercise for that muscle group. This will be the exercise you will do every day, even on the days you don't normally train that muscle group. See table 6.12 for a list of the best exercises to use with the 50–50 method. You will need to perform 100 reps a day of that exercise in two segments in the day. That means you will perform 50 reps at a time, separated by about 8 to 12 hours, with a weight that challenges you but is not so heavy it causes you to fatigue by the 50th rep. For example, if you want to build up your biceps, you will do 50 reps of dumbbell curls in the morning—say at 9:00 a.m.—and again in the evening—maybe at 9:00 p.m. The weight you use is critical to your success. If it's too heavy, then it is likely to lead to overtraining. A good rule is that when you reach the 50th rep you should feel as though you could complete about 10 more reps. Follow this program for no more than eight weeks to see decent results and prevent stagnation. You can, however, switch to other muscle groups and continue the 50–50 method.

RATING

Time	1	2	3	4	5
Length	1	2	3	4	5
Difficulty	1	2	3	4	5
Results	1	2	3	4	5

TABLE 6.12 50–50 Exercises

Muscle group	Best choice of exercises
Chest	Dumbbell bench press (flat or incline)
	Dumbbell fly (flat or incline)
	Push-up
Deltoids	Overhead dumbbell press (standing or seated)
	Dumbbell lateral raise
	Dumbbell upright row
	Bent-over lateral raise
Back	Dumbbell or barbell row
	Pulldown
	Straight-arm pulldown
Triceps	Triceps pressdown
	Lying dumbbell extension
Biceps	Dumbbell curl (standing, seated, or incline)
Forearms	Wrist curl (dumbbell or barbell)
	Reverse wrist curl (dumbbell or barbell)
Quadriceps	Squat
	Leg extension
Hamstrings	Leg curl (lying, seated, standing)
	Romanian deadlift (dumbbell or barbell)
Calves	Standing calf raise
	Donkey calf raise
Abdominals	Crunch

21s

This is an advanced method of training that challenges the working muscle group in three different ranges of motion within a single set. Its name comes from the total number of reps per set you perform with this training technique. In each set, you do a total of 21 repetitions but as three separate sets of 7 reps. You start the set from the start position and do 7 reps through the first half of the range of motion (see table 6.13). After you complete the first 7 reps, you do another 7 reps but only through the last half of the range of motion. When those 7 are complete, you finish with 7 reps through the full range of motion of that exercise. Using the barbell curl as an example, you start with your arms fully extended, holding a barbell across the front of your thighs. First you curl the weight up 7 times only to the point where your arms are parallel with the floor. Then you curl the weight up 7 times from the point where your arms are parallel with the floor to the point where they are close to your shoulders. After these 7 reps, you perform 7 standard barbell curls going through the full range of motion.

The 21s can be done with virtually any exercise but are most practical with single-joint isolation movements. Multijoint exercises, like the bench press and squat, involve so many secondary and stabilizing muscles that straight sets prove the most effective. See table 6.13 for a sample of the best exercises to use with 21s. Regardless of the exercise, you'll need to use lighter resistance than usual when doing 21s, since your muscles are unaccustomed to the increased number of reps. Using cables or machines for this training technique is an excellent way to maintain continuous tension on the muscle. This is especially important, because the tension on the muscle is typically decreased at full flexion when you use free weights.

With 21s you can most effectively work on flexibility within the joint during the first 7 reps, since you begin each rep with the working muscle in a fully stretched position. The middle 7 reps are most productive in terms of muscle growth and development, because you're stronger in the second half of the movement and you can squeeze the contraction at the top for maximum peaking. The last 7 reps essentially serve the purpose of burning out the muscles, which is great for initiating new growth.

To work 21s into your current routine, do three sets of them as the first exercise for a body part (after a proper warm-up, of course), then resume with straight sets for all other movements in that body-part workout. Or do one to three sets of 21s as the last exercise for a particular body part to burn it out. To avoid overtraining, decrease your volume for the body part you're doing 21s with by doing one fewer exercise in that workout. If on chest day you normally do three or four exercises, do two or three if you're doing three sets of 21s. Beginners should start off with only one set of 21s—remember, this is an advanced technique. You can increase to 2 or 3 sets after a couple of sessions. Follow this program for about four to eight weeks, and no more, because it loses its effectiveness after about eight weeks.

RATING

Time	1	2	3	4	5
Length	1	2	3	4	5
Difficulty	1	2	3	4	5
Results	1	2	3	4	5

TABLE 6.13 Dealing 21s

Muscle group	Exercise	Breakdown form for 21s
Chest	Cable crossover	Form for this exercise is the same as for normal cable crossovers, as described in chapter 14. First 7 reps: Start with your hands outside your shoulders and contract your pecs until your arms are about 45 degrees to your torso. Next 7 reps: Go from 45 degrees to hands together, maintaining the same elbow angle from the start, and squeeze. Last 7 reps: Combine previous 2 for 7 complete reps.
Back	Lat pulldown	Form for this exercise is the same as for normal lat pulldown, as described in chapter 16. First 7 reps: Pull the bar toward your upper chest, keeping your elbows back, until your elbows are at approximately 90-degree angles. Next 7 reps: Start at 90 degrees and pull the bar all the way to your upper chest. Last 7 reps: Combine previous 2 for full-range reps.
Shoulders	Cable lateral raise	Form for this exercise is the same as for normal cable lateral raise, as described in chapter 15. First 7 reps: Raise your arm upward and outward, keeping your elbow locked in a slightly bent position, until your arm is at a 45-degree angle to the floor. Next 7 reps: Start at about 45 degrees and pull the weight up until your arm is just past parallel to the floor. Last 7 reps: Combine previous 2.
Quadriceps	Leg extension	Form for this exercise is the same as for normal leg extension, as described in chapter 21. First 7 reps: Extend your knees to where your shins are at 45-degree angles to the floor. Next 7 reps: Start at the 45-degree angle, straighten your legs, and squeeze your quads at the top. Last 7 reps: Combine previous 2.
Hamstrings	Lying leg curl (can also be done on seated leg curl)	Form for this exercise is the same as for normal lying leg curls, as described in chapter 22. First 7 reps: Flex your knees until your shins are just short of perpendicular to the floor. Next 7 reps: The end range is just bringing the pad up to your butt as much as possible. Last 7 reps: Combine previous 2.
Triceps	Triceps pressdown	Because the range of motion on triceps pressdown is relatively small (see chapter 18), increase it when doing 21s by starting with your hands at upper-chest level. Start with your forearms about 30 degrees above horizontal, whereas normally they'd be parallel to the floor. Lock your upper arms and elbows at your sides. First 7 reps: Extend your arms until your elbows are just past parallel to the floor. Next 7 reps: Start at about parallel, extend your arms until your elbows are completely locked out, and squeeze your triceps. Last 7 reps: Combine previous 2.
Biceps	One-arm cable curl	Form for this exercise is the same as for normal one-arm cable curl, as described in chapter 19. First 7 reps: Curl the weight up until your forearm is nearly parallel to the floor. Next 7 reps: Start at about parallel, curl the handle up until your elbow reaches full flexion, and squeeze at the top. Last 7 reps: Combine previous 2.

Four-Rep System

This program involves four different exercises for each muscle group. Each exercise is designed to hit the muscle from a variety of angles and provide a unique stimulus to the muscle. After a thorough warm-up, the first exercise should be a basic exercise (see table 6.14) and done for three sets of four reps. This rep range provides a stimulus for gains in strength. The second exercise can be another basic exercise, preferably a dumbbell version, or it can be an isolation exercise that minimizes the help of assistance muscle groups. Completing three sets of eight reps will provide the best stimulus for muscle growth. The third exercise should be an isolation exercise, performed for three sets of 12 reps. This rep number will provide a potent stimulus for muscle growth and will encourage biochemical changes in the muscle that will enhance muscle growth and endurance (the ability to do more repetitions with a given weight). The last exercise should be done for three sets of 16 reps to provide a significant pump to the muscle. This will drive more fluid into the muscle cells, and the stretch this provides is believed to stimulate muscle growth. This final exercise can be either an isolation exercise or a basic exercise for that given muscle group, depending on what exercise was done for the second exercise.

Because of the higher volume involved with this program, you should split your workouts into three separate body regions. For instance, workout 1 could be chest, shoulders, triceps, and abs; workout 2 could be back and biceps; and workout 3 could be thighs, calves, and abs. Depending on how well you recover, you may consider training each muscle group just once a week on the four-rep system. An alternative way to do the four-rep system is to perform four sets of each exercise. The first set will be done for 4 reps, the second set for 8 reps, the third set for 12 reps, and the last set for 16 reps. Do this with two or three exercises per muscle group. See table 6.15 for a sample back and biceps routine using the alternative four-rep system.

RATING

	1	2	3	4	5
Time	1	2	3	4	5
Length	1	2	3	4	5
Difficulty	1	2	3	4	5
Results	1	2	3	4	5

TABLE 6.14 Four to Grow

Muscle group	Exercises	Sets	Reps
Chest	Incline bench press	3	4
	Dumbbell bench press	3	8
	Decline fly	3	12
	Pec deck	3	16
Shoulders	Standing barbell press	3	4
	Dumbbell lateral raise	3	8
	Upright row	3	12
	Overhead dumbbell press	3	16
Triceps	Close-grip bench press	3	4
	Triceps dip	3	8
	Lying triceps extension	3	12
	Triceps pressdown	3	16
Back	Bent-over row	3	4
	Pulldown	3	8
	Straight-arm pulldown	3	12
	Dumbbell row	3	16
Biceps	Barbell curl	3	4
	Incline dumbbell curl	3	8
	Concentration curl	3	12
	Preacher curl	3	16
Legs	Squat	3	4
	Romanian deadlift	3	8
	Leg extension	3	12
	Leg press	3	16

TABLE 6.15 Alternative Four-Rep System

Muscle group	Exercises	Sets	Reps
Back	Bent-over row	4	4, 8, 12, 16
	Pulldown	4	4, 8, 12, 16
	Straight-arm pulldown	4	4, 8, 12, 16
	Dumbbell row	4	4, 8, 12, 16
Biceps	Barbell curl	4	4, 8, 12, 16
	Incline dumbbell curl	4	4, 8, 12, 16
	Concentration curl	4	4, 8, 12, 16

Forced Repetitions

Forced repetitions allow you to get more reps on a set by having a spotter help you finish the set after you have reached failure. This lets you push your muscles to their limits and beyond, which is important for forcing muscle growth. After you have reached failure on a set, the spotter can help you to perform an extra two or three reps that you wouldn't have been able to get without help. Doing forced reps on the last set of an exercise is all you'll need to get a jump on muscle growth. Researchers suggest that one way that forced reps seem to work so well for pushing muscle growth. A study of 16 male athletes discovered that forced-rep training increased levels of growth hormone after training by almost three times more than a standard workout, as shown in figure 6.1 (Ahtianen, Pakarinen, Kraemer, and Hakkinen 2003). Growth hormone is an important anabolic hormone that is believed to be involved in stimulating the processes that drive muscle growth. Ahtianen and colleagues also studied muscle recovery after forced-rep training. They discovered that up to three days after the forced-rep workout the subjects' trained muscles had not fully recovered. Therefore, when using forced-rep training you should allow the trained muscle groups at least four and up to seven days of rest before training them again. You should use forced-rep training for no more than four weeks for any muscle group.

RATING

	1	2	3	4	5
Time	1	2	3	4	5
Length	1	2	3	4	5
Difficulty	1	2	3	4	5
Results	1	2	3	4	5

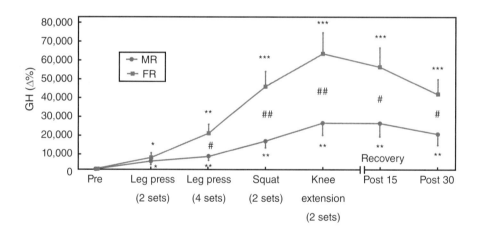

FIGURE 6.1 This graph depicts the response of the elevated growth hormone seen when subjects perform a forced-rep workout versus a normal workout. *Significantly different (* = p < 0.05, ** = p < 0.01, *** = p < 0.001) from corresponding preexercise value. #Statistically significant difference (# = p < 0.05, ## = p < 0.01) between the maximum rep vs. forced rep loadings.

Reprinted, by permission, from J.P. Ahtiainen, A. Pakarinen, W.J. Kraemer, and K. Häkkinen, 2003, "Acute hormonal and neuromuscular responses and recovery to forced vs. maximum repetitions multiple resistance exercises," *International Journal of Sports Medicine*, 24(6): 410-418. ©Georg Thieme Verlag KG.

Negative Repetitions

Like forced reps, negative reps for building size are best used at the end of a set when your muscles have reached failure. After you can no longer complete any more positive reps with a given weight, you can still do several negative reps. This is because muscles are much stronger on the negative portion of an exercise. Negative-rep training lets you take advantage of this fact and the fact that this high-intensity technique can spur new growth when done from time to time. Using negative-rep training for boosting muscle growth is different from using negative-rep training to improve muscle strength. For using negative-rep training to enhance muscle strength, see chapter 9. Resisting the weight down on the eccentric, or negative, portion of an exercise causes definite muscle damage. When muscle fibers are damaged, it sets off a cascade of steps that leads to muscle growth. It also develops protection from further eccentric overloading. That is why you want to use this technique infrequently. Once a tolerance for it has been built, the muscle damage is much less. Therefore, stopping after you have used it once

or twice for a muscle group is the wisest way to add this technique to your training program. Then take a break from it for at least two months. You will need to do only two or three negative reps at the end of the last set for each exercise you do. Have a spotter or two—depending on the amount of weight you use—help you perform the positive portion of each rep. During the negative part of the rep, you should attempt to resist the weight by allowing it to slowly force your muscles through the negative repetition. It should take you no less than about three seconds to lower the weight through the negative rep. If you cannot resist the weight for at least three seconds, do not perform any more negative reps and finish the set.

RATING

Time	1	2	3	4	5
Length	1	2	3	4	5
Difficulty	1	2	3	4	5
Results	1	2	3	4	5

Slow-Repetition Training

Slow-repetition training is a technique in which the repetitions are performed at a very slow speed. Although the term *slow-repetition training* covers a broad spectrum of possibilities, the most popular method is known as superslow training. This method requires you to slow your rep speed down to 10 seconds on the positive portion of the lift and an additional 10 seconds on the negative portion. You should use a weight that is about 50 to 70 percent of the weight you normally lift and attempt to complete 5 to 10 reps per set. Because of the intense nature of slow contractions, you need to perform only about two or three exercises per muscle group and only two sets per exercise. You should also allow five to seven days of rest for all major muscle groups trained with superslow training. Try this workout method for four to six weeks before changing to a different routine that involves normal-speed reps. Another way to incorporate superslow training into your lifting program is to do it every other workout for each muscle group or throw in one superslow rep

set each workout for any muscle group—do it either at the beginning or at the end of the workout. There are many benefits to superslow training that make it an effective technique for adding muscle mass. It minimizes the momentum of the weight to maximize the force placed on the muscle being trained. It helps you to develop the connection between mind and muscle, because the slow movement forces you to concentrate on the muscle contraction. It progressively fatigues all the fibers of the muscles involved. It minimizes the risk of injury from poorly performed exercise movements. And it reduces the stress placed on the joints.

RATING

Time	1	2	3	4	5
Length	1	2	3	4	5
Difficulty	1	2	3	4	5
Results	1	2	3	4	5

Speed-Set Training

By combining fast reps, slow reps, and normal reps into each set, you can do three things: increase strength, increase lean muscle, and decrease fat. The fast reps, like all explosive moves, build power, or the ability to generate strength very quickly. The slow reps build strength by keeping muscles under tension for a longer period. The longer they have to support the weight, the more damaged they get, and hence the more muscle they will develop. And ending each set with the normal reps increases muscular endurance. See table 6.16 for the Speed-Set Training program.

Each set has 15 reps. Reps 1 to 5 are the explosive reps, executed superfast. Reps 6 to 10 are excruciatingly slow, taking five seconds on the positive and another five seconds on the negative. And reps 11 to 15 are done at your normal pace (or roughly 1 to 2 seconds up and the same back down). Because of the intensity of this regimen, you'll pick a weight at which you could normally do 20 to 25 reps.

Avoid unilateral (single-arm or -leg) exercises. Doing 15 reps (five of them ultraslow) per set takes a long time, and if you're doing something like dumbbell rows or presses on each side, it could put too much strain on your stabilizer and core muscle groups. To spare your core muscles,

I recommend incorporating machines, particularly the Smith machine, which also allows you to exert maximum explosive power on the fast reps.

This regimen is ideal for training opposing muscle groups in each workout, pairing chest with back, biceps with triceps, shoulders with calves, and legs with abs. That way, you ensure that each muscle group gets the full benefit of training. Because the rep level is high and the technique is so intense, you could very easily burn out, say, your triceps while training your chest, making it impossible for your triceps to benefit from this type of training on the same day.

Start by doing two sets per exercise during weeks 1 and 2 and build up to three sets per exercise during weeks 3 and 4. Rest should be about one to two minutes between each set. Follow this regimen for four weeks maximum at a time, and then go back to your normal training.

RATING

Time	1	2	3	4	5
Length	1	2	3	4	5
Difficulty	1	2	3	4	5
Results	1	2	3	4	5

TABLE 6.16 Speed-Set Training

WORKOUT 1 (MONDAY): LEGS + ABS

Exercise	Sets Week 1-2/ weeks 3-4	Reps
LEGS		
Smith machine squat*	2/3	15
Leg press	2/3	15
Leg extension	2/3	15
Leg curl	2/3	15
ABS**		
Hanging leg raise	2/3	15
Crunch***	2/3	15

*Back squat or front squat.

** While you can use weights for the ab exercises, if you opt to use only body weight and can do more than five normal-pace reps at the end of the set, continue doing normal-pace reps until you reach failure.

***Or crunch machine.

WORKOUT 2 (TUESDAY): CHEST + BACK

Exercise	Sets Week 1-2/ weeks 3-4	Reps
CHEST		
Smith machine incline press*	2/3	15
Dumbbell bench press**	2/3	15
Cable crossover***	2/3	15
BACK		
Wide-grip pulldown	2/3	15
Seated cable row	2/3	15
Straight-arm pulldown	2/3	15

*Or machine incline press.

**Or machine bench press.

***Or machine fly.

WORKOUT 3 (THURSDAY): SHOULDERS + CALVES

Exercise	Sets Week 1-2/ weeks 3-4	Reps
SHOULDERS		
Smith machine overhead press*	2/3	15
Smith machine upright row	2/3	15
Dumbbell lateral raise**	2/3	15
CALVES		
Standing calf raise	2/3	15
Seated calf raise	2/3	15

*Or machine shoulder press.

**Or machine lateral raise.

WORKOUT 4 (FRIDAY): TRICEPS + BICEPS

Exercise	Sets Week 1-2/ weeks 3-4	Reps
TRICEPS		
Smith machine close-grip bench press	2/3	15
Triceps pressdown*	2/3	15
BICEPS		
Barbell curl	2/3	15
Preacher curl**	2/3	15

*Or machine triceps extension.

**Or machine biceps curl.

Four-Minute Muscle

To do the Four-Minute Muscle technique, you select a weight on each exercise that allows you to perform 15 to 19 reps before reaching muscle failure. You will lift this weight for a total of four minutes, taking short rest breaks each time you reach muscle failure. The goal is to see how many reps you can complete in these four minutes and to progressively increase the total number of reps you can complete over several weeks. You should be able to complete at least 40 reps in four minutes the first week you use this technique. The goal is to complete 60 reps in four minutes after four to six weeks.

The week before taking this journey, use all the exercises as listed and find the weight on each exercise that allows you to complete a minimum of 15 reps and a maximum of 19 reps. The weight you select is critical to your success. A weight that allows you to do fewer than 15 reps will be too heavy to ever get you close to the 60-rep goal in four to six weeks. A weight that allows you to get more than 19 reps will be too easy and will enable you to reach the goal of 60 reps in less than four weeks. Do only enough sets per exercise to determine the proper weight to use and then move on to the next exercise. Do all the exercises in each workout in the order listed.

There are two main ways that you can go about training with the Four-Minute Muscle program. The first way is to go to failure and then rest as little as possible before picking up the weight and going to failure again and continuing in this fashion until the four minutes are up. The problem with this strategy is that there is no way to advance the number of total reps you can complete other than hoping that you will increase muscle endurance each time you train this way, which should allow you to complete more reps in that four-minute window.

A smarter strategy is to pace yourself by sticking with a set amount of rest time between sets. The first time you do this workout, rest 20 seconds between sets each time you hit failure. Do this again in week 2. Then in week 3, drop your rest to 15 seconds between sets each time you hit muscle failure. Do this again in week 4. If you do not hit the goal of 60 reps in week 4, drop to 10 seconds of rest between sets in weeks 5 and 6, and you should hit your goal of 60 reps or at least very close to 60 reps.

If you don't hit the 60-rep mark by the end of the six weeks on all exercises, don't worry about it. Hitting the 60-rep goal is not critical to the results you will have. The results you can you expect in four to six weeks on this program are bigger muscle size, less body fat, and an increase in muscle endurance. Muscle endurance means that you will be able to complete more reps with a given weight. For example, if you can complete 10 reps with 70-pound dumbbells on the dumbbell bench press, you can expect to be getting a solid 12 to 15 reps with that same weight. It also means you'll be able to use heavier dumbbells (say 75- or 80-pounders) to get those same 10 reps.

The reason this program delivers all of this is manifold. For starters, because you are doing an exercise for four minutes with minimal rest between sets, you will be burning many more calories than when you do normal sets with two to three minutes of rest between sets. This will also mean you will still be burning more calories when the workout is over. All of that leads to some serious fat burning. Training this way will also place your muscles under a lot of metabolic stress. That means you'll be creating waste products in your muscles, such as lactate. The metabolic waste products will instigate a higher release of anabolic hormones like growth hormone, testosterone, and insulin-like growth factor-I (IGF-I), which will stimulate muscle growth. Plus dealing with these waste products will train your body to better handle and dispose of them. That will increase your muscle endurance, which will result in strength increases. Going for four minutes with minimal rest like this will also place a lot of mechanical stress on the muscles (muscle damage). That will lead to further gains in muscle size. And training this way is so unique compared to how you have previously trained that it will simply shock your muscles into responding by growing bigger and stronger. That's the principle known as muscle confusion. See table 6.17, Four-Minute Muscle Mayhem, for the full workout.

Try this program for four to six weeks. Rest about two to three minutes between exercises.

RATING

Time	1	2	3	4	5
Length	1	2	3	4	5
Difficulty	1	2	3	4	5
Results	1	2	3	4	5

TABLE 6.17 Four-Minute Muscle Mayhem

WORKOUT 1 (MONDAY): CHEST, BICEPS, ABS

Muscle group	Exercise	Time/rep goal: week 1; week 4
Chest	Smith machine bench press	4 min/40; 60
	Dumbbell bench press	4 min/40; 60
	Incline dumbbell fly	4 min/40; 60
	Cable crossover	4 min/40; 60
Biceps	Barbell curl	4 min/40; 60
	Incline dumbbell curl	4 min/40; 60
	Preacher curl	4 min/40; 60
Forearms	Barbell wrist curl	4 min/40; 60

WORKOUT 2 (TUESDAY): BACK AND TRICEPS

Muscle group	Exercise	Time/rep goal: week 1; week 4
Back	Wide-grip pulldown*	4 min/40; 60
	Seated cable row*	4 min/40; 60
	Reverse-grip pulldown*	4 min/40; 60
	Straight-arm pulldown	4 min/40; 60
Triceps	Smith machine close-grip bench press	4 min/40; 60
	Triceps pressdown	4 min/40; 60
	Cable overhead extension	4 min/40; 60
Abs	Hanging leg raise/knee raise**	4 min/40; 60
	Cable crunch	4 min/40; 60

WORKOUT 3 (THURSDAY): SHOULDERS AND TRAPS

Muscle group	Exercise	Time/rep goal: week 1; week 4
Shoulders	Smith machine shoulder press	4 min/40; 60
	Dumbbell lateral raise	4 min/40; 60
	Dumbbell shoulder press	4 min/40; 60
	Cable high-pulley rear delt raise	4 min/40; 60
Traps	Smith machine shrug*	4-min/40; 60
	Dumbbell shrug*	4-min/40; 60

WORKOUT 4 (FRIDAY): LEGS, CALVES, ABS

Muscle group	Exercise	Time/rep goal: week 1; week 4
Legs	Smith machine squat	4-min/40; 60
	Leg press	4-min/40; 60
	Leg extension	4-min/40; 60
	Romanian deadlift*	4-min/40; 60
	Lying leg curl	4-min/40; 60
Calves	Standing calf raise	4-min/40; 60
	Seated calf raise	4-min/40; 60
Abs	Decline weighted crunch	4-min/40; 60
	Reverse crunch	4-min/40; 60

*Use wrist straps on these exercises.

**If you cannot perform 15 reps of the hanging leg raise with straight legs, do the hanging knee raise; if you can complete more than 15 reps, hold a dumbbell or medicine ball between your feet or knees.

PROGRAMS THAT MANIPULATE LOAD

Because strength training involves lifting weights or resistance, the most fundamental change that can be done to manipulate a training program is to alter the amount of weight used. The following programs do just that—they manipulate the load, or resistance. This can be done by altering sets of heavy weight and light weight within a single workout or on each exercise during a workout. Some of these techniques alter the weight during a set. Regardless of the time line, the result from each of these is greater muscle mass.

Heavy and Light Method

This technique simply incorporates several heavy sets of an exercise followed by several light sets of that same exercise. The theory is that the heavy sets will stimulate the fast-twitch muscle fibers better while the lighter sets promote capillarization of the muscles and induce fatigue. This is often done with just one exercise, as shown in table 6.18. More experienced bodybuilders will sometimes do two exercises but with fewer total sets on each exercise. With this method, the first exercise (which is typically a basic or multijoint movement) is done with heavy weight and low reps, while the second exercise (which is often an isolation-type exercise) is done with very light weight and high reps (see table 6.19). For both programs, the exercises would be completed over a three- or four-day split. For example, workout 1 might be shoulders and thighs; workout 2 could train chest, back, and abs; workout 3 might complete the split with biceps, triceps, and calves.

RATING

Time	1	2	3	4	5
Length	1	2	3	4	5
Difficulty	1	2	3	4	5
Results	1	2	3	4	5

TABLE 6.18 Heavy and Light Single-Exercise Sample Routine

Muscle group	Exercise	Sets	Reps
Shoulders	Shoulder press	4	5
		4	12
Legs	Squat	5	4
		1	15
Chest	Bench press	5	5
		2	12
Back	Barbell row	4	4
		3	15
Abs	Cable crunch	3	10
		3	25
Biceps	Barbell curl	4	5
		4	15
Triceps	Lying triceps extension	4	5
		5	15
Calves	Standing calf raise	4	8
		6	25

TABLE 6.19 Heavy and Light Multiple-Exercise Sample Routine

Muscle group	Exercise	Sets	Reps
Shoulders	Shoulder press	4	5
	Lateral raise	4	15
Thighs	Squat	5	4
	Leg press	5	15
Chest	Bench press	5	4
	Incline fly	4	15
Back	Barbell row	5	4
	Pulldown	5	15
Abdominals	Cable crunch	3	10
	Reverse crunch	3	25
Biceps	Barbell curl	4	5
	Preacher curl	3	15
Triceps	Lying triceps extension	4	5
	Triceps pressdown	3	15
Calves	Standing calf raise	3	8
	Seated calf raise	3	25

Triangle Method

The triangle method is a basic pyramid training system. The term *pyramid* refers to a stepwise increase and decrease in weight used with each set of an exercise. The triangle method starts off with three or four ascending sets. The first two or three are warm-up sets that are not taken to failure. The third or fourth set usually consists of a weight that allows for only four to six reps. After that set the weight is progressively lowered and the reps increase for another two or three sets. See table 6.20 for a sample workout using the triangle method. The benefit of the triangle method is that it allows you to slowly prepare the targeted muscle for very heavy weight. This helps to prevent injury. In addition, this method of training allows for varied rep ranges, which provide different stimuli to the trained muscles.

RATING

Time	1	2	3	4	5
Length	1	2	3	4	5
Difficulty	1	2	3	4	5
Results	1	2	3	4	5

TABLE 6.20 Triangle Chest Using Incline Bench Press

Set	Weight (pounds)	Reps	Rest
1	135	10	2 min
2	185	8	3 min
3	225	6	3 min
4	245	4	3 min
5	185	7	3 min
6	165	8	–

Rack Pyramid Method

This pyramid method is named after the dumbbell rack because it is best used with preset dumbbells found in most gyms. As with the triangle method, you start with a very light weight for 10 reps to warm up. Then you gradually increase the weights of each set by the smallest increase available (usually five pounds each dumbbell) until you can perform only one repetition. After that, if you're really up for punishing your muscles, reverse the order and decline in weight by the smallest decrease possible until you reach your starting point. Rest between sets should be kept to a minimum—about one to two minutes. The benefits of the rack pyramid method are similar to those of the triangle method in that it allows a proper warm-up for preparing the muscle for the intense training task ahead. It also provides a very broad range of reps for a variety of training stimuli to the muscle. It also gives the muscle an intense workout that is sure to kick-start muscle growth. Because this method is rather grueling on the targeted muscles, it's wise to use the rack pyramid method infrequently. It is best thrown into a workout to stimulate a lagging muscle group to grow. One beneficial way to use the rack pyramid method is to use it for one exercise per muscle group. The best exercises to use this method with are the basic dumbbell mass builders and isolation exercises. See table 6.21 for optimal exercises to use with the rack pyramid method. Table 6.22 provides a sample rack pyramid workout for the dumbbell biceps curl.

RATING

Time	1	2	3	4	5
Length	1	2	3	4	5
Difficulty	1	2	3	4	5
Results	1	2	3	4	5

TABLE 6.21 Best Rack Pyramid Exercises

Muscle group	Exercise
Chest	Dumbbell press (flat, incline, decline)
	Dumbbell fly (flat, incline, decline)
Deltoids	Dumbbell press
	Dumbbell raise (front, lateral, rear)
	Dumbbell upright row
Back	Dumbbell row
Traps	Dumbbell shrug
Thighs	Dumbbell lunge
Triceps	Lying dumbbell triceps extension
	Overhead dumbbell triceps extension
Biceps	Dumbbell curls (standing, seated, incline)

TABLE 6.22 Rack It With the Biceps Curl

Set	Weight (pounds)	Reps	Rest
1	30	10	1 min
2	35	10	1 min
3	40	10	1 min
4	45	8	2 min
5	50	6	2 min
6	55	3	2 min
7	60	1	2 min
8	55	2	2 min
9	50	3	2 min
10	45	5	2 min
11	40	6	2 min
12	35	7	2 min
13	30	8	2 min

Inverted Pyramid

This pyramid system is the opposite of the triangle method. You simply start heavy, work down in weight, and then work back up. Because it is so difficult, it is one of the more uncommon methods of pyramid training. One example is that used by professional bodybuilder Dean Tornabane. You begin with a weight you can perform 6 to 10 reps with on your exercise of choice. Perform two more sets, in which you decrease the weight each set just enough to allow you to perform the same number of reps as you did on the first set. After the third set, you will do two more sets, increasing the weight by the same increments by which you decreased the weights previously. Because of the fatigue involved, the last two sets will likely be in the low repetition range of two to four. This is supposed to work synergistically with the higher-rep sets performed in the earlier sets to enhance muscle growth. See table 6.23 for a sample inverted pyramid program. This system can be performed with any exercise for most muscle groups, but it is best performed first in the workout with a basic exercise such as the bench press, shoulder press, squat, barbell curl, or triceps extension. This is best followed with straight sets of one or two isolation exercises for each muscle group.

RATING

Time	1	2	3	4	5
Length	1	2	3	4	5
Difficulty	1	2	3	4	5
Results	1	2	3	4	5

TABLE 6.23 Getting Inverted

Use the shoulder press after two or three warm-up sets.

Set	Weight (pounds)	Repetitions	Rest
1	185	8	2 min
2	175	8	2 min
3	160	8	2 min
4	175	4	2 min
5	185	2	–

Oxford Method

The Oxford descending pyramid technique uses the back half of the triangle pyramid method. The benefit of the Oxford method is that it allows the heaviest weight to be used on the first working set before the muscles are fatigued by previous working sets with lighter weight. With this descending pyramid technique, the first set is done with 100 percent of the 10RM to failure. Of course, this should be preceded by one or two light warm-up sets. On the second and third sets the weight is reduced just enough to allow you to complete 10 reps to failure. The Oxford seems to work well for gaining muscle mass because each set is done to muscle failure. Muscle failure is important for inducing muscle growth. The reason is that reaching muscle failure stimulates the release of growth hormone (GH)

and insulin-like growth factor-I (IGF-I). Although the Oxford method is typically described using 10 reps per set, it can also be used with other rep ranges, such as 6, 8, 12, or even 15 reps per set. See table 6.24 (Oxford Mass) for a sample program using the Oxford descending pyramid technique. This can be followed for four to six weeks before switching to a different training method.

RATING

Time	1	2	3	4	5
Length	1	2	3	4	5
Difficulty	1	2	3	4	5
Results	1	2	3	4	5

TABLE 6.24   Oxford Mass

MONDAY: CHEST AND TRICEPS			
Exercise	Set	Weight	Reps (to failure)
Incline bench press	1	100% 10RM	10
	2	<100% 10RM*	10
	3	<100% 10RM	10
Dumbbell bench press	1	100% 10RM	10
	2	<100% 10RM	10
	3	<100% 10RM	10
Incline dumbbell fly	1	100% 10RM	10
	2	<100% 10RM	10
	3	<100% 10RM	10
Triceps pressdown	1	100% 10RM	10
	2	<100% 10RM	10
	3	<100% 10RM	10
Seated overhead triceps extension	1	100% 10RM	10
	2	<100% 10RM	10
	3	<100% 10RM	10

TUESDAY: LEGS			
Front squat	1	100% 10RM	10
	2	<100% 10RM	10
	3	<100% 10RM	10
Leg press	1	100% 10RM	10
	2	<100% 10RM	10
	3	<100% 10RM	10

TUESDAY: LEGS *(continued)*			
Exercise	Set	Weight	Reps (to failure)
Leg extension	1	100% 10RM	10
	2	<100% 10RM	10
	3	<100% 10RM	10
Leg curl	1	100% 10RM	10
	2	<100% 10RM	10
	3	<100% 10RM	10

THURSDAY: SHOULDERS			
Dumbbell shoulder press	1	100% 10RM	10
	2	<100% 10RM	10
	3	<100% 10RM	10
Lateral raise	1	100% 10RM	10
	2	<100% 10RM	10
	3	<100% 10RM	10
Bent-over lateral raise	1	100% 10RM	10
	2	<100% 10RM	10
	3	<100% 10RM	10
Dumbbell shrugs	1	100% 10RM	10
	2	<100% 10RM	10
	3	<100% 10RM	10

*On second and third sets of each exercise, reduce weight just enough to allow 10 reps to be completed.

Note: Abs can be done at the end of any of these workouts.

> continued

TABLE 6.24 Oxford Mass *(continued)*

FRIDAY: BACK AND BICEPS

Exercise	Set	Weight	Reps (to failure)
Lat pulldown	1	100% 10RM	10
	2	<100% 10RM	10
	3	<100% 10RM	10
Dumbbell row	1	100% 10RM	10
	2	<100% 10RM	10
	3	<100% 10RM	10
Straight-arm pulldown	1	100% 10RM	10
	2	<100% 10RM	10
	3	<100% 10RM	10

FRIDAY: BACK AND BICEPS *(continued)*

Exercise	Set	Weight	Reps (to failure)
Preacher curl	1	100% 10RM	10
	2	<100% 10RM	10
	3	<100% 10RM	10
Alternating dumbbell curl	1	100% 10RM	10
	2	<100% 10RM	10
	3	<100% 10RM	10
Reverse-grip curl	1	100% 10RM	10
	2	<100% 10RM	10
	3	<100% 10RM	10

*On second and third sets of each exercise, reduce weight just enough to allow 10 reps to be completed.

Note: Abs can be done at the end of any of these workouts.

Breakdowns

This technique was devised by Fred Hatfield, PhD, and used successfully by professional bodybuilder Mike Quinn. It involves three distinct repetition ranges for each of the three total sets that are performed. Set 1 works with heavy weight (a weight that limits you to 4 to 6 reps per set to work the fast-twitch muscle fibers). Set 2 is performed using 15 to 20 percent less weight than with set 1. This should allow about 10 to 15 repetitions to be performed and enhances the biochemical milieu within the muscle cells to stimulate muscle growth. The last set, set 3, is performed with about 50 percent less weight than the first set, such that 25 to 30 reps are performed for training the slow-twitch muscle fibers. Rest periods between sets should be about 2 to 3 minutes. See table 6.25 for a sample breakdown workout for triceps.

RATING

Time	1	2	3	4	5
Length	1	2	3	4	5
Difficulty	1	2	3	4	5
Results	1	2	3	4	5

TABLE 6.25 Break Down to Build Up Triceps

Exercise	Weight (pounds)	Set number	Reps
Close-grip bench press	265	1	4
	215	2	12
	135	3	27
Lying triceps extension	135	1	6
	105	2	15
	65	3	30
Triceps pressdown	100	1	6
	80	2	12
	50	3	25

Drop-Set Training

Drop-set training involves an immediate reduction in the amount of weight being used so that you can continue to complete more reps for that given exercise. For example, if you can do 10 reps of barbell curls with 100 pounds on the bar, you would first complete 10 reps and then put the bar down to quickly strip off about 20-30 percent (or about 20-30 pounds). You immediately perform as many reps as possible with that weight before putting it down and stripping another 20-30 percent off the bar and doing more reps. This can continue as many times as you like, although most bodybuilders do one or three drops per drop set. Regardless of how many drops are done per drop set, it is counted as only one set. Most bodybuilders perform about two or three drop sets per exercise. Choose two exercises per muscle group, usually one compound exercise and one isolation exercise, and do three drop sets for each. Another way to use drop-set training is to do the last set of every exercise as a drop set.

The benefit of drop-set training is similar to that of forced-rep training in that it lets you push your muscles beyond their limits. Forcing the muscles to continue contracting with lighter weight will cause an elevated response of growth hormone and IGF-I. The trick is to keep the rest between drops to a minimum. It's a good idea to have a spotter help you strip the weight or use dumbbells for the quickest drops in weight. See table 6.26 for a sample drop-set scheme for shoulder training using dumbbell presses and lateral raises. This is a good way to end a shoulder workout if it is preceded by shoulder presses and upright rows. Follow a similar plan for other muscle groups.

RATING

Time	1	2	3	4	5
Length	1	2	3	4	5
Difficulty	1	2	3	4	5
Results	1	2	3	4	5

TABLE 6.26   Drop-It Delts

Set	Weight (pounds)	Reps	Rest
DUMBBELL PRESS			
1	65	10	None
	45	7	None
	30	5	2 min
2	65	9	None
	45	6	None
	30	4	2 min
3	60	10	None
	40	6	None
	30	3	
LATERAL RAISE			
1	35	12	None
	25	8	None
	15	7	2 min
2	30	12	None
	20	7	None
	10	6	2 min
3	30	10	None
	20	6	None
	10	4	

PROGRAMS THAT MANIPULATE REST PERIODS

Few bodybuilders realize that an effective way to alter training programs to keep their progress involves manipulating the rest periods between sets. This changes the biochemical adaptations the muscles undergo by altering the type of fuel (ATP, creatine phosphate, or glycogen) they rely on during sets and to recover with between sets. The chemicals produced from the use of different fuels can stimulate certain biochemical pathways involved in the process of muscle growth. The following programs change the rest periods between sets in an effort to stimulate muscle growth. This can be done by decreasing the rest between sets from workout to workout or by limiting the amount of rest between sets.

Rest Rundown

This is a program where rest time between sets is reduced by about 15 seconds every consecutive workout. The program starts with three-minute rest periods between sets and progressively drops to about 15 seconds over a 12-week period. The goal is to use the same weight for the same amount of reps each week. While that doesn't seem like progress when looking at the resistance used and the repetitions completed, it is remarkable progress when considering the drastic reductions in rest time. This trains the biochemical pathways in the muscle to allow the muscle to recover faster and allows for more reps to be performed with a given weight. The ability to do the same number of reps with the same weight with less rest time between sets translates to greater muscle growth. In fact, as discussed in chapter 5, research shows that participants following an eight-week strength-training program that decreased the rest period between sets by 15 seconds every week had greater gains in muscle mass than those keeping rest periods steady at two minutes (Souza-Junior et al. 2011). Stay at a rest range if you cannot complete reps in the under-two-minute range. See table 6.27 for a sample weekly progression of the rest rundown program for an athlete who trains each body part once per week. Bodybuilders often use the rest rundown method to prepare for competition. This is believed to help with muscle definition and to decrease body fat because the workout is similar to an aerobic-type workout.

RATING

Time	1	2	3	4	5
Length	1	2	3	4	5
Difficulty	1	2	3	4	5
Results	1	2	3	4	5

TABLE 6.27 Rest Rundown

Week	Rest between sets
1	3 min
2	2 min 45 sec
3	2 min 30 sec
4	2 min 15 sec
5	2 min
6	1 min 45 sec
7	1 min 30 sec
8	1 min 15 sec
9	1 min
10	45 sec
11	30 sec
12	15 sec

Alternating Rest-Pause Program

This variation on Rest-Pause training is a unique way to train using single-arm and single-leg exercises. As you work one side of the body, the opposite side is resting. You cycle back and forth from one side to the other. To do this, choose a weight that allows you to complete about 6 to 8 reps. We will use one-arm dumbbell curls as an example. Do 3 reps of curls on the right arm and immediately switch to the left arm and do 3 reps of curls on the left arm. Then switch to the right arm for 3 more reps of curls. Continue in this fashion resting for 3 reps, then resting for 2 reps, and finally resting for 1 rep. In the end you complete 14 reps per set with a weight you normally could do for only 6 to 8 reps. You basically double the amount of reps you can do with a given weight. That pushes not only muscle growth but muscle strength as well. And because you are using one limb at a time, you are stronger than you are when you use two arms. That is, when you perform single-arm exercises, like a one-arm dumbbell curl, you can curl more weight than half of what you could curl on a barbell using both arms, which leads to even greater gains in muscle strength.

On the last set of each exercise, do as many reps as you can on the final rest that is supposed to be just one rep. Not only will this increase the intensity on the last set, but it will also serve as a barometer for the appropriateness of the weight you selected. If you can do more than one rep on the final rest of the final set of an exercise, increase the weight by 5 to 10 pounds the next workout. If you can complete only one rep on the final rest of the final set, then the weight you selected is perfect. If you can't complete the final rep on the final set, then during the next workout reduce the weight by 5 to 10 pounds. If you can't complete the final rep on any of the first two sets, then reduce the weight by 5 to 10 pounds on the next set.

Follow the Alternating Rest-Pause program in table 6.28 for four weeks and then switch to a new training program.

RATING

	1	2	3	4	5
Time	1	2	3	4	5
Length	1	2	3	4	5
Difficulty	1	2	3	4	5
Results	1	2	3	4	5

TABLE 6.28 Alternating Rest-Pause Program

MONDAY: CHEST, TRICEPS, ABS

Muscle group	Exercise	Sets	Reps
Chest	One-arm dumbbell bench press*	3	3, 3, 3, 2, 2, 1
	Smith machine one-arm incline bench press	3	3, 3, 3, 2, 2, 1
	One-arm low pulley cable crossover	3	3, 3, 3, 2, 2, 1
	One-arm cable crossover	3	3, 3, 3, 2, 2, 1
Triceps	One-arm triceps pressdown	3	3, 3, 3, 2, 2, 1
	One-arm lying triceps extension	3	3, 3, 3, 2, 2, 1
	One-arm dumbbell overhead extension	3	3, 3, 3, 2, 2, 1
Abs*			

* Do your normal ab workout here.

TUESDAY: LEGS

Muscle group	Exercise	Sets	Reps
Legs	One-leg press	3	3, 3, 3, 2, 2, 1
	Smith machine reverse lunge	3	3, 3, 3, 2, 2, 1
	Dumbbell step-up	3	3, 3, 3, 2, 2, 1
	One-leg extension	3	3, 3, 3, 2, 2, 1
	One-leg curl	3	3, 3, 3, 2, 2, 1
Calves	One-leg calf raise	3	3, 3, 3, 2, 2, 1
	One-leg seated calf raise	3	3, 3, 3, 2, 2, 1

> continued

TABLE 6.28 Alternating Rest-Pause Program *(continued)*

THURSDAY: SHOULDERS, TRAPS, ABS

Muscle group	Exercise	Sets	Reps
Shoulders	One-arm dumbbell shoulder press	3	3, 3, 3, 2, 2, 1
	One-arm Smith machine upright row	3	3, 3, 3, 2, 2, 1
	One-arm cable lateral raise	3	3, 3, 3, 2, 2, 1
	One-arm dumbbell bent-over lateral raise	3	3, 3, 3, 2, 2, 1
Traps	One-arm Smith machine shrug	3	3, 3, 3, 2, 2, 1
Abs*			

* Do your normal ab workout here.

FRIDAY: BACK AND BICEPS

Muscle group	Exercise	Sets	Reps
Back	Dumbbell power row	3	3, 3, 3, 2, 2, 1
	One-arm pulldown	3	3, 3, 3, 2, 2, 1
	One-arm seated cable row	3	3, 3, 3, 2, 2, 1
	One-arm straight-arm pulldown	3	3, 3, 3, 2, 2, 1
Biceps	One-arm dumbbell curl	3	3, 3, 3, 2, 2, 1
	One-arm dumbbell incline curl	3	3, 3, 3, 2, 2, 1
	One-arm dumbbell preacher curl	3	3, 3, 3, 2, 2, 1

Quality Training

Quality training is a system that keeps the rest periods between sets at 1 minute or less regardless of the exercise or weight used. Many bodybuilders swear by this technique for adding muscle mass and, therefore, always keep their rest periods under a minute regardless of how heavily they are training. From a physiological standpoint, there is some evidence to support the anecdotal reports. Keeping rest periods between sets to a minimum will cause lactate levels to reach fairly high levels. Since lactate levels are associated with GH levels, the GH response, as well as the IGF-I response (which is associated with GH levels), would be higher with this type of training. See table 6.29 for a sample quality training workout for triceps.

RATING

Time	1	2	3	4	5
Length	1	2	3	4	5
Difficulty	1	2	3	4	5
Results	1	2	3	4	5

TABLE 6.29 Quality Training Workout for Triceps

Exercise	Sets	Reps	Rest between sets
Close-grip bench press	3	8-10	60 seconds
Triceps pressdown	3	8-12	30-45 seconds
One-arm overhead extension	3	10-15	As long as it takes to finish other arm

Power Circuit Training

This is a type of circuit training that involves the use of basic power movements with heavy weight. Typical circuit training involves the use of machines and very light weight. What they both have in common is that the goal is to move from one exercise to the next with no scheduled rest between exercises. Instead of doing several sets for an exercise, you would do only one set of an exercise before moving to a new exercise. In the end, you will complete several sets of each exercise after running through the circuit several times.

Power circuits are designed to increase strength and muscle size while helping decrease body fat. The continuous movement of circuit training keeps your metabolism high through the whole workout. Research studies show that keeping rest periods under 30 seconds burns the most calories regardless of how much weight is used and how many reps are performed. Research also suggests that fat use by the body after exercise is increased more with power circuits than with a traditional weightlifting program. With power circuits the lifter does about 30 total reps for each body part with a weight that is about 75 to 85 percent of the one-rep max (or a weight that could be lifted for 8 to 10 reps). With power circuits it is wise to use either a training partner who can watch the clock or a watch to monitor exercise time. Each exercise in the circuit is performed for 15 seconds. The goal is to complete as many reps as possible in those 15 seconds before moving on to the next exercise without resting. When a total of 30 reps have been completed for an exercise, the exercise is eliminated

from the circuit and a 15-second rest period is set in its place on the following circuit rounds. For example, if you complete 17 reps on the first pass through the circuit and 13 the second time through, on your third trip through the circuit, instead of doing more calf raises, you would stop and rest for that 15 seconds before moving on to the next exercise.

The order of exercises in the circuit will affect the level of muscle fatigue that is reached during the power circuit. It is wise to alternate upper- and lower-body exercises to allow the muscles to recover and delay fatigue when doing power circuits, such as in table 6.30. Whenever possible, push and pull exercises should be alternated as well. For instance, if the power circuit starts with a pulling exercise such as pull-downs and then moves to a lower-body exercise such as the leg press for the quads, the next upper-body exercise should then be a pushing exercise such as the bench press, and the next lower-body exercise could be a leg curl for the hamstrings. Ideally, the power circuit should be completed in less than 25 minutes. Full-body power circuits can be done twice a week as long as at least two days of rest are allowed between workouts.

RATING

Time	1	2	3	4	5
Length	1	2	3	4	5
Difficulty	1	2	3	4	5
Results	1	2	3	4	5

TABLE 6.30 Circuit Breaker

Exercise	CIRCUIT I		CIRCUIT II		CIRCUIT III		CIRCUIT IV	
	Time (seconds)	Reps*	Time (seconds)	Reps*	Time (seconds)	Reps*	Time (seconds)	Reps*
Bent-over row	15	8	15	8	15	8	15	6
Leg press	15	8	15	8	15	8	15	6
Bench press	15	8	15	8	15	8	15	6
Leg curl	15	10	15	8	15	6	15	6
Barbell curl	15	10	15	10	15	10	15	0
Standing calf raise	15	15	15	15	15	0	15	0
Standing military press	15	8	15	8	15	8	15	6
Back extension	15	10	15	8	15	6	15	6
Lying triceps extension	15	10	15	10	15	10	15	0
	Rest 2 min		Rest 2 min		Rest 2 min			

*Reps listed are a suggested goal; do as many as you can in 15 seconds, and do as many passes through the circuit as it takes to reach 30 reps total in each exercise.

Note: For all weighted exercises, use a weight equal to 75 percent to 85 percent of the 1RM (or a weight that normally can be lifted for 8 to 10 reps on that exercise). For example, if you can bench-press 200 pounds for 1 rep, in the circuit you should load the bar with 150 to 170 pounds.

PROGRAMS THAT MANIPULATE EXERCISE SELECTION

There are hundreds of strength training exercises that can be performed (see part V for a complete listing of common strength training exercises). With so many exercises to choose from for each muscle group, it only makes sense that one way to design a training program is through manipulation of exercise choices. This can be done by changing the order of compound and isolation exercises for a given muscle group, making minute changes in the way exercises are performed (changes in grip or spacing of feet), limiting the workout to a specific type of equipment, or performing exercises that train only one side of the body. All such methods can be effective means of increasing your muscle size.

Preexhaust Training

This training method involves performing an isolation exercise before a multijoint exercise for that same muscle group. The point is to fatigue the muscle being trained with the isolation exercise so that it becomes the weak link in the multijoint exercise. For instance, an isolated muscle group such as the deltoids is fatigued (or preexhausted) with a single-joint exercise, such as the dumbbell lateral raise, before training it with a heavier, compound movement such as the dumbbell shoulder press. The reason for this is that the compound exercise involves the targeted muscle as well as at least one assistance muscle. During the shoulder press, the deltoids are assisted by the triceps. While this helps to lift more weight on the compound exercise, it can limit the muscle fatigue the targeted muscle receives. This is especially true if the assistance muscle is much weaker than the targeted muscle. If this is true, then often the exercise ends when the assistance muscle, not the targeted muscle, has fatigued.

Preexhaust works to fatigue the primary muscle group via the isolation exercise so that it can be further fatigued on the compound exercise that follows. Of course, the strength of the targeted muscle will be compromised on the second exercise. This prevents most bodybuilders from using the preexhaust method regularly, yet some use it specifically to limit the amount of weight they can use on the compound exercise. If a bodybuilder has an injury that is aggravated by a specific compound move, preexhaust training will limit the amount of weight he or she can use on the set and thus limit the overall stress placed on the injured muscle or joint. Preexhaust can be followed for four to six weeks or done for each body part once every four to six workouts. See table 6.31 for good exercise choices to pair up for preexhaust training. For a routine, do three sets of 10 to 15 reps on the first exercise and three sets of 6 to 10 reps on the second. Or to use this system as a compound set, do one set of 10 to 15 reps on the first exercise and immediately follow with one set of 6 to 10 reps on the second one. Rest about two to three minutes and repeat this process twice. Regardless of which method you choose, follow the preexhaust pairs with one other exercise for that muscle group done in straight-set fashion.

RATING

Time	1	2	3	4	5
Length	1	2	3	4	5
Difficulty	1	2	3	4	5
Results	1	2	3	4	5

TABLE 6.31 Sample Preexhaust Exercise Pairs

Muscle group	Isolation exercise	Multijoint exercise
Chest	Pec deck	Bench press
	Incline fly	Incline bench press
	Cable crossover	Decline bench press
Shoulders	Dumbbell lateral raise	Dumbbell shoulder press
	Front raise	Barbell shoulder press
Back	Straight-arm pulldown	Pull-down, pull-up, barbell row
Triceps	Triceps pressdown	Triceps dip
	Overhead extension	Close-grip bench press
Biceps	Preacher curl	Close-grip chin-up
Legs	Leg extension	Leg press
	Leg curl	Squat

Extended-Set Training

This is a unique method that uses several variations of one exercise. The variations of that exercise are ordered from hardest to easiest. An example of this can be explained using the dumbbell bench press. The hardest version of the dumbbell bench press is on an incline bench set between 30 and 45 degrees. Doing a dumbbell bench press on a flat bench is easier than doing an incline dumbbell bench press but harder than doing a decline dumbbell bench press. Thus, an example of extended-set training using the dumbbell bench press would be to do one set of incline dumbbell bench press followed immediately by one set of dumbbell bench press on a flat bench using the same amount of weight and finishing with one set of decline dumbbell bench press with the same weight. Because the rest time is minimal between each bench adjustment, these three exercises can be considered one extended set.

Each adjustment with extended-set training places the body in a position that is stronger than the previous position. This makes the weight easier to lift on each successive position change, allowing you to continue doing more reps, when normally you would have failed if your body position had not changed. Not only does this allow you to train with more intensity, but the change in body position also increases the number of muscle fibers targeted in each specific muscle group.

To follow extended-set training, first choose a weight that normally limits you to four or five reps on the first exercise (even though you will attempt no more than four reps). For each change in exercise movement for that extended set, you will attempt two to four reps. Do not do more than four reps on any exercise except on the final movement of the extended set. You can work to failure on the last exercise of all extended sets. If you have three or four exercise changes per extended set, you will have a total of about 7 to 16 reps. So in essence, you are using a weight on each movement that is best for strength gains, but at the end of the extended set the total reps that the muscle group has performed fall in the range that is optimal for muscle growth.

The first exercise movement should be the exercise that your body is weakest at compared to all other exercises in the extended set. Each successive exercise movement in the extended set should be one that your body is stronger at compared to the previous exercise yet weaker than the one that follows. Rest time between sets will always be minimal but can be varied depending on the biomechanical advantage gained in the proceeding set. Some exercises will be dramatically easier than the previous one; for these, rest should involve changing only your body position. Some exercises provide a minimal biomechanical advantage; for these you may rest up to 15 seconds before performing. Rest between extended sets for three to four minutes. Perform between one and three sets for each extended set, depending on the number of exercise movements used in the extended set and the number of years training experience you have.

This is an extremely advanced training technique because it involves heavy weight with very little rest. These two training techniques are usually at opposition to one another, meaning you either train heavy or fast, but rarely ever both—until now.

For most bodybuilders, doing one extended set will suffice. This will depend on the amount of exercise movements you include in each extended set as well as your training experience. Some extended sets involve as few as two different movements (such as with shrugs), while some include as many as nine (such as with the ultimate biceps extended set). See examples of extended sets in table 6.32. The more exercise movements per extended set, the fewer total extended sets you will need. Most lifters will need about two or three extended sets for the trap workout, while many will struggle to finish one ultimate biceps extended set.

You can incorporate extended sets into your training in a number of ways. You can do one extended set per muscle group along with other straight sets for that muscle group. You can do one giant extended set per muscle group. Or you can choose two different extended sets for each muscle group—as long as they complement each other and do not mimic exercise movements. Follow extended-set training for about 4 to 6 weeks, and follow it with a training program that incorporates standard sets and higher reps such as the finish pump method or triangle training method. Do not return to extended-set training for at least 12 weeks. There are several reasons for this. The first is the intensity factor, as described previously. The other problem is exercise order. With this style of training, many of the basic movements are trained toward the end of the extended set. This is the reverse order of a typical bodybuilding workout.

RATING

Time	1	2	3	4	5
Length	1	2	3	4	5
Difficulty	1	2	3	4	5
Results	1	2	3	4	5

TABLE 6.32 Extended Gains

Muscle group	Exercise	Variations
Chest	Dumbbell fly	1. Incline fly: 3-4 reps Rest only long enough to adjust bench.
		2. Flat fly: 2-4 reps Rest only long enough to adjust bench.
		3. Decline fly: 2-4 reps
	Dumbbell press	1. Incline press: 3-4 reps Rest only long enough to adjust bench.
		2. Flat press: 2-4 reps Rest only long enough to adjust bench.
		3. Decline press: 2-4 reps
	Cable crossover	1. Cable crossover from low pulley: 3-4 reps Rest only long enough to change pulley.
		2. Cable crossover from high pulley: 2-4 reps Immediately switch to cable press with no rest.
		3. Cable chest press: 2-4 reps
	Barbell bench press	1. Bench press to neck: 3-4 reps Immediately switch movement without rest.
		2. Bench press to nipple: 2-4 reps Rest only long enough to rack the bar and change body position.
		3. Bench press to lower chest (feet on bench, butt up and off of bench)
		Ultimate declining extended set for chest: Do both the dumbbell fly and dumbbell press extended sets in succession with the same weight.
Back	Pulldown and pull-up	1. Behind-the-neck pulldown or pull-up: 3-4 reps Immediately bring bar to front of head and continue.
		2. Wide-grip pulldown or pull-up to front: 2-4 reps Rest for only 15 seconds.
		3. Close-grip pulldown or pull-up to front: 2-4 reps Rest just long enough to switch grip.
		4. Reverse-grip pulldown or chin-up: 2-4 reps
	Row (barbell or seated cable)	1. Wide-grip (beyond shoulder width) row: 3-4 reps Rest for 15 seconds.
		2. Close-grip (shoulder width) or neutral-grip row: 2-4 reps Rest just long enough to switch grip or handle.
		3. Underhand-grip row: 2-4 reps
Shoulders	Barbell	1. Wide-grip upright row: 3-4 reps Rest only long enough to rack the bar and change body position.
		2. Behind-the-neck press: 2-4 reps Immediately switch to presses in front of neck.
		3. Front press: 2-4 reps
	Dumbbell lateral raise	1. Lateral raise with straight arms and dumbbells at your sides: 3-4 reps Immediately go into next movement with no rest.
		2. Lateral raise with straight arms and dumbbells in front of your thighs: 2-4 reps Immediately go into next movement with no rest.
		3. Lateral raise with arms bent 90 degrees at elbows

Muscle group	Exercise	Variations
Shoulders (continued)	Complete dumbbell delt workout	1. Bent-over laterals: 3-4 reps Immediately go into next movement with no rest.
		2. Front raise: 2-4 reps Immediately go into next movement with no rest.
		3. Lateral raise: 2-4 reps Immediately go into next movement with no rest.
		4. Dumbbell upright row: 2-4 reps Immediately go into next movement with no rest.
		5. Standing dumbbell press: 2-4 reps
Traps	Barbell shrug	1. Behind-the-back barbell shrug: 3-4 reps Rest only long enough to change body position and grip.
		2. Barbell shrug: 2-4 reps
Legs	Squat	1. Front squat narrow stance (feet hip width or closer): 3-4 reps Do not rack the weight; just adjust your stance and immediately continue.
		2. Front squat wide stance (feet wider than shoulder width): 2-4 reps Rack the weight and rest just long enough to switch the bar position.
		3. Back squat narrow stance: 2-4 reps Do not rack the weight; just adjust your stance and immediately continue.
		4. Back squat wide stance: 2-4 reps
	Leg press	1. Single-leg press: 3-4 reps each leg Rack the sled and rest for just 15 seconds.
		2. Feet together: 2-4 reps Rack the sled just long enough to change foot position.
		3. Feet wide (beyond shoulder width): 2-4 reps
Biceps	Reverse-grip dumbbell curl	1. Incline (~45 degrees) reverse-grip dumbbell curl: 3-4 reps
		2. Seated reverse-grip dumbbell curl: 2-4 reps
		3. Standing reverse-grip dumbbell curl: 2-4 reps Perform all 3 movements in succession with no rest and without putting down the dumbbells.
	Dumbbell curl	1. Incline (~45 degrees) dumbbell curl: 3-4 reps
		2. Seated dumbbell curl: 2-4 reps
		3. Standing dumbbell curl: 2-4 reps Perform all 3 movements in succession with no rest and without putting down the dumbbells.
	Hammer curl	1. Incline (~45 degrees) hammer curl: 3-4 reps
		2. Seated hammer curl: 2-4 reps
		3. Standing hammer curl: 2-4 reps Perform all 3 movements in succession with no rest and without putting down the dumbbells.
	Barbell curl	1. Reverse-grip curl: 3-4 reps Rest just long enough to switch grip.
		2. Wide-grip (2-4 inches beyond shoulder width) curl: 2-4 reps Rest for 15 seconds.
		3. Close-grip (hip width) curl: 2-4 reps

Ultimate biceps extended set: Do all three dumbbell extended sets with just 15 seconds of a break between each.

> continued

TABLE 6.32   Extended Gains *(continued)*

Muscle group	Exercise	Variations
Triceps	Lying triceps extension	1. Lying extension to forehead: 3-4 reps Without rest, go into next movement.
		2. Lying extension to nose: 2-4 reps Without rest, go into next movement.
		3. Lying extension to chin (allow elbows to flare out): 2-4 reps Without rest, go into next movement.
		4. Close-grip bench press: 2-4 reps
	Triceps pressdown	1. Reverse-grip pressdown: 3-4 reps Rest only long enough to switch grip and body position.
		2. Overhead extension (from high pulley): 2-4 reps Rest only long enough to switch grip and body position.
		3. Pressdown: 2-4 reps
Abs	Lower abs	1. Hanging leg raise: ~10-15 reps Without rest, go into hanging knee raise.
		2. Hanging knee raise: ~5-10 reps Rest only long enough to get into position.
		3. Reverse crunch straight legs: ~10-15 reps Without rest, switch to bent legs.
		4. Reverse crunch bent legs ~5-10 reps
	Upper abs	1. Decline bench crunch: ~10-15 reps Rest only long enough to switch body position.
		2. Crunch: ~10-15 reps Rest only long enough to get into position.
		3. Standing cable crunch: ~10-15 reps Rest only long enough to switch body position.
		4. Kneeling cable crunch: ~10-15 reps

Because abs are a unique muscle group when it comes to resistance training, reps for abdominal extended sets will typically be much higher than the rep range used for the other muscle groups. As with the other muscle groups, perform each ab movement close to failure.

Small-Angle Training

Small-angle training is similar to extended set in concept. It uses multiple variations of a single exercise to ensure that all muscle fibers in a muscle are adequately trained.

To understand the concept of exercise angles, you need to know the basic structure of muscle. One important but surprising fact is that individual muscle fibers rarely run the entire length of the muscle. Muscles are actually composed of a sequence of one- to four-inch (two-and-a-half- to ten-centimeter) segments of muscle fiber linked together. For that reason, you can't think of muscle fibers as being synonymous with the actual muscle. This is critical, as the growth of each muscle fiber depends on whether it is actually stimulated during a particular exercise. In many cases, muscle fibers remain unused and just go along for the ride during a lifting movement. Whether the fiber is used depends not only on the amount of resistance but also on the angle of the exercise and the specific range of motion used in the exercise. If the angle (such as in the flat bench press versus incline bench press) and the range of motion (such as partial movements versus full range of motion) do not call a specific muscle fiber into action, no growth will occur in that fiber. To make sure you hit each muscle fiber and stimulate it to grow, you have to use a variety of exercises. And even for a given exercise, you must use variety. For example, on dumbbell bench presses, you can adjust the angle of the bench from a 30-degree decline to a 45-degree incline in as many increments as the benches will allow.

See table 6.33 for a sample small-angle training program. This program capitalizes on minute changes in the angles used to work the major muscle groups. Train each muscle group only once per week.

RATING

Time	1	2	3	4	**5**
Length	1	**2**	3	4	5
Difficulty	1	2	3	**4**	5
Results	1	2	3	4	**5**

TABLE 6.33 Small-Angle Workout

WORKOUT 1
CHEST

Exercise	Set number	Reps	Exercise specifics
Flat bench press*	Warm-up	10	Shoulder-width grip
	Warm-up	10	6-8 inches beyond shoulder-width grip
	1	6-8	Natural grip (most comfortable grip)
	2	6-8	Shoulder-width grip
	3	6-8	2 inches beyond shoulder-width grip
	4	4-8	4 inches beyond shoulder-width grip
	5	4-8	6 inches beyond shoulder-width grip
	6	4-8	8 inches beyond shoulder-width grip

*As an alternative, perform the incline bench press with the same grip progression.

Exercise	Set number	Reps	Exercise specifics
Dumbbell fly	1	8-10	45- to 60-degree decline
	2	8-10	15- to 30-degree decline
	3	8-10	Flat
	4	6-10	15- to 30-degree incline
	5	6-10	45-degree incline

As an alternative to flys, try this cable crossover progression:

Exercise	Set number	Reps	Exercise specifics
Cable crossover	1	8-10	From bottom position
	2	8-10	Halfway between bottom and shoulder height
	3	8-10	Shoulder height
	4	8-10	From top pulley

TRICEPS

Exercise	Set number	Reps	Exercise specifics
Extension or pressdown	Warm-up	10	Seated overhead extension (with dumbbell)
	Warm-up	10	Seated pressdown
	1	8-10	Seated overhead extension (with dumbbell)
	2	6-8	Seated overhead extension (with dumbbell)
	3	8-10	Lying triceps extension over top of head (arms angled at 45 degrees)
	4	8-10	Lying triceps extension to forehead
	5	8-10	Pressdown with torso bent slightly forward
	6	8-10	Pressdown with upright torso (rope handle)
	7	6-8	Pressdown with upright torso (straight bar)
Dip	1	6-10	Parallel bars
	2	6-10	Bench

> *continued*

TABLE 6.33 Small-Angle Workout *(continued)*

WORKOUT 1 *(continued)*
ABS

Exercise	Set number	Reps	Exercise specifics
Hanging knee raise to sides	1	15-20	
Hanging knee raise	2	15-20	
Decline bench crunch	3	15-20	
V-up	4	15-20	
Oblique crunch	5	15-20	
Crunch	6	15-20	

Perform all exercises with minimal rest between sets.

WORKOUT 2
BACK

Cable pulldown or row	Warm-up	10	Pulldown behind neck
	Warm-up	10	Pulldown to upper chest
	1	8-10	Pulldown behind neck
	2	8-10	Pulldown to upper chest, wide grip
	3	6-10	Pulldown to upper chest, narrow grip
	4	6-8	Hammer front pulldown or standing row from high pulley
	5	6-8	Standing row from pulley (chest level) or seated row
	6	6-8	Standing row from low pulley
Barbell row	Warm-up	10	Natural grip (most comfortable grip)
	1	6-8	Natural grip
	2	6-8	8 inches beyond shoulder-width grip
	3	6-8	6 inches beyond shoulder-width grip
	4	6-8	4 inches beyond shoulder-width grip
	5	6-8	2 inches beyond shoulder-width grip
	6	6-8	Shoulder-width grip

BICEPS

Curl	Warm-up	10	Supine curl
	Warm-up	10	Standing curl
	1	8-10	Supine curl
	2	8-10	15-degree incline curl
	3	8-10	30-degree incline curl
	4	8-10	45-degree incline curl
	5	8-10	60-degree incline curl
	6	8-10	75-degree incline curl
	7	8-10	Standing dumbbell alternating curl
	8	8-10	Preacher curl
	9	8-10	Scott curl
	10	8-10	Overhead curl (on cable pulldown machine)

As an alternative way to hit biceps, try this barbell curl progression:

Barbell curl	Warm-up	10	Wide grip
	Warm-up	10	Shoulder-width grip
	1	8-10	Natural grip (most comfortable grip)
	2	8-10	6 inches beyond shoulder-width grip

Exercise	Set number	Reps	Exercise specifics
Barbell curl *(continued)*	3	6-10	4 inches beyond shoulder-width grip
	4	6-10	2 inches beyond shoulder-width grip
	5	6-10	Shoulder-width grip
	6	6-10	Narrow grip (hands about 4 inches apart)

WORKOUT 3
SHOULDERS

Exercise	Set number	Reps	Exercise specifics
Dumbbell press	Warm-up set	10	Arnold press
	Warm-up set	10	Palms facing forward
	1	6-8	Arnold press
	2	6-8	Neutral grip
	3	6-8	Palms facing forward
	4	4-8	Palms facing forward
Dumbbell raise	1	8-10	Front raise (with neutral grip) (perform one arm at a time)
	2	8-10	45-degree front raise*
	3	8-10	Lateral raise
	4	8-10	Lateral raise
	5	8-10	30-degree rear raise**
	6	8-10	Bent-over lateral raise
	7	8-10	Bent-over lateral raise

*Perform similar to lateral raise, but raise arm to a point halfway between front raise and lateral raise.

**Perform similar to lateral raise, but raise arm to a point 30 degrees behind lateral raise.

ABS

Exercise	Set number	Reps	Exercise specifics
Hanging knee raise	1	15-20	
Decline bench crossover crunch	2	15-20	
Decline bench crunch	3	15-20	
Exercise-ball pull-in	4	15-20	
Reverse crunch	5	15-20	
Crossover crunch	6	15-20	

Perform all exercises with minimal rest between sets.

WORKOUT 4
LEGS

Exercise	Set number	Reps	Exercise specifics
Squat*	Warm-up	10	Wide stance
	Warm-up	10	Narrow stance
	1	6-10	Shoulder-width stance
	2	6-10	Shoulder-width stance
	3	6-10	Hip-width stance
	4	6-10	4 inches wider than hip-width stance
	5	6-10	6 inches wider than hip-width stance
	6	6-10	8 inches wider than hip-width stance
	7	6-10	10 inches wider than hip-width stance
	8	6-10	12 inches wider than hip-width stance

*As an alternative, perform on leg press or hack squat (though you may be limited by the width of the foot plate).

> *continued*

TABLE 6.33   Small-Angle Workout *(continued)*

WORKOUT 4 *(continued)*
LEGS *(continued)*

As an alternative to the squat, leg press, or hack squat, try this lunge progression:

Exercise	Set number	Reps	Exercise specifics
Lunge	1	10-15	Forward lunge
	2	10-15	45-degree side lunge*
	3	6-10	Side lunge
	4	6-10	45-degree reverse lunge**
	5	6-10	Reverse lunge

*Perform as a cross between a forward lunge and a side lunge. Your foot should land halfway between both points.

**Perform as a cross between the side lunge and the reverse lunge. Your foot should land halfway between the side lunge and the reverse lunge.

Exercise	Set number	Reps	Exercise specifics
Leg extension	1	10-12	Toes straight up
	2	10-12	Toes straight up
	3	8-12	Toes turned out
	4	8-12	Toes turned in
Stiff-leg deadlift	1-3	10-12	Bring barbell just past knees
Lying leg curl*	1	10-12	Toes straight down
	2	10-12	Toes turned in
	3	8-12	Toes turned out

*As an alternative, perform on a seated or standing leg curl machine.

Exercise	Set number	Reps	Exercise specifics
Standing calf raise*	1	10-15	Toes straight forward
	2	10-15	Toes turned out
	3	10-15	Toes turned in

*As an alternative, perform on a leg press, donkey calf machine, or calf slide machine.

Exercise	Set number	Reps	Exercise specifics
Seated calf raise	1	10-15	Toes straight forward
	2	10-15	Toes turned out
	3	8-15	Toes turned in

Note: 1 inch = 2.54 centimeters

Barbell Blasting

The purpose of this training method is to limit all exercise choices to the barbell and use a variety of barbell exercises to stimulate each muscle group from a variety of angles. This serves as a good way to mix up your training for a short while and get creative with the exercises you can perform with a barbell. It's also great if you train at home and do not own dumbbells.

One way to do barbell blasting is by performing all exercises in a power rack, which will save time and provide safety, especially for those who train alone. See table 6.34 for a sample barbell blast program that hits each major muscle group using a three-day training split. This program can be done once or twice per week. Regardless of the frequency, follow it for no more than three weeks straight before switching to a program that offers more variety of exercises. You can also use barbell blasting by throwing it into a workout here or there for some sporadic variety or when the gym is crowded and not much else is available besides a barbell and a power rack.

RATING

	1	2	3	4	5
Time	1	2	3	4	5
Length	1	2	3	4	5
Difficulty	1	2	3	4	5
Results	1	2	3	4	5

TABLE 6.34   Have a Blast

WORKOUT 1: CHEST AND TRICEPS

Exercise	Sets	Reps
Incline barbell bench press (shoulder-width grip)	2	8-10
Incline barbell bench press (wide grip)	2	8-10
Decline barbell bench press	3	6-8
Flat barbell bench press	3	6-8
Reverse-grip barbell bench press	2	8-10
Close-grip barbell bench press	2	6-8
Seated barbell triceps extension	2	10-12
Skull crusher	2	8-10

WORKOUT 2: LEGS, SHOULDERS, TRAPS

Exercise	Sets	Reps
Barbell front squat	3	8-10
Barbell back squat	3	6-8
Barbell hack squat	3	6-8
Barbell lunge	3	8-10
Barbell Romanian deadlift	3	10-12
Barbell standing calf raise	3	10-12
Barbell seated calf raise	3	15-20
Standing barbell shoulder press	3	8-10
Barbell front raise	3	10-12
Barbell upright row (wide grip)	3	8-10
Barbell upright row (close grip)	3	8-10
Barbell shrug	2	6-8
Barbell behind-the-back shrug	2	8-10

WORKOUT 3: BACK, BICEPS, FOREARMS

Exercise	Sets	Reps
Barbell bent-over row (overhand shoulder-width grip)	3	8-10
Barbell bent-over row (overhand wide grip)	3	8-10
Barbell bent-over row (underhand grip)	3	8-10
Barbell decline bench pullover	3	10-12
Barbell curl	3	8-10
Barbell incline bench spider curl	3	10-12
Barbell preacher curl	3	10-12
Barbell reverse-grip curl	2	10-12
Barbell wrist curl	2	10-12
Barbell reverse wrist curl	2	10-12

One-Sided Training

This method of training uses exercises that focus on just one side of the body. This is known as unilateral training. Most training programs neglect unilateral training; at best, some include a one-arm or one-leg exercise here or there, such as the concentration curl or one-leg leg press. This can lead to imbalances in muscle strength and development.

Research shows that you can produce more force on each side of the body when you perform unilateral exercises than you could produce during bilateral exercises, such as the barbell bench press. In addition, because there are crossover effects from training a muscle on one side of the body, one-sided training can encourage better muscle growth on the untrained side. That is, the resting side also receives nervous stimulation from the increased blood flow that is caused by exercising the muscles on the other side of the body. This enhances the delivery of oxygen, nutrients, and hormones to the resting muscles while helping to flush away waste products from the previous workouts. The result may be better muscle regeneration and growth of the muscles.

Another benefit of one-sided training is that it trains the core muscles (the visible and deep muscles of the abdomen and low back) that are important for a better overall strength base. Perhaps the best point about one-sided training, however, is the pure novelty of the stimulus that it places on the body. It stimulates the nervous system and muscle fibers in a more unique way than any other training programs. New stimuli may lead to gains in muscle mass and muscle strength.

One-sided training breaks up workouts into right-side and left-side training days. In other words, muscles on the left side of the body (such as biceps and triceps) are trained on one day, and the same muscles on the right side of the body are trained on a different day. The program (shown in table 6.35) consists of four workouts per week that train the entire body once. Workout 1 consists of the right chest, shoulder, traps, triceps, back, and biceps. Workout 2 consists of the left chest, shoulder, traps, triceps, back, and biceps. On workout 3 you would hit the right quad, hams, glutes, and calves. Workout 4 closes out the body with the left quad, hams, glutes, and calves. Abs can be trained at the end of the first and fourth workout.

The volume of work performed per muscle group is fairly low (two exercises per muscle group for two or three sets per exercise) because this type of training is somewhat shocking on the nervous system. The weight used should be light enough to allow for 10 to 12 reps per set. Follow the one-sided training for only two to four weeks before switching back to normal bilateral training, and do not revisit this alternative training style more than once every four to six months.

In addition to the exercises given in the sample workouts, there are many other unilateral exercises you can perform for each muscle group. Table 6.36 contains a list of options you can try.

RATING

Time	1	2	3	4	5
Length	1	2	3	4	5
Difficulty	1	2	3	4	5
Results	1	2	3	4	5

TABLE 6.35 Side-by-Side Training

WORKOUT 1: RIGHT UPPER BODY (CHEST, SHOULDERS, TRAPS, TRICEPS, BACK, BICEPS)

Muscle group	Exercise	Sets	Reps
Chest	One-arm dumbbell chest press	3	10
	One-arm cable fly	3	12
Shoulder	One-arm dumbbell shoulder press	3	10
	One-arm cable lateral raise	3	12
Trapezius	One-arm Smith machine shrug	3	10
Triceps	Dumbbell kickback	2	12
	One-arm overhead triceps extension	2	12
Back	Dumbbell row	3	10
	One-arm pulldown	3	12
Biceps	One-arm preacher curl	2	12
	Dumbbell concentration curl	2	12

WORKOUT 2: LEFT UPPER BODY (CHEST, SHOULDERS, TRAPS, TRICEPS, BACK, BICEPS)

Muscle group	Exercise	Sets	Reps
Chest	One-arm dumbbell chest press	3	10
	One-arm cable fly	3	12
Shoulder	One-arm dumbbell shoulder press	3	10
	One-arm cable lateral raise	3	12
Trapezius	One-arm Smith machine shrug	3	10

WORKOUT 2: LEFT UPPER BODY (continued)

Muscle group	Exercise	Sets	Reps
Triceps	Dumbbell kickback	2	12
	One-arm overhead triceps extension	2	12
Back	Dumbbell row	3	10
	One-arm pulldown	3	12
Biceps	One-arm preacher curl	2	12
	Dumbbell concentration curl	2	12

WORKOUT 3: RIGHT LOWER BODY (QUADS, HAMSTRINGS, GLUTES, CALVES)

Muscle group	Exercise	Sets	Reps
Legs	One-leg leg press	3	10
	One-leg leg extension	3	12
	One-leg Romanian deadlift	3	10
	One-leg leg curl	3	12
	One-leg calf raise on leg press	2	12
	One-leg seated calf raise	2	12

WORKOUT 4: LEFT LOWER BODY (QUADS, HAMSTRINGS, GLUTES, CALVES)

Muscle group	Exercise	Sets	Reps
Legs	One-leg leg press	3	10
	One-leg leg extension	3	12
	One-leg Romanian deadlift	3	10
	One-leg leg curl	3	12
	One-leg calf raise on leg press	2	12
	One-leg seated calf raise	2	12

TABLE 6.36 Exercises on the Side

Muscle group	Exercise
Chest	One-arm dumbbell incline press
	One-arm dumbbell decline press
	One-arm dumbbell fly (flat, incline, decline)
	One-arm cable crossover
Shoulders	One-arm front raise (dumbbell or cable)
	One-arm dumbbell lateral raise
	One-arm bent-over lateral raise (dumbbell or cable)
	One-arm dumbbell upright row
Traps	One-arm dumbbell shrug
Triceps	Cable kickback
	One-arm triceps pressdown (D-handle or rope)
	One-arm lying triceps extension

Muscle group	Exercise
Back	One-arm seated row
	One-arm straight-arm pulldown
	One-arm straight-arm kickback
Biceps	Cable concentration curl
	One-arm dumbbell curl (seated, incline, standing)
	One-arm cable curl from high pulley
Quads	Step-up
	Lunge
	Squat

Bookend Training

The workouts in Bookend training, found in table 6.37, are bookended by the same exercise. Doing these exercises twice allows you to milk that exercise for all the benefits it offers. And those benefits include increased size, strength, and fat loss.

By doing these exercises at the beginning and end of the workout, you maximize muscle growth and strength. That's because you do the exercise first when you are freshest and strongest, which maximizes your strength and the mechanical overload you place on the muscles. When you do the exercise at the start of the workout you will use heavy weights and lower reps (6-8 per set). This rep range is best for building strength and mass due to the heavier load it places on the muscles, which maximizes muscle damage, and therefore strength gains and growth. When you damage muscle fibers, they are replaced with new ones that grow bigger and stronger in an effort to adapt to the overload placed on them. But that's just one way that muscles grow. Using this rep range also better stimulates the production of the anabolic hormone testosterone.

When you work that same exercise at the very end of the workout, you are preexhausted by the exercises that preceded it. This maximizes the fatigue that you place on the muscles, as does the rep range you will use at these points. You'll do three sets at the end of the workout. Set 1 uses the same weight that you started with. This is to further enhance the muscle damage you started at the beginning of the workout by forcing the muscles to move that weight when they are already fatigued. You'll be able to get only a few reps because of this, but every one of these reps will push muscle damage that much further. You finish with two sets of 12 to 15 reps. This higher rep range will take your muscles to the limits of fatigue, not to mention the fact that you keep the rest between sets in these three final sets to one minute to really fatigue the muscles. Fatigue is also critical for muscle growth due to the biochemical waste products in the muscle cells from the burning of glucose and fat for the energy needed for the muscles to contract. This signals an increase in anabolic hormones and growth factors like growth hormone (GH) and insulin-like growth factor-I (IGF-I). The anabolic factors, along with testosterone, influence muscle growth by enhancing the growth of the new muscle fibers that will replace the damaged ones and by enhancing muscle protein synthesis. Muscle protein synthesis works to build up all of the muscle fibers by providing them with more protein. Since muscle fibers are made of protein, more protein means bigger muscle fibers.

RATING

Time	1	2	3	4	5
Length	1	2	3	4	5
Difficulty	1	2	3	4	5
Results	1	2	3	4	5

TABLE 6.37   Bookend Workouts

WORKOUT 1: CHEST, BICEPS, ABS			
Muscle group	**Exercise**	**Sets/reps**	**Rest**
Chest	Bench press	3/6-8	2-3 min
	Incline dumbbell bench press	3/8-10	2 min
	Incline dumbbell fly	3/10-12	1-2 min
	Cable crossover	2/12-15	1-2 min
	Bench press	1/to failure[1]	1 min
		2/12-15	1 min
Biceps	Barbell curl	3/6-8	2-3 min
	Incline dumbbell curl	3/8-10	2 min
	Cable concentration curl	3/10-12	1 min
	Barbell curl	1/to failure[1]	1 min
		2/12-15	1 min
Abs	Hanging leg raise[2]	2/6-8	1-2 min
	Crunch	3/to failure	1 min
	Hanging leg raise	1/to failure	1 min
		2/to failure[1,3]	1 min

WORKOUT 2: LEGS AND CALVES

Muscle group	Exercise	Sets/reps	Rest
Legs	Squat	3/6-8	2-3 min
	Leg press	3/8-10	2 min
	Dumbbell reverse lunge	3/10-12	1-2 min
	Leg extension	3/12-15	1 min
	Lying leg curl	3/12-15	1 min
	Squat	1/to failure[1] 2/12-15	1 min 1 min
Calves	Standing calf raise	3/6-8	1-2 min
	Seated calf raise	3/15-20	1 min
	Standing calf raise	1/to failure[1] 2/12-15	1 min 1 min

WORKOUT 3: SHOULDERS, TRAPS, ABS

Muscle group	Exercise	Sets/reps	Rest
Shoulders	Barbell shoulder press	3/6-8	2-3 min
	Dumbbell upright row	2/8-10	2 min
	Cable lateral raise	3/10-12	1-2 min
	Rear delt raise	3/12-15	1 min
	Barbell shoulder press	1/to failure[1] 2/12-15	1 min 1 min
Traps	Barbell shrug	3/6-8	2-3 min
	Barbell behind-the-back shrug	2/10-12	1-2 min
	Barbell shrug	1/to failure[1] 2/12-15	1 min 1 min
Abs	Rope cable crunch	2/6-8	1-2 min
	Reverse crunch	3/to failure	1 min
	Rope cable crunch	1/to failure[1] 2/12-15	1 min 1 min

WORKOUT 4: BACK AND TRICEPS

Muscle group	Exercise	Sets/reps	Rest
Back	Barbell row	3/6-8	2-3 min
	Pull-up	3/to failure	2 min
	Seated cable row	3/10-12	1-2 min
	One-arm straight-arm pulldown	3/12-15	1 min
	Barbell row	1/to failure[1] 2/12-15	1 min 1 min
Triceps	Close-grip bench press	3/6-8	2-3 min
	Triceps pressdown	3/8-10	2 min
	Cable overhead extension	3/10-12	1 min
	Close-grip bench press	1/to failure[1] 2/12-15	1 min 1 min

[1]Use same weight as you used on the last set of this exercise.

[2]Hold a dumbbell or medicine ball between your feet.

[3]Use body weight only.

Push–Pull–Angle Training

The push–pull training split (covered in chapter 8) is one of the simplest and most effective splits ever devised. Having been used by competitive bodybuilders and other high-performance athletes, the concept involves categorizing all weight-training exercises down to one of two types—pushing movements and pulling movements—and splitting up workouts accordingly. A typical push day includes exercises for the chest, shoulders, quads, and triceps because these are considered the pushing muscles. And a typical pull day trains the back, biceps, hamstrings, and traps. But weight training is not quite that simple.

For most muscle groups, you can do at least a few exercises that don't fall under the strict definition of either a push exercise or a pull exercise. For example, leg extension, leg curl, biceps curl, triceps extension, lateral raise, and fly are all exercises that are technically neither pushing nor pulling movements. They are actually what we would consider *angular* movements. That is, the movement doesn't follow a straight line but rather the path of an arc. These are always isolation exercises because they involve only a single joint. Pushing or pulling a weight in a straight line involves multiple joints working together. Thus, push and pull exercises are always multijoint exercises.

The push–pull training split works well for powerlifters and strength athletes who rarely do angular (isolation) exercises. But because bodybuilding relies heavily on such movements, I created the push–pull training split into the push–pull–angle split. In it, you'll have one push day in which you hit chest, legs, shoulders, triceps, and calves with multijoint exercises; one pull day in which you hit back, traps, and biceps, again with multijoint moves, as well as abs; and two angle days, which collectively hit all major muscle groups with isolation exercises only.

One angle day trains the chest, legs, shoulders, and triceps, while the other trains back, biceps, forearms, and abs. You'll end up training each muscle group twice per week, once with compound moves (push or pull) and again with isolation moves (angle). This way, you can focus on one heavy basic training day for each muscle group where you use lower reps, and one lighter isolation day where you use higher reps, for a multifaceted approach to overall growth, muscle mass, and strength. Not only is each muscle being trained more frequently, but each is getting different types of stress (heavy and light) each week. Separating the types of exercises into two workouts for each body part will be a welcome change for your muscles, resulting in greater hypertrophy and strength gains.

Follow the four-day push–pull–angle training split as suggested in table 6.38 for four weeks. Feel free to use it longer, but after four weeks on this sample program be sure to make some changes, such as swapping out the exercises listed in table 6.39 in the Push–Pull–Angle Exercises box for others listed as follows. Also, feel free to alter rep ranges and rest periods, depending on your training goals. The routine listed in table 6.38 is a combination of strength and hypertrophy, using low- (4-7), moderate- (8-12), and high-rep schemes (15-20).

RATING

Time	1	2	3	4	5
Length	1	2	3	4	5
Difficulty	1	2	3	4	5
Results	1	2	3	4	5

TABLE 6.38 Push–Pull–Angle Training

PUSH DAY (MONDAY)

Muscle group	Exercise	Sets	Reps	Rest
Chest	Barbell bench press	3	4–6	2 min
	Dumbbell incline press	3	6–8	2 min
	Decline Smith machine press	3	8–10	2 min
Legs	Barbell squat	3	4–6	2 min
	Smith machine front squat	3	6–8	2 min
	Leg press	3	8–10	2 min
Shoulders	Barbell overhead press	4	4–6	2 min
	Dumbbell overhead press	4	6–8	2 min
Triceps	Close-grip bench press	3	6–8	2 min
	Dip	3	8–10	2 min
Calves	Standing calf raise	3	8–10	1 min

PULL DAY (TUESDAY)

Muscle group	Exercise	Sets	Reps	Rest
Back	Deadlift	3	4–6	2 min
	Barbell bent-over row	3	6–8	2 min
	Lat pulldown	3	8–10	2 min
Back and biceps	Reverse-grip pull-up	3	6–8	2 min
	Drag curl	3	8–10	2 min
Traps	Barbell shrug	3	6–8	2 min
	Dumbbell shrug	3	8–10	2 min
Abs	Hanging leg raise	2	10–12	1 min
	Rope crunch	2	10–12	1 min

ANGLE DAY 1 (THURSDAY)

Muscle group	Exercise	Sets ·	Reps	Rest
Chest	Dumbbell incline fly	3	10–12	1 min
	Cable crossover	3	12–15	1 min
	Pec deck	3	15–20	1 min
Quads	Leg extension	4	15–20	1 min
Hamstrings	Lying leg curl	4	15–20	1 min
Shoulders	Cable lateral raise	3	10–12	1 min
	Barbell front raise	2	12–15	1 min
	Dumbbell bent-over lateral raise	2	15–20	1 min
Triceps	Cable pressdown	3	10–12	1 min
	Dumbbell overhead triceps extension	3	12–15	1 min

ANGLE DAY 2 (FRIDAY)

Muscle group	Exercise	Sets	Reps	Rest
Back	Decline dumbbell pullover	4	10–12	1 min
	Straight-arm pulldown	4	12–15	1 min
Biceps	Barbell curl Incline dumbbell curl	3	10–12	1 min
		3	12–15	1 min
Forearms	Barbell wrist curl	3	12–15	1 min
Abs	Reverse crunch	3	15–20	1 min
	Crunch	3	20–25	1 min

Push–Pull–Angle Exercises

Table 6.39 lists virtually every push, pull, and angle exercise for every major body part. Use this catalog to substitute in other exercises to the push–pull–angle sample four-day split.

TABLE 6.39 Push–Pull–Angle Exercises

Muscle group	Push	Pull	Angle
Chest	Flat, incline, or decline barbell press Flat, incline, or decline dumbbell press Flat, incline, or decline Smith machine press Any other machine chest press Push-up	N/A	Flat, incline, or decline dumbbell fly Flat, incline, or decline cable fly Machine fly Cable crossover (high or low pulley) Pec deck Pullover
Back	N/A	Barbell, dumbbell, or straight-arm Smith machine or cable bent-over row Seated cable row Deadlift Lat pulldown Pull-up T-bar row High pulley row	Pulldown Pullover
Shoulders	Barbell, dumbbell, or Smith machine overhead press	Barbell, dumbbell, Smith machine, or cable upright row*	Dumbbell, cable, or machine lateral raise Dumbbell, cable, or barbell front raise Dumbbell or cable bent-over lateral raise Reverse pec deck
Triceps	Barbell, Smith machine, or dumbbell close-grip bench press Dip (includes machine)	N/A	Cable pressdown Barbell or dumbbell lying triceps extension Dumbbell, barbell, or cable overhead extension Dumbbell or cable kickback Machine triceps extension
Biceps	N/A	Reverse-grip pull-up Drag curl	Barbell, dumbbell, or cable curl EZ-bar or dumbbell preacher curl Incline dumbbell curl Concentration curl Machine curl
Quads	Barbell or smith machine squat Leg press Hack squat Barbell or Smith machine front squat Squat machine Barbell or dumbbell lunge	N/A	Leg extension Sissy squat
Hamstrings	Barbell or Smith machine squat Squat machine Barbell or dumbbell lunge	N/A	Lying, seated, or standing leg curl Romanian deadlift

Muscle group	Push	Pull	Angle
Calves	Standing or seated, donkey or leg press calf raise	N/A	N/A
Abs	N/A	N/A	Crunch Reverse crunch Oblique crunch Hanging leg or knee raise Rope crunch
Traps	N/A	N/A	Barbell, dumbbell, or Smith machine shrug Barbell, Smith machine, or cable dumbbell upright row

* Wide-grip barbell, Smith machine, cable, or dumbbell upright row is the one shoulder exercise that is actually a true pulling movement. Though it would technically be inconsistent with the push–pull angle split, feel free to perform upright rows on angle day 1.

Big Band Program

As discussed in chapter 4, resistance bands or strength bands offer a unique type of resistance that is called linear variable resistance, which refers to a increasing resistance progressively with the range of motion. Using the bench press as an example, that means as you press the bar off your chest the resistance gets progressively heavier the farther you press the bar to full arm extension. That increase in resistance necessitates the application of more force toward the top of the lift, which limits the slowing at the top of an exercise that normally occurs to stop the weight.

Bands are also great to travel with because they weigh little yet provide ample resistance. The Big Band program in table 6.40 is a good workout to do even if you have a full weight setup because it will hit the muscles with this unique resistance.

RATING

Time	1	2	3	4	5
Length	1	2	3	4	5
Difficulty	1	2	3	4	5
Results	1	2	3	4	5

TABLE 6.40 Big Band Program

WEEK 1
WORKOUT 1 (MONDAY): CHEST, TRICEPS, ABS

Muscle group	Exercise	Sets/reps	Rest
Chest	Bench press with bands	3/15-20	2 min
	Standing incline chest press	3/15-20	2 min
	Standing one-arm low-band fly	3/15-20	2 min
	Standing one-arm fly with band	3/15-20	2 min
Triceps	Close-grip bench press with bands	3/15-20	2 min
	Overhead triceps extension with band	3/15-20	2 min
	Underhand-grip kickback with band	3/15-20	2 min
Abs	Standing crunch with band	2/15-20	1 min
	Rising knee with band	2/15-20	1 min
	Roundhouse elbow with band	2/15-20	1 min

> *continued*

TABLE 6.40 Big Band Program *(continued)*

WEEK 1 *(continued)*
WORKOUT 2 (TUESDAY): BACK AND BICEPS

Muscle group	Exercise	Sets/ reps	Rest
Back	Barbell row with bands	3/15-20	2 min
	Pulldown with bands	3/15-20	2 min
	Standing one-arm row with band	3/15-20	2 min
	Straight-arm pulldown with bands	3/15-20	2 min
Biceps	Barbell curl with bands	3/15-20	2 min
	Behind-the-back curl with bands	3/15-20	2 min
	High curl with bands	3/15-20	2 min

WORKOUT 3 (THURSDAY): SHOULDERS, TRAPS, ABS

Muscle group	Exercise	Sets/ reps	Rest
Shoulders	Barbell shoulder press with bands	3/15-20	2 min
	Lateral raise with bands	3/15-20	2 min
	Shoulder press with bands	3/15-20	2 min
	Rear delt reverse fly with bands	3/15-20	2 min
Traps	Barbell shrug with bands	3/15-20	2 min
	Barbell behind-the-back shrug with bands	3/15-20	2 min
Abs	Rising knee with band	2/15-20	1 min
	Roundhouse elbow with band	2/15-20	1 min
	Standing twisting crunch with band	2/15-20	1 min

WORKOUT 4 (FRIDAY): LEGS [QUADS AND HAMS], CALVES

Muscle group	Exercise	Sets/ reps	Rest
Quads	Barbell squat with bands	3/15-20	2 min
	Step-up with bands	3/15-20	2 min
	Standing leg extension with bands	3/15-20	1 min
Hamstrings	Barbell Romanian deadlift with bands	3/15-20	2 min
	Standing leg curl with band	3/15-20	1 min
Calves	Barbell standing calf raise with bands	3/15-20	1 min
	Barbell seated calf raise with bands	3/15-20	1 min

WEEK 2
WORKOUT 1 (MONDAY): CHEST, TRICEPS, ABS

Muscle group	Exercise	Sets/ reps	Rest
Chest	Bench press with bands	3/12-15	2 min
	Standing incline chest press	3/12-15	2 min
	Standing one-arm low-band fly	3/12-15	2 min
	Standing one-arm fly with band	3/12-15	2 min
Triceps	Close-grip bench press with bands	3/12-15	2 min
	Overhead triceps extension with bands	3/12-15	2 min
	Underhand-grip kickback with bands	3/12-15	2 min
Abs	Standing crunch with band	2/12-15	1 min
	Rising knee with band	2/12-15	1 min
	Roundhouse elbow with band	2/12-15	1 min

WORKOUT 2 (TUESDAY): BACK AND BICEPS

Muscle group	Exercise	Sets/ reps	Rest
Back	Barbell row with bands	3/12-15	2 min
	Pulldown with bands	3/12-15	2 min
	Standing one-arm row with band	3/12-15	2 min
	Straight-arm pulldown with bands	3/15-20	2 min
Biceps	Barbell curl with bands	3/12-15	2 min
	Behind-the-back curl with bands	3/12-15	2 min
	High curl with bands	3/12-15	2 min

WORKOUT 3 (THURSDAY): SHOULDERS, TRAPS, ABS

Muscle group	Exercise	Sets/ reps	Rest
Shoulders	Barbell shoulder press with bands	3/12-15	2 min
	Lateral raise with bands	3/12-15	2 min
	Shoulder press with bands	3/12-15	2 min
	Rear delt reverse fly with bands	3/12-15	2 min
Traps	Barbell shrug with bands	3/12-15	2 min
	Barbell behind-the-back shrug with bands	3/12-15	2 min

WORKOUT 3 (THURSDAY): SHOULDERS, TRAPS, ABS

Muscle group	Exercise	Sets/ reps	Rest
Abs	Rising knee with band	2/12-15	1 min
	Roundhouse elbow with band	2/12-15	1 min
	Standing twisting crunch with band	2/12-15	1 min

WORKOUT 4 (FRIDAY): LEGS [QUADS AND HAMS], CALVES

Muscle group	Exercise	Sets/ Reps	Rest
Quads	Barbell squat with bands	3/12-15	2 min
	Step-up with band	3/12-15	2 min
	Standing leg extension with bands	3/12-15	1 min
Hamstrings	Barbell Romanian deadlift with bands	3/12-15	2 min
	Standing leg curl with band	3/12-15	1 min
Calves	Barbell standing calf raise with bands	3/12-15	1 min
	Barbell seated calf raise with bands	3/12-15	1 min

WEEK 3
WORKOUT 1 (MONDAY): CHEST, TRICEPS, ABS

Muscle group	Exercise	Sets/ reps	Rest
Chest	Bench press with bands	3/8-12	2-3 min
	Standing incline chest press	3/8-12	2-3 min
	Standing one-arm low-band fly	3/8-12	2-3 min
	Standing one-arm fly with band	3/8-12	2-3 min
Triceps	Close-grip bench press with bands	3/8-12	2-3 min
	Overhead triceps extension with bands	3/8-12	2-3 min
	Underhand-grip kickback with bands	3/8-12	2-3 min
Abs	Standing crunch with bands	3/10-12	1 min
	Rising knee with band	3/10-12	1 min
	Roundhouse elbow with band	3/10-12	1 min

WORKOUT 2 (TUESDAY): BACK AND BICEPS

Muscle group	Exercise	Sets/ reps	Rest
Back	Barbell row with bands	3/8-12	2-3 min
	Pulldown with bands	3/8-12	2-3 min
	Standing one-arm row with band	3/8-12	2-3 min
	Straight-arm pulldown with bands	3/8-12	2-3 min
Biceps	Barbell curl with bands	3/8-12	2-3 min
	Behind-the-back curl with bands	3/8-12	2-3 min
	High curl with bands	3/8-12	2-3 min

WORKOUT 3 (THURSDAY): SHOULDERS, TRAPS, ABS

Muscle group	Exercise	Sets/ reps	Rest
Shoulders	Barbell shoulder press with bands	3/8-12	2-3 min
	Lateral raise with bands	3/8-12	2-3 min
	Shoulder press with bands	3/8-12	2-3 min
	Rear delt reverse fly with bands	3/8-12	2-3 min
Traps	Barbell shrug with bands	3/8-12	2-3 min
	Barbell behind-the-back shrug with bands	3/8-12	2-3 min
Abs	Rising knee with band	3/10-12	1 min
	Roundhouse elbow with band	3/10-12	1 min
	Standing twisting crunch with band	3/10-12	1 min

WORKOUT 4 (FRIDAY): LEGS [QUADS AND HAMS], CALVES

Muscle group	Exercise	Sets/ reps	Rest
Quads	Barbell squat with bands	3/8-12	2-3 min
	Step-up with band	3/8-12	2-3 min
	Standing leg extension with band	3/8-12	2 min
Hamstrings	Barbell Romanian deadlift with bands	3/8-12	2-3 min
	Standing leg curl with band	3/8-12	2 min
Calves	Barbell standing calf raise with bands	3/10-12	1 min
	Barbell seated calf raise with bands	3/10-12	1 min

> continued

TABLE 6.40   Big Band Program *(continued)*

WEEK 4
WORKOUT 1 (MONDAY): CHEST, TRICEPS, ABS

Muscle group	Exercise	Sets/reps	Rest
Chest	Bench press with bands	3/5-8	3 min
	Standing incline chest press	3/5-8	3 min
	Standing one-arm low-band fly	3/5-8	3 min
	Standing one-arm fly with band	3/5-8	3 min
Triceps	Close-grip bench press with bands	3/5-8	3 min
	Overhead triceps extension with bands	3/5-8	3 min
	Underhand-grip kickback with bands	3/5-8	3 min
Abs	Standing crunch with bands	3/8-10	1 min
	Rising knee with band	3/8-10	1 min
	Roundhouse elbow with band	3/8-10	1 min

WORKOUT 2 (TUESDAY): BACK AND BICEPS

Muscle group	Exercise	Sets/reps	Rest
Back	Barbell row with bands	3/5-8	3 min
	Pulldown with bands	3/5-8	3 min
	Standing one-arm row with band	3/5-8	3 min
	Straight-arm pulldown with bands	3/5-8	3 min
Biceps	Barbell curl with bands	3/5-8	3 min
	Behind-the-back curl with bands	3/5-8	3 min
	High curl with bands	3/5-8	3 min

WORKOUT 3 (THURSDAY): SHOULDERS, TRAPS, ABS

Muscle group	Exercise	Sets/reps	Rest
Shoulders	Barbell shoulder press with bands	3/5-8	3 min
	Lateral raise with bands	3/5-8	3 min
	Shoulder press with bands	3/5-8	3 min
	Rear delt reverse fly with bands	3/5-8	3 min
Traps	Barbell shrug with bands	3/5-8	3 min
	Barbell behind-the-back shrug with bands	3/5-8	3 min
Abs	Rising knee with band	3/8-10	1 min
	Roundhouse elbow with band	3/8-10	1 min
	Standing twisting crunch with band	3/8-10	1 min

WORKOUT 4 (FRIDAY): LEGS [QUADS AND HAMS], CALVES

Muscle group	Exercise	Sets/reps	Rest
Quads	Barbell squat with bands	3/5-8	3 min
	Step-up with band	3/5-8	3 min
	Standing leg extension with band	3/5-8	3 min
Hamstrings	Barbell Romanian deadlift with bands	3/5-8	3 min
	Standing leg curl with band	3/5-8	3 min
Calves	Barbell standing calf raise with bands	3/8-10	1 min
	Barbell seated calf raise with bands	3/8-10	1 min

Machine Muscle

Sure, they don't enhance the strength of your stabilizers, but resistance machines do have several benefits:

1. **Ease and convenience** makes them great to use when you're short on time.

2. **Constant tension**: With machines you never lose the stress (or tension) that the weight places on the muscle. (For example, compare the dumbbell fly to the fly machine. You don't lose the stress on the muscle when your hands come together as happens on the dumbbell fly.)

3. **Failure**: You can safely train to all-out muscle failure with or without a spotter and even forced reps on your own on some machines.

The all-machine workout in table 6.41 isn't designed for you to follow for any length of time. Try it for one or two weeks as a change of pace. You'll give your joints some rest from the heavy pounding you normally do with free weights and stimulate some new muscle growth by focusing constant tension on your muscle fibers. Or when you are crunched for time on chest day or arm day, choose the workout for the muscle group you need to train in a hurry.

These workouts take advantage of the machine's ease of changing weight by using drop sets and allow for safety when training past failure, such as with forced reps. Try these workouts and you'll never think about machines as beginner equipment again.

Keep rest periods between sets to a minimum (1-2 minutes).

RATING

Time	1	2	3	4	5
Length	1	2	3	4	5
Difficulty	1	2	3	4	5
Results	1	2	3	4	5

TABLE 6.41 All-Machine Workout

WORKOUT 1: CHEST, SHOULDERS, TRICEPS, ABS

Muscle group	Exercise	Sets/reps
Chest	Seated chest press machine[1]	3/8-10[2]
	Incline press machine[1]	3/8-10[3]
	Pec deck[4]	3/12-15[3]
Shoulders	Shoulder press machine[1]	3/8-10[2]
	Smith machine upright row	3/10-12[3]
	Seated lateral raise machine[4]	3/12-15[3]
Triceps	Seated dip machine[5]	3/8-10[2]
	Seated overhead extension machine[4]	3/12-15[3]
Abs	Crunch machine	3/12-15[3]

WORKOUT 2: QUADS, HAMS, CALVES

Muscle group	Exercise	Sets/reps
Quads	Squat machine[1]	3/8-10[3]
	Leg press	3/8-10[3]
	Leg extension	3/12-15[2]
Hamstrings	Lying leg curl	3/12-15[2]
	Seated leg curl	3/12-15[2]
Calves	Donkey calf raise	3/15-20[3]
	Leg press calf raise	3/10-12[3]

WORKOUT 3: BACK, TRAPS, BICEPS, ABS

Muscle group	Exercise	Sets/reps
Back	Smith machine bent-over row	3/8-10[3]
	Assisted pull-up[5]	3/10-12[2]
	Seated row machine[4]	3/10-12[3]
Traps	Smith machine shrug	3/8-10[3]
Biceps	Preacher curl machine[5]	3/8-10[2]
	Horizontal curl machine[4]	3/10-12[3]
Abs	Lower ab machine[5]	3/12-15[3]

[1]If your gym is not equipped with this machine, do the Smith machine version.

[2]On last set, do 2 or 3 forced reps after reaching failure.

[3]On last set after reaching failure, do one drop set by reducing weight by about 30% and continuing to failure.

[4]If your gym is not equipped with this machine, do the cable version.

[5]If your gym is not equipped with this machine, do the free weight version.

PROGRAMS THAT MANIPULATE TRAINING FREQUENCY

The standard training method for making sound gains in muscle size is to allow a minimum of 48 hours between training sessions for a particular muscle group. This time period allows the processes of muscle recovery to kick in so that the muscle damage inflicted in the previous workout can be repaired and the depleted fuel stores can be replenished. However, on occasion, going against conventional thinking on recovery can be an advantage for making muscle gains. This can be done by training similar muscle groups on consecutive days or even training them twice in one day. Increasing the frequency of training for short periods can lead to more frequent muscle growth.

Back-to-Back Training

Back-to-back training refers to training a muscle group on two consecutive days. It is also referred to in some bodybuilding circles as feeder workouts, because the concept is to train the muscle group again the very next day but with very light weight, higher reps, fewer sets, and very low intensity to help increase blood flow to the muscle tissue. The theory is that this will supply the recovering muscle cells with more nutrients such as amino acids and glucose (both critical for muscle growth and strength), anabolic hormones such as GH and testosterone, and more oxygen for faster recovery. It will also help remove the waste products and cellular debris that were created from the previous workout. It also leads to greater water flow from the blood supply into the muscle—this is the cause of the pump—which is believed to turn on muscle-building pathways because of the stretch that is placed on the muscle cell by the volume overload. While no studies have looked at this effect on muscle growth directly, one study found that the cortisol response on the second workout day is significantly lower and the testosterone levels are slightly higher (Pullinen et al. 2002). Hormonal responses to a resistance exercise performed under the influence of delayed-onset muscle soreness. This means that a greater anabolic environment is created within the muscles, which can enhance the potential for muscle growth and strength gains.

The first back-to-back workout for each muscle group should be very intense. Muscle failure should be reached on all sets and followed with forced reps or drop sets. Volume should also be high (12 to 16 sets per muscle group) to ensure the muscle is thoroughly fatigued. The second workout should be lower in both intensity and volume. Perform only about six to eight sets per muscle group and perform 15 to 20 reps, never reaching muscle failure. See table 6.42 for a sample back-to-back workout program.

RATING

Time	1	2	3	4	5
Length	1	2	3	4	5
Difficulty	1	2	3	4	5
Results	1	2	3	4	5

TABLE 6.42   Back-to-Back Back Attack

Workouts 1 and 2 are performed on two consecutive days.

Exercise	Sets	Reps
WORKOUT 1		
Pull-up	3	6-10*
Barbell row	4	6-10**
Seated cable row	4	6-10**
Pulldown (underhand grip)	4	6-10**
WORKOUT 2		
Pulldown (wide grip)	2	15-20
Barbell row	2	15-20
Seated cable row	1	15-20
Pulldown (underhand grip)	1	15-20

*Perform two or three forced reps at the end of each set.

**Perform each set to failure. At the end of last set, strip the weight down by about 30% and perform as many reps as possible. Then strip another 30% or so off and perform reps until muscle failure is reached.

Twice-a-Day Training

Similar to back-to-back training, twice-a-day training works the same muscle group back to back, just on the same day. The program is based on research that shows that when muscles are trained twice in the same day, the amount of muscle glycogen increases by nearly double the normal value. Since glycogen pulls water into muscle cells, the muscle cells become fuller (more pumped). This causes a stretch on the muscle cells that is believed to trigger muscle growth.

Twice-a-day training also encourages capillary growth in muscle tissue and increases the density of fuel-metabolizing mitochondria in the muscle cells, both of which help the muscle to assimilate nutrients. It also works to boost resting metabolism after the twice-a-day workouts, which can help to encourage fat loss during cutting phases of training.

With twice-a-day training the same exercises should be done for both workouts. This is because different exercises stress different muscle fibers, and it is essential to stress the same muscle fibers in the second workout as were stressed in the first. However, the order of these exercises is not critical. So some bodybuilders begin the first workout with compound movement and then finish with isolation exercises. In the second workout

they reverse that order. This helps to prevent boredom. Repetitions for both workouts should be high (in the range of 12 to 20) to prevent overstressing the targeted muscle group and better deplete muscle glycogen. Rest should be no more than 60 seconds between sets to best deplete glycogen stores, increase caloric expenditure, and facilitate fat loss.

Workouts should be separated by at least three but no more than eight hours of rest. If there is not enough time between sessions, the testosterone response that occurs from training may be blunted, and cortisol levels may increase too much. Muscles should receive about three to seven days of recovery before you train them again. Use the twice-a-day program for no more than six weeks, because using it any longer may actually hinder progress. See table 6.43 for sample twice-a-day workouts.

RATING

Time	1	2	3	4	5
Length	1	2	3	4	5
Difficulty	1	2	3	4	5
Results	1	2	3	4	5

TABLE 6.43 Twice the Workout

Exercise	Sets	Reps
CHEST WORKOUT 1		
Incline barbell press	3	12-15
Dumbbell bench press	3	12-15
Incline dumbbell fly	3	15
CHEST WORKOUT 2		
Incline dumbbell fly	3	15
Dumbbell bench press	3	12-15
Incline barbell press	3	12-15
SHOULDER WORKOUT 1		
Dumbbell shoulder press	3	12-15
Wide-grip upright row	3	12-15
Dumbbell lateral raise	3	15
SHOULDER WORKOUT 2		
Dumbbell lateral raise	3	15
Wide-grip upright row	3	12-15
Dumbbell shoulder press	3	12-15

Exercise	Sets	Reps
BACK WORKOUT 1		
Barbell row	3	12-15
Wide-grip pulldown	3	12-15
Straight-arm pulldown	3	15
BACK WORKOUT 2		
Straight-arm pulldown	3	15
Wide-grip pulldown	3	12-15
Barbell row	3	12-15
LEG WORKOUT 1		
Squat	3	15-20
Leg press	3	15-20
Leg extension	3	15-20
Lying leg curl	3	15-20
Standing calf raise	3	20
Seated calf raise	3	20

> continued

TABLE 6.43 Twice the Workout *(continued)*

Exercise	Sets	Reps
LEG WORKOUT 2		
Lying leg curl	3	15-20
Leg extension	3	15-20
Leg press	3	15-20
Squat	3	15-20
Seated calf raise	3	20
Standing calf raise	3	20
BICEPS WORKOUT 1		
Barbell curl	2	12-15
Seated incline curl	2	12-15
Concentration curl	2	15

Exercise	Sets	Reps
BICEPS WORKOUT 2		
Concentration curl	2	15
Seated incline curl	2	12-15
Barbell curl	2	12-15
TRICEPS WORKOUT 1		
Close-grip bench press	2	12-15
Skull crusher	2	12-15
Triceps pressdown	2	15
TRICEPS WORKOUT 2		
Triceps pressdown	2	15
Skull crusher	2	12-15
Close-grip bench press	2	12-15

CHAPTER 7

Training Cycles for Building Muscle Mass

Once you are familiar with the fundamentals of strength training, including the basic guidelines on designing a training program for building muscle mass as well as having an arsenal of advanced mass-training techniques, it's time to consider the long-term application of your training program. Being able to put this acquired knowledge together in a long-term program is the only way of reaching your desired goals. Whether you're a beginner, intermediate, or advanced weightlifter and just want to add general muscle mass to your frame, or you want to shed body fat while adding muscle, or you have specific muscle groups you want to focus on building up, this chapter has a program for you.

MASS-BUILDING PROGRAMS

Although it is well established that certain exercise choices, orders of exercises, volumes, resistances, and amounts of rest between sets are better than others for developing muscle mass, sticking within those guidelines for too long can actually hinder your progress. This is the foundation of periodization (covered in chapter 3). For instance, although the repetition maximum continuum indicates that using a range of 6 to 12 reps per set is best for muscle hypertrophy, sticking within those confines will lead to stagnation in muscle growth. Therefore, while some of your training should be done with this rep range, you also need to work in both lower- and higher-rep ranges. The question, then, is how and when to do this. This rationale also applies to the other acute variables of training. To ensure that gains in muscle mass are optimized and persistent, smart bodybuilders realize that the frequent cycling of their workouts is as essential to their progress as the acute variables.

Developing a basic cycle that carries your training over the next 6 months or year is much like an insurance policy that protects your progress. This template will serve as a basic guide to steer you through your journey to gain more muscle. If you are a beginner, you should follow this program as prescribed for your first 6 months of serious training. The intermediate (6 to 12 months of training experience) and advanced (over a year of consistent training experience) weightlifters are provided a yearlong training guide. However, at this level you can take a few side roads here or there as long as you mind the overall scheme of the program. In the end, remember that everything works, but nothing works forever.

Beginner Program (First Six Months)

This six-month program breaks down into six four-week segments (see table 7.1). In the first three segments, you follow a whole-body training split and train with weights three days per week, working your entire body each time. The first four weeks you will train one exercise per muscle group. The exercises are the same for each workout and the reps are 15 per set with two- to three-minute rest periods between sets. This helps to train the nervous system during this introductory phase. The second four-week cycle adds a second exercise to each muscle group to increase both volume and variety in the way the muscles are trained. Exercises performed are the same for each workout and reps are 12 to 15 per set with two- to three-minute rest periods. The third four-week cycle changes the exercises at each different workout for the week. This provides three different exercises per muscle group at the end of the week in an effort to target all the muscle fibers in each muscle group.

131

TABLE 7.1 Beginner Basic Program

WEEKS 1-4 (MONDAY, WEDNESDAY, FRIDAY)

Exercise	Sets	Reps
Leg press	3	15
Bench press	3	15
Seated cable row	3	15
Dumbbell shoulder press	3	15
Barbell curl	3	15
Triceps pressdown	3	15
Standing calf raise	3	15
Crunch	3	15

WEEKS 5-8 (MONDAY, WEDNESDAY, FRIDAY)

Exercise	Sets	Reps
Leg press	2	12-15
Lunge	2	15
Bench press	2	12-15
Dumbbell incline fly	2	15
Seated cable row	2	12-15
Lat pulldown	2	15
Dumbbell shoulder press	2	12-15
Dumbbell lateral raise	2	15
Barbell curl	2	12-15
Seated incline curl	2	15
Lying triceps extension	2	12-15
Triceps pressdown	2	15
Standing calf raise	2	15
Seated calf raise	2	15
Hanging knee raise	2	15
Crunch	2	15

WEEKS 9-12 (MONDAY)

Exercise	Sets	Reps
Leg press	4	10-12
Bench press	4	10-12
Seated cable row	4	10-12
Dumbbell shoulder press	4	10-12
Barbell curl	4	10-12
Triceps pressdown	4	10-12
Standing calf raise	4	10-12
Crunch	4	15

WEEKS 9-12 (WEDNESDAY)

Exercise	Sets	Reps
Squat	4	10-12
Decline dumbbell press	4	10-12
Straight-arm pulldown	4	10-12
Rear delt raise	4	10-12
Preacher curl	4	10-12

WEEKS 9-12 (WEDNESDAY) (continued)

Exercise	Sets	Reps
Seated overhead triceps extension	4	10-12
Seated calf raise	4	10-12
Hanging leg raise	4	15

WEEKS 9-12 (FRIDAY)

Exercise	Sets	Reps
Lunge	4	12
Dumbbell incline fly	4	12
Lat pulldown	4	12
Dumbbell lateral raise	4	12
Seated incline curl	4	12
Lying triceps extension	4	12
Leg-press calf raise	4	15
Oblique crunch	4	15

WEEKS 13-16 (MONDAY AND THURSDAY): CHEST, SHOULDERS, TRAPS, BACK, ABS

Muscle group	Exercise	Sets	Reps
Chest	Incline bench press	2	8-10
	Dumbbell bench press	2	8-10
	Cable crossover	2	8-10
Shoulders	Barbell shoulder press	2	8-10
	Cable lateral raise	2	8-10
	Dumbbell rear delt raise	2	8-10
Traps	Barbell shrug	3	8-10
Back	Pull-up	2	8-10
	Dumbbell row	2	8-10
	Underhand-grip pulldown	2	8-10
Abs	Hanging knee raise	3	10-15
	Decline bench crunch	3	8-10

WEEKS 13-16 (TUESDAY AND FRIDAY): LEGS, CALVES, TRICEPS, BICEPS, FOREARMS

Muscle group	Exercise	Sets	Reps
Legs	Squat	2	8-10
	Leg press	2	8-10
	Leg extension	2	8-10
	Lying leg curl	2	8-10
Calves	Standing calf raise	3	8-10
	Seated calf raise	2	8-10
Triceps	Close-grip bench press	2	8-10
	Triceps pressdown	2	8-10
Biceps	Barbell curl	3	8-10
	Preacher curl	2	8-10
Forearms	Wrist curl	2	8-10
	Reverse wrist curl	2	8-10

WEEKS 17-20 (MONDAY): CHEST, SHOULDERS, TRAPS, BACK, ABS

Muscle group	Exercise	Sets	Reps
Chest	Bench press	3	10-12
	Incline cable fly	3	10-12
Shoulders	Dumbbell shoulder press	3	10-12
	Wide-grip upright row	3	10-12
Traps	Barbell shrug	4	10-12
Back	Pulldown	3	10-12
	T-bar row	3	10-12
Abs	Hip thrust	3	10-15
	Exercise-ball crunch	3	10-15

WEEKS 17-20 (TUESDAY): LEGS, CALVES, TRICEPS, BICEPS, FOREARMS

Muscle group	Exercise	Sets	Reps
Legs	Smith machine squat	3	10-12
	Lunge	3	10-12
	Leg extension	2	10-12
	Lying leg curl	2	10-12
Calves	Standing calf raise	3	10-12
	Seated calf raise	3	10-12
Triceps	Dip	3	10-12
	Triceps pressdown	2	10-12
Biceps	EZ-bar curl	3	10-12
	Concentration curl	3	10-12
Forearms	Dumbbell wrist curl	2	10-12
	Standing reverse wrist curl	2	10-12

WEEKS 17-20 (THURSDAY): CHEST, SHOULDERS, TRAPS, BACK, ABS

Muscle group	Exercise	Sets	Reps
Chest	Decline bench press	3	10-12
	Incline dumbbell fly	3	10-12
Shoulders	Barbell shoulder press	3	10-12
	Cable lateral raise	3	10-12
Traps	Dumbbell shrug	4	10-12
Back	Pull-up	3	10-12
	Smith machine row	3	10-12
Abs	Hanging knee raise	3	10-12
	Decline bench crunch	3	10-12

WEEKS 17-20 (FRIDAY): LEGS, CALVES, TRICEPS, BICEPS, FOREARMS

Muscle group	Exercise	Sets	Reps
Legs	Squat	3	10-12
	Hack squat	3	10-12
	One-leg leg extension	2	10-12
	Romanian deadlift	2	10-12

WEEKS 17-20 (FRIDAY): LEGS, CALVES, TRICEPS, BICEPS, FOREARM *(continued)*

Muscle group	Exercise	Sets	Reps
Calves	Donkey calf raise	3	10-12
	Seated calf raise	3	10-12
Triceps	Triceps pressdown	3	10-12
	Dumbbell lying triceps extension	2	10-12
Biceps	Barbell curl	3	10-12
	Scott curl	3	10-12
Forearms	Wrist curl	2	8-10
	Reverse wrist curl	2	8-10

WEEKS 21-24 (MONDAY AND THURSDAY): CHEST, SHOULDERS, TRAPS, BACK, ABS

Muscle group	Exercise	Sets	Reps
Chest	Bench press	3	6-8
	Decline dumbbell press	3	6-8
	Incline dumbbell fly	2	6-8
Shoulders	Dumbbell shoulder press	3	6-8
	Dumbbell lateral raise	2	6-8
	Cable rear delt raise	2	6-8
Traps	Barbell shrug	3	6-8
	Dumbbell shrug	3	6-8
Back	Pull-up	3	6-8
	Barbell row	3	6-8
	Straight-arm pulldown	3	6-8
Abs	Hanging knee raise	3	10-12
	Decline bench crunch	3	10-12

WEEKS 21-24 (TUESDAY AND FRIDAY): LEGS, CALVES, TRICEPS, BICEPS, FOREARMS

Muscle group	Exercise	Sets	Reps
Legs	Leg press	3	6-8
	Leg extension	3	6-8
	Romanian deadlift	3	6-8
Calves	Standing calf raise	3	6-8
	Seated calf raise	3	10-12
Triceps	Triceps pressdown	3	6-8
	Lying triceps extension	3	6-8
Biceps	Barbell curl	3	6-8
	Dumbbell preacher curl	3	6-8
Forearms	Wrist curl	2	8-10
	Reverse wrist curl	2	8-10

For example, chest exercises include flat bench press, incline dumbbell fly, and decline dumbbell press to hit muscle fibers of the lower, middle, and upper pecs. The exercises per muscle group drop back to just one per workout but increase in number of sets. Reps drop down to 10 to 12, while rest periods remain the same at two to three minutes between sets.

In the last three segments, you'll train with a two-day training split for a total of four workouts per week. During the first four weeks exercises will be the same for each muscle group on the two workouts that are done each week. Most major muscle groups will be trained with three exercises for a total of six sets per muscle group. The exceptions are legs, which will be trained with four exercises, and the smaller muscle groups like biceps and triceps are trained with only two exercises per workout. During the second four-week cycle, exercises drop back to about two per major muscle group, but the sets increase to three per exercise. Rest period during this entire phase drops down to one to two minutes between sets. Each muscle group is trained with different exercises on the different workout days. During the last four-week cycle the exercises increase to about three for most major muscle groups, as do the sets for most (three per exercise). After this phase is completed, you can graduate to the intermediate program.

Intermediate Program (Six Months to One Year)

If you are an intermediate lifter, you are at a unique level of weightlifting experience. Because of neurological training, you have surpassed the rapid gains in strength that beginners experience, yet you haven't started to plateau in the gains related to muscle fiber growth. You also have a fair amount of knowledge of and enthusiasm for strength training. This is the stage where the particular training program is not as critical for making continued gains as long as you maintain a periodized plan.

If you are an intermediate lifter, you should follow a basic training program that involves a three-day or four-day split, as discussed in chapter 5. Making frequent changes in exercise selection provides the muscles with resistance from a variety of angles to stress different individual muscle fibers within the targeted muscle. However, the most critical change comes in the form of the resistance, or weight, used and the number of reps performed per set.

The yearlong program found in table 7.2 outlines the rep ranges you should follow throughout the year to graduate to advanced weightlifter status. Because research shows that periodized programs that last a minimum of 8 weeks and a maximum of 20 weeks are the most beneficial (Rhea and Alderman 2004), the intermediate program follows a 20-week linear mass cycle, then an 8-week mass microcycle, and finally a 20-week undulating-mass cycle (which assumes you are using a four-day split). Each phase of the program allows one week of active recovery (where other physical activity outside of weightlifting is encouraged) before moving to the next phase, along with one week of active rest during the undulating phase, for a 52-week program that will keep the muscle gains coming. But feel free to skip these active rest weeks if you prefer to march straight through.

TABLE 7.2   Advancing Intermediate Program

PHASE 1: LINEAR MASS			PHASE 2: MICROMASS		
Week		Rep range	Week		Rep range
1-4		4-6	22		8-10
5-8		6-8	23		5-8
9-12		8-10	24		3-5
13-16		10-12	25		12-15
17-20		12-15	26		3-5
21	Active rest		27		5-8
			28		8-10
			29		10-12
			30	Active rest	

PHASE 3: UNDULATING MASS		
Week		Rep range
31	Workout 1	8-10
	Workout 2	12-15
	Workout 3	6-8
	Workout 4	12-15
32	Workout 1	6-8
	Workout 2	10-12
	Workout 3	8-10
	Workout 4	12-15
33	Workout 1	8-10
	Workout 2	3-5
	Workout 3	6-8
	Workout 4	12-15
34	Workout 1	10-12
	Workout 2	8-10
	Workout 3	6-8
	Workout 4	12-15
35	Workout 1	3-5
	Workout 2	10-12
	Workout 3	6-8
	Workout 4	8-10
36	Workout 1	12-15
	Workout 2	10-12
	Workout 3	6-8
	Workout 4	3-5
37	Workout 1	8-10
	Workout 2	12-15
	Workout 3	6-8
	Workout 4	10-12
38	Workout 1	12-15
	Workout 2	8-10
	Workout 3	3-5
	Workout 4	12-15
39	Workout 1	6-8
	Workout 2	10-12
	Workout 3	12-15
	Workout 4	8-10
40	Workout 1	10-12
	Workout 2	12-15
	Workout 3	6-8
	Workout 4	3-5
41	Active rest	

PHASE 3: UNDULATING MASS *(continued)*		
Week		Rep range
42	Workout 1	8-10
	Workout 2	12-15
	Workout 3	6-8
	Workout 4	12-15
43	Workout 1	10-12
	Workout 2	8-10
	Workout 3	12-15
	Workout 4	10-12
44	Workout 1	3-5
	Workout 2	10-12
	Workout 3	12-15
	Workout 4	6-8
45	Workout 1	8-10
	Workout 2	10-12
	Workout 3	12-15
	Workout 4	3-5
46	Workout 1	6-8
	Workout 2	12-15
	Workout 3	10-12
	Workout 4	8-10
47	Workout 1	12-15
	Workout 2	6-8
	Workout 3	8-10
	Workout 4	10-12
48	Workout 1	3-5
	Workout 2	10-12
	Workout 3	12-15
	Workout 4	6-8
49	Workout 1	8-10
	Workout 2	12-15
	Workout 3	6-8
	Workout 4	10-12
50	Workout 1	12-15
	Workout 2	8-10
	Workout 3	12-15
	Workout 4	6-8
51	Workout 1	3-5
	Workout 2	10-12
	Workout 3	8-10
	Workout 4	12-15
52	Active rest	

If you are an intermediate and are interested in making gains in general mass, you should follow the basic design guidelines in chapter 5 for making exercise selections. Rest periods should be about two to three minutes between exercises, but you should manipulate these on occasion. For example, when reps are in a low phase (4 to 6), allow up to four minutes of rest between sets. When reps are in a high phase (more than 12), limit rest to one minute between sets. For all other rep ranges, keep the rest period between sets to two to three minutes. Cycling the rest periods will further enhance gains in muscle mass.

If you are concerned with gaining muscle while losing body fat, you should limit rest periods to one minute or less. Research suggests that keeping the rest periods below one minute can enhance the number of calories burned during and after a strength training workout, regardless of the rep range used (Falvo et al. 2005). It is also wise to use as many compound exercises as possible. These use more muscle groups than isolation exercises and therefore help to burn more calories. Of course, performing aerobic exercise in addition to strength training is critical to losing body fat along with limiting caloric intake through proper dieting. For more on maximizing fat burning while building muscle and gaining strength, see part IV.

As an intermediate, if you want to use more advanced training techniques during this program, you can find numerous methods in chapter 6 that you can throw in where the rep ranges are appropriate. Several techniques found in the programs that manipulate sets and exercise selection, and even a few in the rep manipulation methods section, are not dependent on rep ranges and can be dropped in where desired. For example, try slow-rep training during weeks 5 to 8, negative training during week 23, and barbell blasting during week 26; throw in superset and forced-rep training where desired during weeks 31 to 51.

Advanced Program (More Than One Year)

If you are an advanced weightlifter, you are at the most difficult level of weightlifting in which to encourage muscle growth. This is because you have spent a long time training and therefore are closer to reaching your genetic ceiling for muscle growth. Because of this, you must frequently train with advanced training techniques that are high in intensity to help stimulate muscle growth. The one-year advanced program in table 7.3 cycles advanced training techniques found in chapter 6 with basic training splits to offer periods of lower intensity in which the muscles can recover before the next advanced technique starts. Feel free to replace any technique with one that better suits your needs at the time. The same can be said about the training splits. Neither the specific techniques nor the specific splits are critical to this yearlong program. What is important is that you cycle four to six weeks of advanced technique training with about four to six weeks of a basic training program that is lower in intensity.

TABLE 7.3 Advanced Growth Program

Week	Technique	Notes
1-4	Basic four- or five-day split	Reps: 10-12; rest: 2-3 min
5-8	5–10–20	Follow 5-day split schedule.
9-12	Advanced whole-body split	Reps: 12-15; rest: 1-2 min
13-16	Superset training	Follow 2- or 3-day split; do it twice per week. Three-day split: Workouts 1 and 4: Chest/back, shoulders/back Workouts 2 and 5: Biceps/triceps Workouts 3 and 6: Legs (quads and hamstrings) Two-day split: Workouts 1 and 3: Chest/back, shoulders/back Workouts 2 and 4: Biceps/triceps, legs (quads and hamstrings) Reps: 8-10
17	Active rest	

Week	Technique	Notes
18-21	Basic four- or five-day split	Reps: 6-8; rest: 2-3 min
22-25	Drop-set training	Follow a five-day split. Reps: 10-12 for start of each drop set; rest: 2-3 min
26-29	Basic two-day split	Choose different exercise for workouts 1 and 2 as well as workouts 3 and 4. Reps: 8-10; rest: 2-3 min
30-31	Power circuit training	Perform twice per week.
32	Tri-set training	Follow a four-day split. Two tri-set groups for chest, shoulders, back, legs. One tri-set group for biceps, triceps, traps, forearms, calves, abs. Reps: 8-10; 3 sets per tri-set; rest: 2-3 min between tri-sets
33	Giant-set training	Follow a five-day split. Do 1 giant set for all muscle groups. Do 4 sets for chest, shoulders, back, legs. Do 3 sets for biceps, triceps, traps, forearms, calves, abs. Reps: 10-12; rest: 2-3 min between tri-sets
34	Active rest	
35-38	Slow-repetition training	Follow a three-day split; train once per week. Reps: 5-10; rest: 2-3 min
39-42	Basic two- or three-day split	Train twice per week. Reps: 12-15; rest: 1-2 min
43-46	Heavy and light multiple-exercise method	Follow a four-day split. Rest: 2-3 min
47	Hundreds training	Follow a two-day split; train twice per week.
48-49	Basic five-day split	Reps: 3-6
50-51	One-sided training	Follow workout split provided on page 110.
52	Active rest	

GOAL TENDING

The long-term programs you just read about are a great start for anyone at any level of experience, as long as the goal is to put on overall muscle size. However, as weightlifters progress, their goals tend to be more specific. Maybe they want to maximize both mass and strength, maybe they want to get lean and large, or maybe they want to develop a specific muscle group. If you are an intermediate or advanced weightlifter and are interested in specific goals, you should follow a long-term program that manipulates the appropriate training variables to enable you to reach those goals. This portion of the chapter has detailed program cycles to match common goals shared by most bodybuilders. More than likely, any goal regarding strength training for muscle mass will be listed here. Try one of the following programs that meets your goals, or design your own personalized program based on the knowledge you have acquired through reading this book.

Lean and Large

Chances are that if you are interested in bodybuilding or strength training for muscle mass, you are also interested in building just lean muscle mass and not adding body fat. Body fat blurs the shape and striations of well-developed muscles.

Although a proper diet and plenty of aerobic exercise are tools to help you shed body fat while gaining muscle, certain strength training programs are better than others for getting lean. This Lean and Large program is composed of three four-week phases that all emphasize compound movements (see table 7.4). Compound exercises use the most muscle fibers and therefore burn the most calories.

TABLE 7.4 Lean and Large Program

PHASE 1: WEEKS 1-4
WORKOUT 1: CHEST AND TRICEPS

Muscle group	Exercise	Sets	Reps
Chest	Incline bench press	2	6
		2	12
	Dumbbell bench press	2	6
		2	12
	Incline fly	4	12
Triceps	Dip	2	6
		2	12
	Close-grip bench press	2	6
		2	12
	Dumbbell overhead triceps extension	2	12

WORKOUT 2: LEGS, CALVES, ABS

Muscle group	Exercise	Sets	Reps
Legs	Squat	2	6
		2	12
	Leg press	2	6
		2	12
	Leg extension	4	12
	Leg curl	4	12
Calves	Standing calf raise	4	12
	Seated calf raise	4	12
Abs	Hanging leg raise	4	12
	Crunch	4	12

WORKOUT 3: SHOULDERS AND TRAPS

Muscle group	Exercise	Sets	Reps
Shoulders	Barbell shoulder press	2	6
		2	12
	Seated dumbbell shoulder press	2	6
		2	12
	Lateral raise	4	12
Traps	Barbell shrug	2	6
		2	12
	Dumbbell shrug	2	6
		2	12

WORKOUT 4: BACK, BICEPS, FOREARMS, ABS

Muscle group	Exercise	Sets	Reps
Back	Deadlift	4	6
	Barbell row	2	6
		2	12
	Lat pulldown	2	6
		2	12
	Straight-arm pulldown	4	12

WORKOUT 4: BACK, BICEPS, FOREARMS, ABS (cont.)

Muscle group	Exercise	Sets	Reps
Biceps	Barbell curl	2	6
		2	12
	Seated incline dumbbell curl	2	6
		2	12
	Hammer curl	2	6
		2	12
Forearms	Wrist curl	2	12
	Reverse wrist curl	2	12
Abs	Reverse crunch	4	15
	Cable crunch	4	12

PHASE 2: WEEKS 5-8
WORKOUT 1: CHEST AND TRICEPS

Muscle group	Exercise	Sets	Reps
Chest	Bench press	2	5
		3	15
	Incline dumbbell press	2	5
		3	15
	Decline fly	4	15
Triceps	Smith machine close-grip bench press	2	5
		3	15
	Machine triceps dip	2	5
		3	15
	Lying triceps extension	2	15

WORKOUT 2: LEGS, CALVES, ABS

Muscle group	Exercise	Sets	Reps
Legs	Smith machine squat	2	5
		3	15
	Lunge	2	5
		3	15
	Leg extension	4	15
	Romanian deadlift	4	15
Calves	Leg press calf raise	4	15
	Seated calf raise	4	15
Abs	Hip thrust	4	15
	Crossover crunch	4	15

WORKOUT 3: SHOULDERS AND TRAPS

Muscle group	Exercise	Sets	Reps
Shoulders	Dumbbell shoulder press	2	5
		3	15
	Smith machine shoulder press	2	5
		3	15
	Wide-grip upright row	4	15
Traps	Barbell shrug	2	5
		3	15
	Dumbbell shrug	2	5
		3	15

PHASE 2: WEEKS 5-8 (continued)
WORKOUT 4: BACK, BICEPS, FOREARMS, ABS

Muscle group	Exercise	Sets	Reps
Back	Deadlift	5	5
	Dumbbell row	2	5
		3	15
	Underhand-grip pulldown	2	5
		3	15
	Straight-arm pulldown	4	15
Biceps	Standing dumbbell curl	2	5
		3	15
	Preacher curl	2	5
		3	15
	Reverse curl	2	5
		2	15
Forearms	Wrist curl	2	15
	Reverse wrist curl	2	15
Abs	Reverse crunch	4	15
	Exercise-ball crunch	4	15

PHASE 3: WEEKS 9-12
WORKOUT 1: CHEST AND TRICEPS

Muscle group	Exercise	Sets	Reps
Chest	Dumbbell bench press	3	4
		3	20
	Smith machine incline bench press	3	4
		3	20
	Cable crossover	4	20
Triceps	Dumbbell close-grip bench press	3	4
		3	20
	Dumbbell overhead triceps extension	2	4
		3	20
	Triceps pressdown	2	20

WORKOUT 2: LEGS, CALVES, ABS

Legs	Squat	3	4
		3	20
	One-leg leg press	3	4
		3	20
	Leg extension	4	20
	Romanian deadlift	4	20
Calves	Standing calf raise	4	20
	Seated calf raise	4	20
Abs	Hanging knee raise	4	20
	Decline crunch	4	20

PHASE 3: WEEKS 9-12 (continued)
WORKOUT 3: SHOULDERS AND TRAPS

Shoulders	Standing dumbbell shoulder press	3	4
		3	20
	Standing barbell shoulder press	3	4
		3	20
	Cable lateral raise	4	20
Traps	Barbell shrug	3	4
		3	20
	Dumbbell shrug	2	4
		3	20

WORKOUT 4: BACK, BICEPS, FOREARMS, ABS

Back	Deadlift	5	4
	T-bar row	3	4
		3	20
	Lat pulldown	3	4
		3	20
	Straight-arm pulldown	4	20
Biceps	Barbell curl	3	4
		3	20
	Concentration curl	3	4
		3	20
	Rope hammer curl	2	4
		2	20
Forearms	Dumbbell wrist curl	2	20
	Standing reverse wrist curl	2	20
Abs	Reverse crunch	4	20
	Crossover crunch	4	20

Training with heavy weight and low reps (4 to 6) keeps the metabolism highest after the workout. Keeping reps high (12 to 20) burns the most calories during the workout. Training heavy in addition to doing high reps has the greatest effect on calorie burn. That's why this program uses heavy weight for half the sets and light weight for the final sets of most exercises. Rest between sets is also critical for burning calories; shorter rest periods lead to greater calorie burn. This program uses rest periods of 30 to 60 seconds between sets and a four-day training split. However, you will be training six days a week to maximize your caloric expenditure. This means you can repeat the four-day split (done on consecutive days), with one rest day between workout 4 and workout 1, a total of six times. For example, you will start with workout 1 on Monday, workout 2 on Tuesday, workout 3 on Wednesday, and workout 4 on Thursday. You rest on Friday and then continue the cycle with workout 1 on Saturday.

In phase 1, you train with 6 reps on the heavy sets and 12 reps on the light sets. You do two heavy sets and two light sets for most exercises. Rest periods during this first phase are 60 seconds between sets.

In phase 2, the reps on the heavy sets drop to 5 per set while reps on the light sets increase to 15 per set. Lighter sets also increase to three per exercise to increase volume and total calories burned during the workout. Rest periods should drop to 30 seconds between sets to further enhance calorie burn during and after the workout.

In phase 3, the reps on the heavy sets drop again to 4 per set, and reps on the light sets increase to 20 per set. In this phase, heavy sets increase to three. Rest periods should remain at 30 seconds between sets.

At the end of phase 3 you can continue the 12-week program if you feel you have more body fat to lose. Take one week off from the gym with an active rest period, in which you do other activities a minimum of six days per week. Then simply start the program over at phase 1.

Big and Strong

For some weightlifters getting big is not the only goal. They are concerned with developing strength and muscle mass at the same time—and with good reason. Generally, as muscles increase in strength, they also increase in size. While there isn't a definite correlation between muscle strength and muscle size, it makes sense that if you can lift more weight or perform more reps with a given amount of weight, you will better stimulate muscle growth. This follows the principle of overload.

The six-month Big and Strong program cycles two pyramid techniques—the DeLorme ascending pyramid method (covered in chapter 9) and the Oxford descending pyramid method (covered in chapter 6). (See table 7.5.) With the DeLorme ascending pyramid technique your first set is done with about 50 percent of your 10-rep max (10RM) for a given exercise, but for just 10 reps. On the second set, you increase the weight to about 75 percent of your 10RM for that exercise and again stop at 10 reps. On the third set you increase the weight to 100 percent of your 10RM for that exercise and complete as many reps as you can until reaching failure. The repetition maximum is not critical, because many powerlifters use this pyramid method with 3RM, 4RM, 5RM, and 6RM to train for strength. In fact, during the second half of this program you will use a 6RM during the DeLorme portion of the training. With the Oxford descending pyramid technique, the first set is done with 100 percent of your 10RM to failure. On the second and third sets you reduce the weight just enough to allow you to complete about 10 reps. Again, the repetition maximum you use is not critical because it is commonly used with 6RM, 8RM, 12RM, and 15RM. In the second half of this program the reps increase to 12 per set. See table 7.5.

The DeLorme method tends to be better for deriving strength gains, while the Oxford method is better for stimulating muscle growth (Fish et al. 2003). This may be due to the amount of times you reach failure on each exercise. With the DeLorme technique, failure is reached only once, whereas the Oxford technique elicits failure on all three sets. Australian researchers have shown that training to failure on just one set increases strength gains better than going to failure on more than one set (Drinkwater et al. 2005). Muscle failure, however, seems to be important for inducing muscle growth. The reason for this is that reaching muscle failure better stimulates the release of growth hormone (GH) and insulin-like growth factor-I (IGF-I). Both are anabolic hormones that stimulate muscles to grow. That is why this program cycles both methods. In the end, you achieve greater strength and muscle growth.

TABLE 7.5 Up and Down for Strength and Size Program

WEEKS 1-6: DELORME 10RM STRENGTH PHASE
MONDAY AND THURSDAY: CHEST, SHOULDERS, TRICEPS

Exercise	Set	Weight	Reps
Incline bench press	1	50% 10RM	10
	2	75% 10RM	10
	3	100% 10RM	10*
Dumbbell bench press	1	50% 10RM	10
	2	75% 10RM	10
	3	100% 10RM	10*
Barbell shoulder press	1	50% 10RM	10
	2	75% 10RM	10
	3	100% 10RM	10*
Upright row	1	50% 10RM	10
	2	75% 10RM	10
	3	100% 10RM	10*
Barbell shrug	1	50% 10RM	10
	2	75% 10RM	10
	3	100% 10RM	10*
Close-grip bench press	1	50% 10RM	10
	2	75% 10RM	10
	3	100% 10RM	10*
Triceps pressdown	1	50% 10RM	10
	2	75% 10RM	10
	3	100% 10RM	10*

TUESDAY AND FRIDAY: LEGS, BACK, BICEPS

Exercise	Set	Weight	Reps
Barbell row	1	50% 10RM	10
	2	75% 10RM	10
	3	100% 10RM	10*
Lat pulldown	1	50% 10RM	10
	2	75% 10RM	10
	3	100% 10RM	10*
Barbell curl	1	50% 10RM	10
	2	75% 10RM	10
	3	100% 10RM	10*
Dumbbell hammer curl	1	50% 10RM	10
	2	75% 10RM	10
	3	100% 10RM	10*
Squat	1	50% 10RM	10
	2	75% 10RM	10
	3	100% 10RM	10*
Leg press	1	50% 10RM	10
	2	75% 10RM	10
	3	100% 10RM	10*

TUESDAY AND FRIDAY: LEGS, BACK, BICEPS (continued)

Exercise	Set	Weight	Reps
Romanian deadlift	1	50% 10RM	10
	2	75% 10RM	10
	3	100% 10RM	10*
Standing calf raise	1	50% 10RM	10
	2	75% 10RM	10
	3	100% 10RM	10*
Seated calf raise	1	50% 10RM	10
	2	75% 10RM	10
	3	100% 10RM	10*

WEEKS 7-12: OXFORD 10RM MASS PHASE
MONDAY: CHEST AND TRICEPS

Exercise	Set	Weight	Reps (to failure)
Incline dumbbell bench press	1	100% 10RM	10
	2	<100% 10RM**	10
	3	<100% 10RM	10
Smith machine bench press	1	100% 10RM	10
	2	<100% 10RM	10
	3	<100% 10RM	10
Incline dumbbell fly	1	100% 10RM	10
	2	<100% 10RM	10
	3	<100% 10RM	10
Triceps pressdown	1	100% 10RM	10
	2	<100% 10RM	10
	3	<100% 10RM	10
Seated overhead triceps extension	1	100% 10RM	10
	2	<100% 10RM	10
	3	<100% 10RM	10

TUESDAY: LEGS

Exercise	Set	Weight	Reps (to failure)
Smith machine squat	1	100% 10RM	10
	2	<100% 10RM	10
	3	<100% 10RM	10
Lunge	1	100% 10RM	10
	2	<100% 10RM	10
	3	<100% 10RM	10
Leg extension	1	100% 10RM	10
	2	<100% 10RM	10
	3	<100% 10RM	10
Leg curl	1	100% 10RM	10
	2	<100% 10RM	10
	3	<100% 10RM	10

Note: Abs can be done at the end of any of these workouts.

*To failure.

**On the second and third sets of each exercise in this phase, reduce weight just enough to allow 10 reps to be completed.

> continued

TABLE 7.5 Up and Down for Strength and Size Program *(continued)*

THURSDAY: SHOULDERS

Exercise	Set	Weight	Reps (to failure)
Dumbbell shoulder press	1	100% 10RM	10
	2	<100% 10RM	10
	3	<100% 10RM	10
Lateral raise	1	100% 10RM	10
	2	<100% 10RM	10
	3	<100% 10RM	10
Bent-over lateral raise	1	100% 10RM	10
	2	<100% 10RM	10
	3	<100% 10RM	10
Dumbbell shrug	1	100% 10RM	10
	2	<100% 10RM	10
	3	<100% 10RM	10

FRIDAY: BACK AND BICEPS

Exercise	Set	Weight	Reps
Lat pulldown	1	100% 10RM	10
	2	<100% 10RM	10
	3	<100% 10RM	10
T-bar row	1	100% 10RM	10
	2	<100% 10RM	10
	3	<100% 10RM	10
Straight-arm pulldown	1	100% 10RM	10
	2	<100% 10RM	10
	3	<100% 10RM	10
Seated incline curl	1	100% 10RM	10
	2	<100% 10RM	10
	3	<100% 10RM	10
Preacher curl	1	100% 10RM	10
	2	<100% 10RM	10
	3	<100% 10RM	10
Reverse-grip curl	1	100% 10RM	10
	2	<100% 10RM	10
	3	<100% 10RM	10

WEEKS 13-18: DELORME 6RM STRENGTH PYRAMID
MONDAY AND THURSDAY: CHEST, SHOULDERS, TRICEPS

Exercise	Set	Weight	Reps
Incline bench press	1	50% 6RM	6
	2	75% 6RM	6
	3	100% 6RM	6*
Dumbbell bench press	1	50% 6RM	6
	2	75% 6RM	6
	3	100% 6RM	6*

MONDAY AND THURSDAY: CHEST, SHOULDERS, TRICEPS *(continued)*

Exercise	Set	Weight	Reps
Barbell shoulder press	1	50% 6RM	6
	2	75% 6RM	6
	3	100% 6RM	6*
Upright row	1	50% 6RM	6
	2	75% 6RM	6
	3	100% 6RM	6*
Barbell shrug	1	50% 6RM	6
	2	75% 6RM	6
	3	100% 6RM	6*
Close-grip bench press	1	50% 6RM	6
	2	75% 6RM	6
	3	100% 6RM	6*
Triceps pressdown	1	50% 6RM	6
	2	75% 6RM	6
	3	100% 6RM	6*

TUESDAY AND FRIDAY: LEGS, BACK, BICEPS

Exercise	Set	Weight	Reps
Barbell row	1	50% 6RM	6
	2	75% 6RM	6
	3	100% 6RM	6*
Lat pulldown	1	50% 6RM	6
	2	75% 6RM	6
	3	100% 6RM	6*
Barbell curl	1	50% 6RM	6
	2	75% 6RM	6
	3	100% 6RM	6*
Dumbbell hammer curl	1	50% 6RM	6
	2	75% 6RM	6
	3	100% 6RM	6*
Squat	1	50% 6RM	6
	2	75% 6RM	6
	3	100% 6RM	6*

Note: Abs can be done at the end of any of these workouts.

*To failure.

**On the second and third sets of each exercise in this phase, reduce weight just enough to allow 10 reps to be completed.

TUESDAY AND FRIDAY: LEGS, BACK, BICEPS (continued)

Exercise	Set	Weight	Reps
Leg press	1	50% 6RM	6
	2	75% 6RM	6
	3	100% 6RM	6*
Romanian deadlift	1	50% 6RM	6
	2	75% 6RM	6
	3	100% 6RM	6*
Standing calf raise	1	50% 6RM	6
	2	75% 6RM	6
	3	100% 6RM	6*
Seated calf raise	1	50% 6RM	6
	2	75% 6RM	6
	3	100% 6RM	6*

WEEKS 19-24: OXFORD 12RM MASS PHASE
MONDAY: CHEST AND TRICEPS

Exercise	Set	Weight	Reps (to failure)
Incline dumbbell bench press	1	100% 12RM	12
	2	<100% 12RM**	12
	3	<100% 12RM	12
Smith machine bench press	1	100% 12RM	12
	2	<100% 12RM	12
	3	<100% 12RM	12
Incline dumbbell fly	1	100% 12RM	12
	2	<100% 12RM	12
	3	<100% 12RM	12
Triceps pressdown	1	100% 12RM	12
	2	<100% 12RM	12
	3	<100% 12RM	12
Seated overhead triceps extension	1	100% 12RM	12
	2	<100% 12RM	12
	3	<100% 12RM	12

TUESDAY: LEGS

Exercise	Set	Weight	Reps (to failure)
Smith machine squat	1	100% 12RM	12
	2	<100% 12RM	12
	3	<100% 12RM	12
Lunge	1	100% 12RM	12
	2	<100% 12RM	12
	3	<100% 12RM	12
Leg extension	1	100% 12RM	12
	2	<100% 12RM	12
	3	<100% 12RM	12

TUESDAY: LEGS (continued)

Exercise	Set	Weight	Reps (to failure)
Leg curl	1	100% 12RM	12
	2	<100% 12RM	12
	3	<100% 12RM	12

THURSDAY: SHOULDERS

Exercise	Set	Weight	Reps (to failure)
Dumbbell shoulder press	1	100% 12RM	12
	2	<100% 12RM	12
	3	<100% 12RM	12
Lateral raise	1	100% 12RM	12
	2	<100% 12RM	12
	3	<100% 12RM	12
Bent-over lateral raise	1	100% 12RM	12
	2	<100% 12RM	12
	3	<100% 12RM	12
Dumbbell shrugs	1	100% 12RM	12
	2	<100% 12RM	12
	3	<100% 12RM	12

FRIDAY: BACK AND BICEPS

Exercise	Set	Weight	Reps (to failure)
Lat pulldown	1	100% 12RM	12
	2	<100% 12RM	12
	3	<100% 12RM	12
T-bar row	1	100% 12RM	12
	2	<100% 12RM	12
	3	<100% 12RM	12
Straight-arm pulldown	1	100% 12RM	12
	2	<100% 12RM	12
	3	<100% 12RM	12
Seated incline curl	1	100% 12RM	12
	2	<100% 12RM	12
	3	<100% 12RM	12
Preacher curl	1	100% 12RM	12
	2	<100% 12RM	12
	3	<100% 12RM	12
Reverse-grip curl	1	100% 12RM	12
	2	<100% 12RM	12
	3	<100% 12RM	12

Note: Abs can be done at the end of any of these workouts.

*To failure.

**On the second and third sets of each exercise in this phase, reduce weight just enough to allow 10 reps to be completed.

With the Big and Strong program you pyramid up in weight on all your exercises during weeks 1 to 6 and again during weeks 13 to 18. The difference in these two phases is the amount of weight you do on the last set of each exercise. During weeks 1 to 6 you end with a weight you can do for 10 reps. During weeks 13 to 18 you end with a weight that you can do for 6 reps. During these parts of the program you will train each muscle group twice per week. That's because you will need less recovery time between workouts because you do fewer total working sets per workout and train to failure on only one set per exercise.

You can use the strength you gain during weeks 1 to 6 and 13 to 18 for lifting heavier weights during weeks 7 to 12 and 19 to 24. Weeks 7 to 12 and 9 to 24 take you down the pyramid as you decrease the weight on each successive set for all exercises. During these phases, you train each muscle group just once per week because they will need the recovery since you will do more total working sets per muscle group, plus you will train to failure on every set.

Shortcut to Size (Micromuscle) Program

One of my most popular training programs is the 12-week Shortcut to Size (a.k.a. Micromuscle) that is featured on bodybuilding.com and detailed in table 7.6. More than a million people have completed the program, and many have gained as much as 20 pounds (about 9 kilograms) of lean muscle. The strength gains with this program are also phenomenal.

The Shortcut to Size program is based on linear periodization using microcycles, as covered in chapter 3. In week 1 your rep range will be 12 to 15. In week 2 you bump up all the weights and drop reps to 9 to 11. Week 3 adds weight again to each exercise to drop the rep range to 6 to 8. And in week 4 you bump the weight up again to drop reps to 3 to 5 per set. Those are the four microcycles that you will repeat. On week 4 you have completed the first phase. On week 5 you drop the weight back down and start all over at 12 to 15 reps per set. This is the start of phase 2. But now you will be able to do each rep range with at least 5 and up to 20 pounds (a little less than 2.5 and as much as about 9 kilograms) more than you could in phase 1. In week 6 (week 2 of

phase 2), you will be back at 9 to 11 reps per set. In week 7, or week 3 of phase 2, weight will go up again to drop your reps down to 6 to 8 per set. And in week 8 (or week 4 of phase 2), weight will increase for 3 to 5 reps per set. That completes phase 2. And in week 9 you start the final phase (phase 3) by dropping back down to 12 to 15 reps per set and run through the four microcycles again until you are back down at 3 to 5 reps per set. Of course, in each phase you will be using 5 to 20 pounds more than you did in phase 2 and 10 to 40 pounds (4.5 to 18 kilograms) more than you used in phase 1. This is how you get stronger—much stronger—over this 12-week program.

The constant increase in weight each week and the recycling of these four phases lead to impressive gains in strength. The microcycles also lead to muscle hypertrophy due to the constant changing of the rep ranges each week. Another reason for the gains in strength and mass has to do with the fact that you keep the weight steady on each exercise for all sets and you are forced to complete the minimum number of reps in that rep range.

Greater gains in strength and muscle mass are guaranteed with this program. I have seen some impressive results with this program. In men, I have seen gains of strength over 90 pounds on the squat and over 50 pounds on the bench press. And for muscle, many guys have gained over 20 pounds of muscle, as I mentioned. Yes, pure muscle, while actually dropping body fat. Speaking of body fat, when maximizing body fat with my training and diet tweaks, some men have lost over 20 pounds of body fat. And women have also seen impressive gains in strength and muscle while losing body fat. Women following my program have increased their squat strength by over 60 pounds and bench press strength by 30 pounds. And they have seen gains in muscle of over 10 pounds and fat loss over 10 pounds.

The first exercise you do for each muscle group (except for abs and calves) will remain constant throughout all 12 weeks. This is the exercise where you focus on increasing your strength. Most of the assistance exercises that follow the first exercise will change in every phase. For abs, the exercises will change each week based on the rep ranges. This is because some ab exercises are easier to do for higher reps, while some are difficult to do for lower reps. So I organized the best ab exercises for the prescribed rep ranges.

TABLE 7.6 Shortcut to Size Program

PHASE 1: WEEK 1
WORKOUT 1: CHEST, TRICEPS, CALVES

Exercise	Sets × reps
Bench press	4 × 12-15
Incline bench press	3 × 12-15
Incline dumbbell fly	3 × 12-15
Cable crossover	3 × 12-15
Triceps pressdown	3 × 12-15
Lying triceps extension	3 × 12-15
Cable overhead triceps extension	3 × 12-15
Standing calf raise	4 × 25-30
Seated calf raise	4 × 25-30

WORKOUT 2: BACK, BICEPS, ABS

Exercise	Sets × reps
Dumbbell bent-over row	4 × 12-15
Wide-grip pulldown	3 × 12-15
Standing pulldown	3 × 12-15
Straight arm pulldown	3 × 12-15
Barbell curl	4 × 12-15
Dumbbell incline curl	3 × 12-15
One-arm high cable curl	3 × 12-15
Hip thrust	3 × 20-30[1]
Crunch	3 × 20-30[1]
Oblique crunch	3 × 20-30[1]

WORKOUT 3: SHOULDERS, TRAPS, CALVES

Exercise	Sets × reps
Dumbbell shoulder press	4 × 12-15
Dumbbell lateral raise	3 × 12-15
One-arm cable front raise	3 × 12-15
High cable reverse fly	3 × 12-15
Dumbbell shrug	4 × 12-15
Seated calf raise	4 × 25-30
Leg press calf raise	4 × 25-30

WORKOUT 4: LEGS AND ABS

Exercise	Sets × reps
Squat	4 × 12-15
One-leg press	3 × 12-15
Leg extension	3 × 12-15
Romanian deadlift	4 × 12-15
Lying leg curl	3 × 12-15
Hip thrust	3 × 20-30[1]
Crunch	3 × 20-30[1]
Plank	3 × 1 minute

PHASE 1: WEEK 2
WORKOUT 1: CHEST, TRICEPS, CALVES

Exercise	Sets × reps
Bench press	4 × 9-11
Incline bench press	3 × 9-11
Incline dumbbell fly	3 × 9-11
Cable crossover	3 × 9-11
Triceps pressdown	3 × 9-11
Lying triceps extension	3 × 9-11
Cable overhead triceps extension	3 × 9-11
Standing calf raise	4 × 15-20
Seated calf raise	4 × 15-20

WORKOUT 2: BACK, BICEPS, ABS

Exercise	Sets × reps
Dumbbell bent-over row	4 × 9-11
Wide-grip pulldown	3 × 9-11
Standing pulldown	3 × 9-11
Straight arm pulldown	3 × 9-11
Barbell curl	4 × 9-11
Dumbbell incline curl	3 × 9-11
One-arm high cable curl	3 × 9-11
Hanging leg raise	3 × 15-19[2]
Weighted crunch	3 × 15-19
Dumbbell side bend	3 × 15-19

WORKOUT 3: SHOULDERS, TRAPS, CALVES

Exercise	Sets × reps
Dumbbell shoulder press	4 × 9-11
Dumbbell lateral raise	3 × 9-11
One-arm cable front raise	3 × 9-11
High cable rear delt fly	3 × 9-11
Dumbbell shrug	4 × 9-11
Seated calf raise	4 × 15-20
Leg press calf raise	4 × 15-20

WORKOUT 4: LEGS AND ABS

Exercise	Sets × reps
Squat	4 × 9-11
One-leg leg press	3 × 9-11
Leg extension	3 × 9-11
Romanian deadlift	4 × 9-11
Lying leg curl	3 × 9-11
Hanging leg raise	3 × 15-19[2]
Weighted crunch	3 × 15-19
Side plank	3 × 1 min

[1]Shoot for 20 to 30 reps, but if you can do more, continue until reaching failure. If you cannot complete 20 reps, do as many as you can, trying to get as close to 20 reps as possible.

[2]If you cannot complete 15 reps, do as many as you can, trying to get as close to 15 reps as possible.

[3]Perform the hip thrust while holding a medicine ball or dumbbell between your feet or while wearing ankle weights.

> continued

TABLE 7.6 Shortcut to Size Program *(continued)*

PHASE 1: WEEK 3
WORKOUT 1: CHEST, TRICEPS, CALVES

Exercise	Sets × reps
Bench press	4 × 6-8
Incline bench press	3 × 6-8
Incline dumbbell fly	3 × 6-8
Cable crossover	3 × 6-8
Triceps pressdown	3 × 6-8
Lying triceps extension	3 × 6-8
Cable overhead triceps extension	3 × 6-8
Standing calf raise	4 × 10-14
Seated calf raise	4 × 10-14

WORKOUT 2: BACK, BICEPS, ABS

Exercise	Sets × reps
Dumbbell bent-over row	4 × 6-8
Wide-grip pulldown	3 × 6-8
Standing pulldown	3 × 6-8
Straight arm pulldown	3 × 6-8
Barbell curl	4 × 6-8
Dumbbell incline curl	3 × 6-8
One-arm high cable curl	3 × 6-8
Weighted hip thrust[3]	3 × 10-14
Cable crunch	3 × 10-14
Cable oblique crunch	3 × 10-14

WORKOUT 3: SHOULDERS, TRAPS, CALVES

Exercise	Sets × reps
Dumbbell shoulder press	4 × 6-8
Dumbbell lateral raise	3 × 6-8
One-arm cable front raise	3 × 6-8
High cable rear delt fly	3 × 6-8
Dumbbell shrug	4 × 6-8
Seated calf raise	4 × 10-14
Leg press calf raise	4 × 10-14

WORKOUT 4: LEGS AND ABS

Exercise	Sets × reps
Squat	4 × 6-8
One-leg press	3 × 6-8
Leg extension	3 × 6-8
Romanian deadlift	4 × 6-8
Lying leg curl	3 × 6-8
Weighted hip thrust[3]	3 × 10-14
Cable crunch	3 × 10-14
Cable woodchopper	3 × 10-14

PHASE 1: WEEK 4
WORKOUT 1: CHEST, TRICEPS, CALVES

Exercise	Sets × reps
Bench press	4 × 3-5
Incline bench press	3 × 3-5
Incline dumbbell fly	3 × 3-5
Cable crossover	3 × 3-5
Triceps pressdown	3 × 3-5
Lying triceps extension	3 × 3-5
Cable overhead triceps extension	3 × 3-5
Standing calf raise	4 × 6-9
Seated calf raise	4 × 6-9

WORKOUT 2: BACK, BICEPS, ABS

Exercise	Sets × reps
Dumbbell bent-over row	4 × 3-5
Wide-grip pulldown	3 × 3-5
Standing pulldown	3 × 3-5
Straight arm pulldown	3 × 3-5
Barbell curl	4 × 3-5
Dumbbell incline curl	3 × 3-5
One-arm high cable curl	3 × 3-5
Smith machine hip thrust	3 × 6-9
Machine crunch	3 × 6-9
Band roundhouse elbow	3 × 6-9

WORKOUT 3: SHOULDERS, TRAPS, CALVES

Exercise	Sets × reps
Dumbbell shoulder press	4 × 3-5
Dumbbell lateral raise	3 × 3-5
One-arm cable front raise	3 × 3-5
High cable rear delt fly	3 × 3-5
Dumbbell shrug	4 × 3-5
Seated calf raise	4 × 6-9
Leg press calf raise	4 × 6-9

WORKOUT 4: LEGS AND ABS

Exercise	Sets × reps
Squat	4 × 3-5
One-leg press	3 × 3-5
Leg extension	3 × 3-5
Romanian deadlift	4 × 3-5
Lying leg curl	3 × 3-5
Smith machine hip thrust	3 × 6-9
Machine crunch	3 × 6-9
Plank	3 × 75 sec

[1]Shoot for 20 to 30 reps, but if you can do more, continue until reaching failure. If you cannot complete 20 reps, do as many as you can, trying to get as close to 20 reps as possible.

[2]If you cannot complete 15 reps, do as many as you can, trying to get as close to 15 reps as possible.

[3]Perform the hip thrust while holding a medicine ball or dumbbell between your feet or while wearing ankle weights.

PHASE 2: WEEK 1	
WORKOUT 1: CHEST, TRICEPS, CALVES	
Exercise	Sets × reps
Bench press	4 × 12-15
Incline dumbbell press	3 × 12-15
Dumbbell fly	3 × 12-15
Incline cable fly	3 × 12-15
Triceps pressdown	3 × 12-15
Dumbbell overhead triceps extension	3 × 12-15
Cable lying triceps extension	3 × 12-15
Standing calf raise	4 × 25-30
Seated calf raise	4 × 25-30
WORKOUT 2: BACK, BICEPS, ABS	
Dumbbell bent-over row	4 × 12-15
Behind-the-neck pulldown	3 × 12-15
Seated cable row	3 × 12-15
Reverse-grip pulldown	3 × 12-15
Barbell curl	4 × 12-15
Preacher curl	3 × 12-15
Behind-the-back cable curl	3 × 12-15
Hip thrust	3 × 20-30[1]
Crunch	3 × 20-30[1]
Oblique crunch	3 × 20-30[1]
WORKOUT 3: SHOULDERS, TRAPS, CALVES	
Dumbbell shoulder press	4 × 12-15
Smith machine upright row	3 × 12-15
One-arm cable lateral raise	3 × 12-15
Bent-over lateral raise	3 × 12-15
Barbell shrug	4 × 12-15
Seated calf raise	4 × 25-30
Leg press calf raise	4 × 25-30
WORKOUT 4: LEGS AND ABS	
Squat	4 × 12-15
Front squat	3 × 12-15
Leg extension	3 × 12-15
Romanian deadlift	4 × 12-15
Seated leg curl	3 × 12-15
Hip thrust	3 × 20-30[1]
Crunch	3 × 20-30[1]
Plank	3 × 75 sec

PHASE 2: WEEK 2	
WORKOUT 1: CHEST, TRICEPS, CALVES	
Exercise	Sets × reps
Bench press	4 × 9-11
Incline dumbbell press	3 × 9-11
Dumbbell fly	3 × 9-11
Incline cable fly	3 × 9-11
Triceps pressdown	3 × 9-11
Dumbbell overhead triceps extension	3 × 9-11
Cable lying triceps extension	3 × 9-11
Standing calf raise	4 × 15-20
Seated calf raise	4 × 15-20
WORKOUT 2: BACK, BICEPS, ABS	
Dumbbell bent-over row	4 × 9-11
Behind-the-neck pulldown	3 × 9-11
Seated cable row	3 × 9-11
Reverse-grip pulldown	3 × 9-11
Barbell curl	4 × 9-11
Preacher curl	3 × 9-11
Behind-the-back cable curl	3 × 9-11
Hanging leg raise	3 × 15-19[2][1]
Weighted crunch	3 × 15-19
Dumbbell side bend	3 × 15-19
WORKOUT 3: SHOULDERS, TRAPS, CALVES	
Dumbbell shoulder press	4 × 9-11
Smith machine upright row	3 × 9-11
One-arm cable lateral raise	3 × 9-11
Bent-over lateral raise	3 × 9-11
Barbell shrug	4 × 9-11
Seated calf raise	4 × 15-20
Leg press calf raise	4 × 15-20
WORKOUT 4: LEGS AND ABS	
Squat	4 × 9-11
Front squat	3 × 9-11
Leg extension	3 × 9-11
Romanian deadlift	4 × 9-11
Seated leg curl	3 × 9-11
Hanging leg raise	3 × 15-19[1]
Weighted crunch	3 × 15-19
Side plank	3 × 75 sec

[1]Shoot for 20 to 30 reps, but if you can do more, continue until reaching failure. If you cannot complete 20 reps, do as many as you can, trying to get as close to 20 reps as possible.

[2]If you cannot complete 15 reps, do as many as you can, trying to get as close to 15 reps as possible.

[3]Perform the hip thrust while holding a medicine ball or dumbbell between your feet or while wearing ankle weights.

> continued

TABLE 7.6 Shortcut to Size Program *(continued)*

PHASE 2: WEEK 3
WORKOUT 1: CHEST, TRICEPS, CALVES

Exercise	Sets × reps
Bench press	4 × 6-8
Incline dumbbell press	3 × 6-8
Dumbbell fly	3 × 6-8
Incline cable fly	3 × 6-8
Triceps pressdown	3 × 6-8
Dumbbell overhead triceps extension	3 × 6-8
Cable lying triceps extension	3 × 6-8
Standing calf raise	4 × 10-14
Seated calf raise	4 × 10-14

WORKOUT 2: BACK, BICEPS, ABS

Exercise	Sets × reps
Dumbbell bent-over row	4 × 6-8
Behind-the-neck pulldown	3 × 6-8
Seated cable row	3 × 6-8
Reverse-grip pulldown	3 × 6-8
Barbell curl	4 × 6-8
Preacher curl	3 × 6-8
Behind-the-back cable curl	3 × 6-8
Weighted hip thrust[3]	3 × 10-14
Cable crunch	3 × 10-14
Cable oblique crunch	3 × 10-14

WORKOUT 3: SHOULDERS, TRAPS, CALVES

Exercise	Sets × reps
Dumbbell shoulder press	4 × 6-8
Smith machine upright row	3 × 6-8
One-arm cable lateral raise	3 × 6-8
Bent-over lateral raise	3 × 6-8
Barbell shrug	4 × 6-8
Seated calf raise	4 × 10-14
Leg press calf raise	4 × 10-14

WORKOUT 4: LEGS AND ABS

Exercise	Sets × reps
Squat	4 × 6-8
Front squat	3 × 6-8
Leg extension	3 × 6-8
Romanian deadlift	4 × 6-8
Seated leg curl	3 × 6-8
Weighted hip thrust[3]	3 × 10-14
Cable crunch	3 × 10-14
Cable woodchopper	3 × 10-14

PHASE 2: WEEK 4
WORKOUT 1: CHEST, TRICEPS, CALVES

Exercise	Sets × reps
Bench press	4 × 3-5
Incline dumbbell press	3 × 3-5
Dumbbell fly	3 × 3-5
Incline cable fly	3 × 3-5
Triceps pressdown	3 × 3-5
Dumbbell overhead triceps extension	3 × 3-5
Cable lying triceps extension	3 × 3-5
Standing calf raise	4 × 6-9
Seated calf raise	4 × 6-9

WORKOUT 2: BACK, BICEPS, ABS

Exercise	Sets × reps
Dumbbell bent-over row	4 × 3-5
Behind-the-neck pulldown	3 × 3-5
Seated cable row	3 × 3-5
Reverse-grip pulldown	3 × 3-5
Barbell curl	4 × 3-5
Preacher curl	3 × 3-5
Behind-the-back cable curl	3 × 3-5
Smith machine hip thrust	3 × 6-9
Machine crunch	3 × 6-9
Band roundhouse elbow	3 × 6-9

WORKOUT 3: SHOULDERS, TRAPS, CALVES

Exercise	Sets × reps
Dumbbell shoulder press	4 × 3-5
Smith machine upright row	3 × 3-5
One-arm cable lateral raise	3 × 3-5
Bent-over lateral raise	3 × 3-5
Barbell shrug	4 × 3-5
Seated calf raise	4 × 6-9
Leg press calf raise	4 × 6-9

WORKOUT 4: LEGS AND ABS

Exercise	Sets × reps
Squat	4 × 3-5
Front squat	3 × 3-5
Leg extension	3 × 3-5
Romanian deadlift	4 × 3-5
Seated leg curl	3 × 3-5
Smith machine hip thrust	3 × 6-9
Machine crunch	3 × 6-9
Plank	3 × 90 sec

[1]Shoot for 20 to 30 reps, but if you can do more, continue until reaching failure. If you cannot complete 20 reps, do as many as you can, trying to get as close to 20 reps as possible.

[2]If you cannot complete 15 reps, do as many as you can, trying to get as close to 15 reps as possible.

[3]Perform the hip thrust while holding a medicine ball or dumbbell between your feet or while wearing ankle weights.

PHASE 3: WEEK 1 WORKOUT 1: CHEST, TRICEPS, CALVES	
Exercise	**Sets × reps**
Bench Press	4 × 12-15
Reverse-grip incline dumbbell press	3 × 12-15
Incline dumbbell fly	3 × 12-15
Cable crossover	3 × 12-15
Triceps pressdown	3 × 12-15
One-arm overhead cable triceps extension	3 × 12-15
Close-grip bench press	3 × 12-15
Standing calf raise	4 × 25-30
Seated calf raise	4 × 25-30
WORKOUT 2: BACK, BICEPS, ABS	
Dumbbell bent-over row	4 × 12-15
Wide-grip pulldown	3 × 12-15
Straight-arm pulldown	3 × 12-15
Seated cable row	3 × 12-15
Barbell curl	4 × 12-15
Incline cable curl	3 × 12-15
Dumbbell concentration curl	3 × 12-15
Hip thrust	3 × 20-30[1]
Crunch	3 × 20-30[1]
Oblique crunch	3 × 20-30[1]
WORKOUT 3: SHOULDERS, TRAPS, CALVES	
Dumbbell shoulder press	4 × 12-15
Dumbbell lateral raise	3 × 12-15
Dumbbell upright row	3 × 12-15
Bent-over lateral raise	3 × 12-15
One-arm Smith machine shrug	4 × 12-15
Seated calf raise	4 × 25-30
Leg press calf raise	4 × 25-30
WORKOUT 4: LEGS AND ABS	
Squat	4 × 12-15
Leg press	3 × 12-15
Leg extension	3 × 12-15
Romanian deadlift	4 × 12-15
Lying leg curl	3 × 12-15
Hip thrust	3 × 20-30[1]
Crunch	3 × 20-30[1]
Plank	3 × 90 sec

PHASE 3: WEEK 2 WORKOUT 1: CHEST, TRICEPS, CALVES	
Exercise	**Sets × reps**
Bench press	4 × 9-11
Reverse-grip incline dumbbell press	3 × 9-11
Incline dumbbell fly	3 × 9-11
Cable crossover	3 × 9-11
Triceps pressdown	3 × 9-11
One-arm overhead cable triceps extension	3 × 9-11
Close-grip bench press	3 × 9-11
Standing calf raise	4 × 15-20
Seated calf raise	4 × 15-20
WORKOUT 2: BACK, BICEPS, ABS	
Dumbbell bent-over row	4 × 9-11
Wide-grip pulldown	3 × 9-11
Straight-arm pulldown	3 × 9-11
Seated cable row	3 × 9-11
Barbell curl	4 × 9-11
Incline cable curl	3 × 9-11
Dumbbell concentration curl	3 × 9-11
Hanging leg raise	3 × 15-19[2]
Weighted crunch	3 × 15-19
Dumbbell side bend	3 × 15-19
WORKOUT 3: SHOULDERS, TRAPS, CALVES	
Dumbbell shoulder press	4 × 9-11
Dumbbell lateral raise	3 × 9-11
Dumbbell upright row	3 × 9-11
Bent-over lateral raise	3 × 9-11
One-arm smith machine shrug	4 × 9-11
Seated calf raise	4 × 15-20
Leg press calf raise	4 × 15-20
WORKOUT 4: LEGS AND ABS	
Squat	4 × 9-11
Leg press	3 × 9-11
Leg extension	3 × 9-11
Romanian deadlift	4 × 9-11
Lying leg curl	3 × 9-11
Hanging leg raise	3 × 15-19[2]
Weighted crunch	3 × 15-19
Side plank	3 × 90 sec

[1]Shoot for 20 to 30 reps, but if you can do more, continue until reaching failure. If you cannot complete 20 reps, do as many as you can, trying to get as close to 20 reps as possible.

[2]If you cannot complete 15 reps, do as many as you can, trying to get as close to 15 reps as possible.

[3]Perform the hip thrust while holding a medicine ball or dumbbell between your feet or while wearing ankle weights.

> continued

TABLE 7.6 Shortcut to Size Program *(continued)*

PHASE 3: WEEK 3
WORKOUT 1: CHEST, TRICEPS, CALVES

Exercise	Sets × reps
Bench press	4 × 6-8
Reverse-grip incline dumbbell press	3 × 6-8
Incline dumbbell fly	3 × 6-8
Cable crossover	3 × 6-8
Triceps pressdown	3 × 6-8
One-arm overhead cable triceps extension	3 × 6-8
Close-grip bench press	3 × 6-8
Standing calf raise	4 × 10-14
Seated calf raise	4 × 10-14

WORKOUT 2: BACK, BICEPS, ABS

Exercise	Sets × reps
Dumbbell bent-over row	4 × 6-8
Wide-grip pulldown	3 × 6-8
Straight-arm pulldown	3 × 6-8
Seated cable row	3 × 6-8
Barbell curl	4 × 6-8
Incline cable curl	3 × 6-8
Dumbbell concentration curl	3 × 6-8
Weighted hip thrust[3]	3 × 10-14
Cable crunch	3 × 10-14
Cable oblique crunch	3 × 10-14

WORKOUT 3: SHOULDERS, TRAPS, CALVES

Exercise	Sets × reps
Dumbbell shoulder press	4 × 6-8
Dumbbell lateral raise	3 × 6-8
Dumbbell upright row	3 × 6-8
Bent-over lateral raise	3 × 6-8
One-arm smith machine shrug	4 × 6-8
Seated calf raise	4 × 10-14
Leg press calf raise	4 × 10-14

WORKOUT 4: LEGS AND ABS

Exercise	Sets × reps
Squat	4 × 6-8
Leg press	3 × 6-8
Leg extension	3 × 6-8
Romanian deadlift	4 × 6-8
Lying leg curl	3 × 6-8
Weighted hip thrust[3]	3 × 10-14
Cable crunch	3 × 10-14
Cable woodchopper	3 × 10-14

PHASE 3: WEEK 4
WORKOUT 1: CHEST, TRICEPS, CALVES

Exercise	Sets × reps
Bench press	4 × 3-5
Reverse-grip incline dumbbell press	3 × 3-5
Incline dumbbell fly	3 × 3-5
Cable crossover	3 × 3-5
Triceps pressdown	3 × 3-5
One-arm overhead cable triceps extension	3 × 3-5
Close-grip bench press	3 × 3-5
Standing calf raise	4 × 6-9
Seated calf raise	4 × 6-9

WORKOUT 2: BACK, BICEPS, ABS

Exercise	Sets × reps
Dumbbell bent-over row	4 × 3-5
Wide-grip pulldown	3 × 3-5
Straight-arm pulldown	3 × 3-5
Seated cable row	3 × 3-5
Barbell curl	4 × 3-5
Incline cable curl	3 × 3-5
Dumbbell concentration curl	3 × 3-5
Smith machine hip thrust	3 × 6-9
Machine crunch	3 × 6-9
Band roundhouse elbow	3 × 6-9

WORKOUT 3: SHOULDERS, TRAPS, CALVES

Exercise	Sets × reps
Dumbbell shoulder press	4 × 3-5
Dumbbell lateral raise	3 × 3-5
Dumbbell upright row	3 × 3-5
Bent-over lateral raise	3 × 3-5
One-arm smith machine shrug	4 × 3-5
Seated calf raise	4 × 6-9
Leg press calf raise	4 × 6-9

WORKOUT 4: LEGS AND ABS

Exercise	Sets × reps
Squat	4 × 3-5
Leg press	3 × 3-5
Leg extension	3 × 3-5
Romanian deadlift	4 × 3-5
Lying leg curl	3 × 3-5
Smith machine hip thrust	3 × 6-9
Machine crunch	3 × 6-9
Plank	3 × 105 sec

[1]Shoot for 20 to 30 reps, but if you can do more, continue until reaching failure. If you cannot complete 20 reps, do as many as you can, trying to get as close to 20 reps as possible.

[2]If you cannot complete 15 reps, do as many as you can, trying to get as close to 15 reps as possible.

[3]Perform the hip thrust while holding a medicine ball or dumbbell between your feet or while wearing ankle weights.

As already mentioned, this program works well for the three main goals that everyone has: increasing muscle strength, boosting muscle size, and enhancing fat loss. Yet, if you want to focus more on one of these three goals, you can also do that and still get the other benefits.

Rest a good 3 minutes or even longer between sets. The key is performing as many reps as possible within that prescribed rep range. More reps equal more work performed each workout, and that equates to greater strength gains over time. During weeks 1 and 2 of each phase of the program, you will do one rest-pause set on the last set of each exercise. To do this, reach muscle failure on the last set, then rack the weight and rest 15 seconds. Then continue the set until you reach muscle failure again. During weeks 3 and 4 of all phases you will do a drop set on the last set of each exercise. To do this, take the last set to muscle failure and then immediately reduce the weight by 20-30%, and continue the set until failure again.

Superman Training

This workout program uses supersets that pair opposing muscle actions. This is a bit different from just pairing opposing (antagonist) muscles because the exercise pairs are ones where the movements are the exact opposites. For example, you will pair the bench press for chest with the barbell row for lats. However, when you perform the lat pulldown for lats, you do not pair it with a chest exercises. Rather, you pair shoulder press for the deltoids with pulldown since these exercises better oppose each other's movement pattern.

The first benefit of supersets done this way is greater strength and power. Research shows that a muscle will contract with more strength and power if preceded by contractions of its antagonist, or opposing muscle group. For example, when you do a superset of barbell rows followed by the bench press, you'll be stronger on the bench press. In fact, Baker and Newton (2005) reported that when trained athletes performed rows before doing the bench press throw, they had significantly more power on the bench press throw than when they did it without first doing the rows. University of Wisconsin at Parkside (Kenosha) researchers (Ebben et al. 2011) found that when subjects did a six-second isometric leg curl to fatigue the hamstrings before doing the vertical jump, quadriceps force production increased by almost 15 percent compared to when they did the vertical jump without first doing the leg curl. This phenomenon may be due to greater inhibition of the antagonist muscles. Normally, the muscle you're working is somewhat limited by its antagonist muscle, much like a brake on a car would limit how fast you can go if you kept it depressed. For example, during the bench press, the strength of the pecs is somewhat limited by the contraction of the back muscles. Doing a set of rows before benching, however, lessens this inhibitory effect, allowing the pecs to contract with more force. Robbins et al. (2010) reported that when participants did three supersets of rows and bench presses using their four-rep max on each exercise, they were able to perform more reps on sets 2 and 3 than when they did traditional sets. This may also be due to the greater inhibition of the antagonist muscles, but it is also likely due to getting a longer rest for each muscle group. When you are training the opposing muscle group, the other muscle group is getting some rest. And when you combine the rest taken between supersets, that equates to greater total rest for each muscle group. For example, if you do three straight sets of the bench press with one minute of rest between sets, you get one minute of rest between each set of the bench press. If you do supersets of the barbell row and the bench press and rested one minute between supersets, then you not only get the one minute of rest between sets of the bench press, but you also get the time it took to do rows as additional rest time between bench press sets. In some cases that could double the amount of rest time between sets for each muscle group. Regardless of the reason, being able to complete more reps with a given weight will lead to greater muscle strength and growth over time.

A second benefit to antagonist superset training is that you will burn more body fat. One study from Syracuse University (Kelleher et al. 2010) found that when participants performed supersets for chest and back, biceps and triceps, and quads and hamstrings, they burned 35 percent more calories during the workout and 35 percent more calories after the workout than when they did straight sets. The big news here is the greater calorie burn after the workout is over. After all, a workout may only last one to two hours, so you can only burn so many extra calories in that time. But burning 35 percent more calories after the workout is over when you are sitting around the rest of the day is where that extra calorie and fat

BISHOP BURTON COLLEGE

burning can really add up. This is the same main reason why high-intensity interval training (or HIIT) outperforms regular steady-state cardio to help you drop fat so much quicker. Superset training allows you to burn more calories and fat the rest of the day, which can make a serious dent on your body fat stores.

A third benefit of doing supersets in this fashion is that you work muscle groups that you've likely neglected. When was the last time that you focused on your tibialis anterior muscle, or your lower traps? Probably never! This not only helps you bring up these often-weaker muscle groups, but it also helps restore balance. Not just balanced muscle development, but it helps to remove strength imbalances that can hold your strength back and predispose you to injury.

A fourth benefit of this style of superset training is time management. You will be able to complete far more sets of exercises in less time. You will complete about 40 to 50 total sets of exercises in each workout. Yes, you read that right: 40 to 50 total sets! That would normally take well over two hours, maybe even close to three hours, to complete so much work doing straight sets. Yet with the Superman training program it will take you only about 60 to 90 minutes. This will really ramp up the fat burning, not to mention muscle growth.

A fifth benefit of this type of training is change. One of my main mottos is *change is good*. Change is critical in making continued progress to get bigger and stronger. That's why I offer so many training programs. So you can keep changing up your training and keep growing bigger, stronger, leaner, and better. Changing up your training in this manner is just what your body needs to finally break through those plateaus that you've been stuck in. When was the last time you did supersets for every muscle group for every workout? Not to mention when was the last time you did supersets where every exercise was an exact opposing motion of the other? Probably never! But I'm not just talking about the change this type of superset provides. There is also the change in your training split. With this program you will work the *entire* body in just two days. Then there's the change in your training frequency. If you've been following my Shortcut to Size (Micromuscle) program, then you've been training each muscle group just once per week (except for abs and calves). And most people train each muscle group just once per week in other programs. In the Superman program you will train each muscle group twice each week. The higher frequency will help to stimulate new muscle growth and strength gains, not to mention greater fat loss.

On top of all the change previously mentioned will be the change in the rep ranges each week of this five-week program. The Superman program in table 7.7 uses an pendulum periodization scheme. Weeks 1 to 3 will be done in a linear periodized scheme where each week the weight gets heavier and the reps get fewer. You will start with 12 to 15 reps per set on most exercises in week 1. Then you will move up in weight to limit you to 8 to 10 reps per set in week 2. And then you bump up the weight again in week 3 to limit your muscles to completing just 4 to 6 reps per set. And week 3 is also the starting point for the next phase of the program because now you will reverse this rep pattern to follow a reverse linear periodization scheme. You already did 4 to 6 reps per set in week 3, so week 4 jumps back up to 8 to 10 reps per set. And then in week 5 you jump back up to where you started with 12 to 15 reps per set. But you will find that you are suddenly much stronger in these rep ranges during weeks 4 and 5 as compared to weeks 1 and 2. That's the magic of periodization.

You'll probably like the bigger, stronger, and leaner you that the 5 weeks of this program delivers. So if you want to continue with this superset plan, you can do another round to extend the Superman training program into a 9-week program.

TABLE 7.7 Superman Workouts

WEEK 1

WORKOUT 1: CHEST/BACK/SHOULDERS, TRAPS, CALVES/TIBIALIS

Exercise	Sets	Reps	Rest
Barbell bent-over row	4	12-15	–
Superset with bench press	4	12-15	1 min
Lat pulldown	4	12-15	–
Superset with dumbbell shoulder press	4	12-15	1 min
Incline dumbbell fly	2	12-15	–
Superset with incline rear delt raise	2	12-15	1 min
Cable crossover	2	12-15	–
Superset with cable lateral raise	2	12-15	1 min
Dumbbell shrug	4	12-15	–
Superset with straight-arm dip	4	12-15	1 min
Standing calf raise	4	12-15	–
Superset with standing toe raise	4	12-15	1 min

WORKOUT 2: LEGS/ABS, BICEPS/TRICEPS, FOREARMS

Exercise	Sets	Reps	Rest
Squat	4	12-15	–
Superset with hanging knee raise	4	12-15*	1 min
Romanian deadlift	4	12-15	–
Superset with crunch	4	12-15	1 min
Leg extension	4	12-15	–
Superset with leg curl	4	12-15	1 min
Side plank reach-through	3	To failure	**
Triceps pressdown	4	12-15	–
Superset with barbell curl	4	12-15	1 min
Cable overhead triceps extension	3	12-15	–
Superset with cable overhead curl	3	12-15	1 min
Barbell reverse wrist curl	3	12-15	–
Superset with barbell wrist curl	3	12-15	1 min

WORKOUT 3: CHEST/BACK/SHOULDERS/TRAPS

Exercise	Sets	Reps	Rest
Reverse-grip bench press	4	12-15	–
Superset with reverse-grip barbell row	4	12-15	1 min
Dumbbell lateral raise	2	12-15	–
Superset with decline dumbbell fly	2	12-15	1 min
Dumbbell upright row	2	12-15	–
Superset with dip	2	12-15*	1 min
Arnold Press	4	12-15	–
Superset with reverse-grip pulldown	4	12-15	1 min
Behind-the-back Smith machine shrug	4	12-15	–
Superset with behind-the-back Smith machine straight-arm dip	4	12-15	1 min
Seated dumbbell toe raise	4	12-15	–
Superset with seated calf raise	4	12-15	1 min

WORKOUT 4: LEGS/ABS, BICEPS/TRICEPS, FOREARMS

Exercise	Sets	Reps	Rest
Barbell roll-out	4	To failure	–
Superset with deadlift	4	12-15	1 min
Roman chair crunch	4	12-15*	–
Superset with back extension	4	12-15	1 min
Leg curl	4	12-15	–
Superset with leg extension	4	12-15	1 min
Leg curl	4	12-15	–
Superset with leg extension	4	12-15	1 min
Oblique crunch	3	To failure	**
Cable lying concentration curl	4	12-15	–
Superset with cable lying triceps extension	4	12-15	1 min
Incline dumbbell curl	3	12-15	–
Superset with bench dip	3	12-15	1 min
Behind-the-back barbell wrist curl	3	12-15	–
Superset with standing barbell reverse wrist curl	3	12-15	1 min

*If you cannot complete the prescribed number of reps, do as many as you can until failure.

**Do not rest between sides and go back and forth from the right side to the left and back until all three sets are completed for both sides.

> continued

TABLE 7.7 Superman Workouts *(continued)*

WEEK 2
WORKOUT 1: CHEST/BACK/SHOULDERS, TRAPS, CALVES/TIBIALIS

Exercise	Sets	Reps	Rest
Bench press	4	8-10	–
Superset with barbell bent-over row	4	8-10	1 min
Dumbbell shoulder press	4	8-10	–
Superset with lat pulldown	4	8-10	1 min
Incline rear delt raise	2	8-10	–
Superset with incline dumbbell fly	2	8-10	1 min
Cable lateral raise	2	8-10	–
Superset with cable crossover	2	8-10	1 min
Straight-arm dip	4	8-10	–
Superset with dumbbell shrug	4	8-10	1 min
Standing toe raise	4	8-10	–
Superset with standing calf raise	4	8-10	1 min

WORKOUT 2: LEGS/ABS, BICEPS/TRICEPS, FOREARMS

Exercise	Sets	Reps	Rest
Hanging knee raise	4	8-10*	–
Superset with squat	4	8-10	1 min
Crunch	4	8-10	–
Superset with Romanian deadlift	4	8-10	1 min
Leg curl	4	8-10	–
Superset with leg extension	4	8-10	1 min
Side plank reach-through	3	To failure	**
Barbell curl	4	8-10	–
Superset with triceps pressdown	4	8-10	1 min
Cable overhead curl	3	8-10	–
Superset with cable overhead triceps extension	3	8-10	1 min
Barbell wrist curl	3	8-10	–
Superset with barbell reverse wrist curl	3	8-10	1 min

WORKOUT 3: CHEST/BACK/SHOULDERS/TRAPS

Exercise	Sets	Reps	Rest
Reverse-grip barbell row	4	8-10	–
Superset with reverse-grip bench press	4	8-10	1 min
Decline dumbbell fly	2	8-10	–
Superset with dumbbell lateral raise	2	8-10	1 min
Dip	2	8-10*	–
Superset with dumbbell upright row	2	8-10	1 min
Reverse-grip pulldown	4	8-10	–
Superset with Arnold press	4	8-10	1 min
Behind-the-back Smith machine straight-arm dip	4	8-10	–
Superset with Arnold press	4	8-10	1 min
Behind-the-back Smith machine shrug seated calf raise	4	12-15	–
Superset with seated dumbbell toe raise	4	12-15	1 min

WORKOUT 4: LEGS/ABS, BICEPS/TRICEPS, FOREARMS

Exercise	Sets	Reps	Rest
Deadlift	4	8-10	–
Superset with barbell roll-out	4	To failure	1 min
Back extension	4	8-10	–
Superset with Roman chair crunch	4	8-10*	1 min
Leg extension	4	8-10	–
Superset with leg curl	4	8-10	1 min
Oblique crunch	3	To failure	**
Cable lying triceps extension	4	8-10	–
Superset with cable lying concentration curl	4	8-10	1 min
Bench dip	3	8-10	–
Superset with incline dumbbell curl	3	8-10	1 min
Behind-the-back barbell reverse wrist curl	3	8-10	–
Superset with behind-the-back barbell wrist curl	3	8-10	1 min

*If you cannot complete the prescribed number of reps, do as many as you can until failure.

**Do not rest between sides and go back and forth from the right side to the left and back until all three sets are completed for both sides.

WEEK 3
WORKOUT 1: CHEST/BACK/SHOULDERS, TRAPS, CALVES/TIBIALIS

Exercise	Sets	Reps	Rest
Barbell bent-over row	4	4-6	–
Superset with bench press	4	4-6	1 min
Lat pulldown	4	4-6	–
Superset with dumbbell shoulder press	4	4-6	1 min
Incline dumbbell fly	2	4-6	–
Superset with incline rear delt raise	2	4-6	1 min
Cable crossover	2	4-6	–
Superset with cable lateral raise	2	4-6	1 min
Dumbbell shrug	4	4-6	–
Superset with straight-arm dip	4	4-6	1 min
Standing calf raise	4	4-6	–
Superset with standing toe raise	4	4-6	1 min

WORKOUT 2: LEGS/ABS, BICEPS/TRICEPS, FOREARMS

Exercise	Sets	Reps	Rest
Squat	4	4-6	–
Superset with hanging knee raise	4	4-6*	1 min
Romanian deadlift	4	4-6	–
Superset with crunch	4	4-6	1 min
Leg extension	4	4-6	–
Superset with leg curl	4	4-6	1 min
Side plank reach-through	3	To failure	**
Triceps pressdown	4	4-6	–
Superset with barbell curl	4	4-6	1 min
Cable overhead triceps extension	3	4-6	–
Superset with cable overhead curl	3	4-6	1 min
Barbell reverse wrist curl	3	4-6	–
Superset with barbell wrist curl	3	4-6	1 min

WORKOUT 3: CHEST/BACK/SHOULDERS/TRAPS

Exercise	Sets	Reps	Rest
Reverse-grip bench press	4	4-6	–
Superset with reverse-grip barbell row	4	4-6	1 min
Dumbbell lateral raise	2	4-6	–
Superset with decline dumbbell fly	2	4-6	1 min
Dumbbell upright row	2	4-6	–
Superset with dip	2	4-6*	1 min
Arnold press	4	4-6	–
Superset with reverse-grip pulldown	4	4-6	1 min
Behind-the-back Smith machine shrug	4	4-6	–
Superset with behind-the-back Smith machine straight-arm dip	4	4-6	1 min
Seated calf raise	4	4-6	–
Superset with seated dumbbell toe raise	4	4-6	1 min

WORKOUT 4: LEGS/ABS, BICEPS/TRICEPS, FOREARMS

Exercise	Sets	Reps	Rest
Barbell Roll-out	4	To failure	–
Superset with deadlift	4	4-6	1 min
Roman chair crunch	4	4-6*	–
Superset with back extension	4	4-6	1 min
Leg curl	4	4-6	–
Superset with leg extension	4	4-6	1 min
Oblique crunch	3	To failure	**
Cable lying concentration curl	4	4-6	–
Superset with cable lying triceps extension	4	4-6	1 min
Incline dumbbell curl	3	4-6	–
Superset with bench dip	3	4-6	1 min
Behind-the-back barbell wrist curl	3	4-6	–
Superset with behind-the-back barbell reverse wrist curl	3	4-6	1 min

*If you cannot complete the prescribed number of reps, do as many as you can until failure.

**Do not rest between sides and go back and forth from the right side to the left and back until all three sets are completed for both sides.

> continued

TABLE 7.7 Superman Workouts *(continued)*

WEEK 4
WORKOUT 1: CHEST/BACK/SHOULDERS, TRAPS, CALVES/TIBIALIS

Exercise	Sets	Reps	Rest
Bench press	4	8-10	–
Superset with barbell bent-over row	4	8-10	1 min
Dumbbell shoulder press	4	8-10	–
Superset with lat pulldown	4	8-10	1 min
Incline rear delt raise	2	8-10	–
Superset with incline dumbbell fly	2	8-10	1 min
Cable lateral raise	2	8-10	–
Superset with cable crossover	2	8-10	1 min
Straight-arm dip	4	8-10	–
Superset with dumbbell shrug	4	8-10	1 min
Standing toe raise	4	8-10	–
Superset with standing calf raise	4	8-10	1 min

WORKOUT 2: LEGS/ABS, BICEPS/TRICEPS, FOREARMS

Exercise	Sets	Reps	Rest
Hanging knee raise	4	8-10*	–
Superset with squat	4	8-10	1 min
Crunch	4	8-10	–
Superset with Romanian deadlift	4	8-10	1 min
Leg curl	4	8-10	–
Superset with leg extension	4	8-10	1 min
Side plank reach-through	3	To failure	**
Barbell curl	4	8-10	–
Superset with triceps pressdown	4	8-10	1 min
Cable overhead curl	3	8-10	–
Superset with cable overhead triceps extension	3	8-10	1 min
Barbell wrist curl	3	8-10	–
Superset with barbell reverse wrist curl	3	8-10	1 min

WORKOUT 3: CHEST/BACK/SHOULDERS/TRAPS

Exercise	Sets	Reps	Rest
Reverse-grip barbell row	4	8-10	–
Superset with reverse-grip bench press	4	8-10	1 min
Decline dumbbell fly	2	8-10	–
Superset with dumbbell lateral raise	2	8-10	1 min
Dip	2	8-10*	–
Superset with dumbbell upright row	2	8-10	1 min
Reverse-grip pulldown	4	8-10	–
Superset with Arnold press	4	8-10	1 min
Behind-the-back Smith machine straight-arm dip	4	8-10	–
Superset with behind-the-back Smith machine shrug	4	8-10	1 min
Seated calf raise	4	12-15	–
Superset with seated dumbbell toe raise	4	12-15	1 min

WORKOUT 4: LEGS/ABS, BICEPS/TRICEPS, FOREARMS

Exercise	Sets	Reps	Rest
Deadlift	4	8-10	–
Superset with barbell roll-out	4	To failure	1 min
Back extension	4	8-10	–
Superset with Roman chair crunch	4	8-10*	1 min
Leg extension	4	8-10	–
Superset with leg curl	4	8-10	1 min
Oblique crunch	3	To failure	**
Cable lying triceps extension	4	8-10	–
Superset with cable lying concentration curl	4	8-10	1 min
Bench dip	3	8-10	–
Superset with incline dumbbell curl	3	8-10	1 min
Behind-the-back barbell reverse wrist curl	3	8-10	–
Superset with behind-the-back barbell wrist curl	3	8-10	1 min

*If you cannot complete the prescribed number of reps, do as many as you can until failure.

**Do not rest between sides and go back and forth from the right side to the left and back until all three sets are completed for both sides.

WEEK 5
WORKOUT 1: CHEST/BACK/SHOULDERS, TRAPS, CALVES/TIBIALIS

Exercise	Sets	Reps	Rest
Barbell bent-over row	4	12-15	–
Superset with bench press	4	12-15	1 min
Lat pulldown	4	12-15	–
Superset with dumbbell shoulder press	4	12-15	1 min
Incline dumbbell fly	2	12-15	–
Superset with incline rear delt raise	2	12-15	1 min
Cable crossover	2	12-15	–
Superset with cable lateral raise	2	12-15	1 min
Dumbbell shrug	4	12-15	–
Superset with dip shrug	4	12-15	1 min
Standing calf raise	4	12-15	–
Superset with standing toe raise	4	12-15	1 min

WORKOUT 2: LEGS/ABS, BICEPS/TRICEPS, FOREARMS

Exercise	Sets	Reps	Rest
Squat	4	12-15	–
Superset with hanging knee raise	4	12-15*	1 min
Romanian deadlift	4	12-15	–
Superset with crunch	4	12-15	1 min
Leg extension	4	12-15	–
Superset with leg curl	4	12-15	1 min
Side plank reach-through	3	To failure	**
Triceps pressdown	4	12-15	–
Superset with barbell curl	4	12-15	1 min
Cable overhead triceps extension	3	12-15	–
Superset with cable overhead curl	3	12-15	1 min
Barbell reverse wrist curl	3	12-15	–
Superset with barbell wrist curl	3	12-15	1 min

WORKOUT 3: CHEST/BACK/SHOULDERS/TRAPS

Exercise	Sets	Reps	Rest
Reverse-grip bench press	4	12-15	–
Superset with reverse-grip barbell row	4	12-15	1 min
Dumbbell lateral raise	2	12-15	–
Superset with decline dumbbell fly	2	12-15	1 min
Dumbbell upright row	2	12-15	–
Superset with dip	2	12-15*	1 min
Arnold press	4	12-15	–
Superset with reverse-grip pulldown	4	12-15	1 min
Behind-the-back Smith machine shrug	4	12-15	–
Superset with behind-the-back Smith machine straight-arm dip	4	12-15	1 min
Seated dumbbell toe raise	4	12-15	–
Superset with seated calf raise	4	12-15	1 min

WORKOUT 4: LEGS/ABS, BICEPS/TRICEPS, FOREARMS

Exercise	Sets	Reps	Rest
Barbell roll-out	4	To failure	–
Superset with deadlift	4	12-15	1 min
Roman chair crunch	4	12-15*	–
Superset with back extension	4	12-15	1 min
Leg curl	4	12-15	–
Leg curl	4	12-15	–
Superset with leg extension	4	12-15	1 min
Oblique crunch	3	To failure	**
Cable lying concentration curl	4	12-15	–
Superset with cable lying triceps extension	4	12-15	1 min
Incline dumbbell curl	3	12-15	–
Superset with bench dip	3	12-15	1 min
Behind-the-back barbell wrist curl	3	12-15	–
Superset with behind-the-back barbell reverse wrist curl	3	12-15	1 min

*If you cannot complete the prescribed number of reps, do as many as you can until failure.

**Do not rest between sides and go back and forth from the right side to the left and back until all three sets are completed for both sides.

Superpumps

For bodybuilders the muscle pump is the ultimate goal of most workouts. The pump is the rapid expansion in the size of muscles during a workout. The pump simply refers to the filling up of muscle cells with water. When you work out, you produce waste products in the muscle cells. These waste products are the result of burning glucose and fat to fuel muscle contractions, and their build-up inside muscle cells draws water (from the blood in the capillaries that feed the muscle and the area surrounding the cells) into the muscle cells. As with a balloon, the more water that the muscle cell can hold, the bigger the pump. The pump essentially places a stretch on the muscle cell. This stretch not only makes muscles momentarily bigger, but it also initiates biochemical pathways that signal the muscle cell to grow.

Training with very high reps causes a greater flow of blood to the trained muscles. It's the muscle contraction that stimulates the blood to be directed in that direction. During the superpump program, workouts focus on just one or two muscle groups per session (see table 7.8). Each muscle group will be trained just once a week with high reps and multiple sets. The workouts focus on isolation exercises and cables for constant tension and employ techniques such as preexhaust, supersets, compound sets, tri-sets, and drop sets. Keep rest to no more than 90 seconds between sets or as specified for each training protocol. Follow this program for no more than six weeks before switching to a program that uses heavier weight and lower reps. After that, you can go back to the superpump program for maximizing muscle pumps during the workout and creating long-term muscle growth.

TABLE 7.8   Superpump Program

MONDAY: CHEST, CALVES			
Exercise	Sets	Reps	Notes
Incline dumbbell fly	4	12	Do each set to failure.
Incline bench press	4	12-15	Drop set on last set. Drop weight 30 percent and continue to failure.
Dumbbell bench press	4	12-15	Drop set on last set. Drop weight 30 percent and continue to failure.
Pec deck	4	20-30	Keep rest between sets to less than 30 seconds.
Standing calf raise	5	20-30	Keep rest between sets to less than 30 seconds.
Seated calf raise	5	20-30	Keep rest between sets to less than 30 seconds.

TUESDAY: BACK, ABS			
Exercise	Sets	Reps	Notes
Straight-arm pulldown	3	12-15	Do each set to failure.
Barbell row	4	12-15	Drop set on last set. Drop weight 30 percent and continue to failure.
Wide-grip and underhand-grip pulldown	4	12-15	Perform these as compound sets.
Straight-arm pulldown	4	20-30	Keep rest between sets to less than 30 seconds.
Hanging leg raise	4	12-15	Keep rest between sets to less than 30 seconds.
Crunch	4	15-25	Keep rest between sets to less than 30 seconds.

WEDNESDAY: QUADS, HAMS, CALVES

Exercise	Sets	Reps	Notes
Leg extension and leg curl	4	12-15	Perform as superset.
Smith machine squat	4	12-15	Drop set on last set. Drop weight 30 percent and continue to failure.
Leg press	4	12-15	Drop set on last set. Drop weight 30 percent and continue to failure.
Leg extension and Romanian deadlift	4	20-30	Perform as superset.
Seated calf raise	5	20-30	Keep rest between sets to less than 30 seconds.
Leg press calf raise	5	20-30	Keep rest between sets to less than 30 seconds.

THURSDAY: SHOULDERS, TRAPS, ABS

Exercise	Sets	Reps	Notes
Dumbbell rear, front, lateral raise	3	12-15	Perform as tri-set.
Dumbbell shoulder press	4	12-15	Drop set on last set. Drop weight 30 percent and continue to failure.
Wide-grip upright row	4	12-15	Drop set on last set. Drop weight 30 percent and continue to failure.
One-arm cable lateral raise	4	20-30	Keep rest between sets to less than 30 seconds.
Dumbbell shrug	4	12-15	Drop set on last set. Drop weight 30 percent and continue to failure.

THURSDAY: SHOULDERS, TRAPS, ABS (continued)

Exercise	Sets	Reps	Notes
Smith machine back and front shrugs	4	12-15	Perform as compound sets.
Reverse crunch	4	15-20	Keep rest between sets to less than 30 seconds.
Cable crunch	4	15-20	Keep rest between sets to less than 30 seconds.

FRIDAY: TRICEPS, BICEPS, FOREARMS

Exercise	Sets	Reps	Notes
Dumbbell kickback	4	12-15	Do each set to failure.
Close-grip bench press	4	12-15	Drop set on last set. Drop weight 30 percent and continue to failure.
Overhead rope extension	4	20-30	Keep rest between sets to less than 30 seconds.
Seated incline curl	4	12-15	Keep rest between sets to less than 30 seconds.
Barbell curl	4	12-15	Drop set on last set. Drop weight 30 percent and continue to failure.
One-arm high cable curl	4	20-30	Keep rest between sets to less than 30 seconds.
Barbell reverse wrist curl	4	15-20	Keep rest between sets to less than 30 seconds.
Barbell wrist curl	4	15-20	Keep rest between sets to less than 30 seconds.

MUSCLE FOCUS

Many bodybuilders are concerned with the development of particular muscle groups, such as biceps, chest, and shoulders. For some, this is due to an imbalance in their overall muscle development—often caused by genetics or improper training. For others, this is due to simple desire for having certain muscle groups (often the biceps) as large as possible. If you have a particular muscle group that you want to concentrate on developing, try one of the following muscle-specific programs. There is a specific program for each major muscle group. Each program is tried and true in application and results.

Big Chest Program

Big pecs are the signature body part of a serious bodybuilder. If your chest is a weak spot on your physique, try following the big chest program shown in table 7.9. It is a 16-week program broken down into four separate phases that alter exercise selection, training techniques used, weight and rep ranges, number of sets, and even rest periods.

During this program you should alternate between a four-day and five-day training split. During weeks 1, 3, 5, 7, 9, 11, 13, and 15 you will train chest twice per week while training all other muscle groups just once. For this you will use a four-day split that trains chest and abs on Monday and Friday; shoulders and triceps on Tuesday; back, biceps, and abs on Wednesday; and legs and calves on Thursday. During weeks 2, 4, 6, 8, 10, 12, 14, 16 you train chest once per week using a five-day split that works chest and abs on Monday; legs and calves on Tuesday; shoulders and abs on Wednesday; back on Thursday; and biceps, triceps, and abs on Friday.

Phase 1 is designed to build mass and strength; therefore, it involves mainly compound exercises done for low reps. Phase 2 develops muscle size and separation by increasing the number of isolation exercises and reps performed per set. Phase 3 is designed to shape and define the muscle you built in the first eight weeks by increasing the reps used again and incorporating compound sets. Phase 4, the final phase, is a combination of the three prior phases. It uses only heavy pressing exercises for two of the workouts during weeks 13

TABLE 7.9   Big Chest Program

PHASE 1: WEEKS 1-4

Rest 60 to 120 seconds between sets.

Exercise	Sets	Reps
Cable crossover (prefatigue)	1	25
Incline barbell bench press	3	6
Flat dumbbell press	4	6
Decline barbell press	4	6
Dumbbell pullovers	3	6

PHASE 2: WEEKS 5-8

Rest about 60 seconds between sets.

Exercise	Sets	Reps
Decline push-up (prefatigue)	1	25
Decline dumbbell press	3	8-10
Incline dumbbell press	4	8-10
Flat dumbbell fly	4	8-10
Cable crossover	3	8-10

PHASE 3: WEEKS 9-12

Rest 30 to 60 seconds between sets.

Exercise	Sets	Reps
Pec deck	1	25
Flat dumbbell press	3	12-15
Incline dumbbell fly	3	12-15
Compound set with cable crossover	3	12-15
Decline barbell press	3	12-15
Compound set with pullover	3	12-15

PHASE 4: WEEKS 13-16

Rest 60 seconds between sets during weeks 13 and 15; 2 minutes between sets during weeks 14 and 16.

MONDAY (WEEKS 13 AND 15)

Exercise	Sets	Reps
Bench press	4	4-6
Incline press	4	6-8
Decline press	4	8-10

FRIDAY (WEEKS 13 AND 15)

Incline fly	4	12-15
Flat fly	4	12-15
Pec deck fly	4	12-15

MONDAY (WEEKS 14 AND 16)

Incline dumbbell fly	4	10-12
Compound set with incline press	4	8-10
Pec deck	4	12-15
Compound set with machine bench press	4	10-12

and 15, lighter isolation for exercises for another two workouts during those weeks, and compound sets with higher volume for the single chest workout during weeks 14 and 16.

Big Wheels Program

Big legs seem to be last on the wish list of many bodybuilders. The lower half of the body seems to get neglected in an effort to focus on the more obvious muscle groups of the upper body, such as the arms and chest. If you've been guilty of neglecting your leg training, or if you are wise enough to realize that muscular legs are just as important as a muscular upper body to produce a balanced physique, try this big wheels program to pack on muscle to your quads and hams.

The 16-week big wheels program (see table 7.10) is broken down into four 4-week phases. Phase 1 kicks off with a high-intensity training (HIT) leg program that uses heavy weight. As discussed in chapter 6, this training method uses high-intensity methods and low volume. Precede each set with one short warm-up set with approximately 50 percent of the weight you will use for the working set. Take each working set to muscle failure. In addition, you should have a spotter help you perform three or four forced reps after reaching muscle failure. Resist the negative portion on every forced rep. Perform the HIT leg workout on Monday and Friday (add abs following the Friday workout). Train chest, back, and abs on Tuesday; train shoulders, biceps, and triceps on Wednesday. Take Thursday off.

Phase 2 training drops the workouts back to one per week as the volume and reps increase dramatically. It also uses supersets and preexhaust techniques to keep the intensity high. This phase should be done as a five-day split, training legs on Monday; chest and abs on Tuesday; shoulders and traps on Wednesday; back on Thursday; and triceps, biceps, and calves on Friday. In addition to this training in the gym, in phase 2 you kick-start the 50–50 method for dumbbell squats (see chapter 6 for details). You will follow the 50–50 program through phase 3 for a total of eight weeks. Use light dumbbells and perform one set of 50 reps of dumbbell squats in the morning and at night, every day.

Phase 3 drops the reps down to 10 to 12 per set, except on leg extensions where you will do three sets of 21 (see chapter 6 for details). Leg training goes back to twice per week as you'll use the same split in weeks 1 to 4.

TABLE 7.10 Big Wheels Program

PHASE 1: WEEKS 1-4		
Exercise	Sets	Reps
Leg extension	1	10-12
Smith machine squat	1	6-8
Leg press	1	6-8
Hack squat	1	6-8
Romanian deadlift	1	6-8
Lying leg curl	1	10-12
Seated leg curl	1	10-12
Standing calf raise	1	12-15
Seated calf raise	1	12-15
Leg press calf raise	1	12-15
PHASE 2: WEEKS 5-8		
Leg extension	5	20
Superset with lying leg curl	5	20
Squats	5	20
Leg press	5	20
Romanian deadlift	5	20
PHASE 3: WEEKS 9-12		
Squat	4	10-12
Hack squat	4	10-12
Leg extension	3	21s
Lying leg curl	4	10-12
Standing calf raise	4	10-12
Compound set with donkey calf raise	4	10-12
PHASE 4: WEEKS 13-16 MORNING: QUADS		
Leg extension	3	8-10
Squat	3	8-10
Leg press	3	8-10
Hack squat	3	8-10
Walking lunge	3	20
One-leg leg extension	3	8-10
EVENING: HAMSTRINGS, CALVES		
Lying leg curl	3	8-10
Romanian deadlift	3	8-10
Standing leg curl	3	8-10
Seated leg curl	3	8-10
Seated calf raise	3	8-10
Donkey calf raise	3	8-10
Standing calf raise	3	8-10
Leg press calf raise	3	8-10

In phase 4 you are back to training legs once per week, but you split the workouts into two per day, with quadriceps on Monday morning and hamstrings and calves on Monday night. Because of this, the volume is very high, with multiple exercises for each muscle group. Follow the same split as done in phase 2. The reps drop back to 8 to 10 per set for optimal muscle gains.

Calves to Cows Program

Calves seem to be the one muscle group of the lower body that few bodybuilders have developed to their satisfaction, and it's also the one muscle group that so many want to develop. Unfortunately, if you aren't genetically predisposed to building big calves, you will have to work extremely hard for every ounce of muscle you can add to them. The calves to cows program (see table 7.11) is for those bodybuilders who need to work their calves hard and diligently. This program is divided into four 4-week phases that change up the rep range and

TABLE 7.11   Calves to Cows Program

PHASE 1: WEEKS 1-4		
Exercise	**Sets**	**Reps**
Standing calf raise	3	25-30
Seated calf raise	3	25-30
PHASE 2: WEEKS 5-8		
Leg press calf raise	4	15-20
Seated calf raise	4	15-20
Standing calf raise	4	15-20
PHASE 3: WEEKS 9-12		
Standing calf raise	4	12-15
Donkey calf raise	4	12-15
Leg press calf raise	4	12-15
Compound set with seated calf raise	4	12-15
PHASE 4: WEEKS 13-16		
Seated calf raise (toes out)	2	8-10*
Seated calf raise (toes in)	2	8-10*
Seated calf raise (toes straight)	2	8-10*
Standing calf raise (toes straight)	2	8-10*
Standing calf raise (toes out)	2	8-10*
Standing calf raise (toes in)	2	8-10*
Leg press calf raise (toes straight)	2	8-10*
Leg press calf raise (toes out)	2	8-10*
Leg press calf raise (toes in)	2	8-10*

*Drop sets

weight used, the volume, and the training frequency in a specific pattern. Each phase reduces the frequency at which you train the calves as well as the rep range, but it increases the volume (number of sets and exercises performed) and weight used.

Phase 1 starts off with training the calves five days a week. Use a basic five-day training split during this phase and train calves at the end of every workout. Reps are extremely high but volume is fairly low. Phase 2 increases the exercise number and the sets performed to four per exercise, but it drops the training frequency back to four days per week. You can use a four- or five-day training split during this phase. Reps decrease to about 15 to 20 per set. In phase 3, the frequency decreases to three times per week, but an extra calf exercise is added and compound-set training is used. Reps drop down to 12 to 15 per set. You can use a three-, four-, or five-day basic training split during this period of calf training. The final phase, phase 4, trains calves only twice per week. Sounds simple, but it increases the number of exercises performed and includes drop sets on the last set of every exercise. After you reach failure on the last set, drop the weight about 30 percent and repeat that twice. You can do this phase with any type of split.

Six Weeks to Sick Arms

Regardless of where you're starting from, this six-week program will put noticeable size on your arms. You might expect to add an inch or more to the arms. This six-week program is a progression that ramps up the training frequency (how often you train arms each week) starting at once per week in week 1, twice per week in week 2, and three times per week in weeks 3 through 5, and then backing way off in the final week 6 to just once per week again. There is a method to this madness.

Week one will annihilate your biceps and triceps. You'll pull out all the stops, using negative-rep training to destroy every single muscle fiber in the arms. You'll need a good week to recover from this. The next week gets involves light weight and high reps. Volume will be low on these workouts because you'll still be recovering from the previous week. These workouts will help you to recover from the previous week and will get you ready for the crazy three weeks that are to come. In weeks 3, 4, and 5 you will be hitting arms three times per week. If you think that sounds like overtraining, you're right. But overtraining does not happen immediately. It takes several weeks to actually become overtrained. The technical term for training that can lead to overtraining is *overreaching*. And what's interesting about overreaching is that research shows that if your diet is adequate in calories, protein, and carbohydrate, as well as the right supplements, then you can actually capitalize on overreaching and turn it into a way to get bigger and stronger. But don't worry. I've got you covered on a diet and supplement plan to ensure that you turn the training into distinct gains. Several studies from the University of Connecticut (Ratamess et al. 2003; Kraemer et al. 2006) have shown that when participants overreach for several weeks, during the two weeks following, they grow significantly bigger and stronger while taking it easy. The key is to stop the overreaching just before it turns into overtraining. That's why you'll be training arms three times per week in weeks 3 through 5 and then switch it up to just once per week in week 6. I also suggest that the week after week 6 you take it fairly easy on your arms and train them just once that week before getting back into any serious training programs.

Not only will the three-day-a-week arm training shock your muscles into growing with frequent and intense workouts that cause overreaching, but it also takes advantage of the staircase effect for building muscle. This refers to the fact that training activates genes in muscle fibers that are responsible for many of the adaptations that take place, such as muscle growth and increased strength. For example, consistent training activates certain genes that result in building more muscle fiber protein, which means more size and strength. These genes are typically activated a few hours, and some remain activated for days. Repeated workouts, if timed appropriately, can build on the activation of the genes to reach an even higher activity level and thus greater muscle growth. This is referred to as the staircase effect. In other words, let's say a certain gene involved in muscle growth is activated by a workout to the point that that its activity is boosted by 100 percent after the workout, then slowly declines in activity over the next few days so that the day after the workout it is still up by 75 percent, and the second day after the workout it is up by 50 percent, then the third day it is up by just 25 percent, and finally on the fourth day after the workout it is back to the original level. If you performed the workout on the fourth day after the first workout or later, then that gene would be bumped back to 100 percent of its original activity. However, if you worked out on the second day after the first workout, when the gene was still up

by 50 percent, then you could potentially bump up its activity to 150 percent. This could lead to even greater muscle growth and strength gains than if you waited to train again after the fourth day or later, such as one week later. This is one reason training a muscle group every 48 hours could lead to even greater muscle growth and strength gains than training every seven days.

Of course, this program is not all about training frequency. While moving to more frequent workouts can help you to build extra size on your arms, to really get them up there in size will require pulling out all the stops. So intensity techniques, like drop sets, forced reps, rest, negative reps, and supersets, will be key in forcing them to grow. These techniques not only put more stress on the muscle, but they are also known to boost growth hormone levels. In fact, one study from Finland (Ahtianen et al. 2003) reported that participants doing forced reps increased GH levels three times higher than when they just stopped after reaching muscle failure. That extra growth hormone will be put to good use initiating muscle recovery and growth. Yarrow et al. (2007) reported that using negative-rep training leads to high GH levels. Another key element to this program is the constant switching up of weight and rep ranges every workout (undulating periodization) to keep your arms growing.

Because you'll be training arms pretty much every other day during weeks 3, 4, and 5, you may be worried about your arms still being sore when you train them. Don't be. Nosaka and Newton (2002) showed that when participants work out intensely to cause muscle pain and train that muscle again just two days later and again four days later when the muscle is still sore, it does not impede recovery. Plus this can actually help muscles grow. Pullinen et al. (2002) found that when participants trained the same muscle group just two days, the catabolic hormone cortisol was lower. Since cortisol competes with testosterone, having lower cortisol levels during and after workouts can make you more anabolic and allow your testosterone to better enhance muscle growth.

To properly hit your arms during these six weeks, you'll need to alternate your training split. Each week you will follow a four-day training split. However, based on the week and number of times you are training arms, you will be training on four days of the week and pairing up different muscle groups each week. Use the training splits in table 7.12 for each week of the Six Weeks to Sick Arms program (see table 7.13).

TABLE 7.12 Six Weeks to Sick Arms Sample Training Split

WEEK 1
USE THIS TRAINING SPLIT DURING WEEK 1

Day	Muscle groups
Monday	Chest, triceps, biceps
Tuesday	Legs, calves
Wednesday	Off
Thursday	Back, abs
Friday	Shoulders, traps
Saturday	Off
Sunday	Off

WEEKS 3-5
USE THIS SPLIT DURING WEEKS 3, 4, AND 5

Day	Muscle groups
Monday	Chest, triceps, biceps
Tuesday	Shoulders, traps, abs
Wednesday	Back, biceps, triceps
Thursday	Off
Friday	Biceps, triceps, legs, calves
Saturday	Off
Sunday	Off

WEEK 2
USE THIS TRAINING SPLIT DURING WEEK 2

Day	Muscle groups
Monday	Chest, triceps, biceps
Tuesday	Legs, calves
Wednesday	Off
Thursday	Back, biceps, triceps
Friday	Shoulders, traps, abs
Saturday	Off
Sunday	Off

WEEK 6
USE THIS TRAINING SPLIT DURING WEEK 6

Day	Muscle groups
Monday	Chest, abs
Tuesday	Back, calves
Wednesday	Off
Thursday	Shoulders, traps
Friday	Triceps, biceps, legs

TABLE 7.13 Six Weeks to Sick Arms Workouts

WEEK 1
MONDAY: CHEST, TRICEPS, BICEPS

Exercise	Sets	Reps	Rest
Bench press	3	8-10	1-2 min
Reverse-grip bench press	3	8-10	1-2 min
Incline dumbbell fly	3	8-10	1-2 min
Cable crossover	3	10-12	1-2 min
Close-grip bench press (negative reps)[1]	3	3-5	2-3 min
Close-grip bench press	3[2]	6-8	2-3 min
Seated dumbbell overhead triceps extension	3[*]	6-8	2-3 min
Triceps pressdown	3[*]	6-8	2-3 min
Barbell curl (negative reps)[1]	3	3-5	2-3 min
Barbell curl	3[2]	6-8	2-3 min
Incline dumbbell curl	3[*]	6-8	2-3 min

TUESDAY: LEGS, CALVES

Exercise	Sets	Reps	Rest
Squat	3	8-10	1-2 min
Leg press	3	10-12	1-2 min
Leg extension	3	12-15	1-2 min
Romanian deadlift	3	8-10	1-2 min

TUESDAY: LEGS, CALVES (continued)

Exercise	Sets	Reps	Rest
Lying leg curl	3	12-15	1-2 min
Standing calf raise	4	12-15	1 min
Seated calf raise	4	12-15	1 min

THURSDAY: BACK, ABS

Exercise	Sets	Reps	Rest
Bent-over barbell row	3	8-10	1-2 min
Wide-grip pulldown	3	8-10	1-2 min
Reverse-grip pulldown	3	8-10	1-2 min
Straight-arm pulldown	3	10-12	1-2 min
Seated cable row	3	10-12	1-2 min
Hanging leg raise	3	To failure	1 min
Standing cable crunch	3	10-12	1 min

FRIDAY: SHOULDERS, TRAPS

Exercise	Sets	Reps	Rest
Barbell shoulder press	4	8-10	1-2 min
Dumbbell upright row	3	8-10	1-2 min
Dumbbell lateral raise	3	10-12	1-2 min
Dumbbell bent-over lateral raise	3	10-12	1-2 min
Barbell shrug	4	8-10	1-2 min

[1]To perform negatives, use a weight that is about 20% more than your one-rep max and have a spotter help you through the positive portion of the rep. You should be able to slowly lower the negative rep for 3 to 5 seconds.

[2]Perform two rests on the last set by resting for 15 seconds after reaching muscle failure and continuing the set and then rest another 15 seconds after reaching muscle failure again, then continue.

[3]Do a drop set on the last set by immediately reducing the weight by 20 to 30% and continuing the set.

WEEK 2
MONDAY: CHEST, TRICEPS, BICEPS

Exercise	Sets	Reps	Rest
Incline bench press	3	8-10	1-2 min
Reverse-grip incline dumb-bell press	3	8-10	1-2 min
Dumbbell fly	3	12-15	1-2 min
Decline dumbbell fly	3	12-15	1-2 min
Triceps pressdown	3	15-20	1 min
Lying triceps extension	3	15-20	1 min
Dumbbell overhead triceps extension	3	15-20	1 min
Incline dumbbell curl	3	15-20	1 min
Dumbbell preacher curl	3	15-20	1 min
Dumbbell hammer curl	3	15-20	1 min

TUESDAY: LEGS, CALVES

Exercise	Sets	Reps	Rest
Front squat	3	8-10	1-2 min
Hack squat	3	8-10	1-2 min
Leg extension	3	8-10	1-2 min
Seated leg curl	3	8-10	1-2 min
Dumbbell Romanian deadlift	3	8-10	1-2 min
Seated calf raise	4	20-25	1 min
Leg press calf raise	4	15-20	1 min

THURSDAY: BACK, BICEPS, TRICEPS

Exercise	Sets	Reps	Rest
Pull-up	3	To failure	1-2 min
One-arm dumbbell row	3	8-10	1-2 min
Wide-grip pulldown	3	10-12	1-2 min

THURSDAY: BACK, BICEPS, TRICEPS (continued)

Exercise	Sets	Reps	Rest
Seated cable row	3	10-12	1-2 min
Straight-arm pulldown	3	12-15	1-2 min
EZ-bar curl	3	20-25	1 min
High cable curl	3	20-25	1 min
Behind-the-back cable curl	3	20-25	[1]
Triceps dip	3	To failure	1 min
Cable overhead triceps extension	3	20-25	1 min
Rope triceps pressdown	3	20-25	1 min

FRIDAY: SHOULDERS, TRAPS, ABS

Exercise	Sets	Reps	Rest
Dumbbell shoulder press	3	8-10	1-2 min
Machine lateral raise	3	12-15	1-2 min
Smith machine upright row	3	12-15	1-2 min
Machine rear delt fly	3	12-15	1-2 min
Dumbbell shrug	4	10-12	1-2 min
Reverse crunch	3	To failure	–
Superset with crunch	3	To failure	1 min

WEEK 3
MONDAY: CHEST, TRICEPS, BICEPS

Exercise	Sets	Reps	Rest
Cable crossover	3	15-20	1-2 min
Bench press	3	15-20	1-2 min
Incline dumbbell fly	3	15-20	1-2 min
Incline dumbbell press	3	15-20	1-2 min

[1]To perform negatives, use a weight that is about 20% more than your one-rep max and have a spotter help you through the positive portion of the rep. You should be able to slowly lower the negative rep for 3 to 5 seconds.

[2]Perform two rests on the last set by resting for 15 seconds after reaching muscle failure and continuing the set and then rest another 15 seconds after reaching muscle failure again, then continue.

[3]Do a drop set on the last set by immediately reducing the weight by 20 to 30% and continuing the set.

> continued

TABLE 7.13   Six Weeks to Sick Arms Workouts *(continued)*

WEEK 3 *(continued)*
MONDAY: CHEST, TRICEPS, BICEPS *(continued)*

Exercise	Sets	Reps	Rest
Close-grip bench press (negative reps)[1]	3	3-5	2-3 min
Close-grip bench press	3[2]	4-6	2-3 min
Seated dumbbell overhead triceps extension	3[3]	4-6	2-3 min
Triceps pressdown	3[3]	4-6	2-3 min
Barbell curl (negative reps)[1]	3	3-5	2-3 min
Barbell curl	3[2]	4-6	2-3 min
Incline dumbbell curl	3[3]	4-6	2-3 min
EZ-bar preacher curl	3[3]	4-6	2-3 min

TUESDAY: SHOULDERS, TRAPS, ABS

Exercise	Sets	Reps	Rest
Cable lateral raise	3	15-20	1-2 min
Smith machine behind-the-neck shoulder press	3	15-20	1-2 min
Smith machine upright row	3	15-20	1-2 min
Face pull	3	15-20	1-2 min
Dumbbell shrug	4	15-20	1-2 min
Bicycle crunch	3	To failure	1 min
Oblique crunch on angled back extension bench	3	To failure	1 min

WEDNESDAY: BACK, BICEPS, TRICEPS

Exercise	Sets	Reps	Rest
Straight-arm pulldown	3	15-20	1-2 min
Wide-grip pulldown	3	15-20	1-2 min
Bent-over barbell row	3	15-20	1-2 min
Seated cable row	3	15-20	1-2 min
Standing cable concentration curl	3	10-12	1-2 min
Behind-the-back cable curl	3	10-12	1-2 min
Machine curl	3	10-12	1-2 min
One-arm dumbbell overhead triceps extension	3	10-12	1-2 min
Triceps pressdown	3	10-12	1-2 min
Bench dip	3	10-12	1-2 min

FRIDAY (TRICEPS, BICEPS, LEGS, CALVES)

Exercise	Sets	Reps	Rest
Lying triceps extension	4	8-10	–
Superset with barbell curl	4	8-10	1-2 min
Triceps pushdown	4	8-10	–
Superset with high cable curl	4	8-10	1-2 min
Leg extension	3	15-20	1-2 min
Squat	3	15-20	1-2 min

FRIDAY (TRICEPS, BICEPS, LEGS, CALVES) *(continued)*

Exercise	Sets	Reps	Rest
Leg press	3	15-20	1-2 min
Lying leg curl	3	15-20	1-2 min
Romanian deadlift	3	15-20	1-2 min
Seated calf raise	4	20-25	1 min
Leg press calf raise	4	15-20	1 min

WEEK 4
MONDAY (CHEST, TRICEPS, BICEPS)

Exercise	Sets	Reps	Rest
Reverse-grip incline bench press	3	10-12	1-2 min
Dumbbell bench press	3	10-12	1-2 min
Machine fly	3	10-12	1-2 min
Cable crossover from low pulley	3	10-12	1-2 min
Close-grip bench press (negative reps)[1]	3	3-5	2-3 min
Close-grip bench press	3[2]	10-12	2-3 min
Seated dumbbell overhead triceps extension	3[3]	10-12	2-3 min
Triceps pressdown	3[3]	10-12	2-3 min
Barbell curl (negative reps)[1]	3	3-5	2-3 min
Barbell curl	3[2]	10-12	2-3 min
Incline dumbbell curl	3[3]	10-12	2-3 min
EZ-bar preacher curl	3[3]	10-12	2-3 min

TUESDAY: SHOULDERS, TRAPS, ABS

Exercise	Sets	Reps	Rest
Dumbbell shoulder press	3	10-12	1-2 min
Cable upright row	3	10-12	1-2 min
Cable lateral raise	3	10-12	1-2 min
Dumbbell bent-over lateral raise	3	10-12	1-2 min
One-arm Smith machine shrug	4	10-12	1-2 min
Hanging leg raise	3	To failure	–
Tri-set with twisting crunch	3	To failure	–
Tri-set with reverse crunch	3	To failure	1 min

WEDNESDAY: BACK, BICEPS, TRICEPS

Exercise	Sets	Reps	Rest
Pull-up	3	10-12	1-2 min
One-arm dumbbell row	3	10-12	1-2 min
Reverse-grip pulldown	3	10-12	1-2 min
Straight-arm pulldown	3	10-12	1-2 min

[1]To perform negatives, use a weight that is about 20% more than your one-rep max and have a spotter help you through the positive portion of the rep. You should be able to slowly lower the negative rep for 3 to 5 seconds.

[2]Perform two rests on the last set by resting for 15 seconds after reaching muscle failure and continuing the set and then rest another 15 seconds after reaching muscle failure again, then continue.

[3]Do a drop set on the last set by immediately reducing the weight by 20 to 30% and continuing the set.

WEEK 4 (continued)
WEDNESDAY: BACK, BICEPS, TRICEPS (continued)

Exercise	Sets	Reps	Rest
Behind-the-back cable curl	3	15-20	1 min
High cable curl	3	15-20	1 min
Rope cable curl	3	15-20	1 min
Triceps pressdown	3	15-20	1 min
Cable overhead triceps extension	3	15-20	1 min
Reverse-grip triceps pressdown	3	15-20	1 min

FRIDAY: TRICEPS, BICEPS, LEGS, CALVES

Lying triceps extension	3	25-30	–
Superset with close-grip bench press	3	25-30	1-2 min
Triceps pushdown (rope handle)	3	25–30	–
Superset with cable overhead triceps extension	3	25-30	1-2 min
Incline dumbbell curl	3	25–30	–
Superset with alternating dumbbell curl	3	25-30	1-2 min
Rope cable curl	3	25-30	–
Superset with cable curl (straight bar)	3	25-30	1-2 min
Lying triceps extension	4	8–10	–
Superset with barbell curl	4	8-10	1-2 min
Triceps pushdown	4	8-10	–
Superset with high cable curl	4	8-10	1-2 min
Front squat	3	10-12	1-2 min
Dumbbell step-up	3	10-12	1-2 min
Leg press	3	10-12	1-2 min
Leg extension	3	10-12	1-2 min
Lying leg curl	3	10-12	1-2 min
Leg press calf raise	4	10-12	1 min
Seated calf raise	4	10-12	1 min

WEEK 5
MONDAY: CHEST, TRICEPS, BICEPS

Exercise	Sets	Reps	Rest
Bench press	3	4-6	2-3 min
Incline dumbbell bench press	3	4-6	2-3 min
Dumbbell fly	3	12-15	1-2 min
Cable crossover from middle pulley	3	12-15	1-2 min

WEEK 5 (continued)
MONDAY: CHEST, TRICEPS, BICEPS (continued)

Exercise	Sets	Reps	Rest
Close-grip bench press (negative reps)[1]	3	3-5	2-3 min
Close-grip bench press	3[2]	8-10	2-3 min
Seated dumbbell overhead triceps extension	3[3]	8-10	2-3 min
Triceps pressdown	3[3]	8-10	2-3 min
Barbell curl (negative reps)[1]	3	3-5	2-3 min
Barbell curl	3[2]	8-10	2-3 min
Incline dumbbell curl	3[3]	8-10	2-3 min
EZ-bar preacher curl	3[3]	8-10	2-3 min

TUESDAY: SHOULDERS, TRAPS, ABS

Barbell shoulder press	3	4-6	2-3 min
Standing dumbbell shoulder press	3	4-6	2-3 min
Dumbbell lateral raise	3	12-15	1-2 min
Machine rear delt fly	3	12-15	1-2 min
Smith machine shrug	2	4-6	2-3 min
Behind-the-back Smith machine shrug	2	12-15	1-2 min
Bicycle crunch	3	To failure	1-2 min
Cable woodchopper	3	15-20	1-2 min

WEDNESDAY: BACK, BICEPS, TRICEPS

Bent-over barbell row	3	4-6	2-3 min
Wide-grip pulldown	3	4-6	2-3 min
Reverse-grip pulldown	3	12-15	1-2 min
Straight-arm pulldown	3	12-15	1-2 min
Preacher curl	3	20-25	1 min
Incline dumbbell curl	3	20-25	1 min
Dumbbell hammer curl	3	20-25	1 min
Triceps pressdown	3	20-25	1 min
Machine triceps extension	3	20-25	1 min
Dumbbell overhead triceps extension	3	20-25	1 min

FRIDAY: TRICEPS, BICEPS, LEGS, CALVES

Close-grip bench press	3	12-15	–
Giant set with lying triceps extension	3	12-15	–
Giant set with dumbbell overhead extension	3	12-15	–
Giant set with bench dip	3	12-15	2-3 min

[1]To perform negatives, use a weight that is about 20% more than your one-rep max and have a spotter help you through the positive portion of the rep. You should be able to slowly lower the negative rep for 3 to 5 seconds.

[2]Perform two rests on the last set by resting for 15 seconds after reaching muscle failure and continuing the set and then rest another 15 seconds after reaching muscle failure again, then continue.

[3]Do a drop set on the last set by immediately reducing the weight by 20 to 30% and continuing the set.

> continued

TABLE 7.13   Six Weeks to Sick Arms Workouts *(continued)*

WEEK 5 *(continued)*
FRIDAY: TRICEPS, BICEPS, LEGS, CALVES *(continued)*

Exercise	Sets	Reps	Rest
Prone incline curl	3	12-15	–
Giant set with incline dumbbell curl	3	12-15	–
Giant set with EZ-bar curl	3	12-15	–
Giant set with dumbbell hammer curl	3	12-15	2-3 min
Squat	3	4-6	2-3 min
Leg press	3	4-6	2-3 min
Leg extension	3	12-15	1-2 min
Romanian deadlift	3	4-6	2-3 min
Seated leg curl	3	12-15	1-2 min
Standing calf raise	4	12-15	1 min
Seated calf raise	4	20-25	1 min

WEEK 6
EASY ARM WORKOUT: HIGHER REPS OR MODERATE REPS
MONDAY: CHEST, ABS

Exercise	Sets	Reps	Rest
Bench press	3	8-10	1-2 min
Reverse-grip incline dumbbell bench press	3	8-10	1-2 min
Incline dumbbell fly	3	15-20	1 min
Smith machine bench press	3	15-20	1-2 min
Hanging leg raise	3	To failure	1 min
Cable crunch	3	15-20	1 min
Oblique cable crunch	3	15-20	1 min

WEEK 6 *(continued)*
TUESDAY: BACK, CALVES

Exercise	Sets	Reps	Rest
Bent-over barbell row	3	8-10	1-2 min
Wide-grip pulldown	3	8-10	1-2 min
Straight-arm pulldown	3	15-20	1-2 min
Seated cable row	3	15-20	1-2 min
Seated calf raise	3	15-20	–
Superset with one-leg standing calf raise (body weight)	3	6-20	1 min

THURSDAY: SHOULDERS, TRAPS

Exercise	Sets	Reps	Rest
Barbell shoulder press	3	8-10	1-2 min
Dumbbell lateral raise	3	8-10	1-2 min
Dumbbell rear delt raise	3	15-20	1-2 min
Machine shoulder press	3	15-20	1-2 min
Barbell shrug	4	8-10	1-2 min
Behind-the-back Smith machine shrug	2	12-15	1-2 min

FRIDAY: TRICEPS, BICEPS, LEGS

Exercise	Sets	Reps	Rest
Close-grip bench press	3	8-10	1-2 min
Dumbbell overhead triceps extension	3	8-10	1-2 min
Triceps pressdown	3	8-10	1-2 min
Barbell curl	3	8-10	1-2 min
Incline dumbbell curl	3	8-10	1-2 min
Dumbbell hammer curl	3	8-10	1-2 min
Squat	3	8-10	1-2 min
Leg press	3	8-10	1-2 min
Leg extension	3	15-20	1 min
Smith machine squat	3	15-20	1 min
Romanian deadlift	3	8-10	1-2 min
Seated leg curl	3	15-20	1 min

Wider Is Better Back Program

Having a wide back makes you look impressive from both the front and back. It's also an important area to develop for strength in all other exercises. This 16-week program can help you build up a weak back (see table 7.14). Phase 1 uses pull-ups as a warm-up and deadlifts, rows, and good mornings to build a strong back. Reps are low to encourage strength gains, and the volume is low because you do this workout twice a week during this phase on Monday and Friday along with abs. Do chest, shoulders, and calves on Tuesday; biceps, triceps, and abs on Wednesday; and legs on Thursday. Phase 2 increases the volume and decreases the frequency to once per week. Train chest, shoulders, and abs on Monday. The compound sets add another level of challenge, which means the back muscles will need a full week of recovery during this phase. Phase 3 is done twice per week with the same training split that is used in phase 1. The Monday and Friday workouts are different. The Monday workout focuses on rowing exercises done with heavier weight and low reps. The Friday workout, on the other hand, focuses on pull-ups and pull-downs with lighter weight and higher reps. This workout should be one giant set cycled through twice. Phase 4 is a cable-ready program that hits the lats from a variety of angles with all cable moves. This keeps maximal tension on

the muscles throughout the full range of motion. Reps are higher, and you should do drop sets on the last set of each cable exercise. Do this workout once per week with a split similar to the one used in phase 2. At the end of phase 4 you can switch to a more basic back workout using the split you typically train with.

TABLE 7.14 Wider Is Better Back Program

PHASE 1: WEEKS 1-4		
Exercise	Sets	Reps
Pull-up	3	8-10
Deadlift	3	4-6
Barbell bent-over row	3	4-6
Lat pulldown	3	4-6
Barbell good morning	3	8-10
PHASE 2: WEEKS 5-8		
Pull-up	2	10-12
Barbell row	3	8-10
Compound set with lat pulldown	3	8-10
T-bar rows	3	8-10
Compound set with straight-arm pulldown	3	8-10
Back extension	3	8-10

PHASE 3: WEEKS 9-12 MONDAY		
Exercise	Sets	Reps
Barbell row	4	6-8
Dumbbell row	4	6-8
Seated cable row	4	6-8
FRIDAY		
Pull-up	2	8-10
Lat pulldown (wide grip)	2	10-12
Lat pulldown (narrow grip)	2	10-12
Lat pulldown (underhand grip)	2	10-12
PHASE 4: WEEKS 13-16		
Lat pulldown	4	12-15
Incline bench cable row from high pulley	4	12-15
Seated cable row	4	12-15
One-arm bent-over cable row	4	12-15
Back extension	3	12-15

Cannonball Delts Program

As with the back, having big, round, muscular shoulders can make your physique appear larger from every angle. Since the deltoid muscle is composed of three heads, a well-balanced shoulder program should target all three heads. The cannonball delts program (see table 7.15) drives growth in all three heads in order to build deltoids that are massive and balanced. Phase 1 starts with a basic strength and mass program done twice per week on Monday and Friday along with traps and abs. The Monday workout is a barbell blasting workout and the Friday workout is done with all dumbbells. Train legs and calves on Tuesday; chest, triceps,

and abs on Wednesday; and back and biceps on Thursday. Both are done with low reps and low volume. Phase 2 drops the frequency back to once per week as the intensity is ratcheted up with high-rep, high-volume training that uses the preexhaust technique. Train chest, triceps, and abs on Monday; shoulders and traps on Wednesday; legs on Thursday; and back, biceps, and abs on Friday. Phase 3 splits the training up into one pressing workout on Monday and one raise workout done as a tri-set on Friday. Do this with the same training split used in phase 1. Phase 4 finishes off the delts with a once-a-week microcycle that blasts the delts with increasing reps each week and plenty of drop sets on the last set of each exercise.

TABLE 7.15 Cannonball Delts Program

PHASE 1: WEEKS 1-4
MONDAY

Exercise	Sets	Reps
Barbell push press	4	3-5
Seated barbell shoulder press	4	4-6
Wide-grip upright row	4	4-6
Barbell front raise	4	6-8
Barbell shrug	4	6-8

FRIDAY

Standing dumbbell shoulder press	3	6-8
One-arm dumbbell lateral raise	3	6-8
Bent-over dumbbell lateral raise	3	6-8
Alternating dumbbell front raise	3	6-8
Dumbbell shrug	3	6-8

PHASE 2: WEEKS 5-8

Cable front raise	4	12-15
Barbell shoulder press	4	8-10
Dumbbell lateral raise	4	10-12
Dumbbell shoulder press	4	8-10
Bent-over lateral raise	4	10-12
One-arm dumbbell shrug*	4	8-10

PHASE 3: WEEKS 9-12
MONDAY

Exercise	Sets	Reps
Standing barbell shoulder press	4	8-10
Seated dumbbell press	4	8-10
Smith machine shoulder press	4	8-10
Behind-the-back barbell shrug	4	8-10

FRIDAY

Bent-over dumbbell lateral raise	4	15-20
Dumbbell lateral raise	4	15-20
Dumbbell front raise	4	15-20
Seated dumbbell shrug	4	10-12

PHASE 4: WEEKS 13-16*

Exercise	WEEK 13		WEEK 14		WEEK 15		WEEK 16	
	Sets	Reps	Sets	Reps	Sets	Reps	Sets	Reps
Barbell shoulder press	4	6	4	10	4	15	4	20
Dumbbell shoulder press	4	6	4	10	4	15	4	20
Dumbbell upright row	4	6	4	10	4	15	4	20
Cable lateral raise	4	6	4	10	4	15	4	20
Standing cable reverse fly	4	6	4	10	4	15	4	20
Dumbbell shrug	4	6	4	10	4	15	4	20

*Alternate right and left arm without resting until each arm has done four sets.

PART III

TRAINING FOR MAXIMAL STRENGTH

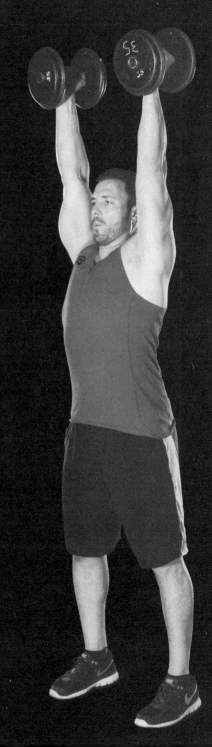

Training for maximal strength is much different from training for muscle mass. From a training standpoint, the total volume and reps performed per set tend to be lower when training for strength compared to the volume and number of reps when training for muscle mass. From a physiological standpoint, muscle growth tends to be more about the aftereffects of training, while muscle strength also has a learning component that develops during the actual workouts. Even though mechanical stress and metabolic stress are important factors for developing muscle strength, there is a large component to strength development that relies on training of the nervous system.

Motor nerves that run from the spinal cord to the muscle fibers are responsible for initiating muscle contractions. Strength training increases muscle strength through several adaptations of the motor nerves. One mechanism involves training the motor nerves to fire at a faster rate. This allows the muscle fibers to contract with more force (that is, greater strength). Strength training also trains the motor nerves to fire at this faster rate for a longer period without fatiguing, This allows more reps to be done with a certain amount of weight. Another mechanism that leads to enhanced strength is synchronization of motor nerves. This refers to the ability of motor nerves that control various muscle fibers within the same muscle to fire at the precise time to allow for the greatest production of muscle force.

What is similar between training programs for maximizing muscle strength and programs for maximizing muscle growth is that both trial and error in the gym and research in the laboratory have defined the training techniques and programs that work best at encouraging strength gains. Part III will teach you how to train for maximal strength. Chapter 8 covers basic workouts for building strength. This chapter starts with a lesson on weekly training splits that are optimal for building strength regardless of your training schedule. From there it progresses to general guidelines for training to maximize strength gains. Finally, it covers training tips and strategies for maximizing muscle strength on the three major strength lifts (bench press, squat, deadlift) as well as rules for training the core.

Chapter 9 introduces you to advanced training techniques that will have you lifting more weight in no time. These techniques work to increase mechanical and metabolic stress as well as enhance the firing rate and synchronicity of motor nerves.

Chapter 10 provides long-term periodized training cycles that will help you continually improve your strength without plateauing. It starts by teaching you how to test your maximal strength, a critical component for assessing your progress over the course of any strength training cycle. From there, you can pick a training cycle that best fits your training experience and follow the sequencing cycles. Or you can follow a cycle that is specific to the exercise in which you want to boost strength. Regardless of your training experience or specific strength goals, this section covers everything you need to know to realize your strength potential.

CHAPTER 8

Tactics for Maximizing Strength

The first step toward getting stronger is learning how to develop workouts and basic training programs with that goal in mind. The variables you will need to consider for developing strength training workouts, as discussed in chapter 2, are the choice of exercises you will perform, the order of those exercises, how many sets of each exercise you will do, how heavy a weight you will use on those exercises, and how much rest you will allow between sets. Furthermore, you will also need to consider how often to train each muscle group and what type of training split you will employ.

This chapter focuses on the common training splits used by lifters interested in maximizing muscle strength. This will help you determine the best weekly schedule to follow for increasing muscle strength. From there the chapter steps back to focus on the variables of each workout. Then it steps back again to focus on the details of the specific exercises. Each step gives you more detail regarding guidelines, techniques, and tips for maximizing your muscle strength.

WEEKLY SPLITS

Regardless of whether your goal is to develop strength or muscle mass, the easiest way to split up your training is to work within the confines of the week. Although the body doesn't specifically follow a seven-day cycle, for practical purposes, a seven-day strength training cycle makes sense with most people's schedules. The following splits for developing strength all follow a seven-day cycle and will fit anyone's schedule and level of strength training experience.

One common denominator of these splits is that they focus on training three major strength lifts—the bench press (the marker for upper-body strength), squats (the marker for lower-body strength), and deadlifts (the marker for overall body strength). These also are the three lifts that are involved in powerlifting competition. Typically, the resistance used on these three exercises is expressed as a percentage of the weightlifter's one-repetition max (1RM), while all other exercises are expressed as an RM target zone—the resistance that limits a lifter to a specific number of repetitions. This is because powerlifters and others interested in training for strength frequently test their 1RM on the three major exercises.

Because training for maximal strength typically involves training with the three major strength exercises, as opposed to training a multitude of muscle groups, there tend to be fewer commonly used training splits. This does not mean that there are a limited number of ways to split up a strength training program. The following training splits are those that are well accepted by the majority of strength experts and athletes.

Whole-Body Strength Training

Whole-body strength training refers to single workouts that stress most major muscle groups of the body. This training split allows for most major muscle groups to be trained three times per week—usually Monday, Wednesday, and Friday. Many experts believe that frequency of training is important for gaining strength. In fact, many strength coaches have their athletes follow a whole-body training system. Not only do they think the frequency of training is important, but most also believe that because the body works as a whole unit, it should be trained accordingly. Therefore, a whole-body strength training split can be an effective means of increasing overall strength.

The frequency offered by whole-body strength training is also beneficial for beginners. As discussed in chapter 5, this is because the initial adaptations made in a strength training program involve the training of the nervous system. The best way for beginners to train to build strength is to use slightly higher repetitions than trained lifters use and more frequent training of the same exercises to program their nervous systems.

The workouts on a whole-body split typically include one exercise per major muscle group. The exercise choices usually include the bench press, squat, and deadlift, or similar exercises that mimic those particular exercises, as well as assistance exercises that help with increasing strength on these particular exercises. Most weightlifters who use a whole-body split do not train small muscle groups (such as traps, forearms, and calves) in order to better concentrate on the muscles that are directly involved in the bench press, squat, and deadlift.

When you are following a whole-body training split, the first exercise of the workout should alternate between the bench press, squat, and deadlift. That way, each major strength exercise is trained once per week when the body is fresh. Some powerlifters also include one extra assistance exercise for the exercise they are focusing on in that workout. For example, in table 8.1, on Monday, leg press is done in addition to the squat.

TABLE 8.1 Whole-Body Strength Training Split

WORKOUT 1 (MONDAY): SQUAT FOCUS		
Exercise	Sets	% 1RM or reps
Squat	4	85%
Leg press	3	8-10
Incline bench press	4	6-8
Dumbbell shoulder press	3	6-8
Barbell row	3	6-8
Stiff-leg deadlift	3	6-8
Close-grip bench press	3	6-8
Dumbbell curl	3	8-10
Hanging leg raise	3	10-12
WORKOUT 2 (WEDNESDAY): BENCH PRESS FOCUS		
Bench press	4	85%
Dumbbell bench press	3	8-10
Barbell hack squat	3	6-8
Barbell shoulder press	3	6-8
Deadlift	3	80%
Dumbbell row	3	8-10
Triceps dip	3	8-10
Barbell curl	3	6-8
Cable woodchopper	3	20
WORKOUT 3 (FRIDAY): DEADLIFT FOCUS		
Deadlift	4	85%
One-arm dumbbell deadlift	3	8-10
Bench press	3	8-10
Upright row	3	6-8
Lat pulldown	3	8-10
Lying triceps extension	3	6-8
Preacher curl	3	8-10
Back extension	3	15-20

Push–Pull Training Split

This split divides the workouts into pushing exercises and pulling exercises. Pushing exercises include any exercise in which the positive (concentric) portion of the exercise involves pushing or pressing the weight away from the body (such as in the bench press and shoulder press) or pushing the body away from the floor or platform (such as in the squat). Pull exercises include any exercise in which the positive (concentric) action involves pulling the weight toward the body (such as in the biceps curl, barbell row, or leg curl) or pulling the body toward a fixed object (such as in the pull-up).

The reason that some weightlifters split their workouts into push-and-pull workouts is that those exercises involve similar muscle groups working together to perform the exercise. For example, the pectoralis, deltoid, and triceps muscles are all used to varying degrees during the bench press and the shoulder press.

Push-and-pull training allows for each workout to be done twice a week for a total of four workouts per week, as shown in table 8.2. On push day, it is wise to alternate between the bench press and the squat as the starting exercise.

TABLE 8.2 Push–Pull Training Split

WORKOUT 1 (MONDAY AND THURSDAY*): PUSH WORKOUT		
Exercise	Sets	% 1RM or reps
Squat*	4	90%
Leg press	3	8-10
Leg extension	3	8-10
Bench press*	4	75%
Incline dumbbell press	3	8-10
Dumbbell shoulder press	4	6-8
Close-grip bench press	4	6-8
Standing calf raise	4	8-10

WORKOUT 2 (TUESDAY AND FRIDAY): PULL WORKOUT		
Deadlift	4	90%
Lying leg curl	3	8-10
Barbell row	4	6-8
Lat pulldown	3	8-10
Barbell curl	4	6-8
Weighted crunch	4	8-10

*On Thursday, perform bench press and incline dumbbell press before squats.

Upper- and Lower-Body Powerlifting Split

This split divides workouts into an upper-body workout day and a lower-body workout day. The upper-body exercises involve all exercises for major muscle groups of the upper body. The lower-body exercises involve all exercises for the major muscle groups of the lower body.

Like push–pull training, upper- and lower-body training allows each workout to be done twice per week for a total of four workouts per week (see table 8.3). Most powerlifters who follow this

TABLE 8.3 Upper- and Lower-Body Powerlifting Split

UPPER-BODY WORKOUT 1 (MONDAY): BENCH PRESS AND PUSHING EXERCISES		
Exercise	Sets	% 1RM or reps
Bench press	4	90%
Dumbbell bench press	3	4-6
Barbell shoulder press	3	4-6
Upright row	3	6-8
Close-grip bench press	3	4-6
Dips	3	6-8
Standing crunch	3	8-10

LOWER-BODY WORKOUT 1 (TUESDAY): SQUAT AND QUADRICEPS EXERCISES		
Squat	5	90%
Leg press	3	4-6
Leg extension	3	6-8
Standing calf raise	4	8-10

UPPER-BODY WORKOUT 2 (THURSDAY): BENCH PRESS AND PULLING EXERCISES		
Bench press	5	75%
Lat pulldown	3	6-8
Barbell row	3	6-8
Barbell curl	4	6-8
Russian twist	3	20

LOWER-BODY WORKOUT 2 (FRIDAY): DEADLIFT AND HAMSTRING EXERCISES		
Deadlift	5	90%
Romanian deadlift	3	6-8
Lying leg curl	3	6-8
Good morning	3	8-10
Seated calf raise	4	10-12

type of split use the two upper-body workouts to emphasize bench press training. In addition, they may use one workout to emphasize the pushing assistance muscles (such as shoulders and triceps), while the other upper-body workout focuses on the pulling assistance muscles (such as back and biceps). For lower-body workouts, most powerlifters split the two workouts into a squat emphasis and quadriceps assistance exercise workout and a deadlift emphasis and hamstring assistance exercise workout.

Max Effort–Dynamic Effort Training Split

This training split is basically a modified version of the upper- and lower-body powerlifting split. Each split trains the entire body in two days, which allows for four workouts per week. The major difference that separates max

effort–dynamic effort from upper- and lower-body training split is the specific amount of resistance used during the max effort–dynamic effort split. For details of the max effort–dynamic effort method, see chapter 9.

With the max effort–dynamic effort training split, the first two workouts of the week are done using the max effort system (see table 8.4). This calls for a gradual buildup of weight on each successive set of the bench press, squat, or deadlift until you reach 90 to 95 percent of 1RM. Some lifters go to 100 percent on some workouts.

During the last two workouts of the week, the weight used on the bench press, squat, and deadlift is only 50 to 60 percent of the 1RM. Although most people can lift this amount of weight for about 20 reps, these sets stop at 3 to 5 reps. The key is in the rep speed at which they are performed. During the dynamic effort workouts, these reps are performed as fast as possible.

TABLE 8.4   Max Effort–Dynamic Effort Training Split

LOWER-BODY WORKOUT 1 (MONDAY): MAX EFFORT			
Exercise	Sets	Reps	% 1RM
Squat	1	5	10%
	1	5	20%
	1	5	30%
	1	3	40%
	1	3	50%
	1	3	60%
	1	1	70%
	1	1	80%
	1	1	90%
	1	1	95%
	1	1	100%
Deadlift	1	5	10%
	1	5	20%
	1	5	30%
	1	3	40%
	1	3	50%
	1	3	60%
	1	1	70%
	1	1	80%
	1	1	90%
	1	1	95%
	1	1	100%

LOWER-BODY WORKOUT 1 (MONDAY): MAX EFFORT (continued)			
Exercise	Sets	Reps	% 1RM
Romanian deadlift	3	4-6	85%
Barbell good morning	3	6-8	80%
Exercise-ball roll-out	3	12-15	Body weight

UPPER-BODY WORKOUT 1 (TUESDAY): MAX EFFORT			
Exercise	Sets	Reps	% 1RM
Bench press	1	5	10%
	1	5	20%
	1	5	30%
	1	3	40%
	1	3	50%
	1	3	60%
	1	1	70%
	1	1	80%
	1	1	90%
	1	1	95%
	1	1	100%
Dumbbell bench press	3	4-6	85%
Barbell shoulder press	3	4-6	85%
Close-grip bench press	3	4-6	85%
Barbell row	3	4-6	85%
Barbell curl	3	6-8	80%
Hanging knee raise	3	10	Body weight

LOWER-BODY WORKOUT 2
(THURSDAY): DYNAMIC EFFORT

Exercise	Sets	Reps	% 1RM
Squat	2	5	10%
	1	5	20%
	1	3	30%
	1	3	40%
	8	3	50%
Deadlift	2	5	10%
	1	5	20%
	1	3	30%
	1	3	40%
	8	3	50%
Romanian deadlift	3	8-10	75%
Barbell good morning	3	8-10	75%
Russian twist	3	15-20	Body weight

UPPER-BODY WORKOUT 2
(FRIDAY): DYNAMIC EFFORT

Exercise	Sets	Reps	% 1RM
Bench press	2	5	10%
	1	5	20%
	1	3	30%
	1	3	40%
	8	3	50%
Dumbbell bench press	3	8-10	75%
Barbell shoulder press	3	8-10	75%
Close-grip bench press	3	8-10	75%
Barbell row	3	8-10	75%
Barbell curl	3	8-10	75%
Decline crunch	3	12	Body weight

Squat–Bench Press–Deadlift Training Split

Some weightlifters split their training into three workouts per week: one squat-focused workout, one bench press-focused workout, and one dead-lift-focused workout. This way each major lift gets an equal amount of training time focused on it. Usually the squat workout is performed first in the week to allow ample time for recovery before the deadlift workout, which also uses the leg muscles to a great extent. The squat workout is usually accompanied by assistance exercises that train the quadriceps, hamstrings, and sometimes the calf muscles. The second workout (performed no sooner than 48 hours after the squat workout) is typically the bench press workout. This workout usually involves assistance pressing exercises that target the chest, shoulders, and triceps muscles. The third workout (performed no sooner than 48 hours after the bench press workout) is the deadlift workout. In addition to the deadlift, this workout often includes assistance pulling exercises that train the back and biceps muscles. See table 8.5 for a sample squat–bench press–deadlift training split.

TABLE 8.5 Squat–Bench Press–Deadlift Training Split

WORKOUT 1 (MONDAY): SQUAT DAY		
Exercise	**Sets**	**Reps**
Squat	4	85%
Leg press	3	6-8
Leg extension	3	8-10
Standing calf raise	3	8-10
Cable woodchopper	3	20
WORKOUT 2 (WEDNESDAY): BENCH PRESS DAY		
Bench press	4	85%
Incline dumbbell press	3	6-8
Barbell shoulder press	4	6-8
Close-grip bench press	4	6-8
Standing crunch	4	8-10
WORKOUT 3 (FRIDAY): DEADLIFT DAY		
Deadlift	4	85%
Good morning	3	6-8
Lying leg curl	3	8-10
Barbell row	4	6-8
Barbell curl	4	6-8

Changing Your Strength Split

The strength training splits covered in the previous section have little differences among them. All focus on training the three major strength lifts; a secondary focus is on training the assistance exercises for these three strength lifts. Because of this, changing the strength training split every few months is one way to institute another form of variation in the training program. However, most competitive powerlifters have one training split that they stick with year round. Therefore, if you find a certain training split that works better for your schedule, you can potentially use it endlessly.

ESSENTIALS OF STRENGTH PROGRAMS

The type of training split you decide to follow is not as critical a factor for successful strength gains as the proper choice of exercises, exercise order, resistance, and volume. Regardless of the split you employ for developing strength, there are certain rules of success to follow. Follow these general rules to ensure that your training is optimal for strength gains. In addition, the three major strength lifts are covered in detail. That's because you can't properly increase your strength on these lifts without being proficient in the proper technique for each. Last but not least, the chapter covers core training. You must have a strong core to transfer strength to the limbs. Once you have these fundamentals of strength training, you will be ready to advance to the techniques for boosting strength (chapter 9).

General Rules of Strength Training

Training for muscle mass uses exercises as a means to an end. Training for maximal strength, on the other hand, does not use exercises merely as tools. Instead, training for strength is about increasing performance on the exercises. For most weightlifters, the exercises they train are the bench press, squat, and deadlift. Therefore, the first and most obvious rule is that you should include these three exercises in your program. You should also include assistance exercises to help you boost strength on the bench press, squat, and deadlift. These choices involve multijoint compound exercises, where appropriate.

Order of exercises is important as well—the bench press, squat, and deadlift should each be performed first in the workout at least once per week. Following the major lift should be the assistance exercises. The second exercise should be a compound exercise that targets the major muscle group used in each of the three exercises. The third exercise and any others that follow should be those that target muscle groups that assist the major strength exercise.

The amount of resistance used is of paramount importance to your strength gains. For the three major strength exercises, the resistance used is typically expressed as a percent of the 1RM. This is convenient because the 1RM for these lifts is frequently tested by those who are interested in increasing their maximal strength. For strength gains, the majority of training time should be spent using a load between 85 and 95 percent of the 1RM. Of course, cycling the training load is wise for making continued gains in strength. In fact, loads as light as 50 percent RM are often used by weightlifters to increase power, which helps to boost strength. The resistance for the assistance exercises is usually expressed as a specific repetition maximum (RM). These will often correspond with the percent RM. For example, if the squat is being trained with 85 percent of the RM, the leg press should be performed using a rep range of about four to six. Regardless of the exercise, muscle failure should be reached only on one set per exercise at the maximum. Many powerlifters rarely, if ever, train to muscle failure. However, research from Australia suggests that training to muscle failure on one set per exercise and no more is better for strength gains than not training to failure or training to failure two or more times per exercise (Drinkwater et al. 2005).

Volume per workout is generally low when training for strength. For the major strength exercises, typically as few as three to as many as eight sets are done per exercise. For assistance exercises, usually three or four sets are performed per exercise. For an entire workout, total volume can be as low as 12 to as high as 30 sets or more, depending on the split being used and the training phase.

When it comes to training rules, nowhere are they more critical than when training for maximal strength. Research and years of experience support a narrow spectrum of exercise choices, exercise order, resistance, volume, and even rest periods that are effective in the quest for strength. Yet, as the saying goes, rules are meant to be broken. As important as it is to follow rules for strength training, breaking from the norm from time to time can be an effective means of improving strength. This is especially true during plateaus, when standard training practices fail to work. The training strategies in chapter 9 will challenge the tried-and-true rules that most strength athletes have adopted as standard training guidelines. Knowing how and when to use them will make a world of difference in the strength gains you can expect from your training program.

Bench Press Training

To many people, strength is all about the bench press. Rarely does a heavily muscled athlete field the question "How much can you squat?" The question everyone wants to know is "How much can you bench-press?" Of course, masculinity is often associated with strong and well-developed upper-body musculature, and the bench press is the marker for this strength. The bench press develops the major muscles of the upper body— chest, shoulders, triceps, and even the back to some extent.

Another reason so many people associate strength solely with the bench press may be the fact that of the three major strength exercises, the bench press is the easiest to perform. Almost anyone can walk into a gym and bench-press with relative ease and safety. Whatever the reason, the bench press is the preeminent strength exercise.

When it comes to training strategies for boosting strength in the bench press, regardless of the training split being used, exercise choice and order are critical factors. Of course, strength in the bench press cannot be optimally enhanced without actually performing the bench press regularly. This is known as the specificity principle. On bench press training days, you should perform the bench press first while the muscle fibers are fully recovered from any previous exercise. This ensures that the muscles can handle the maximal load they are capable of for the specific number of reps prescribed for that workout.

After the bench press, you should do one other chest-pressing assistance exercise, such as the incline or decline barbell press or dumbbell press (flat, incline, or decline). On occasion, you can do chest isolation exercises instead. However, isolation exercises are rarely used unless the weightlifter is in the hypertrophy phase of training. This is because the isolation exercises do not mimic the pressing motion of the bench press. Chest exercises are usually followed with one shoulder exercise and one triceps exercise. These are preferentially compound exercises, such as shoulder press or upright row for shoulders and dips or close-grip bench press for triceps. On occasion these can be isolation exercises. Depending on the split used, one back and one biceps exercise may conclude the bench press workout, or you may train these on separate pull exercise days. See table 8.6 for a sample bench press workout.

Sets performed on the bench press should typically fall in the range of three to five, not including warm-up sets. All assistance exercises are usually limited to three sets per exercise. The weight used on the bench press should start off light (10 to 50 percent RM) and gradually work up to the heavy sets in the range of 85 to 95 percent RM. This is the range that most workouts are performed in,

TABLE 8.6 Big Bench Day

This workout is for a powerlifter who has a maximum bench press of 495 pounds and is training with 90 percent of his or her maximum.

Exercise	Sets	Weight (pounds)	Reps	Rest
Bench press	1	135	10*	1 min
	1	225	8*	1 min
	1	315	6*	2 min
	1	365	5*	2 min
	1	405	3*	3 min
	3	445	3**	3-4 min
Incline bench press	3	375	4-6**	3 min
Barbell shoulder press	3	255	4-6**	3 min
Close-grip bench press	3	385	4-6**	3 min
Standing crunch	4	110	8-10**	1 min

*Warm-up sets.

**Working sets.

Big Bench Tips

Use these tips to help you lift more on the bench press:

SETUP

Lie on a bench-press bench with your feet flat on the ground wider than shoulder-width apart. This helps to stabilize your body. Your knees should be bent at about a 90-degree angle.

Maintain a slight arch in your lower back throughout the exercise and keep your shoulders and glutes pressed into the bench. Keep your glute muscles tightly contracted during the entire exercise.

GRIP

Take a grip that is slightly wider than shoulder width on the bar. To determine the best grip for your arm length, make sure that when the bar reaches your chest there is a 90-degree angle at the shoulder and the elbow.

Be sure to wrap your thumb around the bar. Make sure you squeeze the bar as hard as possible. This creates a solid connection to the bar by allowing the force developed by the chest, shoulder, and triceps muscles to be more effectively transmitted to the bar.

LOWERING THE BAR

Lift the bar off the rack to the point where it is over your upper chest. This is your starting position.

Squeeze your scapulae together while lowering the bar. This stabilizes the shoulder girdle and will help you recruit the lats to push the weight up.

Lower the bar slowly. This allows the stored energy from the descent and the elastic properties of the muscles to produce more force on the lift.

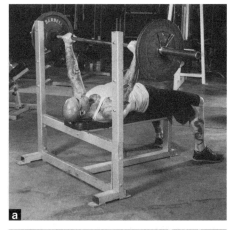

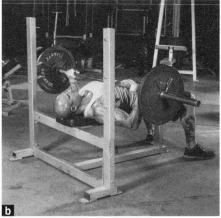

depending on the training phase. Weight may go as high as 100 percent RM to as low as 50 percent RM for some working sets during specific training phases of the cycle. For the assistance exercises, reps typically correspond with the percent RM being used in that workout on the bench press. So reps tend to fall mostly in the range of 2 to 10 reps for assistance exercises, depending on the training phase.

Rest periods between sets should be longer than when training for muscle size. The exact time is not as critical as the fact that the body is mostly recovered from the previous set. When training for strength, fatigue is not as critical as it is for building muscle size. Therefore, resting anywhere from two to five minutes is common

practice. A detailed description of the proper exercise technique for the bench press exercise can be found in the Big Bench Tips box and in chapter 14. Technique is a critical factor when training for strength. The program you follow will not matter much to your strength gains if you do not perfect your technique in the bench press.

Squat Training

The squat is the exercise that defines lower-body strength. Although it's categorized as a leg exercise, the squat technically functions as a whole-body strength and mass builder. It has been estimated that more than 200 muscles are involved in executing the squat. In addition, the surge in growth

ARMS

Your upper arms should form a 45- to 60-degree angle with your torso as you lower and press the weight back up.

TOUCHDOWN

When the bar reaches your chest, it should touch across the nipples, not much lower.

PRESSING THE BAR

Before you push the weight back up, dig your shoulders into the bench and keep your butt on the bench. This stabilizes your shoulder capsule and keeps the bar moving upward in a straight line.

You need to explode the weight off your chest as quickly and powerfully as possible. Think about blasting the bar off your chest as if it weighed just 10 pounds, even though, in reality, the bar will move quite slowly. The neural drive that results from attempting to move the bar as quickly as possible will recruit more high-threshold muscle fibers.

Press the bar straight up or back slightly toward your head. As you press the bar up, try to rip the bar apart by pulling your arms outward without changing your grip on the bar.

LEGS

Although the bench press is an upper-body exercise, don't forget to use your legs. When you press the weight with your arms, you should also drive the weight with your legs to transfer more force to your upper body.

BREATHING

Take a big breath in and hold it as you lower the weight and start it on its return. This causes an increase in pressure in your chest and abdominal cavity, which better supports your body and allows your muscles to produce more force. It also expands the chest, shortening the distance the bar has to travel.

Exhale after passing the most difficult stage of the lift or after you reach the top position.

hormone and testosterone that accompanies the squat as compared to other exercises means it enhances the strength and growth of all muscles. Many great bench pressers espouse the importance of doing squats, if for nothing more than enhancing bench press strength.

To increase squat strength, the first critical component of any training program is the exercise choices and order. Simply stated, you have to actually squat to increase squat strength. On workouts that emphasize squat training, the squat should be the first exercise performed. When you're training for strength, the amount of weight you use is a critical factor for strength gains. Therefore, you should do the squat first, when the muscles are not fatigued and are at their strongest.

You should follow the squat with one assistance squat or leg press exercise (such as the leg press or squat machine) and occasionally an isolation exercise for quadriceps (such as the leg extension). In addition, many weightlifters also perform one or two calf exercises at the end of their squat workouts. This is sensible, since the calf muscles are involved during the squat.

Total sets performed for squats during squat workouts should be about three to five, not including warm-up sets. All assistance exercises are usually limited to three sets per exercise. Weight for the squat exercise should progressively increase from light warm-up sets with weight around 10 to 50 percent RM to heavy working sets of 85 to 95 percent RM. This is the range that most squat workouts are performed in, depending on the training phase the lifter is in. On the upper end, the weight used for training may go as high as 100 percent RM for squats. On the low end, the weight used may be reduced to 30 percent RM or less for working sets, such as during training phases that increase power. For the assistance exercises, reps typically correspond with the percent RM used in that workout on the bench press. So reps tend to fall mostly in the range of 2 to 10 reps for assistance exercises, depending on the training phase. Rest periods between sets usually last about two to five minutes. See table 8.7 for a sample squat training workout. A detailed description of the proper exercise technique during the squat is covered in chapter 21. Proper form is essential for maximal strength on the squat; the Squatter's Rights box presents tips for increasing squat strength.

TABLE 8.7   Squat Day

This squat workout is for a powerlifter who has a maximum squat of 565 pounds and is training with 90 percent of his or her maximum (510 pounds).

Exercise	Sets	Weight (pounds)	Reps	Rest
Squat	1	135	10*	1 min
	1	225	10*	1 min
	1	315	8*	2 min
	1	365	8*	2 min
	1	405	6*	3 min
	1	455	4*	3 min
	3	510	3**	4 min
Leg press	3	720	4-6**	3 min
Leg extension	3	210	4-6**	2 min
Standing calf raise	3	330	8-10**	1 min

*Warm-up sets.

**Working sets.

Squatters' Rights

Closely follow these tips for safe execution of the squat:

SETUP

Position a bar on a squat rack or power rack to about mid-chest height.

Hold the bar with a wide overhand grip and duck under it so that your neck is directly in the middle of the bar. Push your back up into the bar so that the bar is no more than two inches below the top of your shoulders.

Stand up with the bar on your back to unrack it and step back from the rack.

GRIP

Hold the bar with an overhand grip and wrap your thumbs around the bar. Bring your hands in as close to your shoulders as possible.

Use your hands to press the bar against your back and pull your shoulder blades together and your elbows forward to support the bar.

HEAD

Keep your head aligned with your spine by keeping it up and looking straight ahead or slightly up.

TORSO

Maintain the arch in your lower back and pull your shoulders back while pushing your chest up and out.

Isometrically contract your spinal erector muscles and abdominals to keep your core tight.

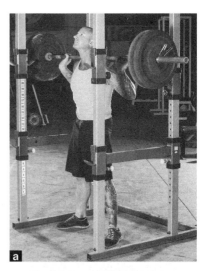

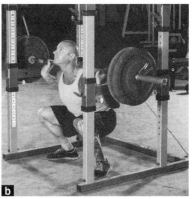

Deadlift Training

The deadlift is considered the best indicator of overall body strength. Because you must hold the bar in the hands while driving it upward from the floor with the legs, it truly involves a majority of the body's musculature. It is called the deadlift because the weight is lifted from the floor. This eliminates the eccentric motion that precedes most exercises such as the squat and bench press. The eccentric motion aids the force that is produced by the muscles during the concentric phase of a lift. Therefore, the deadlift is a much more difficult lift than the squat.

As with the squat and bench press, to increase your strength on the deadlift, you must train the deadlift. This means that you must devote at least one workout per week to specific deadlift training. You should perform the deadlift first in the workout when the muscles are strongest and not fatigued. Many powerlifters follow the deadlift exercise with assistance hamstring exercises such as the Romanian deadlift or leg curl. Depending on the training split used, many powerlifters also train back and sometimes biceps on deadlift day. This strategy makes sense, since these muscle groups are used during the deadlift.

Usually about three to five sets, not including warm-up sets, are performed for the deadlift. All assistance exercises, such as the leg curl, are usually limited to three sets per exercise. As with the other two strength exercises, the weight on the deadlift should progressively increase from very light warm-up sets (weight around 10 to 50 percent RM) to heavy working sets (ranging from 85 to 95 percent RM). This is the range that most lifters use in training the deadlift. However, the weight used during some workouts may go as high as 100 percent RM or as low as 50 percent RM for working sets. For assistance exercises, reps typically correspond

---

STANCE

Place your feet shoulder-width apart or wider—this depends on your preference. Individual bio-mechanics come into play, and you must find the foot position that is most comfortable for you. If your feet are too close together, it makes it difficult for the hamstrings and glutes to properly assist the quads. If your feet are too wide apart, the opposite will occur and your quads will not be able to assist. If you have long legs, going much wider than shoulder width tends to be more comfortable and more biomechanically advantageous. If you are of average height and have legs that are proportional to the length of your upper body, you will likely be comfortable with your feet just slightly wider than shoulder width. If you have short legs, a shoulder-width stance will probably be most comfortable.

Maintain a slight bend in your knees and isometrically contract your quads, hamstrings, and glutes before descending.

DESCENT

To descend, stick your glutes out and descend as if you were to sit down on a chair until your thighs are parallel to the floor or lower.

Keep your hips under the bar as much as possible to avoid excessive forward lean of your torso.

Be sure that your heels do not come off the floor.

ASCENT

Transition from the descent to the ascent by driving forcefully upward with the legs. Concentrate on moving your hips first before your knees. As you push up, force your knees out hard and push out on the sides of your shoes while you squat. This helps to keep the tension in your hips for greater strength.

As you ascend, thrust the head back. Don't lift your chin up; just push your head back to help contract your traps.

BREATHING

Take a big breath in and hold it as you descend into the squat.

Exhale as you pass the most difficult stage of the squat.

Life of the Deadlift

Closely follow these tips to execute the deadlift safely and effectively. Two styles of deadlift—the regular-stance deadlift and the sumo-stance deadlift—are acceptable in competition. The regular-stance version has the feet a little closer than shoulder-width apart, whereas the sumo-stance deadlift has the feet spaced apart much wider than shoulder-width. There is no consensus that has established the clear benefits of one form over the other. Therefore, the choice is pure preference of the individual. Both styles are covered in the following description.

SETUP

Set up a barbell on the floor with the desired amount of weight.

Approach the loaded barbell until your shins are touching the bar.

LEGS

Your stance should be about as wide as your own shoulders or narrower for the regular-stance deadlift. For the sumo-stance deadlift, the feet should be much farther apart than shoulder width.

For the regular-stance deadlift, toes should point straight forward or slightly out (25 degrees at most). For the sumo-stance deadlift, toes should point out to about 30 to 40 degrees.

Squat down to a position that is similar to the bottom position of the squat. However, in the regular-stance deadlift the thighs will be slightly higher than parallel to the floor. With the sumo-stance deadlift, the thighs will be about parallel to the floor. Most of your weight should be on the heels of the feet to facilitate maximal contribution of the glutes and hamstrings.

GRIP

Regardless of the style used, your grip should be a staggered grip. That means one hand should be an underhand grip and the other hand should be an overhand grip. This helps to prevent the bar from slipping out of the hands.

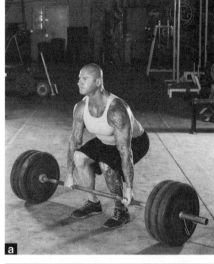

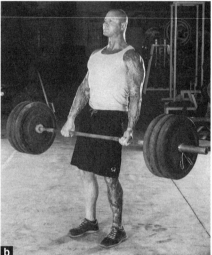

with the percent RM being used in that workout on the deadlift. So reps tend to fall mostly in the range of 2 to 10 for assistance exercises, depending on the training phase. Rest periods between sets usually last about two to five minutes. See table 8.8 for a sample deadlift training workout. A detailed description of the proper exercise technique during the deadlift is covered in chapter 25. Proper form is essential for developing maximal strength in the deadlift. The Life of the Deadlift box presents tips that will ensure you are performing the deadlift most effectively for maximal strength.

TABLE 8.8   Day of the Deadlift

This deadlift workout is for a powerlifter who has a maximum deadlift of 505 pounds and is training with 90 percent of his or her max.

Exercise	Sets	Weight (pounds)	Reps	Rest
Deadlift	1	135	10*	1 min
	1	225	10*	1 min
	1	315	8*	2 min
	1	365	8*	2 min
	1	405	6*	3 min
	1	455	4*	3 min
	3	505	3**	4 min
Romanian deadlift	3	315	4-6**	3 min
Leg curl	3	180	4-6**	2 min

*Warm-up sets.

**Working sets.

For the regular-stance deadlift, the arms will hang straight down and just outside of your thighs. For the sumo-stance deadlift, the arms hang straight down on the insides of the thighs.

TORSO

For the regular-stance deadlift, the upper body should lean slightly forward at about a 45-degree angle to the floor.

For the sumo-stance deadlift, the upper body is slightly more upright than in the regular-stance deadlift (about a 50- to 60-degree angle to the floor).

Regardless of the style used, the shoulder blades should be pulled together tightly throughout the entire exercise.

Isometrically contract your low-back muscles to maintain the natural arch in your lower back. Keep your abs tightly contracted throughout the lift.

HEAD

The head should remain in a straight line with the back. To do this, pick a point on the floor about five to six feet ahead of you and focus on that point.

ASCENT

As you stand up with the weight, imagine pushing the floor away from you with your feet.

Your hips and shoulders should ascend together. During the ascent, the bar will travel as close to the shins and legs as possible

LOCKOUT

You have reached the finish point when you have full extension of the knees, hips, and back. The lockout position should position the front part of your shoulders behind the front part of your hips.

BREATHING

Take a big breath in and hold it as you prepare to ascend.

Exhale as you pass the most difficult stage of the deadlift. Inhale again at the top and hold your breath before the return.

DESCENT

Carefully return the bar to the floor by reversing the techniques used in lifting the weight up.

Abdominal and Low-Back Training

Powerlifters and other strength athletes do train their abs. However, unlike the bodybuilder who is interested in developing the musculature of the abdominals to chisel a well-defined six-pack, the strength athlete is interested in developing the strength of the abdominal musculature. The same can be said about the low back. Both the superficial and deep muscles of the abdominals and low back make up the core musculature of the body. These muscles support the shoulders, spine, and hips during all movements. Building the strength of these muscles not only helps to prevent back injuries but can help to increase strength due to the fact that the body's foundation is stronger. For a complete listing and exercise description of the abdominal and core exercises, see chapter 24. For exercises of the low back, see chapter 16.

You should do core, abdominal, and low-back exercises toward the end of workouts to prevent fatiguing of the core musculature before doing the major strength exercises with heavy weights. Many powerlifters do one or two core, abdominal, and low-back exercises at the end of two to four workouts per week. Some even have a distinct core training day.

Core exercises, if included in a workout, are usually trained first in the series with abdominal and low-back exercises. The number of reps varies depending on the type of exercise. For core and low-back exercises, higher reps in the range of 20 to 30 are acceptable. However, many powerlifters train the good morning exercise with extremely heavy weight and lower reps in the range of 6 to 12. For ab exercises, many powerlifters also prefer to train with heavier weight and lower reps (6 to 10) to increase abdominal muscle strength. See table 8.9 for a sample core program that can be performed twice per week at the end of typical strength workouts, with at least 48 hours of rest between workouts. It includes one core exercise, one low-back exercise, and one abdominal exercise per workout.

TABLE 8.9   Getting to the Core

WORKOUT 1			
Exercise	Sets	Reps	Rest
Dumbbell woodchopper	3	20	1 min
Lying back extension	3	25	1 min
Standing crunch	3	8-10	1 min
WORKOUT 2			
Russian twist	3	25	1 min
Barbell good morning	3	8-10	2 min
Hanging leg raise	3	10-12	1 min

CHAPTER 9

Programs for Maximizing Strength

Training to maximize strength tends to be a much simpler pursuit than training to maximize muscle mass. The basic workout samples provided with the training splits discussed in chapter 8 are from tried-and-true training programs that work exceptionally well when the resistance used and reps performed are cycled. However, as the saying goes, everything works, but nothing works forever. And so, when a standard program fails to deliver the strength gains you expect, it's time to try something out of the ordinary.

This chapter covers strength training methods that are effective for maximizing muscle strength. As in chapter 6, the techniques are categorized by the type of acute variable of training that is being manipulated in each workout. Also as in chapter 6, each technique is rated on a scale of 1 to 5 for four critical areas:

1. **Time**—the amount of time that the specific workout typically takes to complete. This helps you immediately determine if this training technique will fit your training schedule. The higher the number, the longer the workouts for that specific technique will take to complete.

2. **Length**—the amount of time required to follow the program consistently for appreciable results to be noticed. This helps you determine if you have the patience required for a certain program to demonstrate adequate results in strength. The higher the number, the longer this technique must be followed for results to be realized.

3. **Difficulty**—the amount of weightlifting experience required to use the program

effectively. This helps you decide if you have enough training experience to take on specific strength training techniques. The higher the number, the more training experience you should have before attempting that particular technique.

4. **Results**—how effective the program seems to be for strength gains in most people. This helps you estimate how much strength you can expect to gain with each program. The higher the number, the greater the gains in strength you can expect from a particular program.

Each strength training method provides a sample table to show how this particular technique can be used. Some of these tables provide full training programs complete with sample workouts to be followed over several weeks. Others provide only brief details on cycling weight throughout the program. For these you are encouraged to use a basic training program, as shown in chapter 8, but incorporate the weight, rep, set, or rest changes as outlined in the sample program table. Try the advanced strength training programs discussed in chapter 9 by cycling them into your training program along with the basic programs discussed in chapter 8. These advanced programs are great to turn to when your strength gains have reached a plateau. The unorthodox nature of many of these programs will offer a unique stimulus to the muscles, which will encourage strength gains. In the programs, weights are given in pounds; please see appendix for metric conversions.

PROGRAMS THAT MANIPULATE SETS

When it comes to quantifying the strength training workout, the set is the unit that all lifters understand. It signifies how much work you are actually doing. Therefore, manipulating the work in a workout is a logical way to alter workouts in an effort to boost strength. This section covers three strength training techniques that alter the sets during a workout. The first method incorporates sets that are completed only when the muscle is too exhausted to complete another rep. The second method involves using a set system that is based on time. The third method decreases the number of sets it takes to complete a set number of reps.

Failure Training

As defined in chapter 1, muscle failure is the point during an exercise at which the muscles have fully fatigued and can no longer complete an additional rep of that exercise using strict form. While bodybuilders tend to complete all their sets to failure, powerlifters rarely, if ever, train to muscle failure. In fact, the programs in chapter 8 are not meant to be used with muscle failure. Each set is done for a certain number of reps with a certain amount of weight. When the number of reps prescribed for that set are completed, the set is over. In most cases, you will feel as though you could have completed at least one more rep. This is how most powerlifters train to increase muscle strength. Many believe that training to muscle failure can hinder strength gains. However, research from Australia suggests that training to muscle failure may enhance strength gains. The key appears to be the number of sets performed to failure—and that number appears to be one.

Australian researchers discovered that when trained lifters completed one set to failure of the four sets they trained with on the bench press for eight weeks, they had double the strength gains of lifters who did not complete any of the four sets to failure. And in a follow-up study, they discovered that doing more than one set to failure on the bench press for eight weeks offered no additional increase in strength gains. In fact, when comparing the two studies, the strength gains reported in the study using multiple sets to failure were less impressive than the strength gains reported in the study using just one set to failure. The reason may be that performing only one set to failure allows for enough stimulus to be delivered to the muscle fibers without fatiguing the muscle too much, which can limit muscle strength during the workout when training with too many sets to failure.

Taking advantage of this knowledge is rather simple. Choose any basic strength training program offered in chapter 8 and be sure to perform the last set, and only the last set, of every exercise (except the abdominals) to muscle failure. See table 9.1 for a sample training program that takes the last set of each exercise to failure. One caveat about training to failure is safety. For obvious reasons, it is not a method to be used by those who train alone, except when done with exercises that use machines or where it is easy to return the weight to a safe location—such as the deadlift, dumbbell bench press, Smith machine squat, or barbell curl. Under no circumstances should anyone training alone perform any barbell pressing exercises, barbell squat, leg press, or hack squat to failure or close to failure. These exercises all require the help of an adequate spotter to ensure that the last rep is done accurately and safely.

RATING

Time	1	2	3	4	5
Length	1	2	3	4	5
Difficulty	1	2	3	4	5
Results	1	2	3	4	5

TABLE 9.1 Failing for Strength

WORKOUT 1 (MONDAY): SQUAT DAY		
Exercise	Sets	Reps
Squat	1	10 with 50% RM
	1	6 with 60% RM
	1	5 with 75% RM
	3	5 with 85% RM
	1	To failure with 85% RM
Leg press	2	6
	1	To failure with same weight as sets 1 and 2
Leg extension	2	8
	1	To failure with same weight as sets 1 and 2
Standing calf raise	2	8
	1	To failure with same weight as sets 1 and 2
Cable woodchopper	3	20

WORKOUT 2 (WEDNESDAY): BENCH PRESS DAY		
Bench press	1	10 with 50% RM
	1	6 with 60% RM
	1	5 with 75% RM
	3	5 with 85% RM
	1	To failure with 85% RM
Incline dumbbell press	2	6
	1	To failure with same weight as sets 1 and 2

WORKOUT 2 (WEDNESDAY): BENCH PRESS DAY (continued)		
Exercise	Sets	Reps
Barbell shoulder press	2	6
	1	To failure with same weight as sets 1 and 2
Close-grip bench press	2	6
	1	To failure with same weight as sets 1 and 2
Standing crunch	4	8-10

WORKOUT 3 (FRIDAY): DEADLIFT DAY		
Deadlift	1	10 with 50% RM
	1	6 with 60% RM
	1	5 with 75% RM
	3	5 with 85% RM
	1	To failure with 85% RM
Good morning	2	6
	1	To failure with same weight as sets 1 and 2
Lying leg curl	2	8
	1	To failure with same weight as sets 1 and 2
Barbell row	2	6
	1	To failure with same weight as sets 1 and 2
Barbell curl	2	6
	1	To failure with same weight as sets 1 and 2

Time Under Tension

Time under tension (TUT) refers to a different way to define a set. Instead of a set being defined by the number of reps performed, a TUT set is defined by the length of time it takes to complete the set. The time it takes to complete the set is referred to as the time the muscle is under tension. Tension refers to the resistance from the weight being used. The amount of time spent doing each set for an exercise can be a critical component to increasing strength. Consider a set of five reps on the bench press. If the five reps each took about 2 seconds to lower the weight and another 2 seconds to press the weight back up, that's 4 seconds per rep. Five reps at this pace would take a total of about 20 seconds to complete the set. In other

words, the TUT for that set would be 20 seconds. If the time to complete each of those five reps were increased to 6 seconds, the TUT of that set would increase to 30 seconds. Although the number of reps and the amount of weight are the same on each of these sets, the first set with a TUT of 20 seconds is actually better for increasing strength.

Just as it is well established that muscle strength is best developed by training with a rep range of 1 to 6 per set, and muscle growth is best attained with a rep range of about 8 to 12, some strength training experts believe that the total time a set takes to complete may be just as important as the number of reps completed per set. Although no controlled research has yet been done to determine the best TUT ranges for developing strength or muscle mass, anecdotal evidence from strength trainers suggests that the best TUT range for strength is about 4 to 20 seconds per set and about 40 to 60 seconds per set for muscle growth. Table 9.2 shows you the optimal rep range and TUT for the desired muscle adaptation. The last column lists the time per rep range to complete the set within the optimal TUT.

Regardless of the importance of TUT for muscle adaptations, no one has suggested that TUT ranges should replace optimal rep ranges. Instead, combining both TUT and optimal rep ranges within a set may be a more precise way to prescribe how much work should be placed on a muscle to induce the desired adaptations. Using the bench press as an example, if five reps (which is within the optimal rep range for strength gains) were performed at 4 seconds per rep, the entire set would take 20 seconds to complete. That set would meet both the requirements for the optimal rep range and optimal TUT range to stress a muscle for maximizing strength gains. However, training for maximal strength using TUT allows you to increase the rep

range a bit beyond the optimal rep range for maximal strength, as long as the TUT range per set meets the requirements for maximal strength. This allows for more variety in the training program while still staying on target for inducing strength gains.

To train for maximal strength using TUT, keep your rep range at one to eight reps per set and the TUT range at 4 to 20 seconds per set. Both the rep range and TUT range should change frequently, as any good periodized program should. See table 9.3 for a sample TUT strength training program that frequently cycles reps and TUT. Choose a workout program from the training split section in chapter 8 and change the number of reps, rep speed, and TUT weekly as prescribed in the table. The best way to use the TUT method is to train with a stopwatch to monitor the TUT for each set.

RATING

Time	1	2	3	4	5
Length	1	2	3	4	5
Difficulty	1	2	3	4	5
Results	1	2	3	4	5

TABLE 9.2   Rep Time

Muscle adaptation	Optimal rep range	Optimal TUT	Seconds per rep
Strength and power	1-6	4-20 seconds	1 rep: 4-20 2 reps: 2-10 3 reps: 2-6 4 reps: 1-5 5 reps: 1-4 6 reps: 1-3 7 reps: 1-2 8 reps: 1-2
Muscle growth	6-15	40-60 seconds	6 reps: 7-10 7 reps: 6-8 8 reps: 5-7 9 reps: 5-6 10 reps: 4-6 11 reps: 4-5 12 reps: 4-5 13 reps: 4 14 reps: 3-4 15 reps: 3-4

TABLE 9.3   Muscle Countdown

Week	Reps per set	Speed per rep (seconds)	TUT for set (seconds)
1	5	4	20
2	3	4	12
3	8	2	16
4	6	3	18
5	2	10	20
6	4	5	20
7	5	3	15
8	2	4	8

Diminishing-Set Method

The goal of the diminishing-set method is to complete 70 reps of an exercise in four sets. To start, you choose a weight at which you can perform about 20 reps of the exercise of choice. The first time you go through this, it will probably take you about six to eight sets, with two-minute rest periods between sets, to complete 70 repetitions. Your goal is to eventually get the 70 total repetitions done in four sets or fewer. The benefit of this method is that it encourages strength changes and muscle growth by altering the biochemical pathways in the muscle fibers. Over time, the muscles are able to perform more reps per set because they are better at generating energy for muscle contractions. In addition, they are able to recover more fully between sets because of more efficient biochemical pathways. This method is great for developing endurance strength and therefore is best to use during periods in your strength training cycle when reps are on the high end. See table 9.4 for a sample diminishing-set workout for the bench press. A great way to use this method is to do this for two exercises per muscle group using this method for both exercises. For example, follow up the bench press workout with a diminishing-set protocol for one other chest exercise, such as the incline dumbbell bench press.

RATING

Time	1	2	3	4	5
Length	1	2	3	4	5
Difficulty	1	2	3	4	5
Results	1	2	3	4	5

TABLE 9.4 Diminish for Strength

Set	Weight (pounds)	Reps	Rest
WEEK 1			
1	275	20*	2 min
2	275	16*	2 min
3	275	12*	2 min
4	275	9*	2 min
5	275	6*	2 min
6	275	5*	2 min
7	275	2**	2 min
WEEK 2			
1	275	22*	2 min
2	275	17*	2 min
3	275	13*	2 min
4	275	10*	2 min
5	275	7*	2 min
6	275	3**	2 min
WEEK 3			
1	275	23*	2 min
2	275	18*	2 min
3	275	14*	2 min
4	275	10*	2 min
5	275	5**	2 min
WEEK 4			
1	275	24*	2 min
2	275	19*	2 min
3	275	15*	2 min
4	275	10*	2 min
5	275	2**	2 min
WEEK 5			
1	275	24*	2 min
2	275	20*	2 min
3	275	16*	2 min
4	275	10*	2 min

*To failure.

**Stop at repetition 70.

PROGRAMS THAT MANIPULATE REPETITIONS

Maximal strength is all about the single repetition. How strong a person is usually is measured by the amount of weight he or she can lift for one rep. However, it's rare to train for strength by doing single reps. Instead, a variety of rep ranges are used to benefit the one-rep max. This section covers strength training programs that manipulate the repetitions that are performed during each set. This includes programs that alter the number of reps performed per set (such as the 6 by 6 by 6 system, 5 by 10 training, 16-week drop, 5–3–2 method, and higher-strength program) as well as programs that manipulate the way each repetition is performed (such as static strength training, stronger by the inch program, ballistic training, and negative-rep training).

6 by 6 by 6 System

Similar to the other numeral-driven programs, this one involves simply picking a weight that will allow you to perform six sets of six repetitions on an exercise. The ideal weight will take you to failure only on the last set. Because of the higher volume and intensity involved, muscle groups should not be trained more than twice per week. The benefit of using this rep range is that it builds both a good deal of strength and muscle mass. The goal is to increase the weight used on each exercise by the end of the six-week program. Increase the weight when you can do more than six reps on the sixth set. See table 9.5 for a sample six-week 6 by 6 by 6 workout program that follows an upper- and lower-body training split.

RATING

Time	1	2	3	4	5
Length	1	2	3	4	5
Difficulty	1	2	3	4	5
Results	1	2	3	4	5

TABLE 9.5   6 by 6 by 6 Strength

UPPER-BODY WORKOUT 1 (MONDAY): BENCH PRESS AND PUSHING EXERCISES		
Exercise	Sets	Reps
Bench press	6	6
Dumbbell bench press	6	6
Barbell shoulder press	6	6
Upright row	6	6
Close-grip bench press	6	6
Dip	6	6
Standing crunch	6	8-10

LOWER-BODY WORKOUT 1 (TUESDAY): SQUAT AND QUADRICEPS EXERCISES		
Squat	6	6
Leg press	6	6
Leg extension	6	6
Standing calf raise	6	8-10

UPPER-BODY WORKOUT 2 (THURSDAY): BENCH PRESS AND PULLING EXERCISES		
Bench press	6	6
Lat pulldown	6	6
Barbell row	6	6
Barbell curl	6	6
Russian twist	6	20

LOWER-BODY WORKOUT 2 (FRIDAY): DEADLIFT AND HAMSTRING EXERCISES		
Deadlift	6	6
Romanian deadlift	6	6
Lying leg curl	6	6
Good morning	6	6
Seated calf raise	6	10-12

5 by 10 Training

The 5 by 10 training program uses two distinct rep ranges to maximize both strength and muscle-mass gains. The 5 portion of the program comes from the 5 by 5 training method, or five sets of five reps with two-minute rest periods between sets. It is a method for developing strength that dates to the 1950s. The goal of the 5 by 5 workout is to do five sets of five reps with a given weight. On your first workout you should pick a heavy weight that allows you to get only five reps on the first set and possibly five on your second. This should be about 85 percent RM for most exercises. If you can get five reps on the third set, the weight you chose was too light; you'll need to add 5 to 10 pounds depending on the exercise. If, on the other hand, you can't get at least 14 total reps over the five sets, the weight you chose was too heavy; you'll need to drop about 5 to 10 pounds. When you find the right weight for the exercise, stay with that weight over the course of this workout until you can do all five sets for five reps. Then you'll start over and increase the weight again to one that allows you to get only five reps on the first set. Do this on two exercises for each muscle group (for example, bench press and incline dumbbell bench press, squat and leg press, and deadlift and Romanian deadlift). For all other exercises that follow in that workout, do three sets of five to seven reps (except for calf and ab exercises, which can be done at higher reps).

The 10 portion of the 5 by 10 program comes from the 10 by 10 program used in this workout scheme. The goal is to perform 10 sets of 10 reps with a given weight. The reason this is included in a strength program is to stimulate the muscle fibers with a different stimulus in each workout. The schemes of the 5 by 5 and the 10 by 10 are similar, but different weights, reps, and total sets are used for each. This cycling of weight, reps, and sets prevents the muscle fibers from stagnating in the program, and therefore it enhances muscle adaptation.

For the 10 by 10 training, do 10 sets of 10 reps with just one exercise per workout and follow it with three sets of 8 to 10 reps on all the subsequent assistance exercises for that workout (except for calf and ab exercises, which can be done at higher reps). For the 10 by 10 training, choose a weight that you can normally get for about 12 to 15 reps. This should be about 65 to 70 percent RM for most exercises. The first few sets will feel very light. This will serve as a thorough warm-up. Perform these early sets with explosive power on each rep to recruit more of the fast-twitch muscle fibers that are capable of greater gains in strength and power. As the sets continue, the fatigue will start to set in and the number of reps will fall drastically. As with the 5 by 5 program, once you can complete 10 sets of 10 reps, you increase the weight again and start over.

Because you will reach failure several times on each workout, you should train each muscle group only once per week, such as with the squat–bench press–deadlift training split. This split is used in the sample 5 by 10 program outline in table 9.6. Simply follow this split and alternate the weight, reps, and sets every other week. You'll likely reach the 5 by 5 goal first. Increase the weight again and continue progressing until you reach the 10 by 10 goal or eight weeks have passed. Then switch over to a more basic training scheme.

RATING

Time	1	2	3	4	5
Length	1	2	3	4	5
Difficulty	1	2	3	4	5
Results	1	2	3	4	5

TABLE 9.6   5 by 10 Strength

5 × 5 WEEKS
WORKOUT 1 (MONDAY): SQUAT DAY

Exercise	Sets	Reps
Squat	5	5
Leg press	5	5
Leg extension	3	5-7
Standing calf raise	3	8-10
Russian twist	3	10-15

WORKOUT 2 (WEDNESDAY): BENCH PRESS DAY

Exercise	Sets	Reps
Bench press	5	5
Dumbbell bench press	5	5
Barbell shoulder press	3	5-7
Close-grip bench press	3	5-7
Cable crunch	3	10-12

WORKOUT 3 (FRIDAY): DEADLIFT DAY

Exercise	Sets	Reps
Deadlift	5	5
Romanian deadlift	5	5
Lying leg curl	3	5-7
Barbell row	3	5-7
Barbell curl	3	5-7
Hanging leg raise	3	12-15

10 × 10 WEEKS
WORKOUT 1 (MONDAY): SQUAT DAY

Exercise	Sets	Reps
Squat	10	10
Leg press	3	8-10
Lunge	3	8-10
Seated calf raise	3	12-15
Cable woodchopper	3	15-20

WORKOUT 2 (WEDNESDAY): BENCH PRESS DAY

Exercise	Sets	Reps
Bench press	10	10
Dumbbell bench press	3	8-10
Dumbbell shoulder press	3	8-10
Triceps dip	3	8-10
Reverse crunch	3	10-12

WORKOUT 3 (FRIDAY): DEADLIFT DAY

Exercise	Sets	Reps
Deadlift	10	10
Romanian deadlift	3	8-10
Seated leg curl	3	8-10
Pulldown	3	8-10
Dumbbell curl	3	8-10
Weighted crunch	3	8-10

16-Week Drop

This program is a stepwise progression from lighter weight and higher reps to heavy weight and low reps over a 16-week period. The 16-week drop is a great program for beginner and intermediate weightlifters who are interested in peaking maximal strength. Because it starts with lighter weight and higher reps and slowly increases the weight while decreasing the reps over the 16 weeks, it allows the beginner enough time to work with higher reps and lower intensities before jumping into the heavy-weight and low-rep training that is required to boost maximal strength. It works well with any training split, including a whole-body strength training split. This program starts with sets of 12 reps with a weight that is about 70 percent RM for three weeks. Then the reps drop to 10 per set with a weight increase to about 75 percent RM for the next three weeks. Next the weight bumps up to 80 percent RM and the reps drop to 8 per set for the next three weeks. Following that, the weight increases again to 85 percent RM and reps drop to five per set for the next three weeks. This is followed by a bump in weight to 90 percent RM and a corresponding drop in reps to four per set for three more weeks. And finally, the last week is associated with an increase in weight to 95 percent RM as reps drop down to two per set. One-rep max testing on all three exercises can be done after this final week of training. See table 9.7 for a sample 16-week drop program.

RATING

Time	1	2	3	4	5
Length	1	2	3	4	5
Difficulty	1	2	3	4	5
Results	1	2	3	4	5

TABLE 9.7 Sweet 16

WEEKS 1-3
WORKOUT 1 (MONDAY): SQUAT FOCUS

Exercise	Weight (% RM)	Sets	Reps
Squat	70%	5	12
Leg press	70%	3	12
Incline bench press	70%	3	12
Dumbbell shoulder press	70%	3	12
Barbell row	70%	3	12
Stiff-leg deadlift	70%	3	12
Close-grip bench press	70%	3	12
Dumbbell curls	70%	3	12
Hanging leg raise		3	12-15

WORKOUT 2 (WEDNESDAY): BENCH PRESS FOCUS

Exercise	Weight (% RM)	Sets	Reps
Bench press	70%	5	12
Dumbbell bench press	70%	3	12
Barbell hack squat	70%	3	12
Barbell shoulder press	70%	3	12
Deadlift	70%	3	12
Dumbbell row	70%	3	12
Triceps dip	70%	3	12
Barbell curl	70%	3	12
Cable woodchopper		3	20

WORKOUT 3 (FRIDAY): DEADLIFT FOCUS

Exercise	Weight (% RM)	Sets	Reps
Deadlift	70%	5	12
One-arm dumbbell deadlift	70%	3	12
Bench press	70%	3	12
Upright row	70%	3	12
Lat pulldown	70%	3	12
Lying triceps extension	70%	3	12
Preacher curl	70%	3	12
Back extension		3	15-20

WEEKS 4-6
WORKOUT 1 (MONDAY): SQUAT FOCUS

Exercise	Weight (% RM)	Sets	Reps
Squat	75%	5	10
Leg press	75%	3	10
Incline dumbbell press	75%	3	10
Dumbbell shoulder press	75%	3	10
T-bar row	75%	3	10
Romanian deadlift	75%	3	10
Close-grip bench press	75%	3	10
Dumbbell curl	75%	3	10
Reverse crunch		3	12-15

WORKOUT 2 (WEDNESDAY): BENCH PRESS FOCUS

Exercise	Weight (% RM)	Sets	Reps
Bench press	75%	5	10
Incline bench press	75%	3	10
Lunge	75%	3	10
Barbell shoulder press	75%	3	10
Deadlift	75%	3	10
Dumbbell row	75%	3	10
Triceps dip	75%	3	10
Barbell curl	75%	3	10
Dumbbell woodchopper		3	15

WORKOUT 3 (FRIDAY): DEADLIFT FOCUS

Deadlift	75%	5	10
Good morning	75%	3	10
Bench press	75%	3	10
Upright row	75%	3	10
Lat pulldown	75%	3	10
Triceps pressdown	75%	3	10
Preacher curl	75%	3	10
Back extension		3	15

WEEKS 7-9
WORKOUT 1 (MONDAY): SQUAT FOCUS

Exercise	Weight (% RM)	Sets	Reps
Squat	80%	5	8
Leg press	80%	3	8
Incline bench press	80%	3	8
Dumbbell shoulder press	80%	3	8
Barbell row	80%	3	8
Stiff-leg deadlift	80%	3	8
Close-grip bench press	80%	3	8
Dumbbell curls	80%	3	8
Hanging leg raise		3	12-15

WORKOUT 2 (WEDNESDAY): BENCH PRESS FOCUS

Bench press	80%	5	8
Dumbbell bench press	80%	3	8
Barbell hack squat	80%	3	8
Barbell shoulder press	80%	3	8
Deadlift	80%	3	8
Dumbbell row	80%	3	8
Triceps dip	80%	3	8
Barbell curl	80%	3	8
Cable woodchopper		3	12

> continued

TABLE 9.7 Sweet 16 *(continued)*

WEEKS 7-9 *(continued)*
WORKOUT 3 (FRIDAY): DEADLIFT FOCUS

Exercise	Weight (% RM)	Sets	Reps
Deadlift	80%	5	8
One-arm dumbbell deadlift	80%	3	8
Bench press	80%	3	8
Upright row	80%	3	8
Lat pulldown	80%	3	8
Lying triceps extension	80%	3	8
Preacher curl	80%	3	8
Back extension		3	12-15

WEEKS 10-12
WORKOUT 1 (MONDAY): SQUAT FOCUS

Exercise	Weight (% RM)	Sets	Reps
Squat	85%	5	5
Leg press	85%	3	5
Incline dumbbell press	85%	3	5
Dumbbell shoulder press	85%	3	5
T-bar row	85%	3	5
Romanian deadlift	85%	3	5
Close-grip bench press	85%	3	5
Dumbbell curl	85%	3	5
Reverse crunch		3	12-15

WORKOUT 2 (WEDNESDAY): BENCH PRESS FOCUS

Exercise	Weight (% RM)	Sets	Reps
Bench press	85%	5	5
Incline bench press	85%	3	5
Lunge	85%	3	5
Barbell shoulder press	85%	3	5
Deadlift	85%	3	5
Dumbbell row	85%	3	5
Triceps dip	85%	3	5
Barbell curl	85%	3	5
Dumbbell woodchopper		3	15

WORKOUT 3 (FRIDAY): DEADLIFT FOCUS

Exercise	Weight (% RM)	Sets	Reps
Deadlift	85%	5	5
Good morning	85%	3	5
Bench press	85%	3	5
Upright row	85%	3	5
Lat pulldown	85%	3	5
Triceps pressdown	85%	3	5
Preacher curl	85%	3	5
Back extension		3	15

WEEKS 13-15
WORKOUT 1 (MONDAY): SQUAT FOCUS

Exercise	Weight (% RM)	Sets	Reps
Squat	90%	5	4
Leg press	90%	3	4
Incline bench press	90%	3	4
Dumbbell shoulder press	90%	3	4
Barbell row	90%	3	4
Stiff-leg deadlift	90%	3	4
Close-grip bench press	90%	3	4
Dumbbell curl	90%	3	4
Hanging leg raise		3	10

WORKOUT 2 (WEDNESDAY): BENCH PRESS FOCUS

Bench press	90%	5	4
Dumbbell bench press	90%	3	4
Barbell hack squat	90%	3	4
Barbell shoulder press	90%	3	4
Deadlift	90%	3	4
Dumbbell row	90%	3	4
Triceps dip	90%	3	4
Barbell curl	90%	3	4
Cable woodchopper		3	10

WORKOUT 3 (FRIDAY): DEADLIFT FOCUS

Deadlift	90%	5	4
One-arm dumbbell deadlift	90%	3	4
Bench press	90%	3	4
Upright row	90%	3	4
Lat pulldown	90%	3	4
Lying triceps extension	90%	3	4
Preacher curl	90%	3	4
Back extension		3	10

WEEK 16
WORKOUT 1 (MONDAY): SQUAT FOCUS

Exercise	Weight (% RM)	Sets	Reps
Squat	95%	5	2
Leg press	95%	3	2
Incline dumbbell press	95%	3	2
Dumbbell shoulder press	95%	3	2
T-bar row	95%	3	2
Romanian deadlift	95%	3	2
Close-grip bench press	95%	3	2
Dumbbell curl	95%	3	2
Reverse crunch		3	12-15

WEEK 16 *(continued)*
WORKOUT 2 (WEDNESDAY): BENCH PRESS FOCUS

Exercise	Weight (% RM)	Sets	Reps
Bench press	95%	5	2
Incline bench press	95%	3	2
Lunge	95%	3	2
Barbell shoulder press	95%	3	2
Deadlift	95%	3	2
Dumbbell row	95%	3	2
Triceps dip	95%	3	2
Barbell curl	95%	3	2
Dumbbell woodchopper		3	10

WORKOUT 3 (FRIDAY): DEADLIFT FOCUS

Exercise	Weight (% RM)	Sets	Reps
Deadlift	95%	5	2
Good morning	95%	3	2
Bench press	95%	3	2
Upright row	95%	3	2
Lat pulldown	95%	3	2
Triceps pressdown	95%	3	2
Preacher curl	95%	3	2
Back extension		3	10

5-3-2 Method

This 10-week maximal-strength peaking program is best used by those with at least one year of solid training experience. It starts off heavy and gets even heavier throughout the program. It is a simple program to follow because the rep ranges correspond with the number of weeks you should train with that rep range. The first five weeks is a 5 by 5 program where you stick with a weight that allows you to get five sets of five reps. Then for the next three weeks you bump it up to a weight that allows you to get three sets of three reps, or a 3 by 3 program. You finish with two weeks of training with a weight that allows you to get only two sets of two reps, or a 2 by 2 program. Similar to other weight progression schemes for increasing strength, this program works because it slowly increases the weight until a weight close to the one-rep max is being used. See table 9.8 for a sample 10-week 5–3–2 program that will boost strength on all three major lifts. This sample program uses a push–pull training split.

RATING

Time	1	2	3	4	5
Length	1	2	3	4	5
Difficulty	1	2	3	4	5
Results	1	2	3	4	5

TABLE 9.8   5–3–2 Strength Program

WEEKS 1-5
WORKOUT 1 (MONDAY AND THURSDAY): PUSH

Exercise	Weight (% RM)	Sets	Reps
Squat[1]	85%	5	5
Leg press	85%	5	5
Leg extension	85%	5	5
Bench press[1]	85%	5	5
Incline dumbbell press	85%	5	5
Dumbbell shoulder press	85%	5	5
Close-grip bench press	85%	5	5
Standing calf raise[2]		5	10-12

WORKOUT 2 (TUESDAY AND FRIDAY): PULL

Exercise	Weight (% RM)	Sets	Reps
Deadlift	85%	5	5
Lying leg curl	85%	5	5
Barbell row	85%	5	5
Lat pulldown	85%	5	5
Barbell curl	85%	5	5
Weighted crunch[3]		5	10-12

> continued

TABLE 9.8 5-3-2 Strength Program *(continued)*

WEEKS 6-8
WORKOUT 1 (MONDAY AND THURSDAY): PUSH

Exercise	Weight (% RM)	Sets	Reps
Squat[1]	90%	3	3
Leg press	90%	3	3
Split squat	90%	3	3
Bench press[1]	90%	3	3
Incline bench press	90%	3	3
Barbell shoulder press	90%	3	3
Dips	90%	3	3
Standing calf raise[2]		4	8-10

WORKOUT 2 (TUESDAY AND FRIDAY): PULL

Exercise	Weight (% RM)	Sets	Reps
Deadlift	90%	3	3
Good morning	90%	3	3
Seated cable row	90%	3	3
Lat pulldown	90%	3	3
Barbell curl	90%	3	3
Standing crunch[4]		4	8-10

[1]Thursday perform bench press and incline dumbbell press before squat.

[2]Thursday perform seated calf raise.

WEEKS 9-10
WORKOUT 1 (MONDAY AND THURSDAY): PUSH

Exercise	Weight (% RM)	Sets	Reps
Squat[1]	95%	2	2
Front squat	95%	2	2
Leg press	95%	2	2
Bench press[1]	95%	2	2
Dumbbell bench press	95%	2	2
Barbell shoulder press	95%	2	2
Close-grip bench press	95%	2	2
Standing calf raise[2]		3	6-8

WORKOUT 2 (TUESDAY AND FRIDAY): PULL

Exercise	Weight (% RM)	Sets	Reps
Deadlift	95%	2	2
Romanian deadlift	95%	2	2
Barbell row	95%	2	2
Lat pulldown	95%	2	2
Barbell curl	95%	2	2
Standing crunch[5]		3	6-8

[3]Friday perform hanging leg raise.

[4]Friday perform Russian twist.

[5]Friday perform dumbbell woodchopper.

Higher-Strength Program

This program is based on research from Japan that has discovered when one set of very high reps is added to the last set of each exercise, strength gains are better than when training with just low reps. They studied leg strength in subjects on a 10-week program of leg presses and leg extensions. One group trained with five sets of three to five reps while the second group added one set of 25 to 30 reps at the end of each exercise. The group that added the 25 to 30 reps had a 5 percent greater increase in strength, as well as greater increases in muscle size, than the group performing just five sets of 3 to 5 reps. Although the scientists were unsure of the exact mechanism for the additional strength gains, it appears that the single set of higher reps provides an additional training stimulus that affects strength gains. The higher levels of growth hormone associated with the higher-rep training may have affected adaptations in muscle fibers that could have increased the strength of the muscle fibers. Taking advantage of this information is as simple as adding one set of 25 to 30 reps with a weight that is only about 45 to 50 percent RM to a program that incorporates a 5 by 5 strength training system. Be sure to take this final set to muscle failure. Since this program is fairly demanding on the muscle fibers, you should train each muscle group just once per week while using this program in table 9.9. Follow it for no more than eight weeks.

RATING

Time	1	2	3	4	5
Length	1	2	3	4	5
Difficulty	1	2	3	4	5
Results	1	2	3	4	5

TABLE 9.9   Get High for Strength

WORKOUT 1 (MONDAY): SQUAT DAY				WORKOUT 3 (FRIDAY): DEADLIFT DAY			
Exercise	Sets	Reps	Weight (% RM)	Exercise	Sets	Reps	Weight (% RM)
Squat	5	5	85%	Deadlift	5	5	85%
	1	25-30	45-50%		1	25-30	45-50%
Leg press	5	5	85%	Romanian deadlift	5	5	85%
	1	25-30	45-50%		1	25-30	45-50%
Leg extension	5	5	85%	Lying leg curl	5	5	85%
	1	25-30	45-50%		1	25-30	45-50%
Standing calf raise	5	25-30		Barbell row	5	5	85%
Cable woodchopper	5	25-30			1	25-30	45-50%
WORKOUT 2 (WEDNESDAY): BENCH PRESS DAY				Barbell curl	5	5	85%
Bench press	5	5	85%		1	25-30	45-50%
	1	25-30	45-50%	Incline reverse crunch	5	15-20	
Incline bench press	5	5	85%				
	1	25-30	45-50%				
Barbell shoulder press	5	5	85%				
	1	25-30	45-50%				
Close-grip bench press	5	5	85%				
	1	25-30	45-50%				
Standing crunch	5	8-10					

Static Strength Training

This method involves holding a heavy weight at the end of the positive phase of a rep for up to 20 seconds. Although using a full range of motion (ROM) is typically a smart thing to do, there are occasions when going against the norm is warranted, such as when strength gains have come to a halt regardless of the programs you have tried. When this is the case, it's time to pull out all the stops and use something quite unorthodox—such as static strength training. The term *static* means lack of movement, as in an isometric contraction. And as this term implies, with static training you take a weight and hold it in a fixed position for several seconds. This concept is based on the idea that by forcing the muscle to work only when it is maximally contracted and using the heaviest weight possible, you can optimize its strength potential.

Although there is no published research to support its effectiveness, anecdotal reports on static strength training are quite impressive. In fact, Bob Hoffman, founder of the York Barbell Company and former U.S. Olympic weightlifting coach, had

members of the U.S. team use a similar training system with much success in the early 1960s. The late Mike Mentzer, professional bodybuilder, also touted the effectiveness of static contractions for building both muscle size and strength. It appears to work because of the overload that is placed on the muscle. When you train using a full ROM, the amount of weight you can use is limited by your sticking point—the point in the exercise ROM where you're weakest. You can use only as much weight as you can lift through that sticking point. With static contractions, the sticking point is eliminated, so you can overload the muscle fibers with as much weight as you can hold for at least 10 seconds in the strongest position of the particular muscle.

To use static strength training properly, be sure to start each workout with a thorough warm-up. Do two light sets of each exercise you're training statically. On each rep, stop and hold for a count of three at about two to four inches from the end of the full contraction. Hit a third warm-up set with a weight you can do for about six reps, but do only one rep—being sure to hold it for a count of three before ending the set. Do two static sets per exercise with two minutes of rest in between sets. The weight you choose should be light enough to allow you to hold it statically at about two to four inches from the full contraction point of the movement for at least 10 seconds but heavy enough so that you can't hold it for more than 20 seconds. See the following sample photos of static contraction hold positions for common exercises. Once you can hold a weight for more than 20 seconds, it's time to increase the weight. After the second set, drop the weight and do three full-ROM sets of that exercise.

You'll need a reliable training partner to help you with this training method. Your training partner will need to help you move the weight to the static position but should apply only enough force as needed to help you get the weight there. That will help to prepare your muscles to resist the weight during the static contraction. The training partner should also watch the clock during your static sets to make sure you are within the time window of 10 to 20 seconds per set. A Smith machine makes a good tool to use for many of the static contraction exercises because it is easier to set the weight in the correct position.

Try the static strength training program outlined in table 9.10 for eight weeks before returning to full-ROM training. The goal is to progress to heavier weights for the static contraction sets over the eight weeks. This should carry over to greater strength when you return to full-ROM training. This sample static strength training workout uses an upper- and lower-body powerlifting split.

RATING

Time	1	2	3	4	5
Length	1	2	3	4	5
Difficulty	1	2	3	4	5
Results	1	2	3	4	5

TABLE 9.10 Static King Workout

UPPER-BODY WORKOUT 1 (MONDAY): BENCH PRESS AND PUSHING EXERCISES

Exercise	Sets	Reps
Bench press	2 static sets/ 10-20 sec	
	3	6 with 80%
Dumbbell bench press	2 static sets/ 10-20 sec	
	3	6 with 80%
Barbell shoulder press	2 static sets/ 10-20 sec	
	3	6 with 80%
Dumbbell lateral raise	2 static sets/ 10-20 sec	
	3	6 with 80%
Close-grip bench press	2 static sets/ 10-20 sec	
	3	6 with 80%
Triceps pressdown	2 static sets/ 10-20 sec	
	3	6 with 80%
Standing crunch	3	8-10

LOWER-BODY WORKOUT 1 (TUESDAY): SQUAT AND QUADRICEPS EXERCISES

Exercise	Sets	Reps
Squat	2 static sets/ 10-20 sec	
	3	6 with 80%
Leg press	2 static sets/ 10-20 sec	
	3	6 with 80%
Leg extension	2 static sets/ 10-20 sec	
	3	6 with 80%
Standing calf raise	2 static sets/ 10-20 sec	
	3	10-12

UPPER-BODY WORKOUT 2 (THURSDAY): BENCH PRESS AND PULLING EXERCISES

Exercise	Sets	Reps
Bench press	5	75%*
	2 static sets/ 10-20 sec	
Seated cable row	3	6 with 80%
Lat pulldown	2 static sets/ 10-20 sec	
	3	6 with 80%

*Light bench press day—no static contractions.

> continued on page 202

Static Contraction Hold Positions

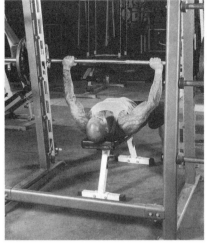
Static bench press.

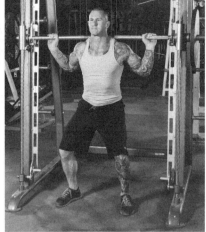
Static squat.

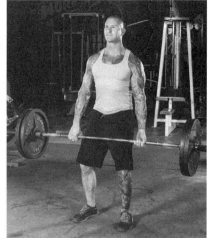
Static deadlift.

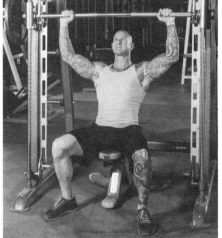
Static shoulder press.

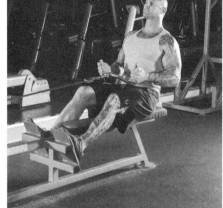
Static seated row.

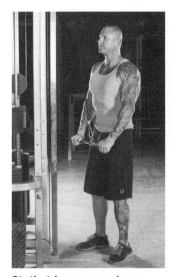
Static triceps pressdown.

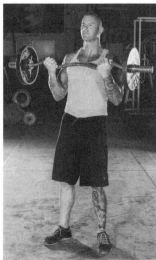
Static barbell curl.

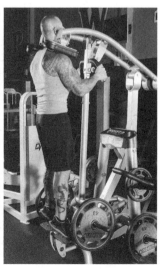
Static standing calf raise.

TABLE 9.10 Static King Workout *(continued)*

UPPER-BODY WORKOUT 2 (THURSDAY): BENCH PRESS AND PULLING EXERCISES *(continued)*

Exercise	Sets	Reps
Barbell curl	2 static sets/ 10-20 sec	
	3	6 with 80%
Russian twist	3	15-20

LOWER-BODY WORKOUT 2 (FRIDAY): DEADLIFT AND HAMSTRING EXERCISES

Exercise	Sets	Reps
Deadlift	2 static sets/ 10-20 sec	
	3	6 with 80%

LOWER-BODY WORKOUT 2 (FRIDAY): DEADLIFT AND HAMSTRING EXERCISES *(continued)*

Exercise	Sets	Reps
Romanian deadlift	2 static sets/ 10-20 sec	
	3	6 with 80%
Lying leg curl	2 static sets/ 10-20 sec	
	3	6 with 80%
Seated calf raise	2 static sets/ 10-20 sec	
	3	12-15
Back extension	3	10-12

Stronger by the Inch Program

This strength training program takes advantage of overload by starting with a weight that is greater than the lifter's 1RM. This weight is performed for partial-ROM reps that gradually increase in ROM until the full ROM is completed. It is a method to use sparingly, such as when all other strength training methods have failed to provide sufficient gains in strength. This method of using progressive partial reps to grow stronger works best for compound movements such as the three major strength lifts: bench press, squat, and deadlift. To follow the stronger by the inch program safely and effectively, you should perform the lifts in a power rack. This allows you to accurately measure the ROM and keep it limited to where you want it. The pins will also act as a safety net for when you fail. See the Rack It Up box for setting up properly in the rack.

You start the program with about 10 percent more weight than your current one-rep max (1RM) for the lift on which you wish to increase your strength. For example, if your max bench press is 250 pounds, you should use about 275 for the Stronger by the Inch program. The program works best if you concentrate on using it for one lift at a time and train each major lift just once per week. The first week, start by doing a four-inch partial rep: Lower the bar only four inches (10 centimeters) from the top position of the exercise, near lockout. Each week you'll attempt to lower the ROM by lowering the pins in the rack by two inches (five centimeters). If you get stuck at a setting and can't get one rep, increase the pin height by two inches and complete the workout from there. Next week, lower the pin by two inches and try again. If you don't stick it at

this point, strip off some plates to find a weight at which you can complete the partial rep. This is the new weight with which you'll finish the program. The goal is to lower the weight an additional two inches each week until you're about four inches above the bottom position. If you don't progress to this point by eight weeks, stop where you are and test your 1RM. You should still show some improvement on your strength in the full ROM for that lift.

This method of progressive partials works because of overload. By using a weight that's heavier than you could normally handle for full-range reps, you overload the majority of the muscle fibers that perform the full-ROM version of the exercise. Although your strength increase will be mainly in the small ROM you're using, some of this will carry over into the lower portions of the ROM. By slowly lowering the ROM in two-inch increments, you allow the muscle fibers to adapt to the heavier weight and slowly increase the ROM to which your new strength can be applied.

Table 9.11 shows a sample bench press program set up for a lifter with an 18-inch range of motion and a 275-pound 1RM using 300 as his or her new weight. Table 9.12 shows a sample program for incorporating partial rep training on the bench press into a workout program.

RATING

Time	1	2	3	**4**	5
Length	1	2	**3**	4	5
Difficulty	1	2	3	4	**5**
Results	1	2	**3**	4	5

TABLE 9.11 Inching Along on the Bench Press

Week	Pin setting
1	4 inches from top
2	6 inches from top
3	8 inches from top
4	10 inches from top (if you can't make without assistance, do it again)
5	10 inches from top
6	12 inches from top
7	14 inches from top
8*	Full-ROM 1RM with 300 pounds

*Always retest your 1RM on week 8, regardless of how far you've progressed down the rack. You may be able to do the weight for a full-ROM rep, even if you haven't gotten below 10 or 12 inches from the top. Even if you can't do a full ROM with the new weight, you should be able to do at least 5% more than your original 1RM.

Note: 1 inch = 2.54 centimeters.

TABLE 9.12 Full-Rep Program

Exercise	Set	ROM	Weight (% 1RM)	Reps
Bench press	Warm-up	Full	50%	10
	Warm-up	Full	70%	6
	Warm-up	Partial	90%	2
	Warm-up	Partial	100%	1
	1	Partial	110%	1-3
	2	Partial	110%	1-3
	3	Full	90%	2-3
	4	Full	85%	5-6
	5	Full	75%	10
Dumbbell bench press	1	Full	80%	6-8
	2	Full	80%	6-8
	3	Full	80%	6-8
Barbell shoulder press	1	Full	80%	6-8
	2	Full	80%	6-8
	3	Full	80%	6-8
Close-grip bench press	1	Full	80%	6-8
	2	Full	80%	6-8
	3	Full	80%	6-8
Hanging leg raise	4 sets	Full	Body weight	12-15

Rack It Up

Follow these steps to get set up in the power rack for progressive partials.

- Measure the distance between safety pin settings (holes) on the rack. Most racks will have holes spaced every 2 to 4 inches (5 to 10 centimeters).
- Determine the top position in your ROM, just before lockout. Use the pinhole just below this to designate your top point.
- Determine the bottom position of your ROM and designate it with the lower pinhole.
- Count the number of pin settings between the top and bottom positions. The distance will probably range from 12 to 24 inches (30.5 to 61 centimeters), depending on your limb length and the exercise you're doing. Therefore, the number of pin settings will likely range from 2 to 10 holes. Your progression scheme will be based partly on this number.
- Subtract 4 inches from the top, meaning you won't use the first one or two pin settings.
- Subtract 4 inches from the bottom, meaning you won't work below 4 inches from the bottom position. (Once you're close to this point, you'll likely be able to perform a full rep with the weight.) In other words, you won't work down to the last one or two pegs.
- Now count the number of pin settings between these two settings. This should be somewhere from one to seven holes.
- If the rack you're using has setting increments larger than 2 inches, you'll need to modify it so that you make 2-inch progressions over the course of the program. You can use bar pads, towels, or 2.5-pound plates (most have about a 2-inch radius).

Ballistic Strength Training

This training method develops explosive power, which can increase strength. This is because each strength exercise has a natural biomechanical sticking point that occurs at a spot in the range of motion where primary muscle groups are changing. For example, in the bench press, the sticking point for many lifters is where the primary force is being changed from the pectoralis major to the deltoids and triceps. Ballistic training uses explosive movements that power you through these sticking points.

The major benefit of ballistic training has to do with acceleration. In a traditional rep, you typically accelerate the weight on the concentric portion only during the first third of the range of motion. During the other two-thirds, the weight is actually being decelerated. If deceleration did not take place, you wouldn't be able to hold onto the weight at the end of the rep. Yet, when you train ballistically, the weight is accelerated through the whole range of motion and starts to decelerate only after you've let go of the bar. This allows you to develop much more power through the rep.

Ballistic training also forces your body to trigger fast-twitch muscle fibers. This is important because these fibers have the greatest potential for strength gains. Because ballistic training forces the muscles to adapt to contracting very quickly and forcefully, it trains the fast-twitch fibers to produce a great amount of force in a very short period. This is very useful when applying a great amount of force such as during a max bench press, squat, or deadlift.

Ballistic training is most commonly performed with bench press throws and squat jumps, often using a Smith machine, which guides the bar securely along metal rods. Yet, ballistic training is not confined to these exercises. In fact, ballistic training can be done for almost any muscle group.

See table 9.13 for a list of ballistic exercises that can be performed in any gym.

Regardless of the exercise, ballistic training should be done with a weight that is about 30 to 50 percent of the 1RM for that exercise. This weight is used because research has shown that optimal power is produced at about 30 to 50 percent RM. For example, if your max bench press is 300 pounds, you would do bench press throws on the Smith machine with about 90 to 150 pounds. The number of reps performed with ballistic training is three to five reps, never any more. This is to keep every rep a max effort and prevent fatigue. Fatigue does not benefit the development of power and can actually increase the risk of injury when training ballistically. Therefore, rest time should be ample between sets. Take at least three minutes of rest before doing another set.

A great way to work ballistic training into your regimen is to use a max effort–dynamic effort training split and perform the ballistic training during the dynamic effort portion of the split. An example of this is outlined in table 9.14 to be done on the third and fourth workouts (usually on Thursday and Friday) of a max effort–dynamic effort training split. Another way to train ballistically is to follow a squat, bench press, and deadlift training split on a full-body ballistic workout performed on a fourth day. An example of such a workout is presented in table 9.15.

RATING

Time	1	2	3	4	5
Length	1	2	3	4	5
Difficulty	1	2	3	4	5
Results	1	2	3	4	5

TABLE 9.13 Ballistic Bounty

Muscle group	Exercise	Execution
Chest	Smith machine bench press throw	On the Smith machine, lower the bar to your chest just as you would during a normal set. Then, press the weight off your chest explosively so that you throw it up as high as possible. Keep your arms extended with a slight bend in the elbows and catch the weight as it comes back down. Reset your hands so they're even before doing the next rep.
Legs	Jump squat	Stand with your feet about shoulder-width apart. Drop into a squat until your thighs are about parallel to the ground, then explode up as fast as you can so that your feet leave the floor at the top of the motion. Land with soft knees and go down into your next rep. Research shows that doing jump squats with just your body weight develops more power than using additional weight from a barbell.
Legs and back	Dumbbell deadlift jump	Squat to grab dumbbells that are placed just outside your feet. As with the jump squat, you will explode up as fast as you can so that your feet leave the ground at the top of the motion. Land with soft knees and immediately go down to return the weight to the floor.
Back	One-arm Smith machine power row	Place the bar at the very bottom of the Smith machine and stand sideways to it with your right foot 12 to 18 inches (30.5 to 46 centimeters) away to provide the bar with plenty of clearance when you release it. Grasp the bar with your right hand, bend your knees slightly, and keep your back flat. Using your back muscles, pull the weight up forcefully and let go of the bar as you pull your shoulder blade back. Let the weight fall to the start; it will be cushioned by the bumper springs. Repeat for 3 to 5 reps and then switch arms.
Shoulders	Smith machine overhead press throw	Get on your knees or sit on a low-back bench while holding the bar of the Smith machine at upper chest level. Push the weight up forcefully overhead, releasing your grip at the top of the movement and catching the weight when it comes back down.
Triceps	Smith machine close-grip bench throw	This movement will be the same as for the bench throw, except that you'll grasp the bar with a shoulder-width grip. After catching the bar on the way down, be sure to reset your hands so they're even and close together.
Biceps	Smith machine curl throw	Because the Smith machine limits you to a fixed path, the range of motion here will be shorter than on a free-weight barbell curl. Start just below halfway (arms at about 45 degrees to the floor) with a shoulder-width grip. Explode the weight up so that it leaves your hands before you're able to squeeze the contraction, as you normally would when curling. Again, catch the bar on the way down and reset your grip.

TABLE 9.14 Going Ballistic

LOWER-BODY WORKOUT 2: SQUAT, DEADLIFT			
Exercise	Sets	Reps	%1RM
Squat jump	3	3-5	30-50%
Dumbbell deadlift jump	3	3-5	30-50%
Romanian deadlift	3	3-5	75%
Barbell good morning	3	3-5	75%
Russian twist	3	15-20	Body weight
UPPER-BODY WORKOUT 2: BENCH PRESS			
Smith machine bench press throw	3	3-5	30-50%
Smith machine overhead press throw	3	3-5	30-50%
Smith machine close-grip bench throw	3	3-5	30-50%
One-arm Smith machine power row	3	3-5	30-50%
Smith machine curl throw	3	3-5	30-50%
Decline crunch	3	12	Body weight

TABLE 9.15 Power Play Day

Exercise	Sets	Reps	%1RM
Squat jump	3	3-5	30-50%
Smith machine bench press throw	3	3-5	30-50%
One-arm Smith machine power row	3	3-5	30-50%
Dumbbell deadlift jump	3	3-5	30-50%
Smith machine overhead press throw	3	3-5	30-50%
Smith machine close-grip bench throw	3	3-5	30-50%
Smith machine curl throw	3-4	3-5	

Negative-Rep Strength Training

Negative-rep training refers to training that emphasizes the negative, or eccentric, portion of the exercise. Unlike negative-rep training to build muscle mass, negative-rep strength training does not come as an afterthought at the end of a workout but as the first and foremost method used in the workout. Doing negative reps as the first sets of an exercise allows for greater than 100 percent RM to be used as weight. Most lifters can resist about 130 percent of their 1RM on the negative portion of the rep. Training with this much weight even on the negative motion of an exercise can cause real strength gains on the positive portion of the exercise as well. This has to do with muscle fiber and nerve adaptations. The overload that the excess weight places on the muscle fiber induces muscle damage and influences the nerves that cause the muscles to recruit more fast-twitch muscle fibers. These two factors result in muscle regeneration that leads to larger and stronger muscle fibers as well as a greater number of fast-twitch muscle fibers.

When training with negative reps, the key is to perform the rep slowly. You should attempt a weight that is about 130 percent of your 1RM for the exercises you are training and resist it at a rate

that takes three to five seconds to complete the negative rep. If you can resist the weight for longer than five seconds, add more weight. If you can't resist the weight for at least three seconds, reduce the weight. Perform three sets of four to six negative reps for each major lift—bench press, squats (should be done on Smith machine), and deadlift. Follow the negatives with two sets of regular reps using a weight that is about 75 to 80 percent RM.

Because of the intensity of negative-rep training, you'll need more time to recover between sets, at least three minutes. The same holds true for recovery between workouts, because you should allow a full seven days of rest between workouts. That makes the squat–bench press–deadlift training split a popular one to use when training with negative-rep training. See table 9.16 for a sample negative-rep training week using that split. Follow this for no more than six weeks.

To use negative-rep training safely and effectively, you should have the help of a training partner. Those who train alone can do unilateral negatives with the help of a Smith machine. To do this, load the Smith machine with about 70 percent RM for the bench press, squat, or deadlift. Lift the weight through the positive, or concentric, portion of the lift, but resist the weight through the negative portion with only one limb. Switch the limb that takes the negative rep every other rep until each limb has performed four to six negative reps.

Finally, you should be aware of delayed-onset muscle soreness (DOMS) that usually accompanies negative-rep training. For those unaccustomed to negative-rep training, DOMS can be severe. The more often you use the technique, the less severe the soreness will be. Some people may be at risk for developing a rare condition known as rhabdomyolysis. This sometimes-fatal condition can occur after severe muscle damage. When muscles break down, they release potassium, enzymes, and myoglobin into the blood. Myoglobin can accumulate in the kidneys and cause them to collapse. This can escalate into dangerously high blood potassium levels and may result in heart failure. To prevent rhabdomyolysis while using negative-rep training, drink plenty of water (up to one gallon per day), limit alcohol consumption, avoid training with negatives for several weeks after a viral infection, and go to the hospital immediately if your urine turns dark brown.

RATING

Time	1	2	3	4	5
Length	1	2	3	4	5
Difficulty	1	2	3	4	5
Results	1	2	3	4	5

TABLE 9.16 Accentuate the Positive

WORKOUT 1 (MONDAY): SQUAT DAY			
Exercise	Sets	Reps	Weight (% RM)
Smith machine squat	3	4-6	130%
Barbell squat	2	6-8	80%
Leg press	3	6-8	80%
Leg extension	3	8-10	75%
Standing calf raise	3	8-10	75%
Crunch	3	20	
WORKOUT 2 (WEDNESDAY): BENCH PRESS DAY			
Bench press	3	4-6	130%
	2	6-8	80%
Incline dumbbell press	3	6-8	80%
Barbell shoulder press	3	6-8	80%
Close-grip bench press	3	6-8	80%
Hanging leg raise	3	12-15	
WORKOUT 3 (FRIDAY): DEADLIFT DAY			
Deadlift	3	4-6	130%
	2	6-8	80%
Good morning	3	6-8	80%
Lying leg curl	3	8-10	75%
Barbell row	4	6-8	80%
Barbell curl	4	6-8	80%
Russian twist	4	15-20	

PROGRAMS THAT MANIPULATE LOAD

Strength is all about weight. The amount of weight you can lift defines your level of strength. Because of this, it is only logical that strength training programs that vary the weight you lift are successful strategies for building muscle strength. This section discusses strength training techniques that alter the load, or amount of weight, used during workouts. Some techniques work through mechanisms involving the nervous system, such as the max-out for muscle strength method and wave training method. The 5 percent method works by systematically increasing and decreasing the weight over time, while the DeLorme ascending pyramid progressively increases the weight on each successive set. One program—the same-weight training method—uses the same weight for all sets. Modifying the weight you train with by following any of these programs will work to increase the total amount of weight you can lift.

Max-Out for Muscle Strength Method

This method takes advantage of a phenomenon known formally as postactivation potentiation, or simply potentiation. This refers to the ability of one exercise to immediately enhance the performance of a second exercise that is performed shortly after the first exercise. Although there are many ways to do this, the max-out for muscle strength method uses the same exercise but different weights to achieve the same effect. More precisely, this method uses a one-rep set with 90 percent RM to enhance the number of reps that can be performed with a subsequent set using 80 percent RM.

Although the exact mechanism for this phenomenon has not been pinpointed, scientists currently believe that it may be due to enhanced excitation of the central nervous system or to molecular events in the muscle fibers themselves. In simpler terms, performing the heavy set "tricks" your nervous system into preparing for another heavy set. When you suddenly drop the weight, it feels lighter than it normally would because your nervous system is calling in more muscle fibers to do the job than it normally would for the lighter weight. This is the reason baseball players swing with a weighted bat before hitting with a much lighter bat. Regardless of the mechanism, the bottom line is that it may increase your strength on lighter sets by close to 10 percent.

To perform this method in the gym, you do one set using 90 to 95 percent RM for just one rep. Then you rest three minutes and perform a set with about 10 percent more than 80 percent RM (a weight you can normally lift for about eight reps). The potentiation from the previous set should allow you to complete about eight reps with the heavier weight. For example, if your 1RM on the bench press is 300, the first set you do (after two or three warm-up sets) is for one rep with about 275 to 285 pounds. The second set you do would be with 260 pounds for about eight reps. Normally you would be able to lift only 240 pounds for eight reps, but the potentiation increased your strength by roughly 10 percent.

The best way to use this technique is to reserve it for major lifts and train those lifts just once per week. Do not use the max-out for muscle strength technique for more than eight weeks consecutively for any exercise. See table 9.17 for a sample squat workout using the max-out for muscle strength technique. This workout is for a lifter whose 1RM on the squat is 365 pounds, whose 90% RM is about 330 pounds, and whose 80% RM (what he or she can normally complete for eight reps) is about 290 pounds. This workout should be followed with the typical squat assistance exercises.

RATING

Time	1	2	3	4	5
Length	1	2	3	4	5
Difficulty	1	2	3	4	5
Results	1	2	3	4	5

TABLE 9.17   Fast Strength

Exercise	Set	Weight (pounds)	Reps	Rest (minutes)
Squat	Warm-up	135	10	2
	Warm-up	225	7	2
	Warm-up	275	5	2
	Warm-up	315	1	3
	Set 1	330	1	3-5
	Set 2	310*	8	5
	Set 3	330	1	3-5
	Set 4	310*	8	3

*Although the lifter normally can squat only 290 pounds for eight reps, the potentiation allows for two sets of eight reps with 310 pounds.

5 Percent Method

This program follows a set pattern of progression in the amount of weight lifted. Basically, in each workout the weight lifted is increased by about 5 percent and the number of reps performed is decreased by one. Although the 5 percent program is a little more complicated than that, the result is simply an increase in strength of about 10 percent after only six successive workouts. The 5 percent program is best used on basic exercises such as the bench press, incline bench press, squat, deadlift, leg press, shoulder press, barbell row, and pulldown. It can also be adapted to basic arm exercises such as close-grip bench press, triceps pressdown, triceps extension, and the barbell curl. Perform no more than three exercises per muscle group and provide each with five to seven days of rest between workouts. To start the 5 percent program, pick a weight for each exercise that allows you to perform four sets of six reps with three- to four-minute rest periods between sets. We'll use the squat, with a weight of 300 pounds, as an example. In workout 1 you would perform four sets of the squat, each for six reps using 300 pounds. For workout 2 you increase the weight by 5 percent—or to 315 pounds—and finish four sets of five reps. At workout 3 you increase the weight by 5 percent again (from the original 300 pounds)—or 330 pounds—and do four sets of four reps. Workout 4 has a slight change. Here you drop 5 percent of the weight from the previous workout—back to 315 pounds—but you do four sets of six reps. At workout 5 you bump up the weight again by 5 percent to 330 pounds and do four sets of five reps. In workout six you increase the weight again by 5 percent—or 345 pounds—and do four sets of four reps. During the next workout, you should be able to get four sets of six reps using 330 pounds—a nice 10 percent increase in strength.

See table 9.18 for a sample leg workout using the 5 percent method. Follow the leg press with other assistance exercises performed for three sets of four to six reps each.

The best way to use the 5 percent method is by training each muscle group only once per week to provide adequate recovery. The squat–bench press–deadlift training split fares well for this technique.

RATING

Time	1	2	3	4	5
Length	1	2	3	4	5
Difficulty	1	2	3	4	5
Results	1	2	3	4	5

TABLE 9.18   5 Percent Squat Workout

Workout	Exercise	Weight (pounds)	Sets	Reps
1	Squat	300	4	6
	Leg press	700	4	6
2	Squat	315	4	5
	Leg press	735	4	5
3	Squat	330	4	4
	Leg press	770	4	4
4	Squat	315	4	6
	Leg press	735	4	6
5	Squat	330	4	5
	Leg press	770	4	5
6	Squat	345	4	4
	Leg press	805	4	4
7	Squat	330	4	6
	Leg press	770	4	6

Same-Weight Training Method

With this method the weight is maintained through all sets for that particular exercise. The key is starting with a weight at which you can get more repetitions than you will perform. For example, you should start with a weight at which you can get seven or eight reps on your exercise of choice (about 80 percent RM), but you'd perform only six reps. Rest only one to two minutes between sets. By the third to fifth set you will struggle to be able to complete six reps. You end the exercise once you fail to complete six reps. Your goal is to complete five sets of six reps. Once you are able to do more than five sets of six reps with a weight, increase the weight by 5 to 10 percent the next time and start the progression over. See table 9.19 for a sample same-weight training program for the bench press. In this example the lifter has a bench press 1RM of 315 pounds. This lifter's 80% RM for the bench press is 250 pounds. It takes the lifter seven weeks to finish two cycles of same-weight training. Each of these workouts can be followed with assistance exercises such as dumbbell bench press, barbell shoulder, press, and triceps dip.

Reserve same-weight training for just the major lifts and follow these lifts with assistance exercises for three sets of six to eight reps. Do two complete cycles for each exercise you are training with the same weight training method. That is, make it through one cycle of five sets of six reps and increase the weight. Then continue to that cycle until you can do five sets of six reps with the new weight. After that, switch back to a more basic training method. The same-weight training method works well with almost any training split, particularly the squat–bench press–deadlift training split.

RATING

Time	1	2	3	4	5
Length	1	2	3	4	5
Difficulty	1	2	3	4	5
Results	1	2	3	4	5

TABLE 9.19 Same-Weight Program

Weight	Set	Reps	Rest
WORKOUT 1			
250	1	6	1 min
	2	6	1 min
	3	6	1 min
	4	4	
WORKOUT 2			
250	1	6	1 min
	2	6	1 min
	3	6	1 min
	4	6	1 min
	5	4	
WORKOUT 3			
250	1	6	1 min
	2	6	1 min
	3	6	1 min
	4	6	1 min
	5	6	
WORKOUT 4			
265	1	6	1 min
	2	6	1 min
	3	5	
WORKOUT 5			
265	1	6	1 min
	2	6	1 min
	3	6	1 min
	4	4	
WORKOUT 6			
265	1	6	1 min
	2	6	1 min
	3	6	1 min
	4	6	1 min
	5	5	
WORKOUT 7			
265	1	6	1 min
	2	6	1 min
	3	6	1 min
	4	6	1 min
	5	6	

Wave Training Method

This training method can boost your strength by up to 10 percent in only six to eight weeks. This is due to the small progressions in weight that take place with each wave. The waves actually allow you to lift up to 102 percent of your current max right off the bat. While that may equate to only a few extra pounds, over six to eight weeks the total expected strength boost is somewhere around 10 percent.

For this program, you'll perform a few warm-up sets, then two or three waves of three sets each, with four minutes of rest between waves and between each set. During wave 1, your first set will consist of three reps with 90 percent RM (a weight you can normally lift for about four reps). Set 2 consists of two reps with 95 percent RM. And on set 3, you'll do one rep with 100 percent RM. On wave 2 you'll increase the weight used on each set by about 1 percent. In other words, set 1 will be about 91 percent RM, set 2 will be 96 percent RM, and set 3 will be 101 percent RM. Because this increment is so small and the smallest Olympic plates are 1.25 pounds, this will equal a 2.5-pound jump on any weight under 400 pounds. For weights of 400 pounds or more, add 5 pounds. In either case, on the third set of wave 2, you'll be lifting more than your current max. If you're up for it, go for a third wave. To do so, simply increase the weight another 1 percent for each set and go for the same number of reps on each set. That means 102 percent of your max on that third set.

The goal of wave training is to increase the weight used on each wave by 1 to 2 percent every workout. Bit by bit, you can notch up your overall strength. But if you aren't successful completing the last set of the last wave of a workout, start the next workout with the same weights you used the previous time and really push to break through on this round. Then you can raise the weight on the next workout.

The reason wave training works has to do with potentiation—similar to the potentiation discussed in the max-out for muscle strength method. The earlier sets prime the nervous system, or the contractile fibers of the muscle, in such a way that the muscle is able to contract with more force on later sets. As most of the strength techniques suggest, reserve this strength training method for the prime strength movements or the exercises you substitute for them. Follow the wave training with three sets of four to six reps on assistance exercises.

Because of the high intensity of this program, you shouldn't train each major lift or muscle group more than once per week. Therefore, the squat–bench press–deadlift training split is ideal to use with wave training. See table 9.20 for a sample wave training deadlift program, set up for a person who can currently deadlift 405 pounds for one rep and wants to get up to 445 pounds. Follow this program for no more than eight weeks.

RATING

Time	1	2	3	4	5
Length	1	2	3	4	5
Difficulty	1	2	3	4	5
Results	1	2	3	4	5

TABLE 9.20 Strong Waves

WARM-UP			
Set	Weight (pounds)	Reps	Rest
1	135 (~30% 1RM)	10	2 min
2	225 (~55% 1RM)	8	2 min
3	315 (~75% 1RM)	5	4 min
WAVE 1			
1	365 (90% 1RM)	3	4 min
2	385 (95% 1RM)	2	4 min
3	405 (100% 1RM)	1	4 min
WAVE 2			
1	367.5 (91% 1RM)	3	4 min
2	387.5 (96% 1RM)	2	4 min
3	410 (101% 1RM)	1	4 min
WAVE 3 (IF POSSIBLE)			
1	370 (92% 1RM)	3	4 min
2	390 (97% 1RM)	2	4 min
3	415 (102% 1RM)	1	4 min

DeLorme Ascending Strength Pyramid

This program increases weight on each successive set for three sets total until you are doing the appropriate weight for the rep range you are using. For example, on set 1 you perform 10 reps with 50 percent of your 10RM. On set 2 you perform 10 reps with 75 percent of your 10RM. On set 3 you perform 10 reps (or as many reps as it takes to reach failure) with the actual 10RM. The first two sets function as warm-up sets because the weight is relatively light given the number of reps you have to perform. It is just the last set that can be considered a working set.

Although this method may seem like little work to many lifters, this one-working-set scheme may be the reason it works so well to increase strength. It provides a thorough warm-up and allows only one set to failure. This corresponds to research from Australia that supports the notion that one set to failure is superior to no sets to failure as well as more than one set to failure. In fact, a study that investigated the strength gains after following the DeLorme ascending strength pyramid or the Oxford descending pyramid (covered in chapter 6) found that the DeLorme method led to greater strength gains than the Oxford method.

When using the DeLorme technique, the repetition maximum is not critical, because many powerlifters use this pyramid method with 3RM, 4RM, 5RM, and 6RM to train for strength. In fact, one way to use this technique is to routinely change the RM. Because there is only one working set per exercise, this program works well with a push–pull training split or an upper- and lower-body powerlifting split. See table 9.21 for a sample DeLorme training program that follows a typical push–pull training split.

RATING

Time	1	2	3	4	5
Length	1	2	3	4	5
Difficulty	1	2	3	4	5
Results	1	2	3	4	5

TABLE 9.21 DeLorme Strength Pyramid

WORKOUT 1 (MONDAY AND THURSDAY): PUSH			
Exercise	Set	Weight	Reps
Squat*	1	50% 5RM	5
	2	75% 5RM	5
	3	100% 5RM	5
Leg press	1	50% 5RM	5
	2	75% 5RM	5
	3	100% 5RM	5
Leg extension	1	50% 5RM	5
	2	75% 5RM	5
	3	100% 5RM	5
Bench press*	1	50% 5RM	5
	2	75% 5RM	5
	3	100% 5RM	5
Incline dumbbell press	1	50% 5RM	5
	2	75% 5RM	5
	3	100% 5RM	5
Dumbbell shoulder press	1	50% 5RM	5
	2	75% 5RM	5
	3	100% 5RM	5
Close-grip bench press	1	50% 5RM	5
	2	75% 5RM	5
	3	100% 5RM	5
Standing calf raise	4 sets		8-10
WORKOUT 2 (TUESDAY AND FRIDAY): PULL			
Deadlift	1	50% 5RM	5
	2	75% 5RM	5
	3	100% 5RM	5
Lying leg curl	1	50% 5RM	5
	2	75% 5RM	5
	3	100% 5RM	5
Barbell row	1	50% 5RM	5
	2	75% 5RM	5
	3	100% 5RM	5
Lat pulldown	1	50% 5RM	5
	2	75% 5RM	5
	3	100% 5RM	5
Barbell curl	1	50% 5RM	5
	2	75% 5RM	5
	3	100% 5RM	5
Weighted crunch	4 sets		8-10

*Thursday perform bench press and incline dumbbell press before squat.

PROGRAMS THAT MANIPULATE REST PERIODS

When it comes to training for strength, rest periods are pretty standard. Most lifters rest a full three minutes between sets and rarely veer from this standard. However, altering rest periods can have a significant impact on strength gains when properly executed. This section covers strength training programs that systematically alter the rest periods involved. This can be done by implementing short rest periods between each rep (as with the rest–pause technique), by progressively lowering the rest between sets every week (as with one-rep to one-set method), or by progressively losing rest time between sets because of an increase in the number of reps performed each week (as found in the density training technique).

Rest–Pause Technique

Rest–pause is a lifting technique that involves stopping during a set, resting for a short period, and then continuing with the set. Its major advantage is that it allows for more total reps to be done with a given weight. That's because it takes advantage of the muscles' ability to recover rapidly. In simple terms, it allows the muscles time to replenish phosphocreatine (PCr)—the same molecule that creatine supplements boost. With this shot of extra energy, the muscle can contract more strongly, producing greater force and getting more reps. The greater the force your muscle can produce and the more reps you can perform, the greater the stimulus the muscles receive and the greater the gains in strength that you can expect.

The concept behind rest–pause training for strength gains is not necessarily to get more total reps or reach a higher state of fatigue but to optimize the force produced on each rep. To prioritize strength gains with rest–pause, you typically use a weight that allows you to get only three to five reps (3- to 5RM). The most common form of rest–pause training is to choose a weight that you can perform at only about three reps. Do one rep and rack the weight. Rest 15 seconds and then pump out another rep. Repeat this process until you have completed three to five reps total. That concludes one rest–pause set. This technique has been shown to be effective at producing decent strength gains, but it may not be the most effective.

In the laboratory it was discovered that an even better rest–pause technique for building strength involved shorter rest periods—about 3 to 5 seconds. Instead of racking the weight and resting 15 seconds between each rep, you simply hold the weight and rest for 3 to 5 seconds then complete another rep. Do this for a total of three reps. Stopping at three reps allows you to do three sets at the same weight, which maximizes the stimulus the muscle receives. Rest–pause training can work with any training split. To get appreciable results from rest–pause training, you will need to use it consistently for four to six weeks.

Table 9.22 gives a sample bench press routine. Do all three sets using this rest–pause technique and then follow them up with a second exercise for chest (such as incline bench press or dumbbell bench press) for another three sets of rest–pause. You will find that you can use considerably more weight than usual on the second exercise because you will not be as fatigued as you would be with three regular sets.

RATING

Time	1	2	3	4	5
Length	1	2	3	4	5
Difficulty	1	2	3	4	5
Results	1	2	3	4	5

TABLE 9.22 A Pause for Strength

Exercise	Weight	Set	Reps	Rest	Comments
Bench press	260	1, 2, 3	1, 1, 1	3 min	Do 3 reps total, each separated by 5 seconds of rest in top position.

One-Rep to One-Set Method

This method takes advantage of time by slowly decreasing the time rested between each exercise until you are doing one continuous set. Doing 10 sets of one rep with the same weight each set is the same amount of work as one set of 10 reps with that same weight. The difference is that doing the work as a single set is harder because of the fatigue that sets in—partly from the increasing levels of lactic acid. If you slowly, over time, reduce the amount of rest between those 10 sets, you will train the muscle to be better at producing the quick energy you need and to deal with the lactic acid—and this obviously will help the muscles grow stronger. The best way to go about this is to start with a weight at which you can do 10 sets of one rep with 90-second rest periods between sets. You then attempt to shave 15 seconds off of the rest periods with each successive workout.

How this works is simple: Consider that you can lift the weight for 10 reps—just not 10 reps in a row. See table 9.23 for a sample program. This program can be used with any training split.

RATING

Time	1	2	3	4	5
Length	1	2	3	4	5
Difficulty	1	2	3	4	5
Results	1	2	3	4	5

TABLE 9.23   Bench Rundown

Follow the bench press workout with standard assistance exercises for three sets of four to six reps.

Workout	Exercise	Sets	Reps	Rest (seconds)
1	Bench press	10	1	90
2	Bench press	10	1	75
3	Bench press	10	1	60
4	Bench press	10	1	45
5	Bench press	10	1	30
6	Bench press	10	1	15
7	Bench press	10	1	10
8	Bench press	10	1	5
9	Bench press	1	10	0

Density Training

Density training is a great way to trick your muscles into lifting more weight for more reps. This is particularly good for increasing strength on body-weight exercises, such as pull-ups, dips, and push-ups (since you can't change your body weight easily), but it can be used for any exercise. Density training begins by doubling the volume of work you want to accomplish. If your goal is to complete 12 reps with a certain amount of weight, then you start off with 12 sets of 2 reps (or 24 total reps) in 12 minutes. So rest is about 50 seconds between sets. Basically you have 1 minute to complete each set and rest before the next set. The more reps you do each set, the less rest you are allowed. After this becomes easy, move to 8 sets of 3 reps in 8 minutes. When this becomes easy, move to 6 sets of 4 reps in 6 minutes, then 5 sets of 5 reps in 5 minutes, then 4 sets of 6 reps in 4 minutes. When this becomes easy, move to 3 sets of 8 reps in 3 minutes. When you've mastered this, you should be able to get 1 set of 12 straight reps. By performing the same overall amount of work (24 reps) and progressively decreasing the amount of rest time, you are increasing the amount of work done during a given amount of time or increasing the density of the work. Density training works because of biochemical adaptations within the muscle cells during the progression of the program.

RATING

Time	1	2	3	4	5
Length	1	2	3	4	5
Difficulty	1	2	3	4	5
Results	1	2	3	4	5

TABLE 9.24 Density Workout

Workout	Sets*	Reps	Rest (seconds)	Total set time (minutes)
1	12	2	50	12
2	8	3	45	8
3	6	4	40	6
4	5	5	35	5
5	4	6	30	4
6	3	8	25	3
7	1	12		1

*As the number of sets decreases, you may find that you cannot complete all the reps. The first time this happens, stay with the same sets and reps on your next workout. If you still cannot complete the full number of reps, move forward anyway. Decrease the sets accordingly and do as many reps as you can. Allow yourself to repeat the same workout only twice.

PROGRAMS THAT MANIPULATE EXERCISE SELECTION

There are countless exercises that you can use to enhance muscle strength. Using the proper exercises can make a huge difference in your strength gains. This section discusses strength training methods that alter the exercises that are used to increase muscle strength. Some of these techniques focus solely on specific types of exercises, such as unilateral training and the dumbbell power program, while others use specific types of exercises in a particular order, such as the three-step strength method, front-to-back training, and ECO training method.

Unilateral Training

Unilateral training refers to training one side of the body at a time. Unlike one-sided training for building muscle mass (covered in chapter 6), unilateral training does not separate training days into left- and right-side workouts. Unilateral training simply uses exercises that are performed with one limb at a time—such as the one-arm dumbbell bench press, the one-leg squat, and even the one-leg, one-arm dumbbell deadlift. Although this approach to training is nothing revolutionary, few powerlifters actually train using unilateral exercises. This is unfortunate, since research confirms that when you train unilaterally the muscles are able to produce more force, and more muscle fibers (particularly fast-twitch muscle fibers) are active. One study comparing unilateral biceps curls to bilateral (both arms) biceps curls reported that the force produced on bilateral biceps curls was up to about 20 percent less than the sum of the force produced from the left- and right-arm unilateral curls. In other words, if you could curl 100 pounds with a barbell for one rep, you would expect to be able to curl only a 50-pound dumbbell with each arm for one rep. In reality, you may be able to curl a 60-pound dumbbell with each arm for one rep. Adding the weight of those dumbbells together would mean that you could curl a total of 120 pounds, or 20 percent more than with both arms at the same time.

To take advantage of the added strength that unilateral training offers, you should periodically do one-arm and one-leg exercises. See table 9.25 for a list of one-arm and one-leg exercises that can be added to a strength training program. Descriptions of how to perform these exercises correctly are found in part V. A great way to incorporate these exercises into your current strength training program is to include two sets of unilateral versions of the strength lifts after you have completed the working sets of the strength lifts. For assistance exercises, do two sets of the unilateral version followed by two sets of the bilateral version for each exercise. See table 9.26 for a sample strength training program that heavily incorporates unilateral exercises into an upper- and lower-body powerlifting split.

RATING

Time	1	2	3	4	5
Length	1	2	3	4	5
Difficulty	1	2	3	4	5
Results	1	2	3	4	5

TABLE 9.25 Unilateral Exercises

Muscle group	Exercise
Chest	One-arm dumbbell bench press (flat, incline, decline)
	One-arm dumbbell fly (flat, incline, decline)
Shoulders	One-arm dumbbell overhead press
	One-arm dumbbell upright row
	One-arm dumbbell lateral raise
Back	One-arm dumbbell row
	One-arm cable lat pulldown
Legs	One-leg squat
	One-leg leg press
	One-leg leg extension
	One-leg leg curl
	One-leg, one-arm deadlift
	One-leg Romanian deadlift
Triceps	One-arm dumbbell triceps extension
	One-arm triceps pressdown
	One-arm lying triceps extension
Biceps	One-arm dumbbell curl
	Dumbbell concentration curl
	One-arm dumbbell preacher curl

TABLE 9.26 One Strong Program

UPPER-BODY WORKOUT 1 (MONDAY): BENCH PRESS AND PUSHING EXERCISES

Exercise	Sets	Reps
Bench press	4	5 with 85% RM
One-arm dumbbell bench press	2	4-6
Dumbbell bench press	2	4-6
One-arm dumbbell shoulder press	2	4-6
Dumbbell shoulder press	2	4-6
One-arm dumbbell upright row	2	6-8
Dumbbell upright row	2	6-8
One-arm dumbbell triceps press	2	4-6
Dumbbell close-grip bench press	2	4-6
Standing crunch	3	8-10

LOWER-BODY WORKOUT 1 (TUESDAY): SQUAT AND QUADRICEPS EXERCISES

Squat	4	5 with 85% RM
One-leg squat	2	4-6
One-leg leg press	2	4-6
Leg press	2	4-6
One-leg leg extension	2	6-8
Leg extension	2	6-8
Standing calf raise	4	8-10

UPPER-BODY WORKOUT 2 (THURSDAY): BENCH PRESS AND PULLING EXERCISES

Bench press	4	75%
One-arm dumbbell row	2	4-6
Barbell row	2	4-6
One-arm cable lat pulldown	2	6-8
Lat pulldown	3	6-8
One-arm dumbbell curl	2	6-8
Dumbbell curl	2	6-8
Russian twist	3	20

LOWER-BODY WORKOUT 2 (FRIDAY): DEADLIFT AND HAMSTRING EXERCISES

Deadlift	4	5 with 85% RM
One-leg, one-arm dumbbell deadlift	2	4-6
One-leg Romanian deadlift	2	6-8
Romanian deadlift	2	6-8
One-leg lying leg curl	2	6-8
Lying leg curl	2	6-8
Seated calf raise	4	10-12

Three-Step Strength Method

This training method incorporates dumbbell, barbell, and machine versions of one exercise in that specific order to enhance muscle strength. While one benefit of this training method is the variety of exercises, the main benefit stems from the order in which you do these exercises. The major reason for this has to do with the stabilizer muscles.

The stabilizer muscles generally lie deep under your major muscle groups (the prime movers). Though the stabilizers are often much smaller and weaker, they're important for securing the joints during various movements. When you train with equipment that's fairly unstable—such as dumbbells—the stabilizer muscles become fatigued much sooner than the muscle group you're trying to work because the stabilizers are weaker. When the stabilizers are fatigued, the brain limits the nervous input to the prime movers in order to prevent injury from occurring. In other words, the stabilizers limit the amount of force the prime movers can produce.

One unorthodox way to train that prevents the stabilizers from being the weak link in your training is to order your exercises in a manner that moves from the least stable exercise to the most stable. This way, as the stabilizer muscles fatigue, you change the exercises to ones that require less activity of the stabilizers. This allows the prime movers to train with heavy weights that are not limited by the fatigue of the stabilizer muscles. The three-step strength method follows this order by starting the workout with dumbbell exercises, which require the most help from the stabilizers because each arm is allowed to move in all directions that the joints will allow. For leg exercises, one-leg exercises would take the place of dumbbell exercises. The workout then moves to a barbell exercise. Because it is a free-weight exercise, you still require some use of stabilizer muscles. But because these exercises are done bilaterally with both arms locked in place on the bar (upper-body exercises) or both legs locked in place on the floor (leg exercises), there is less use of the stabilizers than with dumbbell or unilateral leg exercises. The last type of exercise on the list is a machine exercise. This type of exercise requires barely any help from the stabilizers because the movement of the machine forces your body to follow a predetermined path that doesn't permit deviation. Since the machine is designed to target particular prime movers, the stabilizers are basically not needed.

As an example of a three-step strength method workout for a bench press-focused workout, you would start with the dumbbell bench press, then move to the barbell bench press, and finish with the machine bench press. For a squat-focused workout, you could start with the one-leg squat as the first exercise, then move to the barbell squat as the second exercise, and finish with the leg press. Using this training method for a deadlift-focused workout is not ideal but can be done. For this workout, start with the one-leg, one-arm dumbbell deadlift, then move to the standard deadlift, and finish with a horizontal leg press machine (but start the movement from the down position, which mimics the deadlift).

This training method should not take the place of standard strength training methods that organize the major strength exercises first in the workout. Instead, the best way to use the three-step strength method is to train with it on a second workout for that lift later in the week. For instance, you can do a standard bench press workout early in the week and then do a three-step strength method bench press workout later in the week. This works well with the squat–bench press–deadlift training split by adding a three-step strength method workout on Saturday. An example of this is shown in the workout in table 9.27. Each exercise should be done for 3 working sets. The amount of weight used and the reps performed can be cycled to correspond with your training phase.

RATING

Time	1	2	3	4	5
Length	1	2	3	4	5
Difficulty	1	2	3	4	5
Results	1	2	3	4	5

TABLE 9.27   Three-Stepping for Strength

WORKOUT 1 (MONDAY): SQUAT DAY

Exercise	Sets	Reps
Squat	4	5 with 85% RM
Leg press	3	6-8
Leg extension	3	8-10
Standing calf raise	3	8-10
Cable woodchopper	3	20

WORKOUT 2 (WEDNESDAY): BENCH PRESS DAY

Bench press	4	5 with 85% RM
Incline dumbbell press	3	6-8
Barbell shoulder press	4	6-8
Close-grip bench press	4	6-8
Standing crunch	4	8-10

WORKOUT 3 (THURSDAY): DEADLIFT DAY

Exercise	Sets	Reps
Deadlift	4	5 with 85% RM
Good morning	3	6-8
Lying leg curl	3	8-10
Barbell row	4	6-8
Barbell curl	4	6-8
Hanging leg raise	4	10-12

WORKOUT 4 (SATURDAY): THREE-STEP STRENGTH WORKOUT FOR BENCH PRESS AND SQUAT

Dumbbell bench press	3	6-8
Bench press	3	5 with 80% RM
Machine bench press	3	6-8
One-leg squat	3	6-8
Barbell squat	3	5 with 80% RM
Leg press	3	6-8

Dumbbell Power Program

This is a basic strength training program that uses only dumbbell exercises. Training this way is not any more beneficial than using barbells, but it can work to pull you out of a training slump and get your strength gains climbing again for several reasons. The first reason is the change. Changing your training with different exercises, such as those found in the dumbbell power program, can affect your overall strength by recruiting different muscle fibers that you may have neglected from doing the usual exercises in your routine. Then there's the strength imbalance that most lifters have. Some experience up to a 10 percent difference between their stronger side and weaker side. Unilateral training with dumbbells forces the weaker side to gain strength since that side must lift the dumbbell on its own.

Another benefit of dumbbells is that they can improve the strength of your stabilizer muscles. This can actually enhance overall muscle strength while reducing the risk of injury to your joints. Dumbbell strength training is also great for those who train at home. Dumbbells take up little room, and you can perform a variety of exercises in a minimal amount of space. These exercises are also great for those with shoulder, elbow, or wrist injuries because they allow a freer ROM compared to the ROM allowed with barbells.

The dumbbell power program is a six-week program that involves many multijoint and multimovement exercises that increase overall body strength. See table 9.28 for the outline of the program. Detailed descriptions on how to perform these exercises can be found in part V. Each workout is done three days per week—usually Monday, Wednesday, and Friday. If you want, you can include one extra training day that hits the squat, bench press, and deadlift. In weeks 1 and 2, you'll train with three sets of 10 to 12 reps with 90 seconds of rest between sets. During weeks 3 and 4, the weight increases and the reps drop to six to eight per set. Increase the rest to two minutes between sets. For the final two weeks (weeks 5 and 6), you increase the weight again and drop the reps to four to six per set. Increase the rest periods again to three minutes between sets to allow ample recovery time. The abdominal and core exercises, however, increase in reps. For these, the weight should stay the same or even increase over the six weeks, and rest should be constant at one minute between sets.

RATING

Time	1	2	3	4	5
Length	1	2	3	4	5
Difficulty	1	2	3	4	5
Results	1	2	3	4	5

TABLE 9.28 Six-Week Dumbbell Power Workout

Exercise	WEEKS 1-2		WEEKS 3-4		WEEKS 5-6	
	Sets	Reps	Sets	Reps	Sets	Reps
Dumbbell clean and press	3	10-12	3	6-8	3	4-6
Dumbbell push-up + row	3	10-12	3	6-8	3	4-6
Dumbbell squat + overhead press	3	10-12	3	6-8	3	4-6
Dumbbell pullover + press	3	10-12	3	6-8	3	4-6
Dumbbell deadlift + upright row	3	10-12	3	6-8	3	4-6
Dumbbell kickback	3	10-12	3	6-8	3	4-6
Standing alternating dumbbell curl	3	10-12	3	6-8	3	4-6
Dumbbell woodchopper	3	10-12	3	12-15	3	15-20
Dumbbell V-sit	3	10-12	3	12-15	3	15-20

Front-to-Back Training

This training method involves training opposing muscle groups and exercise movements to increase muscle strength. With this method, you train exercises that are opposing movements and train opposing muscle groups back to back. That is, you do one set of the first exercise and follow it with one set of an exercise that is the opposite movement of that first exercise. This is similar to superset training with a longer rest period allowed between the opposing exercises. For example, during front-to-back training you will train the bench press and barbell row together.

The advantage of training opposing muscle groups back to back is that you'll be stronger in the second exercise. Research has found that a muscle will be stronger if preceded immediately by a contraction of its antagonist, or opposing muscle group. For example, when you do a superset of barbell row and bench press in that order, you'll be stronger on the bench press—as long as you don't train to failure on the row. The reason for this phenomenon is that, to some degree, the agonist muscle is limited by its antagonist. When bench-pressing using straight sets, for example, the back muscles inhibit the contraction of the pectoral muscles to a certain extent. Doing a set of rows shortly before benching, however, lessens this inhibitory effect, allowing your pecs to contract more forcefully.

The front-to-back training routine presented in table 9.29 uses an upper- and lower-body training split for a total of four workouts per week. The upper-body workout is done on Mondays and Thursdays, and the lower-body workouts are done on Tuesdays and Fridays. On the Thursday upper-body workout, you should switch the order of the exercise pair on all exercises except the bench press. The Tuesday lower-body workout focuses on the squat, and the Friday lower-body workout focuses on the deadlift. You will do five sets of each exercise pair. The first exercise should be done for no more than five reps with a weight that is about 50 to 70 percent RM (a weight that allows you to complete about 12 to 20 reps) for that exercise. The key is doing these reps explosively and not fatiguing the muscles. Rest no more than 60 seconds between exercises and do four to six reps on the second exercise. Normally that would be a weight that is about 85 to 90 percent RM. However, the additional strength you get from the antagonist exercise may allow you to complete four to six reps with up to 95 percent RM. After completing the fifth set of the second exercise, do one set to failure of the first exercise with a weight that normally allows you to complete about 8 to 10 reps. Follow this program for no more than six weeks before cycling back to standard straight-set training.

RATING

Time	1	2	3	4	5
Length	1	2	3	4	5
Difficulty	1	2	3	4	5
Results	1	2	3	4	5

TABLE 9.29 Front-to-Back Strength

UPPER-BODY WORKOUT (MONDAY AND THURSDAY)		EXERCISE 1	EXERCISE 2	
Exercise pair	Sets	Reps	Reps	
Barbell row and bench press	5	2-3	4-6	
Lat pulldown and overhead press	5	2-3	4-6	
Barbell curl and triceps dip	5	2-3	4-6	
Back extension and weighted crunch	5	5-6	8-10	
LOWER-BODY WORKOUT (TUESDAY): SQUAT				
Hanging leg raise (with dumbbell) and squat	5	2-3	4-6	
Seated or lying leg curl and leg extension	5	3-4	6-8	
Seated toe raise and seated calf raise	5	5-6	6-8	
LOWER-BODY WORKOUT (FRIDAY): DEADLIFT				
Hanging leg raise (with dumbbell) and deadlift	5	2-3	4-6	
Leg raise and Romanian deadlift	5	5-6	6-8	
Leg extension and seated or lying leg curl	5	3-4	6-8	
Standing toe raise and standing calf raise	3	5-6	6-8	

ECO Training Method

This method of training incorporates three different types of exercises that all offer a distinct benefit to build strength. The acronym ECO stands for explosive exercise, closed-chain exercise, open-chain exercise. Explosive exercises are plyometric, or ballistic-type movements (discussed earlier in ballistic strength training), such as the squat jump and bench press throw. Closed-chain exercises are those where your hands or feet remain stationary and your body moves, such as squats, push-ups, and pull-ups. Open-chain exercises are those where the resistance is in your hands or at your feet, such as leg extensions and most dumbbell upper-body exercises. The ECO workout progresses in that exact order—the explosive exercise is done first, followed by the closed-chain exercise, and finishing with the open-chain exercise.

You must do the explosive exercises first while the muscle fibers are fresh. If the muscle fibers are fatigued when you do them, they won't be able to contract as quickly and explosively. In addition, because these moves are performed with such quick movements, there could be a higher risk of injury if you are fatigued. Explosive moves target the fast-twitch muscle fibers. Gaining explosive strength or power from these exercises translates to greater strength on other exercises, such as the

squat and bench press. You will do no more than three reps on the explosive exercises. The point is to be explosive on all three sets of three reps, not to tire the muscle. You will use a very light weight (just your body weight or a weight with which you can perform about 25 to 30 normal reps on the exercise, or about 30 to 50 percent RM).

The closed-chain exercises force your body to move while your hands or feet are stationary. These types of exercises are great for building strength in the muscle you are training. They also develop functional strength because they require balance and the use of stabilizers to move your body. Because the only true closed-chain chest exercise is the push-up, the bench press is substituted in this ECO program. The problem with the push-up is that it's difficult to increase the resistance to fall in the proper rep range of four to six. If you are willing, however, you can do weighted push-ups by having someone sit on your back or load plates on your back, or you can do push-ups with the bar of a Smith machine loaded on your back.

An open-chain exercise is anything that involves holding the weight in your hands (dumbbell fly) or having the weight at your feet (leg extension). In the ECO program closed-chain exercises are used as isolation exercises to focus the force onto the muscle of interest for enhancing muscle growth. For the open-chain exercises, perform 8 to 10 reps per set.

The best split to use with the ECO program is the upper- and lower-body training split as shown in table 9.30. Follow the program for four weeks and then return to your standard form of training.

RATING

Time	1	2	3	4	5
Length	1	2	3	4	5
Difficulty	1	2	3	4	5
Results	1	2	3	4	5

TABLE 9.30   ECO-Friendly Strength Program

UPPER-BODY WORKOUT 1 (MONDAY): BENCH PRESS AND PUSHING EXERCISES			
Muscle group	**Exercise**	**Sets**	**Reps**
Chest	E: Power push-up	3	3
	C: Bench press	3	4-6
	O: Dumbbell fly	3	8-10
Shoulders	E: Overhead press throw (Smith machine)	3	3
	C: Barbell shoulder press	3	4-6
	O: Dumbbell lateral raise	3	8-10
Triceps	E: Close-grip bench press throw	3	3
	C: Dips	3	4-6
	O: Skull crusher	3	8-10
LOWER-BODY WORKOUT 1 (TUESDAY): SQUAT AND QUADRICEPS EXERCISES			
Quadriceps	E: Jump squat	3	3
	C: Barbell squat	3	4-6
	O: Leg extension and leg curl*	3	8-10
Calves	Standing calf raise	3	8-10
Abs	Standing crunch	3	8-10
UPPER-BODY WORKOUT 2 (THURSDAY): BENCH PRESS AND PULLING EXERCISES			
Chest	E: Bench press throw (Smith machine)	3	3
	C: Weighted push-up	3	4-6
	O: Incline dumbbell fly	3	8-10
Back	E: One-arm power row (Smith machine)	3	3
	C: Pull-up	3	4-6
	O: Straight-arm pulldown	3	8-10
Biceps	E: Biceps curl throw	3	3
	C: Close-grip chin-up	3	4-6
	O: Incline dumbbell curl	3	8-10
LOWER-BODY WORKOUT 2 (FRIDAY): DEADLIFT AND HAMSTRING EXERCISES			
Quadriceps	E: Dumbbell deadlift jump	3	3
	C: Deadlift	3	4-6
	O: Leg curl	3	8-10
Calves	Standing calf raise	3	8-10
Abs and core	Russian twist	3	12-15

*Perform as a superset.

PROGRAMS THAT MANIPULATE TRAINING FREQUENCY

This section covers strength training methods that modify the frequency of training. There are only two programs covered here because few lifters interested in training for strength view training frequency as an important variable to cycle in an effort to increase muscle strength. However, changing the frequency of your training can have a dramatic effect on gains in muscle strength. The overreaching method and the up-and-down strength method are two programs that are effective at enhancing strength by manipulating the frequency of training.

Overreaching Method

This program actually causes you to overtrain in an effort to increase strength. The program design is based on research investigating overtraining in athletes. But the concept is not all that new. It originated from training principles from the Eastern Bloc countries. Overreaching is basically overtraining without suffering from the negative effects of overtraining. The trick is backing off at the right time. The difference between overtraining and overreaching is mainly time. Overtraining is a more chronic situation. It's not something that can just happen in a couple of days; it may take two to four weeks of training too heavily or too long to become truly overtrained. By then hormonal perturbations usually have surfaced and so will the classic signs: fatigue, loss of appetite, lack of strength, muscle loss, insomnia, and depression.

Overreaching is similar to overtraining in that the training is the same. The difference is that overreaching is for a short period and ends before the catastrophic changes in your body's physiology have taken place. In other words, overreaching is overtraining before the overtrained state is reached. For four weeks you will train all muscle groups five days per week. See table 9.31 for the outline of the overreaching training split. You will do three sets per exercise; each week the weight increases and the reps decrease. The exception is the Friday workout, where you train using maximal effort (up to 100 percent RM) on the squat, bench press, and deadlift. At the end of the four weeks, you back off on the training frequency as well as the weight and slow it down to training each muscle group just once per week with a squat–bench press–deadlift training split. During this back-off phase your strength will increase dramatically. In fact, in the study that the overreaching method is based on, researchers discovered that after two weeks on the back-off phase, the trained lifters had increases in 1RM strength of more than 10 percent on both the bench press and squat.

RATING

Time	1	2	3	4	5
Length	1	2	3	4	5
Difficulty	1	2	3	4	5
Results	1	2	3	4	5

TABLE 9.31 Overreaching for Strength

	WEEKS 1-4 MONDAY AND WEDNESDAY								
	WEEK 1		WEEK 2		WEEK 3		WEEK 4		Rest between sets (minutes)
Exercise	Sets	Reps	Sets	Reps	Sets	Reps	Sets	Reps	
Squat	3	10-12	3	8-10	3	6-8	3	4-6	3
Lunge	3	10-12	3	8-10	3	6-8	3	4-6	2
Bench press	3	10-12	3	8-10	3	6-8	3	4-6	3
Barbell shoulder press	3	10-12	3	8-10	3	6-8	3	4-6	2
Lat pulldown	3	10-12	3	8-10	3	6-8	3	4-6	2
Dumbbell curl	3	10-12	3	8-10	3	6-8	3	4-6	2
Lying triceps extension	3	10-12	3	8-10	3	6-8	3	4-6	2
Standing calf raise	3	15-20	3	12-15	3	10-12	3	8-10	1
Hanging leg raise	3	15-20	3	15-20	3	15-20	3	15-20	1

TUESDAY AND THURSDAY

Exercise	WEEK 1 Sets	WEEK 1 Reps	WEEK 2 Sets	WEEK 2 Reps	WEEK 3 Sets	WEEK 3 Reps	WEEK 4 Sets	WEEK 4 Reps	Rest between sets (minutes)
Bench press	3	10-12	3	8-10	3	6-8	3	4-6	3
Deadlift	3	10-12	3	8-10	3	6-8	3	4-6	3
Leg press	3	10-12	3	8-10	3	6-8	3	4-6	3
Upright row	3	10-12	3	8-10	3	6-8	3	4-6	2
Barbell row	3	10-12	3	8-10	3	6-8	3	4-6	2
Barbell curl	3	10-12	3	8-10	3	6-8	3	4-6	2
Dips	3	10-12	3	8-10	3	6-8	3	4-6	2
Seated calf raise	3	15-20	3	12-15	3	10-12	3	8-10	1
Crunch	3	20	3	20	3	20	3	20	1

FRIDAY

Exercise	Sets	Reps	% 1RM
Follow this set, rep, and % 1RM scheme for the squat, bench press, and deadlift	1	5	10%
	1	5	20%
	1	5	30%
	1	3	40%
	1	3	50%
	1	3	60%
	1	1	70%
	1	1	80%
	1	1	90%
	1	1	95%
	1	1	100%

WEEKS 5-6
WORKOUT 1 (MONDAY): SQUAT DAY

Exercise	Sets	Reps	% 1RM
Squat	4	8-10	75%
Leg press	3	8-10	
Leg extension	3	8-10	
Standing calf raise	3	8-10	
Cable woodchopper	3	20	

WORKOUT 2 (WEDNESDAY): BENCH PRESS DAY

Bench press	4	8-10	75%
Incline dumbbell press	3	8-10	
Barbell shoulder press	4	8-10	
Close-grip bench press	4	8-10	
Standing crunch	4	8-10	

WORKOUT 3 (FRIDAY): DEADLIFT DAY

Deadlift	4	8-10	75%
Good morning	3	8-10	
Lying leg curl	3	8-10	
Barbell row	4	8-10	
Barbell curl	4	8-10	

Up-and-Down Strength Program

This six-week strength training program cycles the training frequency every week by switching up training splits. The program, shown in table 9.32, starts with a whole-body strength training split, which works each muscle group three times per week. The second week switches to a push–pull training split, which trains each muscle group twice per week. The third week uses a squat–bench press–deadlift training split, which trains each muscle group once per week. At the fourth week the cycle starts all over but the reps change from about six to eight per set or 80 percent RM for the

major strength lifts to two or three reps or 95 percent RM for the major strength lifts. This program works to increase strength by gradually increasing the recovery time the muscles receive each week.

RATING

Time	1	2	3	4	5
Length	1	2	3	4	5
Difficulty	1	2	3	4	5
Results	1	2	3	4	5

TABLE 9.32   Strong Split

WEEK 1
WORKOUT 1 (MONDAY): SQUAT FOCUS

Exercise	Sets	% 1RM or reps
Squat	4	6-8 with 80% RM
Leg press	3	6-8
Incline bench press	4	6-8
Dumbbell shoulder press	3	6-8
Barbell row	3	6-8
Stiff-leg deadlift	3	6-8
Close-grip bench press	3	6-8
Dumbbell curl	3	6-8
Hanging leg raise	3	10-12

WORKOUT 2 (WEDNESDAY): BENCH PRESS FOCUS

Exercise	Sets	% 1RM or reps
Bench press	4	6-8 with 80% RM
Dumbbell bench press	3	6-8
Barbell hack squat	3	6-8
Barbell shoulder press	3	6-8
Deadlift	3	6-8 with 80% RM
Dumbbell row	3	6-8
Triceps dip	3	6-8
Barbell curl	3	6-8
Cable woodchopper	3	20

WORKOUT 3 (FRIDAY): DEADLIFT FOCUS

Exercise	Sets	% 1RM or reps
Deadlift	4	6-8 with 80% RM
One-arm dumbbell deadlift	3	6-8
Bench press	3	6-8
Upright row	3	6-8
Lat pulldown	3	8-10
Lying triceps extension	3	6-8

WORKOUT 3 (FRIDAY): DEADLIFT FOCUS (continued)

Exercise	Sets	% 1RM or reps
Preacher curl	3	6-8
Back extension	3	15-20

WEEK 2
WORKOUT 1 (MONDAY AND THURSDAY): PUSH

Exercise	Sets	% 1RM or reps
Squat*	4	6-8 with 80% RM
Leg press	3	6-8
Leg extension	3	6-8
Bench press*	4	6-8 with 80% RM
Incline dumbbell press	3	6-8
Dumbbell shoulder press	4	6-8
Close-grip bench press	4	6-8
Standing calf raise	4	8-10

WORKOUT 2 (TUESDAY AND FRIDAY): PULL

Exercise	Sets	% 1RM or reps
Deadlift	4	6-8 with 80% RM
Lying leg curl	3	6-8
Barbell row	4	6-8
Lat pulldown	3	6-8
Barbell curl	4	6-8
Weighted crunch	4	8-10

WEEK 3
WORKOUT 1 (MONDAY): SQUAT DAY

Exercise	Sets	% 1RM or reps
Squat	4	6-8 with 80% RM
Leg press	3	6-8
Leg extension	3	6-8
Standing calf raise	3	12-15
Cable woodchopper	3	12

WEEK 3 (continued)
WORKOUT 2 (WEDNESDAY): BENCH PRESS DAY

Exercise	Sets	% 1RM or reps
Bench press	4	6-8 with 80%
Incline dumbbell press	3	6-8
Barbell shoulder press	4	6-8
Close-grip bench press	4	6-8
Standing crunch	4	8-10

WORKOUT (FRIDAY) 3: DEADLIFT DAY

Exercise	Sets	% 1RM or reps
Deadlift	4	6-8 with 80% RM
Good morning	3	6-8
Lying leg curl	3	6-8
Barbell row	4	6-8
Barbell curl	4	6-8

WEEK 4
WORKOUT 1 (MONDAY): SQUAT FOCUS

Exercise	Sets	% 1RM or reps
Squat	4	2-3 with 95% RM
Leg press	3	2-3
Incline bench press	4	2-3
Dumbbell shoulder press	3	2-3
Barbell row	3	2-3
Stiff-leg deadlift	3	4-6
Close-grip bench press	3	2-3
Dumbbell curl	3	4-6
Hanging leg raise	3	12-15

WORKOUT 2 (WEDNESDAY): BENCH PRESS FOCUS

Exercise	Sets	% 1RM or reps
Bench press	4	2-3 with 95% RM
Dumbbell bench press	3	2-3
Barbell hack squat	3	2-3
Barbell shoulder press	3	2-3
Deadlift	3	2-3 with 95% RM
Dumbbell row	3	2-3
Triceps dip	3	4-6
Barbell curl	3	4-6
Cable woodchopper	3	25

WORKOUT 3 (FRIDAY): DEADLIFT FOCUS

Exercise	Sets	% 1RM or reps
Deadlift	4	2-3 with 95% RM
One-arm dumbbell deadlift	3	2-3
Bench press	3	2-3
Upright row	3	4-6
Lat pulldown	3	4-6
Lying triceps extension	3	4-6

WEEK 4 (continued)
WORKOUT 3 (FRIDAY): DEADLIFT FOCUS (continued)

Exercise	Sets	% 1RM or reps
Preacher curl	3	4-6
Back extension	3	15-20

WEEK 5
WORKOUT 1 (MONDAY AND THURSDAY): PUSH

Exercise	Sets	% 1RM or reps
Squat*	4	2-3 with 95% RM
Leg press	3	2-3
Leg extension	3	4-6
Bench press*	4	2-3 with 95% RM
Incline dumbbell press	3	2-3
Dumbbell shoulder press	4	2-3
Close-grip bench press	4	2-3
Standing calf raise	4	6-8

WORKOUT 2 (TUESDAY AND FRIDAY): PULL

Exercise	Sets	% 1RM or reps
Deadlift	4	2-3 with 95% RM
Lying leg curl	3	4-6
Barbell row	4	2-3
Lat pulldown	3	4-6
Barbell curl	4	4-6
Weighted crunch	4	6-8

WEEK 6
WORKOUT 1 (MONDAY): SQUAT DAY

Exercise	Sets	% 1RM or reps
Squat	4	2-3 with 95% RM
Leg press	3	2-3
Leg extension	3	4-6
Standing calf raise	3	10-12
Cable woodchopper	3	15

WORKOUT 2 (WEDNESDAY): BENCH PRESS DAY

Exercise	Sets	% 1RM or reps
Bench press	4	2-3 with 95% RM
Incline dumbbell press	3	2-3
Barbell shoulder press	4	2-3
Close-grip bench press	4	2-3
Standing crunch	4	6-8

WORKOUT 3 (FRIDAY): DEADLIFT DAY

Exercise	Sets	% 1RM or reps
Deadlift	4	2-3 with 95% RM
Good morning	3	2-3
Lying leg curl	3	4-6
Barbell row	4	2-3
Barbell curl	4	4-6

*Thursday perform bench press and incline dumbbell press before squat.

BISHOP BURTON COLLEGE

CHAPTER 10

Training Cycles for Gaining Maximal Strength

The fundamentals of strength training covered in part I will help you understand how to design effective strength training programs. This chapter is designed to help you take the information you have learned from chapter 8 (basic program design for training programs that build maximal strength) and chapter 9 (advanced training techniques) and put it together to build a long-term training program that works to continually build strength.

This chapter starts by teaching you how to test your 1RM. Regardless of your training level, you need to assess your strength level accurately for best results from your training. The first training program offered in this chapter is a beginner program. If you have little experience in strength training, this program will enable you to take on the basic strength programs that are most effective for gaining strength. Once you have followed a strength training program consistently for at least six months, you are ready to take on an effective program based on the splits discussed in chapter 8. If you are at the intermediate level, these programs use the percentage method of training. This is a training system that gradually increases the weight used by a percentage of the 1RM.

Advanced lifters, those with over a year of strength training experience, can begin using the methods and techniques covered in chapter 9. One cycle found in the following section is an advanced program that alters these techniques throughout the different phases. Finally, if you are interested in increasing your strength in one lift, you can refer to the sections that focus on just one lift.

TESTING ONE-REPETITION MAXIMUM

Regardless of where they are starting from, all lifters interested in training to build maximal strength have one goal in common—more strength! With the exception of powerlifters, who commonly test their 1RM strength in competition, most lifters do not routinely test their strength by maxing out. *Maxing out,* a slang term, means to test your strength by seeing how much weight you can lift for one ultimate rep on an exercise (usually on the three strength moves: bench press, squat, and deadlift). Anyone who is interested in developing muscle strength needs to routinely test 1RM strength on the bench press, squat, and deadlift.

Assessing your strength on the bench press, squat, and deadlift is important for several reasons. Because the bench press represents upper-body strength, the squat represents lower-body strength, and the deadlift represents whole-body strength, knowing your maximal strength on each of these lifts will give you an indication of your overall body strength as well as indicate any strength imbalances you may have. Norms have been established that indicate how strong a person should be on each of these lifts. For strength norms relative to body weight, refer to table 10.1. Testing your 1RM on the bench press, squat, and deadlift and comparing your relative strength on each to the established norms will indicate how your strength levels compare to the strength levels of others. You can do this by dividing your 1RM in pounds on each lift by your body weight in pounds. For example, if your bench press 1RM is 300 pounds and you weigh 150 pounds (68 kilograms), your relative strength on the bench press is 2. The Balanced Strength box provides a ratio of squat to deadlift to bench press strength. Comparing your own 1RM strength ratios of these three lifts can indicate whether you have balanced strength or whether you are particularly weak or strong on a particular lift. Knowing whether you have an imbalance can help you tailor your training to work toward improving the weaker lifts.

Another important reason to assess your 1RM strength on the bench press, squat, and deadlift is to determine the training weights that will correspond to each phase of your strength training program. When training for strength, you will train using a percentage of your 1RM on the major lifts—such as 85 percent of the 1RM or 85 percent RM. The only way to know how much weight you should train with is to know how much your 1RM is. For example, if your current 1RM on the squat is 400 pounds and you are in a training phase that requires 85 percent RM, then you should train with 340 pounds on the squat. This requires frequent retesting because your strength will increase while you are training with effective strength programs. You should plan on testing your 1RM about once every four to six weeks to keep your training weights accurate with your current level of strength.

Last and most obvious, it's important to test your 1RM strength to assess the effectiveness of each program you use in your strength training

TABLE 10.1   Relative Strength

Values listed as "good" represent 1RM that is greater than the general population. Values listed as "excellent" represent observed 1RM values for advanced lifters. Values listed as "elite" represent observed 1RM values for competitive-level powerlifters.

Rating	Male	Female
BENCH PRESS		
Good	>1.25 × body weight	>0.8 × body weight
Excellent	≥1.75 × body weight	1 × body weight
Elite	≥2 × body weight	≥1.25 × body weight
SQUAT		
Good	>2 × body weight	>1.5 × body weight
Excellent	≥2.5 × body weight	≥2 × body weight
Elite	≥3 × body weight	≥2.5 × body weight
DEADLIFT		
Good	≥2 × body weight	≥1.5 × body weight
Excellent	≥2.5 × body weight	≥2 × body weight
Elite	≥3 × body weight	≥2.5 × body weight

regimen. Knowing your 1RM for the bench press, squat, and deadlift (or any other exercise you want to increase your strength on) before you start a program and after you finish it is the only way to determine how effective a strength training program is and whether you should consider using the same program in the future.

To test your maximal strength on an exercise, you must have a capable spotter to assist you,

---

Balanced Strength

Here I list the suggested ratio of bench press to squat to deadlift 1RM weight. This can be used to determine whether your upper-body, lower-body, and overall strength are balanced. Having a ratio on a lift that is much higher or lower than the suggested ratios would indicate areas in which you should work on bringing your strength up to par with the others.

A balanced ratio of bench to squat to deadlift is 1:1.5:1.5.*

For example, if your bench press is 300 pounds, your squat is 450 pounds, and your deadlift is 425 pounds (300:450:425), your ratio would be 1:1.5:1.4.

This would suggest your strength in these three lifts is balanced.

If your bench press is 300 pounds, your squat is 700 pounds, and your deadlift is 650 pounds (300:700:650), your ratio would be 1:2.33:2.17.

This would suggest your strength on the bench press is well below your squat and deadlift strength. This means your training should focus on bringing up your bench press and upper-body strength.

*In practice the weight for the deadlift tends to be slightly less than the weight for the squat.

because to determine a true 1RM, you must reach muscle failure. The first step to testing your 1RM is to do several light warm-up sets starting with the bar itself and gradually move up in weight over those several sets until you are close to your true 1RM weight. Rest three minutes after your final warm-up before testing your 1RM. Estimate a conservative 1RM weight and try it for one rep. Rest three to four minutes before making another attempt. If you failed on the second attempt, subtract 5 to 10 pounds and try again. If you were successful on the attempt, add 5 to 10 pounds and try another attempt. Keep doing this, resting three to four minutes between sets until you fail an attempt. The weight you lifted on the prior set is your true 1RM.

Although not considered nearly as accurate, it is possible to estimate your 1RM without doing a true 1RM test. There are several equations that you can use to estimate 1RM based on how many reps you can complete with a certain amount of weight. This is a good option if you have an injury that could be worsened by training with extremely heavy weight or if you want to avoid doing a true 1RM for whatever reason. The most commonly used equation is the Epley formula, also known as the Nebraska formula:

$$1RM = [1 + (0.0333 \times \text{reps completed})] \times \text{weight lifted}$$

Using this equation, if you completed 10 reps on the bench press with 225 pounds, then

$$1RM = [1 + (0.0333 \times 10)] \times 225 \text{ pounds}$$

$$1RM = 1.333 \times 225 \text{ pounds}$$

$$1RM = 300 \text{ pounds}$$

After estimating your 1RM with the Nebraska formula, use that weight to determine your relative strength, your training weight, or how much progress you have made with a particular strength program.

BEGINNER OVERALL STRENGTH PROGRAM

If you have more than six months of consistent lifting experience, you can take on the majority of basic strength training programs that are designed to build maximal strength. The reason is that most programs for developing maximal strength start with lighter weight and higher reps and gradually increase the weight and decrease the reps performed. This systematic progression can prepare you to hoist heavy weights. However, if you have less than six months of experience, you are a special case because of the immaturity of your nervous system in regard to the specific exercises that you perform in your training regimen. Any time the body learns a new movement pattern—such as the barbell squat—it requires time for nerve connections to be strengthened and muscle fiber contractions to be synchronized. These adaptations of the nervous system can have a dramatic effect on strength gains in a short period of time. It is these adaptations that make up the majority of the strength gains that beginners make. Therefore, you should design a beginner strength training program to enhance these adaptations.

To enhance the neural adaptations that you need as a beginning lifter, this program emphasizes repetition—that is in the number of reps performed per set and the frequency of training. The training split used is a whole-body strength training split done on Monday, Wednesday, and Friday, or any three days per week allowing one full day of rest between workouts (see table 10.2). In each workout a different strength exercise is emphasized and performed as the first exercise of the workout. Training the same exercises three times per week helps the nervous system to "learn" the movement patterns of the exercise, strengthening the nerve connections that are required. During the first three months of the program, the assistance exercises stay the same for every workout (except for abdominal and core exercises). In the last three months, the assistance exercises are switched up in each workout to provide better variety in an effort to stimulate different muscle fibers, which may help to enhance strength on the three lifts.

The repetitions start out very high (20 per set for the first four weeks) and progressively drop every four weeks as the weight increases. This first four-week phase starts with weights equal to 55 percent RM on most lifts. This is a great starting weight if you are unaccustomed to doing particular exercises. The high reps further enhance the nerve connections and synchronicity of muscle fiber contractions that you need to develop to perform the exercises with correct form and maximal force. Sets start out at three per exercise for all exercises for the first three months. During the fourth and fifth months, you will perform all exercises for four sets.

TABLE 10.2　Beginnings of Strength

WORKOUT 1 (MONDAY): SQUAT FOCUS

Exercise	WEEKS 1-4			WEEKS 5-8			WEEKS 9-12		
	Sets	Reps	Weight	Sets	Reps	Weight	Sets	Reps	Weight
Squat	3	20	55% RM	3	15	65% RM	3	12	70% RM
Bench press	3	20	55% RM	3	15	65% RM	3	12	70% RM
Barbell shoulder press	3	20		3	15		3	12	
Deadlift	3	20	55% RM	3	15	65% RM	3	12	70% RM
Barbell row	3	20		3	15		3	12	
Close-grip bench press	3	20		3	15		3	12	
Barbell curl	3	20		3	15		3	12	
Hanging leg raise	3	12		3	15		3	15-20	

WORKOUT 2 (WEDNESDAY): BENCH PRESS FOCUS

Exercise	Sets	Reps	Weight	Sets	Reps	Weight	Sets	Reps	Weight
Bench press	3	20	55% RM	3	15	65% RM	3	12	70% RM
Squat	3	20	55% RM	3	15	65% RM	3	12	70% RM
Barbell shoulder press	3	20		3	15		3	12	
Deadlift	3	20	55% RM	3	15	65% RM	3	12	70% RM
Barbell row	3	20		3	15		3	12	
Close-grip bench press	3	20		3	15		3	12	
Barbell curl	3	20		3	15		3	12	
Cable woodchopper	3	12		3	15		3	15-20	

WORKOUT 3 (FRIDAY): DEADLIFT FOCUS

Exercise	Sets	Reps	Weight	Sets	Reps	Weight	Sets	Reps	Weight
Deadlift	3	20	55% RM	3	15	65% RM	3	12	70% RM
One-arm dumbbell deadlift	3	20		3	15		3	12	
Bench press	3	20	55% RM	3	15	65% RM	3	12	70% RM
Upright row	3	20		3	15		3	12	
Lat pulldown	3	20		3	15		3	12	
Lying triceps extension	3	20		3	15		3	12	
Preacher curl	3	20		3	15		3	12	
Back extension	3	12		3	15		3	15-20	

WORKOUT 1 (MONDAY): SQUAT FOCUS

Exercise	WEEKS 13-16			WEEKS 17-20			WEEKS 21-24		
	Sets	Reps	Weight	Sets	Reps	Weight	Sets	Reps	Weight
Squat	4	10	75% RM	4	8	80% RM	5	6	85% RM
Leg press	4	10		4	8		4	6	
Bench press	4	10	75% RM	4	8	80% RM	4	6	85% RM
Dumbbell shoulder press	4	10		4	8		4	6	
Barbell row	4	10		4	8		4	6	
Deadlift	4	10	75% RM	4	8	80% RM	4	6	85% RM
Close-grip bench press	4	10		4	8		4	6	
Dumbbell curl	4	10		4	8		4	6	
Standing crunch	4	12		4	10		4	8	

WORKOUT 2 (WEDNESDAY): BENCH PRESS FOCUS								
	WEEKS 13-16			WEEKS 17-20			WEEKS 21-24	
Exercise	Sets	Reps	Weight	Sets	Reps	Weight	Sets	Reps	Weight
Bench press	4	10	75% RM	4	8	80% RM	5	6	85% RM
Incline dumbbell press	4	10		4	8		4	6	
Squat	4	10	75% RM	4	8	80% RM	4	6	85% RM
Barbell shoulder press	4	10		4	8		4	6	
Deadlift	4	10	75% RM	4	8	80% RM	4	6	85% RM
Dumbbell row	4	10		4	8		4	6	
Triceps dip	4	10		4	8		4	6	
Barbell curl	4	10		4	8		4	6	
Russian twist	4	12		4	15		4	15-20	
WORKOUT 3 (FRIDAY): DEADLIFT FOCUS								
Deadlift	4	10	75% RM	4	8	80% RM	5	6	85% RM
One-arm dumbbell deadlift	4	10		4	8		4	6	
Bench press	4	10	75% RM	4	8	80% RM	4	6	85% RM
Upright row	4	10		4	8		4	6	
Lat pulldown	4	10		4	8		4	6	
Squat	4	10	75% RM	4	8	80% RM	4	6	85% RM
Lying triceps extension	4	10		4	8		4	6	
Preacher curl	4	10		4	8		4	6	
Good morning	4	10		4	8		4	6	

Then in the last month, you will bump up the sets to five on the three major lifts—but just on the workout in which you perform that exercise first. In the other workouts, sets remain at four. During the second phase the weight increases to 65 percent RM and reps drop to 15 per set. The third phase increases weight to 70 percent RM and drops reps to 12 per set. In phase 4, weight increases to 75 percent RM and reps are 10 per set. Phase 5 uses weights that are 80 percent RM for reps of 8 per set. In the final four weeks, weights are increased to 85 percent RM as reps drop down to 6 per set.

During this program 1RM testing should take place during the last week of each phase. Each of the three exercises will be tested on the workout in which you perform them first. After testing for the 1RM on that exercise, finish with three sets of that exercise with the prescribed weight and rep scheme for that phase. At the end of this six-month program, you are ready to progress to any of the other training programs discussed in this chapter. However, you should pick up with the intermediate strength training cycles.

INTERMEDIATE STRENGTH TRAINING CYCLES

Once you have been training consistently for more than six months, you are ready to take on most of the basic strength programs that follow a sound progression of increases in weight. Most strength programs follow some form of gradually increasing the percent RM used for training. This method is known as the percentage method of training and is the most commonly used method for increasing strength. The major differences between most training programs for developing strength involve the training split, the length of the program, the starting percent RM, and the finishing percent RM. The three training cycles that follow do not provide exercise choices. They list only the time line, the number of sets per exercise, the number of reps per set, the working weight (as percent RM), and the rest allowed between sets. Choose any training split provided in chapter 8 (to provide exercise choices and order as well as workouts per week) and apply it to these cycles.

Small-Step Cycle

You can use this 20-week basic periodized scheme with any training split. It follows the classical periodization format but increases the weight in very small increments each week—usually just 2 to 3 percent of the 1RM. See table 10.3 for the details of the small-step cycle. Depending on the weight of your 1RM, these increments may be as small as 2.5 pounds (the smallest increment available with weight plates) or as high as 25 pounds (for elite powerlifters with lifts up to 800 pounds). This constant and small increase in weight used each week is often referred to as *microloading*. It is believed that constantly challenging the muscle with progressively heavier weights forces the muscles to adapt by increasing their capacity to produce force (that is, muscle strength). This follows the principle of progressive overload. In addition to the prescribed percent RM used each week, this cycle has scheduled retesting of the 1RM. This allows for fine-tuning of the percent RM as the 1RM will increase over the course of the training cycle.

TABLE 10.3   Small Steps to Strength

Week	Sets	Reps	Weight (% RM)	Rest (minutes)
HYPERTROPHY PHASE				
1*	5	15	55%	1-2
2	4	15	57%	1-2
3	3	12	60%	1-2
4	3	12	62%	1-2
5*	3	10	65%	1-2
STRENGTH PHASE				
6	5	10	67%	2
7	5	8	70%	2
8	4	8	73%	2
9*	4	7	75%	2
10	3	6	77%	2
POWER PHASE				
11	3	6	80%	3
12	3	4	82%	3
13*	3	4	85%	3
14	3	3	87%	3
PEAKING CYCLE				
15	3	3	90%	4
16	2	2	92%	4
17*	2	1	95%	5
18	2	1	97%	5
19	Off or active rest			
20*	Competition or testing of 1RM			

*1RM test week.

Countdown Cycle

Although all the basic strength training programs have some form of gradual progression where the reps performed at each workout decrease over time, the countdown cycle uses a corresponding system that matches sets, reps, and weeks that each phase is followed in a 6, 5, 4, 3, 2, 1 countdown progression. See table 10.4 for the weekly progression of the countdown cycle. To expand on this, the first phase lasts six weeks and uses six sets of six reps for each exercise. The next phase lasts five weeks and uses five sets of five reps. This pattern continues with each phase dropping one week, one set, and one rep until the final week, where one set of one maximal rep is performed for each exercise. As with all the basic percentage method strength programs, this works well with any split discussed in chapter 8.

TABLE 10.4   Strength Countdown

Week	Sets	Reps	Weight (% RM)	Rest (minutes)
PHASE 6				
1*	6	6	55%	1-2
2	6	6	55%	1-2
3	6	6	55%	1-2
4	6	6	60%	1-2
5*	6	6	60%	1-2
6	6	6	60%	1-2
PHASE 5				
7	5	5	65%	2
8	5	5	65%	2
9*	5	5	65%	2
10	5	5	70%	2
11	5	5	70%	2
PHASE 4				
12	4	4	75%	3
13*	4	4	75%	3
14	4	4	80%	3
15	4	4	80%	3
PHASE 3				
16	3	3	85%	4
17*	3	3	85%	4
18	3	3	85%	4
PHASE 2				
19	2	2	90%	5
20	2	2	95%	5
PHASE 1				
21*	1	1	100%	5

*1RM test week.

9 to 5 Cycle

This training cycle is simple in that it uses two rep ranges—nine reps per set and five reps per set. This is great for those who like to keep rep ranges fairly constant. However, training weights do change each week over the 15-week program while the reps are kept constant throughout each of the two phases. As the weight increases, the number of sets decreases and rest between sets increases. See table 10.5 for the specifics of the 9 to 5 cycle. Weight increments are small, similar to the small-step cycle, but this one stops at 85 percent and doesn't go higher. Many believe that going much higher isn't necessary for building maximal strength.

TABLE 10.5 Getting Strong 9 to 5

Week	Sets	Reps	Weight (% RM)	Rest (minutes)
PHASE 1: 9 REPS				
1*	8	9	50%	2
2	8	9	53%	2
3	8	9	55%	2
4	7	9	57%	2
5*	7	9	60%	2
6	7	9	62%	2
7	6	9	65%	3
8	6	9	67%	3
9*	6	9	70%	3
10	5	9	73%	3
PHASE 2: 5 REPS				
11	5	5	75%	4
12*	4	5	77%	4
13	4	5	80%	4
14	3	5	82%	4
15	3	5	85%	4
16*	1RM test			

*1RM test week.

One-Year-Plus Intermediate Program

If you are an intermediate lifter you should consider following the previous cycles in the order presented—starting with the small-step cycle, following with the countdown cycle, and finishing with the 9 to 5 cycle. This will carry you through over 55 weeks—just over a solid year—of well-planned strength training. With the conclusion of this year plan you will be ready to progress into more advanced training cycles. One great advanced training cycle to follow the 9 to 5 cycle that concludes the year of intermediate training cycles is the 85-plus strength cycle found in the advanced training cycles section that follows. See table 10.6 for a sample training cycle progression that puts you in the rank of advanced weightlifter.

TABLE 10.6 Strength Calendar

Weeks	Cycle	Notes
1-20	Small-step cycle	
21	Active rest	Stay out of gym but take up other activities
22-43	Countdown cycle	
44	Active rest	Stay out of gym but take up other activities
45-60	9 to 5 cycle	
61	Active rest	Stay out of gym but take up other activities
62-	85-plus strength	

ADVANCED STRENGTH TRAINING CYCLES

The cycles that follow are advanced in the sense that they require greater skill and training experience in order to be used safely and properly. These programs are considered advanced for several reasons—they may start off at a heavier weight or they may require the use of advanced techniques. This does not imply that the training cycles covered in the basic strength training cycles are not useful for advanced weightlifters. Those programs may be basic in their progression; however, many elite competitive powerlifters use them. These advanced programs are designed for the advanced trainer who has a more difficult time continuing to make large strength gains, since basic programs may not always do the trick.

85-Plus Strength Cycle

Unlike the intermediate programs, which all start with very light weight in the 50 to 60 percent RM range, this program starts off at 85 percent RM and progressively builds up to 95 percent RM. This is depicted in table 10.7. It also increases the reps as time progresses with each percent RM. This is good for more advanced trainers or as a second leg to a previous program that started with a lighter phase. The 9 to 5 cycle, for instance, is a good cycle to use before this cycle. Another advanced technique that this cycle uses is negative-rep training. However, instead of doing it at the beginning of the working sets for bench press and squat, you would do these as the final working set for each major lift on working days.

TABLE 10.7 85-Plus Strength

Day	Exercise	Sets	Reps	Weight (% RM)
	WEEK 1*			
1	Squat	5	3	85%
		1	3	120% (negative set)
	Leg press	3	3	
	Leg extension	3	3	
	Bench press	5	2	80%
	Standing calf raise	3	6	
3	Bench press	5	3	85%
		1	3	120% (negative set)
	Dumbbell bench press	3	3	
	Squat	5	2	80%
	Barbell shoulder press	3	3	
	Close-grip bench press	3	3	
5	Deadlift	5	3	85%
	Good morning	3	3	
	Lying leg curl	3	3	
	Standing crunch	3	6	
	WEEK 2			
8	Squat	5	4	85%
		1	3	120% (negative set)
	Leg press	3	4	
	Leg extension	3	4	
	Bench press	5	2	80%
	Standing calf raise	3	8	
10	Bench press	5	4	85%
		1	3	120% (negative set)
	Dumbbell bench press	3	4	
	Squat	5	2	80%
	Barbell shoulder press	3	4	
	Close-grip bench press	3	4	
12	Deadlift	5	4	85%
	Good morning	3	4	
	Lying leg curl	3	4	
	Standing crunch	3	8	

*1RM test week.

WEEK 3

Day	Exercise	Sets	Reps	Weight (% RM)
15	Squat	5	5	85%
		1	3	120% (negative set)
	Leg press	3	5	
	Leg extension	3	5	
	Bench press	5	2	80%
	Standing calf raise	3	10	
17	Bench press	5	5	85%
		1	3	120% (negative set)
	Dumbbell bench press	3	5	
	Squat	5	2	80%
	Barbell shoulder press	3	5	
	Close-grip bench press	3	5	
19	Deadlift	5	5	85%
	Good morning	3	5	
	Lying leg curl	3	5	
	Standing crunch	3	10	

WEEK 4

Day	Exercise	Sets	Reps	Weight (% RM)
22	Squat	5	6	85%
		1	3	120% (negative set)
	Leg press	3	6	
	Leg extension	3	6	
	Bench press	5	2	80%
	Standing calf raise	3	12	
24	Bench press	5	6	85%
		1	3	120% (negative set)
	Dumbbell bench press	3	6	
	Squat	5	2	80%
	Barbell shoulder press	3	6	
	Close-grip bench press	3	6	
26	Deadlift	5	6	85%
	Good morning	3	6	
	Lying leg curl	3	6	
	Standing crunch	3	12	

WEEK 5*

Day	Exercise	Sets	Reps	Weight (% RM)
29	Squat	3	2	90%
		1	3	120% (negative set)
	Leg press	3	3	
	Leg extension	3	3	
	Bench press	5	2	80%
	Standing calf raise	3	6	

*1RM test week.

> continued

TABLE 10.7 85-Plus Strength *(continued)*

Day	Exercise	Sets	Reps	Weight (% RM)
	WEEK 5* *(continued)*			
31	Bench press	3	2	90%
		1	3	120% (negative set)
	Dumbbell bench press	3	3	
	Squat	5	2	80%
	Barbell shoulder press	3	3	
	Close-grip bench press	3	3	
33	Deadlift	3	2	90%
	Good morning	3	3	
	Lying leg curl	3	3	
	Standing crunch	3	6	
	WEEK 6			
36	Squat	3	3	90%
		1	3	120% (negative set)
	Leg press	3	3	
	Leg extension	3	3	
	Bench press	5	2	80%
	Standing calf raise	3	6	
38	Bench press	3	3	90%
		1	3	120% (negative set)
	Dumbbell bench press	3	3	
	Squat	5	2	80%
	Barbell shoulder press	3	3	
	Close-grip bench press	3	3	
40	Deadlift	3	3	90%
	Good morning	3	3	
	Lying leg curl	3	3	
	Standing crunch	3	6	
	WEEK 7			
43	Squat	3	4	90%
		1	3	120% (negative set)
	Leg press	3	4	
	Leg extension	3	4	
	Bench press	5	2	80%
	Standing calf raise	3	8	
45	Bench press	3	4	90%
		1	3	120% (negative set)
	Dumbbell bench press	3	3	
	Squat	5	2	80%
	Barbell shoulder press	3	4	
	Close-grip bench press	3	4	

*1RM test week.

WEEK 7 (continued)				
Day	Exercise	Sets	Reps	Weight (% RM)
47	Deadlift	3	4	90%
	Good morning	3	4	
	Lying leg curl	3	4	
	Standing crunch	3	8	
WEEK 8				
No assistance exercises are performed from here out, just the major lifts.				
50	Squat	3	2	95%
		1	3	120% (negative set)
	Bench press	5	2	80%
52	Bench press	3	2	95%
		1	3	120% (negative set)
	Squat	5	2	80%
54	Deadlift	3	2	95%
WEEK 9*				
62	Squat	1	1	100%
	Bench press	1	1	100%
	Deadlift	1	1	100%

*1RM test week.

Advanced Six Cycle

For some advanced weightlifters, strength gains no longer come easily. After all, the longer you train, the stronger you get; the stronger you get, the harder it is to get stronger. This is because trained lifters with greater strength are close to reaching the height of their genetic strength ceiling. This advanced program is designed to encourage strength gains in even the most seasoned lifter. In each of the six phases, the cycle uses an advanced training technique to encourage strength gains. The constant cycling of weight and reps, along with the specialized training techniques, prevents stagnation and promotes continual strength gains throughout the eight-month cycle.

This cycle uses a squat–bench press–deadlift training split that is meshed with a push–pull training split. That is, the workouts are divided into three separate workouts—squat, bench press, and deadlift with upper-body pushing exercises (shoulders and triceps exercises) done with the bench press day and the upper-body pulling exercises (back and biceps exercises) done with the deadlift day. For variety, each phase alters the order of the training split. See table 10.8, Advanced Six, for details.

During the first phase (weeks 1 to 5), the training technique used is density training. This will increase the amount of weight you can perform 10 reps with on the squat, bench press, and deadlift. This will carry over into greater strength on the 1RM for each of these lifts as well. This will be apparent when you test your 1RM in week 6. That is the only gym workout you will do in week 6.

In phase 2 (weeks 7 to 9), the training days are reorganized so that the deadlift day is first and the squat day is last. The bench press workout still is left in the middle to separate the two workouts that both use lower-body muscles to allow for better recovery. You will do working sets with 80 percent RM—however, this will be heavier than you could previously lift because of the boost in strength from the density training. The technique for this phase is forced-rep training. This is a mass-training technique covered in chapter 6. The reason it is included here in a strength cycle is to encourage some growth in muscle fibers—which can lend itself to greater force production and therefore muscle strength. In addition, the procedure of forcing extra reps can lead to direct increases in muscle strength. This phase lasts just three weeks because of the high intensity of the forced-rep training.

Phase 3 (weeks 11 to 17) starts off using about 80 to 85 percent RM or a weight you can do for four sets of six reps. This will kick off the 5 percent method that will carry this phase through the next seven weeks. Use the 5 percent method for each major lift and one assistance exercise that mimics the lift. In phase 4 (weeks 19 to 22) you will use a static contraction technique that calls on potentiation to enhance muscle strength on the second set. You will do working sets with 90 percent RM. Phase 5 (weeks 24 to 27) uses another potentiation technique known to boost your power on the three lifts. For each strength exercise (squat, deadlift, and bench press), you will perform one rep with 95 percent of your 1RM weight as quickly as possible. Rest for three minutes and downshift to 50 percent of your 1RM weight and perform five reps as explosively as possible. Repeat this three times to develop explosive strength. The final phase is yet another potentiation program. This is basically the reverse of the technique of the previous phase because it uses explosive movements to enhance maximal strength. At the climax of this program your 1RM on all three moves will be dramatically enhanced. Follow this final phase with one or two weeks of active rest before starting the cycle over or moving on to a new strength training cycle.

TABLE 10.8 Advanced Six

PHASE 1: WEEKS 1-5 WORKOUT 1: SQUAT				
Exercise	**Sets**	**Reps**	**%1RM**	**Notes**
Squat	10	2 (week 1)	80%	Follow the density training method found in chapter 9 for a goal of 10 reps.
	6	3 (week 2)		
	5	4 (week 3)		
	4	5 (week 4)		
	3	6 (week 5)		
Leg press	3	10		
Leg extension	3	10		
Leg curl	3	10		
Standing calf raise	4	20		
WORKOUT 2: BENCH PRESS AND PUSH				
Bench press	10	2 (week 1)	80%	Follow the density training method found in chapter 9 for a goal of 10 reps.
	6	3 (week 2)		
	5	4 (week 3)		
	4	5 (week 4)		
	3	6 (week 5)		
Incline dumbbell press	2	10		Perform the last set of each exercise to muscle failure.
Flat dumbbell press	2	10		
Barbell shoulder press	3	10		
Lying triceps extensions	3	10		
Hanging leg raise	4	12-15		
WORKOUT 3: DEADLIFT AND PULL				
Deadlift	10	2 (week 1)	80%	Follow the density training method found in chapter 9 for a goal of 10 reps.
	6	3 (week 2)		
	5	4 (week 3)		
	4	5 (week 4)		
	3	6 (week 5)		

PHASE 1: WEEKS 1-5 *(continued)*
WORKOUT 3: DEADLIFT AND PULL *(continued)*

Exercise	Sets	Reps	%1RM	Notes
Barbell row	2	10		Perform the last set of each exercise to muscle failure.
Lat pulldown	2	10		
Barbell curl	3	10		
Standing cable crunch	3	12		

PHASE 1: WEEK 6
WORKOUT 1: PERFORM MID- TO LATE WEEK

Test your 1RM on the squat, bench press, and deadlift in that order.

PHASE 2: WEEKS 7-9
WORKOUT 1: DEADLIFT AND PULL

Exercise	Sets	Reps	%1RM	Notes
Deadlift	5	8	80%	For the last set of each exercise, perform forced reps where you perform 2 or 3 reps with the assistance of a spotter or a training partner after you reach failure. The exception is ab exercises.
Pull-up	3	8		
Barbell row	3	8		
Barbell curl	3	8		
Reverse crunch	3	12-15		

WORKOUT 2: BENCH PRESS AND PUSH

Bench press	5	8	80%	
Incline dumbbell press	3	8		
Dumbbell shoulder press	2	8		
Lateral raise	2	8		
Seated overhead triceps extension	2	8		
Dip	3	8		
Cable crunch	3	12-15		

WORKOUT 3: SQUAT

Squat	5	8	80%	
Leg press	2	8		
Leg extension	2	8		
Leg curl	2	8		
Leg press calf raise	3	15-20		

PHASE 2: WEEK 10
WORKOUT 1: PERFORM MID- TO LATE WEEK

Test your 1RM on the squat, bench press, and deadlift in that order.

PHASE 3: WEEK 11
WORKOUT 1: SQUAT

Exercise	Sets	Reps	%1RM	Notes
Squat	4	6	~80-85%	
Leg press	4	6	~80-85%	
Leg extension	3	6		
Leg curl	3	6		
Standing calf raise	3	15-20		

> continued

TABLE 10.8   Advanced Six *(continued)*

PHASE 3: WEEK 11 *(continued)*
WORKOUT 2: BENCH PRESS AND PUSH

Exercise	Sets	Reps	% 1RM	Notes
Bench press	4	6	~80-85%	
Incline bench press	4	6	~80-85%	
Barbell shoulder press	3	6		
Close-grip bench press	3	6		
Weighted crunch	3	12-15		

WORKOUT 3: DEADLIFT AND PULL

Exercise	Sets	Reps	% 1RM	Notes
Deadlift	4	6	~80-85%	
Romanian deadlift	4	6	~80-85%	
Barbell row	3	6		
Barbell curl	3	6		
Reverse crunch	3	12-15		

PHASE 3: WEEK 12
WORKOUT 1: SQUAT

Exercise	Sets	Reps	% 1RM	Notes
Squat	4	5	~80-85% + 5%	
Leg press	4	5	~80-85% + 5%	
Leg extension	3	5		
Leg curl	3	5		
Standing calf raise	3	15-20		

WORKOUT 2: BENCH PRESS AND PUSH

Exercise	Sets	Reps	% 1RM	Notes
Bench press	4	5	~80-85% + 5%	
Incline bench press	4	5	~80-85% + 5%	
Barbell shoulder press	3	5		
Close-grip bench press	3	5		
Weighted crunch	3	12-15		

WORKOUT 3: DEADLIFT AND PULL

Exercise	Sets	Reps	% 1RM	Notes
Deadlift	4	5	~80-85% + 5%	
Romanian deadlift	4	5	~80-85% + 5%	
Barbell row	3	5		
Barbell curl	3	5		
Reverse crunch	3	12-15		

PHASE 3: WEEK 13
WORKOUT 1: SQUAT

Exercise	Sets	Reps	% 1RM	Notes
Squat	4	4	~80-85% + 10%	
Leg press	4	4	~80-85% + 10%	
Leg extension	3	4		
Leg curl	3	4		
Seated calf raise	3	20		

WORKOUT 2: BENCH PRESS AND PUSH

Exercise	Sets	Reps	% 1RM	Notes
Bench press	4	4	~80-85% + 10%	
Incline bench press	4	4	~80-85% + 10%	
Barbell shoulder press	3	4		
Close-grip bench press	3	4		
Cable crunch	3	10		

PHASE 3: WEEK 13 *(continued)*
WORKOUT 3: DEADLIFT AND PULL

Exercise	Sets	Reps	% 1RM	Notes
Deadlift	4	4	~80-85% + 10%	
Romanian deadlift	4	4	~80-85% + 10%	
Barbell row	3	4		
Barbell curl	3	4		
Russian twist	3	12-15		

PHASE 3: WEEK 14
WORKOUT 1: SQUAT

Exercise	Sets	Reps	% 1RM	Notes
Squat	4	6	~80-85% + 5%	
Leg press	4	6	~80-85% + 5%	
Leg extension	3	6		
Leg curl	3	6		
Seated calf raise	3	25		

WORKOUT 2: BENCH PRESS AND PUSH

Exercise	Sets	Reps	% 1RM	Notes
Bench press	4	6	~80-85% + 5%	
Incline bench press	4	6	~80-85% + 5%	
Barbell shoulder press	3	6		
Close-grip bench press	3	6		
Cable crunch	3	12		

WORKOUT 3: DEADLIFT AND PULL

Exercise	Sets	Reps	% 1RM	Notes
Deadlift	4	6	~80-85% + 5%	
Romanian deadlift	4	6	~80-85% + 5%	
Barbell row	3	6		
Barbell curl	3	6		
Russian twist	3	12-15		

PHASE 3: WEEK 15
WORKOUT 1: SQUAT

Exercise	Sets	Reps	% 1RM	Notes
Squat	4	5	~80-85% + 10%	
Leg press	4	5	~80-85% + 10%	
Leg extension	3	5		
Leg curl	3	5		
Leg press calf raise	3	12		

WORKOUT 2: BENCH PRESS AND PUSH

Exercise	Sets	Reps	% 1RM	Notes
Bench press	4	5	~80-85% + 10%	
Incline bench press	4	5	~80-85% + 10%	
Barbell shoulder press	3	5		
Close-grip bench press	3	5		
Cable crunch	3	15		

WORKOUT 3: DEADLIFT AND PULL

Exercise	Sets	Reps	% 1RM	Notes
Deadlift	4	5	~80-85% + 10%	
Romanian deadlift	4	5	~80-85% + 10%	
Barbell row	3	5		
Barbell curl	3	5		
Dumbbell woodchopper	3	12-15		

> continued

TABLE 10.8   Advanced Six *(continued)*

PHASE 3: WEEK 16
WORKOUT 1: SQUAT

Exercise	Sets	Reps	% 1RM	Notes
Squat	4	4	~80-85% + 15%	
Leg press	4	4	~80-85% + 15%	
Leg extension	3	4		
Leg curl	3	4		
Seated calf raise	3	25		

WORKOUT 2: BENCH PRESS AND PUSH

Exercise	Sets	Reps	% 1RM	Notes
Bench press	4	4	~80-85% + 15%	
Incline bench press	4	4	~80-85% + 15%	
Barbell shoulder press	3	4		
Close-grip bench press	3	4		
Cable crunch	3	12		

WORKOUT 3: DEADLIFT AND PULL

Exercise	Sets	Reps	% 1RM	Notes
Deadlift	4	4	~80-85% + 15%	
Romanian deadlift	4	4	~80-85% + 15%	
Barbell row	3	4		
Barbell curl	3	4		
Russian twist	3	12-15		

PHASE 3: WEEK 17
WORKOUT 1: SQUAT

Exercise	Sets	Reps	% 1RM	Notes
Squat	4	6	~80-85% + 10%	
Leg press	4	6	~80-85% + 10%	
Leg extension	3	6		
Leg curl	3	6		
Standing calf raise	3	15-20		

WORKOUT 2: BENCH PRESS AND PUSH

Exercise	Sets	Reps	% 1RM	Notes
Bench press	4	6	~80-85% + 10%	
Incline bench press	4	6	~80-85% + 10%	
Barbell shoulder press	3	6		
Close-grip bench press	3	6		
Weighted crunch	3	12-15		

WORKOUT 3: DEADLIFT AND PULL

Exercise	Sets	Reps	% 1RM	Notes
Deadlift	4	6	~80-85% + 10%	
Romanian deadlift	4	6	~80-85% + 10%	
Barbell row	3	6		
Barbell curl	3	6		
Reverse crunch	3	12-15		

PHASE 3: WEEK 18
WORKOUT 1: PERFORM MID- TO LATE WEEK

Test your 1RM on the squat, bench press, and deadlift in that order.

PHASE 4: WEEKS 19-22
WORKOUT 1: DEADLIFT AND PULL

Exercise	Sets	Reps	% 1RM	Notes
Static-drive deadlift	3	3	120% +	Alternate between static-drive deadlifts and regular heavy deadlifts, resting 30 seconds after static-drive deadlifts and resting 3 minutes after heavy deadlifts. Complete 3 sets of each deadlift and rest for 1 minute before continuing with the remaining exercises.
Alternated with heavy deadlift	3	4	90%	
Pull-up	3	6-8		
Barbell row	3	3-4		
Barbell curl	3	3-4		
Preacher curl	3	3-4		
Reverse crunch	3	12-15		

WORKOUT 2: BENCH PRESS AND PUSH

Exercise	Sets	Reps	% 1RM	Notes
Static-drive bench press	3	3	120% +	Alternate between static-drive bench presses and regular heavy bench presses, resting 30 seconds after static-drive bench presses and resting 3 minutes after heavy bench presses. Complete 3 sets of each bench press and rest for 1 minute before continuing with the remaining exercises.
Alternated with heavy bench press	3	4	90%	
Incline dumbbell press	3	3-4		
Dumbbell shoulder press	3	3-4		
Dip	3	3-4		Add weight as needed to reach failure in the 3- to 4-rep range.
Cable crunch	3	8-10		

WORKOUT 3: SQUAT

Exercise	Sets	Reps	% 1RM	Notes
Static-drive squat	3	3	120% +	Alternate between static-drive squats and regular heavy squats, resting 30 seconds after static-drive squats and resting 3 minutes after heavy squats. Complete 3 sets of each squat and rest for 1 minute before continuing with the remaining exercises.
Alternated with heavy squat	3	4	90%	
Leg press	3	3-4		
Leg extension	3	6-8		Add weight as needed to reach failure in the 6- to 8-rep range.
Leg curl	3	6-8		
Leg-press calf raise	3	12-15		

PHASE 4: WEEK 23
WORKOUT 1: PERFORM MID- TO LATE WEEK

Test your 1RM on the squat, bench press, and deadlift in that order.

> continued

TABLE 10.8   Advanced Six *(continued)*

PHASE 5: WEEKS 24-27
WORKOUT 1: SQUAT

Exercise	Sets	Reps	% 1RM	Notes
Squat	3	1	95%	After a thorough warm-up, do the first set with 1 rep (no more or you will fatigue the muscle) with 95% of your 1RM weight. Rest for 3 minutes and then do the next set with 3 to 5 reps with 50% of your 1RM weight. Alternate between the weights 3 times for a total of 6 sets.
	3	5	50%	
Leg press	3	5	50%	
Leg extension	3	5	50%	
Leg curl	3	5	50%	
Leg press calf raise	3	5	50%	

WORKOUT 2: BENCH PRESS

Exercise	Sets	Reps	% 1RM	Notes
Bench press	3	1	95%	After a thorough warm-up, do the first set with 1 rep (no more or you will fatigue the muscle) with 95% of your 1RM weight. Rest for 3 minutes and then do the next set with 3 to 5 reps with 50% of your 1RM weight. Alternate between the weights 3 times for a total of 6 sets.
	3	5	50%	
Dumbbell bench press	3	5	50%	
Barbell shoulder press	3	5	50%	
Dumbbell upright rows	3	5	50%	
Close-grip bench press	3	5	50%	
Hanging leg raise	3	12-15		

WORKOUT 3: DEADLIFT

Exercise	Sets	Reps	% 1RM	Notes
Deadlift	3	1	95%	After a thorough warm-up, do the first set with 1 rep (no more or you will fatigue the muscle) with 95% of your 1RM weight. Rest for 3 minutes and then do the next set with 3 to 5 reps with 50% of your 1RM weight. Alternate between the weights 3 times for a total of 6 sets.
	3	5	50%	
Pulldown	3	5	50%	
Barbell row	3	5	50%	
Barbell curl	3	5	50%	
Reverse crunch	3	12-15		

PHASE 5: WEEK 28
WORKOUT 1: PERFORM MID- TO LATE WEEK

Test your 1RM on the squat, bench press, and deadlift in that order.

PHASE 6: WEEKS 29-32
WORKOUT 1: DEADLIFT

Exercise	Sets	Reps	% 1RM	Notes
Dumbbell deadlift jump	3	3	30%	
Alternated with deadlift	3	2-3	95%	
Barbell row	3	2-3	95%	
Barbell curl	3	2-3	95%	
Standing cable crunch	3	6-8		

WORKOUT 2: BENCH PRESS

Exercise	Sets	Reps	% 1RM	Notes
Power push-up	3	3	Body weight	
Alternated with bench press	3	2-3	95%	
Barbell incline press	3	2	95%	
Barbell shoulder press	3	2	95%	
Close-grip bench press	3	2	95%	
Hanging leg raise	3	15-20		

WORKOUT 3: SQUAT

Exercise	Sets	Reps	% 1RM	Notes
Barbell squat jump	3	3	30%	
Alternated with squat	3	2-3	95%	
Leg press	3	2	95%	
Standing calf raise	3	2	95%	

PHASE 6: WEEK 33
WORKOUT 1: PERFORM MID- TO LATE WEEK

Test your 1RM on the squat, bench press, and deadlift in that order.

LIFT-SPECIFIC CYCLES

Training to build overall strength should be every weightlifter's major goal. However, after you have a strong base of overall strength from lifting for a good while, you may want to build up strength in certain lifts. This may be due to an imbalance of strength in a certain area. Or you may just have an affinity for a particular lift and want to excel at it. This is often common with the bench press. The following programs are designed to build up your strength in one lift and only one lift. However, this does not mean that you shouldn't work on increasing your strength in the other lifts. These programs emphasize the bench press, squat, or deadlift. However, they are designed to fit in with regular training splits. One way to use these cycles is to alternate the three of them so that you emphasize bench press strength at one phase in your training cycle, squat strength in another, and deadlift strength in another before cycling back to bench press-focused training.

Bench Press Booster Cycle

This 10-week cycle involves using an upper- and lower-body split so that you can train chest twice each week (once on Monday with a heavy day and once on Thursday with a light day of bench press work). See table 10.9, Big Bench Routine, for details. On the heavy chest day, all you do is bench press. Weight increases and therefore repetitions decrease every three weeks until you reach the last week where you max out with your new record weight. Allow three to five minutes of rest between sets on your heavy bench day to keep your strength up. On the light chest day you do the bench press along with the other upper-body assistance exercises. In this workout, you'll perform light bench presses as well as dumbbell bench presses (incline or flat) and flys (incline or flat). Rotate the incline and flat version of these exercises so that when you do incline dumbbell presses, you follow with flat flys and vice versa. Allow two to three minutes of rest between sets on the light chest day.

Finish the chest workout with power push-ups to develop explosive power that will help you throw up more weight on the bench press. This light day is important because it keeps the muscle from losing its memory of how strong it was at the previous training session, enhances the blood circulation in the areas that are important to the bench, keeps your muscle size up, and reinforces your groove—that unique lifting path that you'll discover to be the best way to push the bar up to completion. Follow the light chest routine with one exercise for shoulders, back, triceps, and biceps.

Follow this routine for 9 weeks. On the 10th week, you max out on your specified heavy chest day. You'll be amazed at your newfound strength. Do no other lifting this week; you should be at your peak. After you peak, take a period of active recovery in which you perform some form of light exercise. Try other activities that involve both upper- and lower-body movements such as swimming, racket sports, or rock-wall climbing.

TABLE 10.9   Big Bench Routine

MONDAY: HEAVY BENCH PRESS DAY

Exercise	Sets	Reps	Weight (% RM)
Bench press	1	10	50%
	1	6	60%
	1	4	70%
Weeks 1-3	4	6	85%
	3	Muscle failure	60%
Weeks 4-6	4	4	90%
	3	Muscle failure	60%
Weeks 7-9	4	2	95%
	3	Muscle failure	60%
Week 10	1	1RM max	New 100%

THURSDAY: LIGHT BENCH PRESS DAY

Exercise	Sets	Reps	Weight (% RM)
Bench press	1	10	50%
	1	6	60%
	3	4	75%
	1	8	55%
Dumbbell bench press	2	10	70%
Incline dumbbell fly	2	10	70%
Power push-up	3	Failure	Body weight
Barbell overhead press	3	6	80%
Barbell row	3	6	80%
Close-grip bench press	3	6	80%
Barbell curl	3	6	80%

Squat-Building Cycle

This six-week squat program is a modified version of what is known as the Russian squat routine. It will increase your squat weight 5 to 10 percent in just six weeks. However, it does require you to squat for three days per week (see table 10.10). That makes the squat–bench press–deadlift training split the best split to use with this program, but with one modification: You will squat first on all three workout days. On Monday do a full squat workout with just two extra assistance exercises for quads (the leg press and leg extension) as well as one calf exercise. On Wednesday you will perform just the prescribed number of squats and no other leg work before your bench press workout. On Friday you will do the same thing before your deadlift workout. Some lifters opt to train their squats in the morning on Wednesdays and Fridays and their bench presses and deadlifts in the evening. This can help prevent the fatigue that may hinder your other lifts after performing several sets of squats.

The program starts at 80 percent RM and cycles over the 18-day program to reach 100 percent by the 16th workout. Then it drops back to 80 percent for the 17th workout to give the legs a rest before the 18th workout, where you will test your 1RM with at least 105 percent of your original 1RM before this program.

TABLE 10.10 Russian Squat Strength

Before each workout, do several warm-up sets to get up to working set weight.

WEEK 1
MONDAY: SQUAT WORKOUT DAY

Exercise	Sets	Reps	Weight (% RM)
Squat	6	2	80%
Leg press	3	6	
Leg extension	3	6	
Standing calf raise	3	10	

WEDNESDAY: BENCH PRESS WORKOUT DAY

Squat	6	3	80%
Bench press workout (immediately after squats or later in day)			

FRIDAY: DEADLIFT WORKOUT DAY

Squat	6	2	80%
Deadlift workout (immediately after squats or later in day)			

WEEK 2
MONDAY: SQUAT WORKOUT DAY

Squat	6	4	80%
Leg press	3	6	
Leg extension	3	6	
Standing calf raise	3	10	

WEDNESDAY: BENCH PRESS WORKOUT DAY

Squat	6	2	80%
Bench press workout (immediately after squats or later in day)			

FRIDAY: DEADLIFT WORKOUT DAY

Squat	6	5	80%
Deadlift workout (immediately after squats or later in day)			

WEEK 3
MONDAY: SQUAT WORKOUT DAY

Squat	6	2	80%
Leg press	3	6	
Leg extension	3	6	
Standing calf raise	3	10	

WEDNESDAY: BENCH PRESS WORKOUT DAY

Squat	6	6	80%
Bench press workout (immediately after squats or later in day)			

FRIDAY: DEADLIFT WORKOUT DAY

Squat	6	2	80%
Deadlift workout (immediately after squats or later in day)			

WEEK 4
MONDAY: SQUAT WORKOUT DAY

Exercise	Sets	Reps	Weight (%RM)
Squat	5	5	85%
Leg press	3	6	
Leg extension	3	6	
Standing calf raise	3	10	

WEDNESDAY: BENCH PRESS WORKOUT DAY

Squat	6	2	80%
Bench press workout (immediately after squats or later in day)			

FRIDAY: DEADLIFT WORKOUT DAY

Squat	4	4	90%
Deadlift workout (immediately after squats or later in day)			

WEEK 5
MONDAY: SQUAT WORKOUT DAY

Squat	6	2	80%
Leg press	3	6	
Leg extension	3	6	
Standing calf raise	3	10	

WEDNESDAY: BENCH PRESS WORKOUT DAY

Squat	3	3	95%
Bench press workout (immediately after squats or later in day)			

FRIDAY: DEADLIFT WORKOUT DAY

Squat	6	2	80%
Deadlift workout (immediately after squats or later in day)			

WEEK 6
MONDAY: SQUAT WORKOUT DAY

Squat	2	2	100%
Leg press	3	6	
Leg extension	3	6	
Standing calf raise	3	10	

WEDNESDAY: BENCH PRESS WORKOUT DAY

Squat	6	2	80%
Bench press workout (immediately after squats or later in day)			

FRIDAY: DEADLIFT WORKOUT DAY

No squats, just deadlift workout			

WEEK 7

Test new 1RM.

Deadlift Raising Cycle

This 10-week program is effective for boosting strength in the deadlift in even the most experienced lifters. In fact, this program is similar to one used by many elite deadlifters, including Mark Phillipi. This program works well with a squat–bench press–deadlift training split, as long as you do the deadlift workout first in the week and the squat workout last (see table 10.11). It consistently uses just one set of heavy weight for very low reps (one or two) as the first working set of each workout. Over the 10 weeks the weight for this set moves from 75 percent to 100 percent. Following the heavy set are several sets of light deadlifts done explosively. This builds up the power you will need to explode the weight off the floor at the start of the deadlift. The first four weeks use a circuit program for the assistance exercises. This helps to condition the muscles to prevent fatigue. The last six weeks use straight sets for all assistance exercises.

TABLE 10.11 Raising the Dead

Before each workout, do several warm-up sets to get up to working-set weight. Do the assistance circuit in a circuit format—rest 90 seconds between each exercise and rest 3 minutes between the end of the circuit and beginning the circuit again. Do three circuits, totaling eight reps on each exercise.

WEEK 1				
Exercise	Sets	Reps	Weight (% RM)	Rest
Deadlift	1	2	75%	3 min
	8	3	60%	90 sec
ASSISTANCE CIRCUIT				
Romanian deadlift	3	8		90 sec
Barbell row	3	8		90 sec
Lat pulldown	3	8		90 sec
Good morning	3	8		90 sec
WEEK 2				
Deadlift	1	2	80%	3 min
	8	3	65%	90 sec
ASSISTANCE CIRCUIT				
Romanian deadlift	3	8		90 sec
Barbell row	3	8		90 sec
Lat pulldown	3	8		90 sec
Good morning	3	8		90 sec
WEEK 3				
Deadlift	1	2	85%	3 min
	6	3	70%	2 min
ASSISTANCE CIRCUIT				
Romanian deadlift	3	8		90 sec
Barbell row	3	8		90 sec
Lat pulldown	3	8		90 sec
Good morning	3	8		90 sec

WEEK 4				
Exercise	Sets	Reps	Weight (% RM)	Rest
Deadlift	1	2	90%	3 min
	5	3	70%	2 min
ASSISTANCE CIRCUIT				
Romanian deadlift	3	8		90 sec
Barbell row	3	8		90 sec
Lat pulldown	3	8		90 sec
Good morning	3	8		90 sec
WEEK 5				
Deadlift	1	2	80%	3 min
	3	3	65%	2 min
Power shrug	3	5	60%	2 min
Romanian deadlift	3	5		2 min
Barbell row	3	5		2 min
Lat pulldown	3	5		2 min
Good morning	3	5		2 min
WEEK 6				
Deadlift	1	2	85%	3 min
	3	3	70%	2 min
Power shrug	3	5	65%	2 min
Romanian deadlift	3	5		2 min
Barbell row	3	5		2 min
Lat pulldown	3	5		2 min
Good morning	3	5		2 min

WEEK 7

Exercise	Sets	Reps	Weight (% RM)	Rest
Deadlift	1	2	90%	3 min
	3	3	75%	2 min
Power shrug	2	5	70%	2 min
Romanian deadlift	2	5		2 min
Barbell row	2	5		2 min
Lat pulldown	2	5		2 min
Good morning	2	5		2 min

WEEK 8

Exercise	Sets	Reps	Weight (% RM)	Rest
Deadlift	1	2	95%	3 min
	3	3	70%	2 min
Power shrug	2	5	75%	2 min
Romanian deadlift	2	5		2 min
Barbell row	2	5		2 min
Lat pulldown	2	5		2 min
Good morning	2	5		2 min

WEEK 9

Exercise	Sets	Reps	Weight (% RM)	Rest
Deadlift	1	1	97.5%	3 min
	2	3	70%	2 min
Power shrug	2	5	75%	2 min
Romanian deadlift	2	5		2 min

WEEK 10

Exercise	Sets	Reps	Weight (% RM)	Rest
Deadlift	1	1	100%	3 min
	2	3	60%	2 min
Power shrug	2	5	75%	2 min
Romanian deadlift	2	5		2 min

WEEK 11

Test 1RM for deadlift.

PART IV

TRAINING FOR MAXIMAL FAT LOSS

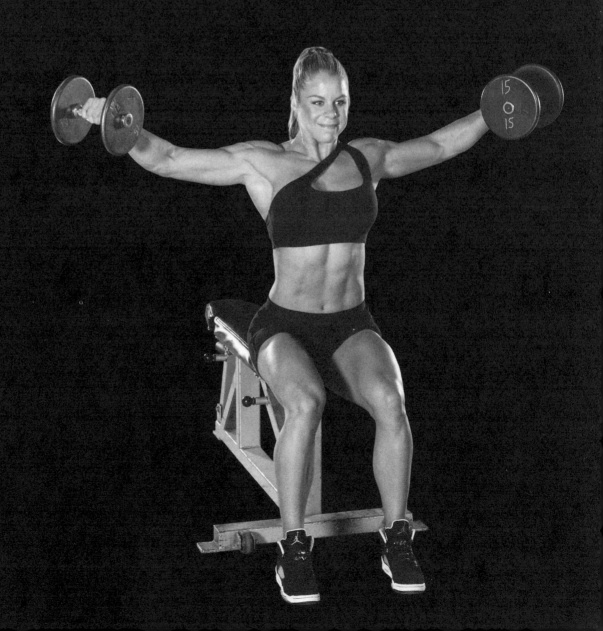

Strength training for fat loss does not have to be all that much different from strength training for muscle mass or for maximal strength. In fact, many of the programs in this section actually maximize fat loss while increasing muscle mass and increasing muscle strength. The real key to fat loss comes from the cardio techniques you employ (covered in chapter 12) and the diet you follow (covered in chapter 28). That being said, you can use a few tricks with your strength training to enhance fat loss, such as manipulating rest periods, weight and reps used, and exercises selected.

Chapter 11 covers the basics of creating strength training programs for maximizing fat loss. This chapter covers the training variables that you want to manipulate and the reasons for doing so to enhance fat loss through strength training.

Chapter 12 gets into various cardio techniques to use along with a strength training program. It discusses the science behind high-intensity interval training (HIIT) and covers several HIIT techniques and tips for including them in your overall training program.

Chapter 13 concludes this section with specific training programs that maximize fat loss. This chapter covers programs for beginners as well as those for intermediate and advanced lifters.

CHAPTER 11

Tactics for Maximizing Fat Loss

Unless you are a strength athlete with the goal of lifting as much weight as possible, then your pursuit for a fitter, more muscular, and stronger physique should not be just about building total mass but about building lean muscle. After all, if the muscle that you have spent so much effort building is not readily visible, then what's the point of all that hard work? Sure, weight training has many health benefits and will improve your quality of life, but those are all nice fringe benefits of the main reason you weight train—to look better. And looking better makes you feel better.

The best way to enhance fat loss is with a proper combination of weight training and cardio along with diet. Techniques to employ in weight training and cardio workouts are covered later in this chapter. Nutrition advice for promoting fat loss is covered in chapter 28.

STRENGTH TRAINING TECHNIQUES THAT ENHANCE FAT LOSS

The very act of weightlifting can affect fat loss by increasing both the number of calories your body burns during the workout and how many calories your body burns after the workout is long over. And it can now be argued that the body of someone who weight trains is better equipped at burning more fat throughout the day and storing less fat. Yet years of research have proven that manipulating certain acute training variables can have an even bigger impact on the calories burned during workouts and the calories burned the rest of the day after the workout is over.

Exercise Selection

While a variety of exercises is always best, there are certain types of exercises that you will want to include in workouts to aid in fat loss. Research suggests that using multijoint, free-weight exercises, such as the squat, bench press, shoulder press, and bent-over row, will maximize the number of calories burned more than machine exercises or single-joint isolation exercises. This is likely because multijoint exercises use more muscle groups, such as those that assist the target muscle and stabilizer muscles, which stabilize the joints involved. And the more muscles you use, the more calories you burn. In fact, one study found that when participants did the barbell squat, they burned 50 percent more calories than when they did the leg press (Tower et al. 2005).

Resistance and Rep Range

The weight you train with and the number of reps you complete can have a big impact on your calorie burn. To burn more calories during the workout, higher reps do the trick. College of New Jersey researchers found that when participants used a weight that allowed them to complete 10 reps on the bench press, they burned about 10 percent more calories than when they used a weight that limited them to 5 reps (Ratamess et al. 2007). The more reps you do, the more calories you burn. On the flip side of that, several studies have shown that while using heavier weight for fewer reps burns fewer calories during the workout, it burns more calories when the workout is over and you go about the rest of your day. In fact, research has shown that when you work out with heavy weights that limit you to 6 reps per set, the boost in your metabolic rate for 2 days after the workout more than doubles the boost you get when you work out with light weight that allows you to complete 12 reps per set (Borshein and Bahr 2003). So some combination of both heavy weight for low reps and light weight for high reps is the best way to take advantage of both benefits. This can be achieved by either using both low and high rep ranges in each workout or periodizing the rep ranges of the program.

Volume

The total number of sets you do for each muscle group and per workout (volume) will affect the number of calories you burn in the workout. The more sets you perform, the more work you are doing, and the more calories you end up burning. So increasing total volume of workouts is not only a strategy that can help to increase muscle growth, as discussed in chapter 2, but it can also increase the number of calories burned. As a general rule, keeping workouts to a minimum of 20 sets and ideally closer to 30 or more sets per workout can lead to significantly greater fat loss than workouts that are under 20 sets.

Rep Speed

A fourth variable to consider is the speed of the reps that you perform. Research has shown that doing reps in a fast and explosive manner can increase the number of calories you burn both during and after the workout. Researchers from Ball State University had weight-trained males do a squat exercise using 60 percent of their one-rep max at a normal pace (2 seconds on the positive part of the rep and 2 seconds on the negative part of the rep) or a very fast pace (1 second on the positive part of the rep and 2 seconds on the negative part of the rep). For both workouts, they did 4 sets of 8 reps, during which they were hooked up to a metabolic instrument to measure the number of calories they burned. The researchers discovered that when the participants did the 4 sets of squats with fast reps, they burned over 11 percent more calories during the workout and over 5 percent more calories at rest after the workout compared to when they used slower reps (Mazzetti et al. 2007).

While you don't want to do every exercise with fast and explosive reps, a better plan is to start your workouts with one exercise for each muscle group done in an explosive manner. For example, for chest you can start the workout with three or four sets of power push-ups or Smith machine bench press throws. This will help you build muscle power in the chest, which can help you gain muscle strength as you burn fat. And since ballistic exercises like this are done with light weight, they serve as a good warm-up to the heavier working sets that will follow, such as the bench press.

Rest

One of the more critical variables for increasing fat loss is the rest period you allow between sets. Generally speaking, the less rest you allow, the greater the number of calories you burn in a workout.

Research from the College of New Jersey has shown that if you cut your rest periods from the standard 3 minutes between sets to just 30 seconds between sets, you can increase the number of calories you burn during the workout by over 50 percent (Ratamess et al. 2007). These shorter rest periods, compared to longer rest periods, also lead to a bigger increase in the metabolic rate boost that follows the workout. Research also shows a similar response to supersets, which basically eliminates any rest periods between sets. This is covered in more detail in the following section.

While you should keep rest periods between sets to a minimum, the one time to hold the rest period between sets to at least one minute, if not longer, is when using the cardio technique of cardioacceleration, where instead of truly resting between sets you do cardio between sets. To learn more about cardioacceleration, see chapter 12.

Intensity Techniques

Another thing to consider regarding weight training for maximizing fat loss is the use of intensity techniques that allow you to take sets past the point of normal muscle failure. For example, with forced reps the assistance from a partner helps you go past muscle failure by continuing to do more reps than you would be able to complete on your own. Research shows that this technique leads to a higher increase in growth hormone levels than by simply ending the set at muscle failure (Ahtiainen et al. 2003). Since growth hormone (GH) increases lipolysis, the release of fat from the fat cells, having higher GH levels can lead to more fat being freed up from the fat cells so that it can be burned away as fuel during the workout and after.

One study on collegiate football players found that those following a high-intensity weight program, which consisted of just one set per exercise done for 6 to 10 reps per exercise done to failure along with forced reps and finally a static contraction for several seconds, lost more body fat over 10 weeks than those using a lower-intensity program, which consisted of three sets of 6 to 10 reps per exercise taken to just muscle failure (Fincher 2004).

Using the intensity technique, supersets also can enhance calorie burning and therefore fat loss. One study from Syracuse University reported that participants supersetting chest and back, biceps and triceps, and quads and hamstrings increased the number of calories burned during the workout and the hour after the workout by 35 percent more than those performing the same chest and back exercises as straight sets (Kelleher et al. 2010). While this may be because an athlete uses more muscle fibers by supersetting different muscle groups, the fact that rest periods between supersets are minimal is likely to be a big factor as well. The influence that rest periods have between sets is discussed earlier in this chapter. This would likely mean that using techniques such as tri-sets and giant sets, in which you train three and four or more exercises, respectively, back to back, would provide a similar effect, if not an even bigger one.

Training Frequency

How often you train muscle groups can also have an impact on fat loss. The most obvious reason for this is that when you train muscle groups more frequently you tend to train more often during the week. More workouts during the week equate to more total calories burned throughout the weeks.

Another reason more frequent workouts lead to greater fat loss is that when you train muscle groups more frequently, you need to train more muscle groups per workout. This means that you have more muscle tissue that is recovering after the workout is over. After workouts your body is in a state known as oxygen debt. That means it needs more oxygen to replenish ATP and phosphocreatine stores. It needs that oxygen to burn more fuel (calories) to recover from the workout. With more muscle fibers needed to recover, the calorie burn stays higher for longer.

SUMMARY

The way in which you design your weight training program can significantly affect fat loss. Generally speaking, programs that use many multijoint movements, incorporate explosive and ballistic training exercises, use heavy weight for fewer reps, use lighter weight for higher reps, keep rest periods very short, combine techniques such as supersets, employ intensity techniques such as forced reps, train muscle groups more frequently, or have you in the gym more often all seem to be effective ways to keep fat burning maximized.

Of course, you can't employ all of these techniques into every workout, but a good strategy is to employ a multitude of these techniques in each program you design and swap out techniques as you change up programs. You will also need to add some form of cardio to these strength programs in order to maximize fat loss. Cardio techniques that work best are covered in chapter 12.

If you are not keen at designing your own training programs, turn to chapter 13, which has several fat-loss programs. Not only have these programs been shown to be effective for fat loss, but trainees often have gains in muscle size and strength. These programs also serve as a good template for combining the techniques discussed in this chapter.

CHAPTER 12

Cardio Training for Maximizing Fat Loss

Cardio is the intimate word we give to aerobic exercise. *Aerobic exercise* refers to the energy system used. With weight training, which is done with high intensity for short bursts followed by a short rest period, you tend to rely more on the anaerobic energy systems to fuel muscle contractions. With aerobic exercise, which typically refers to rhythmic movement at a low to moderate intensity for prolonged periods, such as jogging or bicycling, the energy systems that fuel this type of activity require oxygen.

Although it is possible to lose fat with just weight training, especially certain types of programs, to truly maximize fat loss you need to incorporate some form of cardio in your training regimen. Plus, cardio provides health benefits, such as improved cardiovascular health, reduced risk of diabetes and other metabolic diseases, and reduced risk of certain types of cancer. It can also help to enhance recovery from weight training. This chapter covers the most effective forms of cardio for fat loss while maintaining muscle and building muscle.

HIIT VERSUS STEADY-STATE CARDIO

There was a time when bodybuilders would only consider doing low- to moderate-intensity, steady-state cardio, such as fast walking or pedaling a stationary bike at a moderate intensity. Anything more intense would be considered a no-no. There were two main reasons for this. The first was that they believed that more intense cardio would burn up muscle tissue (meaning that muscle tissue would be broken down to fuel the exercise). The second belief was that lower-intensity cardio was reported to put a person in an optimal fat-burning zone.

Today, we know that both of those lines of thinking are flawed. The concept that high-intensity cardio will burn up muscle while low-intensity cardio will spare muscle is quite wrong. In fact, if you just compared the muscle mass of longer-distance runners (who spend a good deal of their training at a slower pace for longer periods) to the muscle mass of sprinters (who spend a good deal of their training at higher intensities for short periods), you could see how that logic is flawed.

When you train at a slow and steady pace for a longer period, you train your muscle fibers to be more aerobic and have greater endurance. There is some evidence that suggests that muscle fibers adapt to becoming more aerobic and to increasing endurance by becoming smaller and weaker. This is because the smaller a muscle fiber is, the less time it takes for nutrients to travel within the muscle fiber. This speeds up the rate that nutrients can be burned for fuel.

Another way to consider the misconception that low-intensity cardio done for longer periods will better spare muscle mass than high-intensity cardio for shorter periods is to compare a higher-intensity squat workout done for 5 sets with a weight that limits you to 10 reps per set and a lower-intensity squat workout done with a weight that allows you to complete 100 reps per set. Would the higher-intensity leg workout of 10 rep sets burn up muscle tissue while the lower-intensity leg workout of 100 rep sets would better maintain muscle? No. If anything, it would be quite the opposite. In fact, doing higher-intensity cardio, particularly HIIT (discussed later in this chapter), may actually help to increase muscle mass.

While lower-intensity cardio has been shown to burn a higher percentage of calories from fat, you actually burn fewer total calories with lower-intensity cardio. So to burn an equivalent amount of calories and fat as higher-intensity cardio, you would have to exercise for considerably longer. One obvious problem with doing excessive cardio is time. Most people barely have time to fit in a 60-minute weight workout, let alone another 60 minutes or longer of cardio. However, another problem with excessively long cardio, particularly for men, is that it has been found to lower testosterone levels.

Focusing on just how many calories you burn and how many calories you burn from fat during a workout is also flawed. The real benefit of cardio for fat loss is the amount of calories (and calories from fat) that you burn the rest of the day after the workout is over. This is due to the process known as EPOC (excess postexercise oxygen consumption). It refers to the boost in your metabolism, or calorie burning that comes after the workout is over. When you work out, you burn calories to fuel your muscles. But when the workout is over, your body keeps burning more calories than normal, despite the fact that you are doing nothing. This is due to the processes involved in recovery from exercise. After exercise, your body must repair damaged muscle fibers, restock muscle glycogen levels, remove lactic acid from the muscles, and so on. All these processes require calories, and a lot of those calories come from fat. And when it comes to EPOC, this is where HIIT really destroys steady-state cardio done at a lower intensity.

Science Behind HIIT

High-intensity interval training (HIIT) is a form of cardio that involves intervals of high-intensity exercise (such as running at a very fast pace) interspersed with intervals of low-intensity activity (walking at a slow pace) or complete rest. This is in sharp contrast to the typical continuous steady-state (slow and steady) exercise that is done at a moderate intensity, such as walking at a fast pace or jogging for 30 to 60 minutes.

Although HIIT seems to have gained popularity in the last few years, the concept is actually quite old. The origin of HIIT can be traced back many decades to a technique called Fartlek training that was used by track coaches to better prepare runners. *Fartlek* is actually Swedish for *speed* (fart) and *play* (lek),

so it means speed play, which is essentially what HIIT is. Today HIIT has crossed over to the fitness industry because of its beneficial results that have been established through both anecdotal reports and published research studies. In fact, studies comparing HIIT to continuous steady-state cardio have shown that HIIT is far superior for fat loss, despite the fact that it requires much less time.

One of the first studies to discover that HIIT was more effective for fat loss was a 1994 study by researchers at Laval University in Ste-Foy, Quebec, Canada (Tremblay et al. 1994). They reported that young men and women who followed a 15-week HIIT program lost significantly more body fat than those following a 20-week continuous steady-state endurance program, despite the fact that the steady-state program burned about 15,000 calories more during exercise than the HIIT program. A 2001 study from East Tennessee State University demonstrated similar findings with participants who followed an 8-week HIIT program (participants dropped 2 percent body fat) compared to those who followed a continuous steady-state program (participants had no drop in body fat) on a treadmill (King 2001). A study from Australia reported that females following a 20-minute HIIT program that consisted of 8-second sprints followed by 12 seconds of rest lost 6 times more body fat than the group who followed a 40-minute cardio program performed at a constant intensity of 60 percent of their maximum heart rate (Trapp 2008).

A study from the University of Western Ontario suggests that you can burn off more body fat with even less than 15 minutes of HIIT than with slow and steady cardio (Macpherson 2011). The research team had male and female participants follow one of two cardio programs for six weeks. One group ran slow and steady for 30 to 60 minutes three times per week. The other group did four to six 30-second sprints with a 4-minute rest period between sprints three times per week. That's basically HIIT with an extended rest interval between the high-intensity exercise intervals. The group doing the sprint intervals lost more than twice as much body fat as the slow-and-steady group despite the fact that they did only 2 to 3 minutes of total cardio exercise per day and just 6 to 9 minutes per week! The sprint interval group also gained over one pound of muscle. So this type of cardio not only burns off body fat and spares muscle, but it also may even help to build it.

One of the major reasons HIIT works so well in reducing body fat to a greater degree than continuous steady-state cardio appears to be due to the greater increase in resting metabolism after HIIT. Researchers at Baylor College of Medicine reported that participants who followed a HIIT workout on a stationary cycle burned significantly more calories during the 24 hours after the workout than those who cycled at a moderate steady-state intensity (Treuth, 1996). The East Tennessee State University study mentioned earlier also found that participants following the HIIT program burned more calories during the 24 hours after exercise than the steady-state cardio group did. A study presented at the 2007 annual meeting of the American College of Sports Medicine by Florida State University researchers reported that participants who performed HIIT burned about 10% more calories during the 24 hours after exercise as those who performed continuous steady-state exercise, despite the fact that the total calories burned during the workouts were the same (Meuret et al. 2007).

In addition to the increase in resting metabolism, research confirms that HIIT is effective at enhancing the metabolic machinery in muscle cells that promote fat burning and blunt fat production. Researchers in the Laval University study that found a decrease in body fat with HIIT discovered that the HIIT participants' muscle fibers had significantly higher markers for fat oxidation (fat burning) than those in the continuous steady-state exercise group. A study of young females who performed seven HIIT workouts over a two-week period showed a 30 percent increase in both fat oxidation and levels of muscle enzymes that enhance fat oxidation (Talanian et al. 2007). Research shows that this may be due to an increase in mitochondria, the machinery in muscle cells and other cells that burns fat to produce energy. Scalzo and colleagues (2014) found that both men and women completing four to eight bouts of 30-seocnd sprints on a stationary cycle had significant boosts in mitochondrial biogenesis. In a study from the Norwegian University of Science and Technology, participants with metabolic syndrome who followed a 16-week HIIT program had a 100 percent greater decrease in content of the fat-producing enzyme fatty acid synthase compared to participants who followed continuous moderate-intensity exercise. In other words, HIIT enhances the body's ability to burn fat and prevent the storage of fat (Tjonna 2007).

Another way that HIIT appears to work has to do with getting the fat to where it will be burned away for good. Talanian and colleagues (2010) shed some light on another way that HIIT burns more body fat: 6 weeks of HIIT increased the amount of special proteins in muscle cells that are responsible for carrying fat into the mitochondria (where fat is burned for fuel) by up to 50 percent. Having more of these proteins in muscle means that more fat can be burned up for fuel during workouts and when resting.

HIIT, done at a higher intensity for a shorter time, will not only help you maintain your muscle but can actually help you build muscle mass. In a study by Smith and colleagues (2009), male participants following a six-week HIIT program (done for 15 minutes per day, 3 days a week, at a ratio of 2:1 for exercise to rest) while supplementing with beta-alanine gained over 2 pounds of muscle despite the fact that they never lifted weights during the program. The 2011 study on sprinting from the University of Western Ontario discussed earlier reported that those performing 30-second sprint intervals actually gained some muscle mass, while the slow-and-steady cardio group did not. A study from the UK reported that obese participants following a low-carbohydrate diet lost muscle mass, yet those performing HIIT along with the low-carbohydrate diet were able to maintain muscle mass (Sartor 2010). This makes sense when you consider that weight training is technically a form of HIIT— short periods of high-intensity exercise are interspersed with periods of rest.

One reason HIIT can lead to greater gains in muscle mass may be an increase in muscle protein synthesis. The Colorado State University study showing an increase in mitochondrial biogenesis also reported a significant increase in muscle protein synthesis after the sprints. The results were greater in male than in female participants. Another reason for greater gains in muscle mass with HIIT may be the anabolic hormone testosterone. New Zealand researchers (Paton et al. 2009) had competitive cyclists complete 4 weeks of HIIT training involving 30-second sprints on a stationary cycle separated by 30 seconds of rest. One group sprinted with high resistance on the pedals, making it harder to pedal, while the other group used a lighter resistance, which was easier to pedal. Both groups pedaled as fast as they could during the 30-second sprints. The men pedaling at the highest resistance increased their testosterone levels by almost 100 percent, while the group pedaling at a lighter resistance increased testosterone levels by only about 60 percent.

Another reason for both the health benefits of HIIT and its benefits on muscle mass, not to mention fat loss, has to do with improved insulin sensitivity. When you improve insulin sensitivity, not only does this help you keep lean and prevent diabetes, but it can also aid muscle growth. Insulin is an anabolic hormone that acts on the muscle cells to increase muscle protein synthesis, decrease muscle protein breakdown, and drive more glucose, amino acids, and creatine and carnitine into muscle cells. Researchers at Watt University in Edinburgh had participants follow a two-week training program with workouts consisting of just four to six 30-second sprints on stationary cycles (Babraj et al. 2009). Sprints were separated by 4 minutes of rest. They discovered that at the end of the two weeks the participants' blood glucose and insulin levels were reduced by almost 15 and 40 percent, respectively, after the consumption of 75 grams of glucose. Insulin sensitivity, which is the measurement of how well insulin does its job at the muscle cells, improved by about 25 percent. In a more recent study by Racil and colleagues (2013), young females following a 12-week HIIT program had positive changes in insulin sensitivity as well as reduced waist size, lower total cholesterol, lower LDL cholesterol, and higher HDL cholesterol.

This does not mean that you should never do steady-state cardio. If you enjoy jogging, hiking, or cycling, then by all means include that exercise in your program. However, you should still consider adding a few days of HIIT into your routine. This not only will improve your physique but will also improve your performance when you do steady-state cardio.

Cardio Frequency

Many weight training enthusiasts ask about the minimum amount of cardio that needs to be done each week to result in fat loss? This question usually comes from those who think that cardio is only the slow-and-steady type done on a treadmill or stationary bike. Most people who enjoy weightlifting tend to loathe cardio. Of course, once they realize that cardio can be done with weights in HIIT style, they end up asking how much is too much. At any rate, there is some evidence both from research and anecdotal reports that the minimum amount of cardio that you should do each week is three workouts.

One study placed 90 male and female participants on an eight-week program that consisted of 30 minutes of straight cardio (Willis et al. 2009). They divided the participants into groups based on how often they exercised each week. One group served as a control and did no exercise, a second group did the cardio workout fewer than two times a week, a third group did the workouts two or three times per week, and the fourth group did cardio four or more times per week. They discovered that at the end of the eight weeks only the last group performing cardio four or more times per week lost a decent amount of body fat (almost 15 pounds of it). Of course, the participants were not weight training in addition to doing cardio, and they also weren't doing HIIT, so it's hard to say from this study precisely how many days of cardio you need in addition to weight training.

Anecdotal reports suggest a minimum of three HIIT cardio sessions per week in addition to weight training. But obviously, the more you do each week, the greater the expected fat loss. In fact, you can do seven days of cardio per week if you prefer. And that can be seven days of HIIT. Some are worried that doing HIIT every day will lead to overtraining. However, as long as you switch up the exercises, you can do HIIT every day of the week. After all, it is typically done for only 15 to 30 minutes, and that is not total exercise time. Research on athletes suggests that those using HIIT every day had no decrement in performance. Hatle et al. (2014) found that those performing eight sessions of HIIT per week for 3 weeks had similar increases in $\dot{V}O_2max$ as those doing three sessions per week for 8 weeks. This supports an earlier study in Alpine skiers (Breil et al. 2010) that showed a 6 percent increase in $\dot{V}O_2max$ after 15 sessions of HIIT performed for 11 days. Both studies, however, reported that the increase in $\dot{V}O_2max$ was not apparent until several days after stopping the frequent HIIT. This suggests that performing HIIT every day could overtax the body and lead to overtraining. So if improving aerobic performance is one of your goals, you should provide at least one rest day, if not three or four, per week. However, doing two or three weeks of HIIT every day can lead to quicker improvements in endurance as long as you back off on the frequency later on. For the best fat loss, do three to six sessions of HIIT per week, leaving a minimum of one day of rest.

Timing of Cardio

Whether you do your cardio immediately before you lift weights, immediately after, or even during weight workouts (such as cardioacceleration discussed at the end of this chapter), or at a different time of day or completely different day, matters little to the effect it will have on fat loss. The most critical aspect of scheduling your cardio is when you will be most consistent doing it.

If you find that you tend to skip your cardio workouts when you leave it to after your weight workout, then you should consider doing it before or during your weight training workout or at a completely different time or day. There are two options when it comes to doing cardio during your weight training workouts. The first option is to do cardio-acceleration, which involves a 30- to 90-second bout of high-intensity cardio in between every set. Or you can do a bout of HIIT in between muscle groups. For example, if you train back, biceps, and calves in one workout, you could do 10 minutes of HIIT in between back and biceps, in between biceps and calves, and after calves for a total of 30 minutes of HIIT. Several studies have reported that breaking up your cardio into several shorter sessions allows you to burn more calories during the workout as well as more calories after the workout is over (Altena 2003; Almuzaini 1998; Kaminsky 1990). This has also been shown to allow people to lose significantly more total fat over a prolonged period.

Fasted Cardio

Another misconception about cardio is that the best time to do it is first thing in the morning on an empty stomach. Research does in fact show that you burn more total fat when you do cardio fasted than you would if you ate first. Some research shows that you can burn 20 percent more fat when you do cardio in the morning on an empty stomach (Gonzalez et al. 2013). However, as mentioned earlier, how many calories—and specifically the number you burn from fat—during the exercise should not be the major focus. When you burn carbohydrate during exercise, you burn more fat after the exercise is over, and when you burn more fat during exercise, you burn more carbohydrate after (Deighton 2012). In other words, it's more about the total amount of calories and fat you burn throughout the day, not just during exercise. Research also suggests that whether you exercise first thing in the morning fasted or fed, you end up burning the same amount of calories throughout the day (Hansen 2005).

So, generally speaking, your best bet is to not worry about doing cardio first thing in the morning or fasted. If doing cardio first thing in the morning is best for your schedule, then by all means do your cardio then. But it is advisable to have at least a protein shake—ideally a protein shake and some carbohydrate, such as fruit—before the workout. If you are trying to limit carb intake, then you may want to avoid the carbohydrate until after the workout.

There is one time when fasted cardio may be a strategy you want to employ. I have found that when a male's body fat is in the low single digits (somewhere around 5 to 6 percent) or a female's body fat is in the low teens (somewhere around 13 to 14 percent), but they have one body area that they cannot trim, then the fasted cardio seems to be beneficial for dropping the stubborn fat. For example, many males, especially older males, tend to hold fat on the lower back and obliques. Many females tend to hold fat on the hips and thighs. Once they have dropped the majority of the subcutaneous fat on the rest of the body, fasted cardio does seem to work well to rid that last bit of fat. Although there are no direct data, it may be that when a person is so low in body fat, encouraging the body to burn more fat during exercise is one way to burn off the stubborn body fat that otherwise won't go.

FORMS OF HIIT

HIIT can take on many forms and be done with virtually any equipment or absolutely none. You can do it while running on a track or a treadmill, riding a stationary bike or climbing a stair stepper, or doing calisthenics and using your body weight or explosive exercises and free weights. Chapters 25 (whole-body exercises) and 26 (calisthenic exercises) are good resources for exercises to use for HIIT.

There is almost no wrong way to use HIIT other than not doing it at all. And while there are numerous exercises that you can do with HIIT, there are also numerous ways to employ HIIT. Following are some of the more effective ways to use HIIT.

Standard HIIT

Standard HIIT refers to scheduling a block of time for just HIIT. Some evidence suggests that when doing HIIT, a ratio of 2:1 of high-intensity exercise to low-intensity exercise, or work to rest, provides the best benefits in performance, fat loss, and health. For example, you could sprint as fast as possible for 30 seconds and walk for 15 seconds. Or you could jump rope for 1 minute and rest for 30 seconds. Of course, studies like the University of Western Ontario study on sprinting for 30 seconds and resting for 4 minutes suggest that results are still substantial even with a HIIT work-to-rest ratio of 1:8. Despite that, I would still recommend shooting for a 2:1 ratio. If that is too much for you to handle at first, start off with a 1:2, or a 1:4, or even a 1:8 ratio of work to rest and gradually increase the ratio over time.

The intensity of the high-intensity exercise intervals can be something that is tightly prescribed, such as a certain percent of your maximum heart rate, or loosely determined based on what feels intense to you. Because I prefer to do a variety of exercises, such as dumbbell cleans, kettlebell swings, and bench step-ups, checking your heart rate manually or even on a heart rate monitor is pretty impractical. So I prefer to use a simple RPE (rating of perceived exertion) scale of 1 to 10, as shown in table 12.1. During the high-intensity exercise intervals you should be somewhere from 6 to

TABLE 12.1   Rating of Perceived Exertion (RPE) Scale

Use the following scale when rating your HIIT intervals.

Rate	Description
0	Nothing at all
1	Very easy
2	Easy
3	Moderate
4	Somewhat hard
5	Hard
6	
7	Very hard
8	
9	
10	Very, very hard
Maximal	

9. Stick with the lower end of that range when just beginning with the goal of increasing your RPE as you go. If you are not taking complete rest between the high-intensity exercise intervals, then your RPE during the low-intensity exercise intervals should be somewhere in the range of 1 to 3.

You should also shoot to increase the block of total time spent doing HIIT as you progress. Even if you start with just 10 to 15 minutes, that is fine. But your goal should be to slowly increase your total time.

Beginner to Advanced HIIT Program

The HIIT program in table 12.2 will progress you from the beginner level to the intermediate level of HIIT proficiency. This can be done with any equipment, such as a treadmill, jump rope, pair of dumbbells, kettlebell, exercise bands, medicine ball, TRX, or just your body weight and calisthenics.

The suggested time of each phase is not carved in stone. If you feel you need to spend more than two weeks at a particular phase before moving up, then do so. Or if a phase seems too easy and you want to jump right up to the next phase, then do so. It starts with a work-to-rest ratio of 1:4 in phase 1 for a total workout time of just under 15 minutes. Then in phase 2, it bumps up the amount of time in the work phase to bring the ratio up to 1:2 and the total workout time to 17 minutes. In phase 3, the rest is cut in half to bring the ratio up to 1:1, and the total workout time increases to 18.5 minutes. And finally in phase 4, the rest is cut in half again to get the ratio to 2:1 and the total time at 20 minutes.

Tabata Intervals

Tabata intervals use a 2:1 ratio of work to rest. But specifically you alternate 20 seconds of high-intensity exercise with 10 seconds of rest done for eight cycles in this fashion for a total of 4 minutes per exercise. The point is to not fall into a specific heart rate range but to just go as intensely as possible. So shoot for an RPE of about 9 to 10.

Tabatas are named after the Japanese scientist who designed them, Dr. Izumi Tabata. He was actually looking for a way to better train athletes. The story is that he was analyzing the training of the Japanese speed skating team in an effort to enhance their performance. He discovered that when he had athletes perform eight cycles of

TABLE 12.2 Beginner to Advanced HIIT Program

PHASE 1 (1:4): WEEKS 1-2

Time	Activity
15 sec	High-intensity exercise
1 min	Rest or low-intensity exercise
15 sec	High-intensity exercise
1 min	Rest or low-intensity exercise
15 sec	High-intensity exercise
1 min	Rest or low-intensity exercise
15 sec	High-intensity exercise
1 min	Rest or low-intensity exercise
15 sec	High-intensity exercise
1 min	Rest or low-intensity exercise
15 sec	High-intensity exercise
1 min	Rest or low-intensity exercise
15 sec	High-intensity exercise
1 min	Rest or low-intensity exercise
15 sec	High-intensity exercise
1 min	Rest or low-intensity exercise
15 sec	High-intensity exercise
1 min	Rest or low-intensity exercise
15 sec	High-intensity exercise
1 min	Rest or low-intensity exercise
15 sec	High-intensity exercise
Total time: 14 minutes	

PHASE 2 (1:2): WEEKS 3-4

Time	Activity
30 sec	High-intensity exercise
1 min	Rest or low-intensity exercise
30 sec	High-intensity exercise
1 min	Rest or low-intensity exercise
30 sec	High-intensity exercise
1 min	Rest or low-intensity exercise
30 sec	High-intensity exercise
1 min	Rest or low-intensity exercise
30 sec	High-intensity exercise
1 min	Rest or low-intensity exercise
30 sec	High-intensity exercise
1 min	Rest or low-intensity exercise
30 sec	High-intensity exercise
1 min	Rest or low-intensity exercise

PHASE 2 (1:2): WEEKS 3-4 (continued)

Time	Activity
30 sec	High-intensity exercise
1 min	Rest or low-intensity exercise
30 sec	High-intensity exercise
1 min	Rest or low-intensity exercise
30 sec	High-intensity exercise
1 min	Rest or low-intensity exercise
30 sec	High-intensity exercise
1 min	Rest or low-intensity exercise
30 sec	High-intensity exercise
Total time: 17 min	

PHASE 3 (1:1): WEEKS 5-6

Time	Activity
30 sec	High-intensity exercise
30 sec	Rest or low-intensity exercise
30 sec	High-intensity exercise
30 sec	Rest or low-intensity exercise
30 sec	High-intensity exercise
30 sec	Rest or low-intensity exercise
30 sec	High-intensity exercise
30 sec	Rest or low-intensity exercise
30 sec	High-intensity exercise
30 sec	Rest or low-intensity exercise
30 sec	High-intensity exercise
30 sec	Rest or low-intensity exercise
30 sec	High-intensity exercise
30 sec	Rest or low-intensity exercise
30 sec	High-intensity exercise
30 sec	Rest or low-intensity exercise
30 sec	High-intensity exercise
30 sec	Rest or low-intensity exercise
30 sec	High-intensity exercise
30 sec	Rest or low-intensity exercise
30 sec	High-intensity exercise
30 sec	Rest or low-intensity exercise
30 sec	High-intensity exercise
30 sec	Rest or low-intensity exercise

> continued

TABLE 12.2 Beginner to Advanced HIIT Program *(continued)*

PHASE 3 (1:1): WEEKS 5-6 *(continued)*

Time	Activity
30 sec	High-intensity exercise
30 sec	Rest or low-intensity exercise
30 sec	High-intensity exercise
30 sec	Rest or low-intensity exercise
30 sec	High-intensity exercise
30 sec	Rest or low-intensity exercise
30 sec	High-intensity exercise
30 sec	Rest or low-intensity exercise
30 sec	High-intensity exercise

Total time: 18.5 min

PHASE 4 (2:1): WEEKS 7-8

Time	Activity
30 sec	High-intensity exercise
15 sec	Rest or low-intensity exercise
30 sec	High-intensity exercise
15 sec	Rest or low-intensity exercise
30 sec	High-intensity exercise
15 sec	Rest or low-intensity exercise
30 sec	High-intensity exercise
15 sec	Rest or low-intensity exercise
30 sec	High-intensity exercise
15 sec	Rest or low-intensity exercise
30 sec	High-intensity exercise
15 sec	Rest or low-intensity exercise
30 sec	High-intensity exercise
15 sec	Rest or low-intensity exercise
30 sec	High-intensity exercise
15 sec	Rest or low-intensity exercise
30 sec	High-intensity exercise
15 sec	Rest or low-intensity exercise
30 sec	High-intensity exercise
15 sec	Rest or low-intensity exercise
30 sec	High-intensity exercise

PHASE 4 (2:1): WEEKS 7-8 *(continued)*

Time	Activity
15 sec	Rest or low-intensity exercise
30 sec	High-intensity exercise
15 sec	Rest or low-intensity exercise
30 sec	High-intensity exercise
15 sec	Rest or low-intensity exercise
30 sec	High-intensity exercise
15 sec	Rest or low-intensity exercise
30 sec	High-intensity exercise
15 sec	Rest or low-intensity exercise
30 sec	High-intensity exercise
15 sec	Rest or low-intensity exercise
30 sec	High-intensity exercise
15 sec	Rest or low-intensity exercise
30 sec	High-intensity exercise
15 sec	Rest or low-intensity exercise
30 sec	High-intensity exercise
15 sec	Rest or low-intensity exercise
30 sec	High-intensity exercise
15 sec	Rest or low-intensity exercise
30 sec	High-intensity exercise
15 sec	Rest or low-intensity exercise
30 sec	High-intensity exercise
15 sec	Rest or low-intensity exercise
30 sec	High-intensity exercise
15 sec	Rest or low-intensity exercise
30 sec	High-intensity exercise

Total time: 20 min

these 20-second high-intensity exercise intervals followed by 10 seconds of rest, they increased both their aerobic (endurance) capacity and their anaerobic (quick power) capacity—the two things that speed skaters need (Tabata et al. 1996; 1997). In other words, whether you're an endurance athlete like a cyclist or a power athlete like a weightlifter, Tabata offers you benefits because it trains both

the major metabolic pathways that give you endurance and those that give you explosive energy. That's why so many athletes do Tabata intervals. And, of course, they work very well for fat loss.

You can either choose anywhere from 4 to 8 exercises and do them as a block of Tabatas for a total cardio workout time of 16 to 32 minutes. Or you can do one or two exercises Tabata style in between muscle groups. For example, if you trained chest, triceps, and abs in one workout, you could start with Tabata rope jumping for 4 minutes to warm up. Then after finishing chest, do Tabata kettlebell swings for 4 minutes and Tabata bench step-ups for another 4 minutes before training triceps. After triceps, you could do 4 minutes of Tabata dumbbell cleans and Tabata jumping jacks before training abs. Then you do more two more Tabata-style exercises after abs for a total time of 28 minutes of Tabata HIIT.

A typical Tabata exercise would look like this, using kettlebell swings as an example:

Time	Activity
20 seconds	Kettlebell swings
10 seconds	Rest
20 seconds	Kettlebell swings
10 seconds	Rest
20 seconds	Kettlebell swings
10 seconds	Rest
20 seconds	Kettlebell swings
10 seconds	Rest
20 seconds	Kettlebell swings
10 seconds	Rest
20 seconds	Kettlebell swings
10 seconds	Rest
20 seconds	Kettlebell swings
10 seconds	Rest
20 seconds	Kettlebell swings
10 seconds	Rest

Power HIIT

Power HIIT involves doing intervals of explosive exercises with short intervals of rest. These exercises could include power cleans, snatches, squat jumps, power push-ups, and kettlebell swings. These exercises are typically done to develop explosive power, strength, and speed for sport performance. Combining them with HIIT allows you to build more muscle power while increasing fat loss and cardiorespiratory conditioning.

With Power HIIT, both the exercise intervals and the rest intervals last 20 seconds. So it works on a 1:1 ratio of exercise to rest. This time frame typically allows you to complete about 3 or 4 reps during each exercise interval. This rep range is perfect for building power. Then you get an equal amount of time to recover to help you better maintain power on the next exercise interval. This 1:1 work-to-rest ratio can also help to build muscle size, strength, and power by boosting testosterone levels. The New Zealand study discussed earlier found that cyclists performing 30-second high-powered sprints separated by 30 seconds of rest (1:1 work-to-rest ratio) increased their testosterone levels by up to 100 percent.

For each exercise you do three exercise-to-rest intervals and then move on to the next exercises. This way you have worked at building power on that exercise without completely exhausting the specific muscles used on that move.

The power exercises in Power HIIT are very fast and explosive. These fast reps primarily recruit the fast-twitch muscle fibers, which grow the biggest, strongest, and fastest. So it's easy to understand how using HIIT workouts can help you build muscle and power. But the fast-twitch muscle fibers also burn the most calories when you use them, as discussed in chapter 11. Plus, most of the exercises in Power HIIT use so many muscle groups that they also burn more calories that way, as also discussed in chapter 11.

Power HIIT Workouts

Start each Power HIIT workout with a 5-minute HIIT warm-up of rope jumping or jumping jacks. This warm-up should be done in typical HIIT fashion at a 2:1 ratio of jumping to rest. In this case, it's 30 seconds of jumping followed by 15 seconds of rest. You do 7 cycles of this for a total of 5 minutes. If you do the Power HIIT workouts after weight training, then you do not need to do the 5-minute HIIT warm-up.

After the jump rope HIIT warm-up (see table 12.3), go right into the Power HIIT workout (see table 12.4). You do three 20-second sets of each exercise, taking 20 seconds of rest between sets and exercises. In workout A, start with squat jumps (chapter 21) for building leg power. Then you move into power push-ups (chapter 14) for building power in the chest and triceps. Next power cleans (chapter 25) are done with dumbbells or a barbell. Then it's on to medicine ball overhead throws (chapter 25). If you don't have a medicine ball, you can simply do band shoulder presses (chapter 15) or even barbell or dumbbell push presses (chapter 25). Finish with the band standing crunch (chapter 24) to build strength and power in the midsection.

If bands are a problem, you can do a medicine ball crunch throw (chapter 24) or even a regular crunch with explosive reps on the positive rep.

Because you'll want to repeat this workout several times a week, I've provided a workout B so you can alternate between the workouts without hitting the same exercises in the same order every time. In workout B, you start with the kettlebell snatch (chapter 25). You can also do this with a dumbbell as well if kettlebells are not an option for you. Then you move into the band sprint (chapter 26) and then calf jumps (chapter 23) to build strength and power in the calves. Then do kettlebell swings (chapter 25), which can also be done with a dumbbell, and finish with the band woodchopper (chapter 24) (or you can use a cable or a dumbbell) to build rotational power in the upper body and strengthen the core. Since you have to do both sides of the body, instead of doing three sets of 20 seconds each, do two 20-second sets on each side for a total of four sets.

In both workouts A and B you do five exercises for three 20-second sets each (except in workout B where you have an extra set for woodchoppers) with 20-second rest periods; this totals 10 minutes. With the jump rope HIIT work for 5 minutes and the 10 minutes of Power HIIT, that's a total of 15 minutes of intense cardio that not only burns fat and enhances cardiorespiratory fitness and health but also builds overall muscle strength, power, and mass. If your goal is to maximize muscle mass, strength, and power, and cardio is more of an afterthought, then keep it at this duration. Work on increasing the weight on the exercises or the number of reps you can bang out in those 20 seconds. If fat loss is your primary goal, as well as the cardiorespiratory benefits that this novel form of cardio offers, then you'll want to progressively bump up your total time of Power HIIT. I've offered three stages to work up to; each stage increases total Power HIIT time. Go at your own pace, and

when the 15-minute workout no longer is much of a challenge, start on phase 2, which brings your total HIIT workout to almost 20 minutes. Then when that becomes less of a challenge, it's time to get serious and jump into phase 3, which brings your total HIIT workout time to 25 minutes.

You can do the Power HIIT either at the beginning or the end of your workouts or on a separate day. It all depends on your major goals. If you're using Power HIIT to boost muscle power and athletic performance, do this workout at the start of your weight training or on a separate day from your usual weight training altogether. If fat loss is the primary goal with Power HIIT, you can do it either at the beginning or at the end of your weight workouts or on a separate day from weights.

TABLE 12.3 Jump Rope or Jumping Jacks Workout

Do this workout at the start of each Power HIIT workout, regardless of the phase you are in.

Time	Exercise
30 sec	Jump rope or jumping jacks
15 sec	Rest
30 sec	Jump rope or jumping jacks
15 sec	Rest
30 sec	Jump
15 sec	Rest
30 sec	Jump
15 sec	Rest
30 sec	Jump
15 sec	Rest
30 sec	Jump
15 sec	Rest
30 sec	Jump
15 sec	Rest
30 sec	Jump
Total time: 300 sec (5 min)	

TABLE 12.4 Power Cardio Workouts

PHASE 1, WORKOUT A	
Time	Exercise
20 sec	Squat jump
20 sec	Rest
20 sec	Squat jump
20 sec	Rest
20 sec	Squat jump
20 sec	Rest
20 sec	Power push-up
20 sec	Rest
20 sec	Power push-up
20 sec	Rest
20 sec	Power push-up
20 sec	Rest
20 sec	Power clean
20 sec	Rest
20 sec	Power clean
20 sec	Rest
20 sec	Power clean
20 sec	Rest
20 sec	Medicine ball overhead throw
20 sec	Rest
20 sec	Medicine ball overhead throw
20 sec	Rest
20 sec	Medicine ball overhead throw
20 sec	Rest
20 sec	Band standing crunch
20 sec	Rest
20 sec	Band standing crunch
20 sec	Rest
20 sec	Band standing crunch
Total time: 9 min, 40 sec	

PHASE 1, WORKOUT B	
20 sec	Kettlebell snatch
20 sec	Rest
20 sec	Kettlebell snatch
20 sec	Rest
20 sec	Kettlebell snatch
20 sec	Rest
20 sec	Band sprint
20 sec	Rest
20 sec	Band sprint
20 sec	Rest

PHASE 1, WORKOUT B *(continued)*	
Time	Exercise
20 sec	Band sprint
20 sec	Rest
20 sec	Calf jump
20 sec	Rest
20 sec	Calf jump
20 sec	Rest
20 sec	Calf jump
20 sec	Rest
20 sec	Kettlebell swing
20 sec	Rest
20 sec	Kettlebell swing
20 sec	Rest
20 sec	Kettlebell swing
20 sec	Rest
20 sec	Band woodchopper (right)
20 sec	Rest
20 sec	Band woodchopper (left)
20 sec	Rest
20 sec	Band woodchopper (right)
20 sec	Rest
20 sec	Band woodchopper (left)
Total time: 10 min, 20 sec	

PHASE 2, WORKOUT A	
20 sec	Squat jump
20 sec	Rest
20 sec	Squat jump
20 sec	Rest
20 sec	Squat jump
20 sec	Rest
20 sec	Power push-up
20 sec	Rest
20 sec	Power push-up
20 sec	Rest
20 sec	Power push-up
20 sec	Rest
20 sec	Power clean
20 sec	Rest
20 sec	Power clean
20 sec	Rest
20 sec	Power clean
20 sec	Rest

> continued

TABLE 12.4 Power Cardio Workouts *(continued)*

PHASE 2, WORKOUT A *(continued)*	
Time	Exercise
20 sec	Medicine ball overhead throw
20 sec	Rest
20 sec	Medicine ball overhead throw
20 sec	Rest
20 sec	Medicine ball overhead throw
20 sec	Rest
20 sec	Heavy bag work
20 sec	Rest
20 sec	Heavy bag work
20 sec	Rest
20 sec	Heavy bag work
20 sec	Rest
20 sec	Band standing crunch
20 sec	Rest
20 sec	Band standing crunch
20 sec	Rest
20 sec	Band standing crunch
20 sec	Rest
20 sec	Medicine ball reach and slam
20 sec	Rest
20 sec	Medicine ball reach and slam
20 sec	Rest
20 sec	Medicine ball reach and slam
Total time: 13 min, 40 sec	

PHASE 2, WORKOUT B	
20 sec	Kettlebell snatch
20 sec	Rest
20 sec	Kettlebell snatch
20 sec	Rest
20 sec	Kettlebell snatch
20 sec	Rest
20 sec	Band sprint
20 sec	Rest
20 sec	Band sprint
20 sec	Rest
20 sec	Band sprint
20 sec	Rest
20 sec	Calf jump
20 sec	Rest
20 sec	Calf jump
20 sec	Rest
20 sec	Calf jump

PHASE 2, WORKOUT B *(continued)*	
Time	Exercise
20 sec	Rest
20 sec	Kettlebell swing
20 sec	Rest
20 sec	Kettlebell swing
20 sec	Rest
20 sec	Kettlebell swing
20 sec	Rest
20 sec	Kettlebell clean and jerk
20 sec	Rest
20 sec	Kettlebell clean and jerk
20 sec	Rest
20 sec	Kettlebell clean and jerk
20 sec	Rest
20 sec	Medicine ball underhand throw
20 sec	Rest
20 sec	Medicine ball underhand throw
20 sec	Rest
20 sec	Medicine ball underhand throw
20 sec	Rest
20 sec	Band woodchopper (right)
20 sec	Rest
20 sec	Band woodchopper (left)
20 sec	Rest
20 sec	Band woodchopper (right)
20 sec	Rest
20 sec	Band woodchopper (left)
Total time: 14 min, 20 sec	

PHASE 3, WORKOUT A	
20 sec	Squat jump
20 sec	Rest
20 sec	Squat jump
20 sec	Rest
20 sec	Squat jump
20 sec	Rest
20 sec	Power push-up
20 sec	Rest
20 sec	Power push-up
20 sec	Rest
20 sec	Power push-up
20 sec	Rest
20 sec	Power clean
20 sec	Rest

Time	Exercise
20 sec	Power clean
20 sec	Rest
20 sec	Power clean
20 sec	Rest
20 sec	Medicine ball overhead throw
20 sec	Rest
20 sec	Medicine ball overhead throw
20 sec	Rest
20 sec	Medicine ball overhead throw
20 sec	Rest
20 sec	Heavy bag work
20 sec	Rest
20 sec	Heavy bag work
20 sec	Rest
20 sec	Heavy bag work
20 sec	Rest
20 sec	Power clean
20 sec	Rest
20 sec	Power clean
20 sec	Rest
20 sec	Power clean
20 sec	Rest
20 sec	Medicine ball overhead throw
20 sec	Rest
20 sec	Medicine ball overhead throw
20 sec	Rest
20 sec	Medicine ball overhead throw
20 sec	Rest
20 sec	Heavy bag work
20 sec	Rest
20 sec	Heavy bag work
20 sec	Rest
20 sec	Heavy bag work
20 sec	Rest
20 sec	Band standing crunch
20 sec	Rest
20 sec	Band standing crunch
20 sec	Rest
20 sec	Band standing crunch
20 sec	Rest
20 sec	Medicine ball reach and slam
20 sec	Rest

Time	Exercise
20 sec	Medicine ball reach and slam
20 sec	Rest
20 sec	Medicine ball reach and slam
Total time: 19 min, 40 sec	

PHASE 3, WORKOUT B

Time	Exercise
20 sec	Kettlebell snatch
20 sec	Rest
20 sec	Kettlebell snatch
20 sec	Rest
20 sec	Kettlebell snatch
20 sec	Rest
20 sec	Band sprint
20 sec	Rest
20 sec	Band sprint
20 sec	Rest
20 sec	Band sprint
20 sec	Rest
20 sec	Calf jump
20 sec	Rest
20 sec	Calf jump
20 sec	Rest
20 sec	Calf jump
20 sec	Rest
20 sec	Kettlebell swing
20 sec	Rest
20 sec	Kettlebell swing
20 sec	Rest
20 sec	Kettlebell swing
20 sec	Rest
20 sec	Kettlebell clean and jerk
20 sec	Rest
20 sec	Kettlebell clean and jerk
20 sec	Rest
20 sec	Kettlebell clean and jerk
20 sec	Rest
20 sec	Medicine ball underhand throw
20 sec	Rest
20 sec	Medicine ball underhand throw
20 sec	Rest
20 sec	Medicine ball underhand throw
20 sec	Rest
20 sec	Kettlebell snatch

> *continued*

TABLE 12.4 Power Cardio Workouts *(continued)*

Time	Exercise
20 sec	Rest
20 sec	Kettlebell snatch
20 sec	Rest
20 sec	Kettlebell snatch
20 sec	Rest
20 sec	Kettlebell swing
20 sec	Rest
20 sec	Kettlebell swing
20 sec	Rest
20 sec	Kettlebell swing
20 sec	Rest
20 sec	Kettlebell clean and jerk
20 sec	Rest

PHASE 3, WORKOUT B *(continued)*

Time	Exercise
20 sec	Kettlebell clean and jerk
20 sec	Rest
20 sec	Kettlebell clean and jerk
20 sec	Rest
20 sec	Band woodchopper (right)
20 sec	Rest
20 sec	Band woodchopper (left)
20 sec	Rest
20 sec	Band woodchopper (right)
20 sec	Rest
20 sec	Band woodchopper (left)

Total time: 20 min, 20 sec

Cardioacceleration

Cardioacceleration refers to doing intervals of cardio (anywhere from 30 to 90 seconds) in between sets of resistance exercise. So, for example, on chest day, you would do one set of the bench press; then instead of sitting on the bench for 2 to 3 minutes resting, you perform 30 to 90 seconds of high-intensity cardio. Then you go do the next set of bench presses and continue in this manner throughout the entire workout.

Multiply those 30 to 90 seconds of cardio by the number of sets you complete in each workout, and it adds up. If you train chest, triceps, and abs, and do 12 sets for chest, 9 sets for triceps, and 9 sets for abs (30 total sets), and complete 60 seconds of cardio between each set, then you just completed 30 minutes of high-intensity cardio *during* your chest, triceps, and ab workout. That means that you don't have to spend extra time doing cardio after the weight workout is over or on a separate day. You can rest assured you've done your weight training *and* your cardio, all in one fell swoop.

Although it may not be readily apparent, cardioacceleration is a form of HIIT. You are doing 30- to 90-second intervals of cardio and then moving on to a set of weightlifting. Then you go back to the cardio interval, and then back to the weight training interval.

Cardioacceleration is based on a study by University of California at Santa Cruz researchers. Trained participants completing 30 to 60 seconds of cardio in between sets of weight training for over two months recovered better than those resting normally between sets (Davis et al. 2008). Not only does this method of HIIT allow for better recovery after workouts, but it allows for greater recovery between sets. It is surprising that this technique works so well in aiding recovery between sets. In fact, in my programs it has helped thousands of men and women break PRs while getting leaner at the same time. Many worry that doing cardio in between sets will decrease strength in weightlifting, but as I have found, once the body adapts to the cardioacceleration, it appears to enhance strength and recovery between sets.

Another nice thing about cardioacceleration is that it does not mean that you have to use the treadmill or other typical form of cardio equipment. You can do the cardio interval right there at the station where you are weight training. So, for example, if you are doing the bench press, you can do 30 to 90 seconds of bench step-ups on the bench-press bench. If you're doing dumbbell flys, then do dumbbell cleans for cardio right next to your bench. Or the simplest exercise of all is to run in place. This way you do not lose your spot in a busy gym. For good exercises to use for cardioacceleration, see chapter 26. Many exercises in chapter 25 also work well for cardioacceleration.

Start at on the low end of scale with 30 seconds of cardio in between sets. Over time, you can increase that by 15 seconds until you are up to doing 90 seconds of cardioacceleration in between sets. For a sample training program that uses cardioacceleration, see the TRX Cardioacceleration program (table 12.5) and Shortcut to Shred program in chapter 13.

TABLE 12.5   TRX Cardioacceleration Workout

The TRX allows you to add body-weight resistance to maximize fat loss. Since TRX exercises involve using the body as resistance, they not only strengthen the core and stabilizer muscles, but they also burn a lot of calories. Adding cardioacceleration to the TRX workout burns even more calories. Choose any exercise you prefer in between sets of every exercise and between every exercise.

Exercise	Sets/reps
TRX push-up	3/15-20
TRX inverted row	3/15-20
TRX one-leg squat	3/15-20
TRX pike push-up	3/15-20
TRX biceps curl	3/15-20
TRX triceps extension	3/15-20
TRX knee tuck	3/15-20

SUMMARY

While there is much confusion regarding cardio, this chapter should clarify the best type of cardio to do and why, the best times to do it, and the frequency of it. The sample HIIT workouts will help you put that knowledge into practice and maximize fat loss while optimizing performance and gains in muscle mass. The variety of HIIT forms will allow you to find a HIIT program that best suits you. Now all that you have to do is get out there and do it.

CHAPTER 13

Programs for Maximizing Fat Loss

The training programs in this chapter employ a variety of the strength training techniques covered in chapter 11 combined with the cardio techniques covered in chapter 12. Many of these programs have become very popular on the Internet. Over the years I have received feedback from hundreds of thousands of people following these plans. The transformations have been nothing but spectacular, and many drop their percentage of body fat by up to 10 percent while increasing their muscle mass, strength, and endurance.

These programs are best suited for intermediate to advanced weightlifters and not typically for beginners. Beginners should focus on the fundamentals of weight training with any of my beginner programs along with the Beginner to Advanced HIIT program. In fact, beginners will shed significant body fat just from consistently following a weight training program.

Feel the Burn Workout

This workout program uses techniques covered in chapter 11 for increasing fat loss. Each workout starts with an explosive movement using fast-twitch muscle fibers that burn the most calories. The workouts also incorporate a lot of multijoint exercises to burn more calories before and after the workout. They also employ both heavy weight for low reps to boost metabolic rate after the workout and lighter weight for high reps to boost calorie burn during the workout. Rest periods are kept short to keep the calorie burn up during and after the workout,

and some supersets are used to further the calorie burn during the workout and after.

This workout program follows a four-day training split (see table 13.1). However, to truly maximize fat loss, do all four workouts back to back over four days and rest on the fifth day. Then start over on the sixth day and continue in this fashion. Be sure to add some form of HIIT to this program, whether it's a block of standard HIIT done separately from the workouts, cardioacceleration, or some form of HIIT in between muscle groups.

TABLE 13.1   Feel the Burn Workout

WORKOUT 1: CHEST, TRICEPS, ABS

Exercise	Sets/reps	Rest
Power push-up	3/5-8	30 sec
Bench press	3/6-8	1-2 min
Incline dumbbell press	3/6-8	–
Superset with incline dumbbell fly	3/20	1 min
Cable crossover	3/25	30 sec
Smith machine close-grip bench press throw	3/5-8	30 sec
Close-grip bench press	3/6-8	1-2 min
Cable lying triceps extension	3/20	–
Superset with triceps pressdown	3/20	30 sec
Hip thrust	4/to failure	–
Superset with crossover crunch	4/to failure	30 sec

WORKOUT 2: LEGS, CALVES

Exercise	Sets/reps	Rest
Squat jump	3-3/5	30 sec
Squat	4/6-8	1-2 min
Leg press	3/20	30 sec
Leg extension	3/25	–
Superset with leg curl	3/25	30 sec
Romanian deadlift	3/25	30 sec
Standing calf raise	4/10	–
Superset with seated calf raise	4/30	30 sec

WORKOUT 3: SHOULDERS, TRAPS, ABS

Exercise	Sets/reps	Rest
Squat jump	2-3/5	30 sec
Medicine ball overhead throw	2-3/5	30 sec
Smith machine overhead press	3/6-8	1-2 min
Dumbbell overhead press	3/6-8	–
Superset with dumbbell lateral raise	3/20	1 min
Dumbbell bent-over lateral raise	3/25	30 sec
Barbell shrug	4/6-8	1-2 min
Cable crunch	3/10	–
Superset with plank	3/to failure	30 sec
Oblique cable crunch	3/20	–

WORKOUT 4: BACK, BICEPS, CALVES

Exercise	Sets/reps	Rest
Dumbbell power row	3/8	30 sec
Barbell bent-over row	4/6-8	1-2 min
Pulldown	4/6-8	–
Superset with straight-arm lat pulldown	4/20	1 min
Seated cable row	3/25	30 sec
Smith machine curl throw	3/8	30 sec
Barbell curl	3/6-8	1-2 min
Incline dumbbell curl	3/20	–
Superset with prone incline dumbbell curl	3/20	30 sec
Seated calf raise	4/10	–
Superset with leg press calf raise	4/20	30 sec

Shortcut to Shred Program

This program uses periodization in a microcycle fashion. It also uses two forms of periodization: linear and reverse linear. The program splits each muscle group into two workouts each week. The first half of the week (Monday, Tuesday, and Wednesday) you train using mainly multijoint exercises. For example, for chest you will only do presses using both barbell and dumbbells. The second half of the week (Thursday, Friday, and Saturday), when you train each muscle group for the second time, use mainly single-joint (isolation) exercises. For example, on chest you will do only fly exercises such as dumbbell flys and cable crossovers.

The multijoint-focused workouts in the first half of the week follow the linear periodized scheme and get heavier each week. However, the single-joint-focused workouts in the second half of the week follow a reverse linear periodization scheme and therefore get lighter each week.

There are a few exceptions for obvious reasons. For starters, there aren't any really useful multijoint exercises for biceps. So the first biceps workout each week you use barbell exercises, such as barbell curls and barbell preacher curls, while the second half of the week you use dumbbell and cable biceps exercises. Another issue is that there aren't many single-joint exercises for back, except the straight-arm pulldown and similar movements. So the first time you train your back each week, use rowing exercises, such as the barbell bent-over row and seated cable row. Then the second time you train your back that week, use only pulldown exercises as well as the single-joint straight-arm pulldown. The other exceptions are abdominals, calves, and forearms.

The weight workouts also enhance fat burning because of the exercise selection and rep ranges. The multijoint exercises increase the amount of calories you burn during the workout. The higher-rep workouts also increase the number of calories burned during the workout. The heavy-weight and low-rep workouts, on the other hand, help to boost calorie and fat burn after the workout.

There are two three-week phases to this six-week program (see table 13.2). In phase 1 you start with reps in the range of 9 to 11 for the multijoint-focused training in the first half of week 1. For the single-joint-focused work in the second half of the week, you do reps in the range of 12 to 15. In week 2 for the multijoint-focused training

in the first half of the week, the weight increases to drop the rep range down to 6 to 8 per set. The second half of the week when you are doing the single-joint-focused work, the weight is reduced to allow reps to increase to 16 to 20 per set. Then in the third and final week of phase 1, weight increases again to drop reps down to just 2 to 5 per set on the multijoint-focused workouts in the first half of the week. And in the second half of the week during the single-joint-focused workouts, weight decreases again and reps go up to 21 to 30 per set.

In phase 2 the cycle repeats again. So in the first week, which is week 4 of the program, the weight is reduced to allow the reps to go back to 9 to 11 per set during the first half of the week for the multijoint-focused workouts. And the weight increases for the single-joint-focused work in the second half of the week to bring the reps back down to 12 to 15 per set. And each week it follows just as in phase 1. However, the major difference in phase 2 is that the majority of exercises are different except for a few of the staple exercises that are key for strength. Changing up the exercises allows you to target slightly different fibers in the muscles for the best overall gains in size.

To enhance fat loss, not to mention aid recovery, this program uses cardioacceleration in between each set in every workout. If you keep moving from exercise to exercise without taking any rest before or after the cardioacceleration, you can complete most of these workouts in under an hour. That's less than an hour for both weight training and cardio.

I've also included an intensity technique that I call cardioaccelerated rest-pause/drop sets. On the last set of each exercise you take that set to muscle failure. Then you rack the weight and "rest" 15 to 20 seconds. I say "rest" because you won't really rest. You will do cardioacceleration by running in place for those 15 to 20 seconds. Then you pick up the weight again and continue doing reps for that exercises until you reach muscle failure again. But you're not finished yet. Now you immediately decrease the weight you are using by 20 to 30 percent and continue doing reps of that exercise until you reach muscle failure again. Now you are finally finished with that exercise and can move on to the next one. For body-weight exercises, or exercises where the weight is so light that you cannot do a drop set, you will do two cardioaccelerated rest-pause/drop sets. So after reaching muscle failure on the last set of an exercise, immediately go into 15 to 20 seconds of running in place. Then continue doing reps of that exercise until you reach muscle failure again.

Then immediately do another 15 to 20 seconds of running in place, and then immediately do more reps of that exercise until you reach muscle failure yet again. Now you are finally finished with that exercise.

TABLE 13.2   Shortcut to Shred Program

WEEK 1
WORKOUT 1: CHEST, TRICEPS, ABS (MULTIJOINT)

Exercise	Sets	Reps
Bench press	4*	9-11
Incline dumbbell press	3*	9-11
Decline Smith machine press	3*	9-11
Dip	4*	9-11
Close-grip bench press	4*	9-11
Cable crunch	3*	9-11
Smith machine hip thrust	3*	9-11

WORKOUT 2: SHOULDERS, LEGS, CALVES

Exercise	Sets	Reps
Barbell shoulder press	4*	9-11
Alternating dumbbell shoulder press (standing)	3*	9-11
Smith machine one-arm upright row	3*	9-11
Squat	4*	9-11
Deadlift	3*	9-11
Walking lunge	3*	9-11
Standing calf raise	3*	9-11
Seated calf raise	3*	9-11

WORKOUT 3: BACK, TRAPS, BICEPS

Exercise	Sets	Reps
Barbell bent-over row	4*	9-11
Dumbbell bent-over row	3*	9-11
Seated cable row	3*	9-11
Barbell shrug	4*	9-11
Barbell curl	3*	9-11
Barbell or EZ-bar preacher curl	3*	9-11
Reverse-grip barbell curl	3*	9-11
Barbell wrist curl	3*	9-11

WORKOUT 4: CHEST, TRICEPS, ABS (SINGLE JOINT)

Exercise	Sets	Reps
Incline dumbbell fly	4*	12-15
Dumbbell fly	3*	12-15
Cable crossover	3*	12-15
Triceps pressdown	3*	12-15
Overhead dumbbell extension	3*	12-15

WORKOUT 4: CHEST, TRICEPS, ABS (SINGLE JOINT) *(cont.)*

Exercise	Sets	Reps
Cable lying triceps extension	3*	12-15
Crunch	3*	12-15
Standing oblique cable crunch	3*	12-15

WORKOUT 5: SHOULDERS, LEGS, CALVES

Exercise	Sets	Reps
Dumbbell lateral raise	4*	12-15
Barbell front raise	3*	12-15
Dumbbell bent-over lateral raise	3*	12-15
Leg extension	4*	12-15
Leg curl	4*	12-15
Seated calf raise	3*	12-15
Donkey or leg press calf raise	3*	12-15

WORKOUT 6: BACK, TRAPS, BICEPS

Exercise	Sets	Reps
Lat pulldown	4*	12-15
Reverse-grip pulldown	3*	12-15
Straight-arm pulldown	3*	12-15
Smith machine behind-the-back shrug	4*	12-15
Incline dumbbell curl	3*	12-15
High cable curl	3*	12-15
Rope cable curl	3*	12-15
Dumbbell reverse wrist curl	3*	12-15

WEEK 2
WORKOUT 1: CHEST, TRICEPS, ABS (MULTIJOINT)

Exercise	Sets	Reps
Bench press	4*	6-8
Incline dumbbell press	3*	6-8
Decline smith machine press	3*	6-8
Dip	4*	6-8
Close-grip bench press	4*	6-8
Cable crunch	3*	7-8
Smith machine hip thrust	3*	7-8

WORKOUT 2: SHOULDERS, LEGS, CALVES

Exercise	Sets	Reps
Barbell shoulder press	4*	6-8
Alternating dumbbell shoulder press (standing)	3*	6-8

*On the last set do cardioaccelerated rest-pause/drop sets.

WEEK 2 (continued)
WORKOUT 2: SHOULDERS, LEGS, CALVES (continued)

Exercise	Sets	Reps
Smith machine one-arm upright row	3*	6-8
Squat	4*	6-8
Deadlift	3*	6-8
Walking lunge	3*	6-8
Standing calf raise	3*	7-8
Seated calf raise	3*	7-8

WORKOUT 3: BACK, TRAPS, BICEPS

Exercise	Sets	Reps
Barbell bent-over row	4*	6-8
Dumbbell bent-over row	3*	6-8
Seated cable row	3*	6-8
Barbell shrug	4*	6-8
Barbell curl	3*	6-8
Barbell or EZ-bar preacher curl	3*	6-8
Reverse-grip barbell curl	3*	6-8
Barbell wrist curl	3*	6-8

WORKOUT 4: CHEST, TRICEPS, ABS (SINGLE JOINT)

Exercise	Sets	Reps
Incline dumbbell fly	4*	16-20
Dumbbell fly	3*	16-20
Cable crossover	3*	16-20
Triceps pressdown	3*	16-20
Overhead dumbbell extension	3*	16-20
Cable lying triceps extension	3*	16-20
Crunch	3*	16-20
Standing oblique cable crunch	3*	16-20

WORKOUT 5: SHOULDERS, LEGS, CALVES

Exercise	Sets	Reps
Dumbbell lateral raise	4*	16-20
Barbell front raise	3*	16-20
Dumbbell bent-over lateral raise	3*	16-20
Leg extension	4*	16-20
Leg curl	4*	16-20
Seated calf raise	3*	16-20
Donkey or leg press calf raise	3*	16-20

*On the last set do cardioaccelerated rest-pause/drop sets.

WORKOUT 6: BACK, TRAPS, BICEPS

Exercise	Sets	Reps
Lat pulldown	4*	16-20
Reverse-grip pulldown	3*	16-20
Straight-arm pulldown	3*	16-20
Smith machine behind-the-back shrug	4*	16-20
Incline dumbbell curl	3*	16-20
High cable curl	3*	16-20
Rope cable curl	3*	16-20
Dumbbell reverse wrist curl	3*	16-20

WEEK 3
WORKOUT 1: CHEST, TRICEPS, ABS (MULTIJOINT)

Exercise	Sets	Reps
Bench press	4*	2-5
Incline dumbbell press	3*	2-5
Decline Smith machine press	3*	2-5
Dip	4*	2-5
Close-grip bench press	4*	2-5
Cable crunch	3*	5-6
Smith machine hip thrust	3*	5-6

WORKOUT 2: SHOULDERS, LEGS, CALVES

Exercise	Sets	Reps
Barbell shoulder press	4*	2-5
Alternating dumbbell shoulder press (standing)	3*	2-5
Smith machine one-arm upright row	3*	4-5
Squat	4*	2-5
Deadlift	3*	2-5
Walking lunge	3*	4-5
Standing calf raise	3*	5-6
Seated calf raise	3*	5-6

WORKOUT 3: BACK, TRAPS, BICEPS

Exercise	Sets	Reps
Barbell bent-over row	4*	2-5
Dumbbell bent-over row	3*	2-5
Seated cable row	3*	2-5
Barbell shrug	4*	2-5
Barbell curl	3*	2-5
Barbell or EZ-bar preacher curl	3*	4-5
Reverse-grip barbell curl	3*	4-5
Barbell wrist curl	3*	4-5

> continued

TABLE 13.2 Shortcut to Shred Program *(continued)*

WEEK 3 *(continued)*
WORKOUT 4: CHEST, TRICEPS, ABS (SINGLE JOINT)

Exercise	Sets	Reps
Incline dumbbell fly	4*	21-30
Dumbbell fly	3*	21-30
Cable crossover	3*	21-30
Triceps pressdown	3*	21-30
Overhead dumbbell extension	3*	21-30
Cable lying triceps extension	3*	21-30
Crunch	3*	21-30
Standing oblique cable crunch	3*	21-30

WORKOUT 5: SHOULDERS, LEGS, CALVES

Exercise	Sets	Reps
Dumbbell lateral raise	4*	21-30
Barbell front raise	3*	21-30
Dumbbell bent-over lateral raise	3*	21-30
Leg extension	4*	21-30
Leg curl	4*	21-30
Seated calf raise	3*	21-30
Donkey or leg press calf raise	3*	21-30

WORKOUT 6: BACK, TRAPS, BICEPS

Exercise	Sets	Reps
Lat pulldown	4*	21-30
Reverse-grip pulldown	3*	21-30
Straight-arm pulldown	3*	21-30
Smith machine behind-the-back shrug	4*	21-30
Incline dumbbell curl	3*	21-30
High cable curl	3*	21-30
Rope cable curl	3*	21-30
Dumbbell reverse wrist curl	3*	21-30

WEEK 4
WORKOUT 1: CHEST, TRICEPS, ABS (MULTIJOINT)

Exercise	Sets	Reps
Bench press	4*	9-11
Incline bench press	3*	9-11
Decline dumbbell press	3*	9-11
Dip	4*	9-11
Close-grip bench press	4*	9-11
Smith machine crunch	3*	9-11
Hanging leg raise	3*	9-11

*On the last set do cardioaccelerated rest-pause/drop sets.

WORKOUT 2: SHOULDERS, LEGS, CALVES

Exercise	Sets	Reps
Barbell shoulder press	4*	9-11
Dumbbell shoulder press (seated)	3*	9-11
Dumbbell upright row	3*	9-11
Squat	4*	9-11
Deadlift	3*	9-11
Leg press	3*	9-11
Standing calf raise	3*	9-11
Seated calf raise	3*	9-11

WORKOUT 3: BACK, TRAPS, BICEPS

Exercise	Sets	Reps
Barbell bent-over row	4*	9-11
Incline dumbbell row	3*	9-11
Seated cable row	3*	9-11
Barbell shrug	4*	9-11
Barbell curl	3*	9-11
Seated barbell curl	3*	9-11
Reverse-grip barbell or EZ-bar curl	3*	9-11
Behind-the-back wrist curl	3*	9-11

WORKOUT 4: CHEST, TRICEPS, ABS (SINGLE JOINT)

Exercise	Sets	Reps
Cable crossover from low pulley	4*	12-15
Cable crossover	3*	12-15
Dumbbell fly	3*	12-15
Overhead cable triceps extension	3*	12-15
Lying triceps extension	3*	12-15
Rope triceps pressdown	3*	12-15
Crossover crunch	3*	12-15
Cable woodchopper	3*	12-15

WORKOUT 5: SHOULDERS, LEGS, CALVES

Exercise	Sets	Reps
Dumbbell lateral raise	4*	12-15
Cable front raise	3*	12-15
Lying cable rear delt fly	3*	12-15
Leg extension	4*	12-15
Leg curl	4*	12-15
Seated calf raise	3*	12-15
Donkey or leg press calf raise	3*	12-15

WEEK 4 (continued)
WORKOUT 6: BACK, TRAPS, BICEPS

Exercise	Sets	Reps
Lat pulldown	4*	12-15
Behind-the-neck pulldown	3*	12-15
Rope straight-arm pulldown	3*	12-15
Dumbbell shrug	4*	12-15
EZ-bar cable curl	3*	12-15
Incline dumbbell curl	3*	12-15
Dumbbell hammer curl	3*	12-15
Dumbbell reverse wrist curl	3*	12-15

WEEK 5
WORKOUT 1: CHEST, TRICEPS, ABS (MULTIJOINT)

Exercise	Sets	Reps
Bench press	4*	6-8
Incline bench press	3*	6-8
Decline dumbbell press	3*	6-8
Dip	4*	6-8
Close-grip bench press	4*	6-8
Smith machine crunch	3*	7-8
Hanging leg raise**	3*	7-8

WORKOUT 2: SHOULDERS, LEGS, CALVES

Exercise	Sets	Reps
Barbell shoulder press	4*	6-8
Dumbbell shoulder press (seated)	3*	6-8
Dumbbell upright row	3*	6-8
Squat	4*	6-8
Deadlift	3*	6-8
Leg press	3*	6-8
Standing calf raise	3*	7-8
Seated calf raise	3*	7-8

WORKOUT 3: BACK, TRAPS, BICEPS

Exercise	Sets	Reps
Barbell bent-over row	4*	6-8
Incline dumbbell row	3*	6-8
Seated cable row	3*	6-8
Barbell shrug	4*	6-8
Barbell curl	3*	6-8
Seated barbell curl	3*	6-8
Reverse-grip barbell or EZ-bar curl	3*	6-8
Behind-the-back wrist curl	3*	6-8

WORKOUT 4: CHEST, TRICEPS, ABS (SINGLE JOINT)

Exercise	Sets	Reps
Cable crossover from low pulley	4*	16-20
Cable crossover	3*	16-20

WORKOUT 4: CHEST, TRICEPS, ABS (SINGLE JOINT) (cont.)

Exercise	Sets	Reps
Dumbbell fly	3*	16-20
Overhead cable triceps extension	3*	16-20
Lying triceps extension	3*	16-20
Rope triceps pressdown	3*	16-20
Crossover crunch	3*	16-20
Cable woodchopper	3*	16-20

WORKOUT 5: SHOULDERS, LEGS, CALVES

Exercise	Sets	Reps
Dumbbell lateral raise	4*	16-20
Cable front raise	3*	16-20
Lying cable rear delt fly	3*	16-20
Leg extension	4*	16-20
Leg curl	4*	16-20
Seated calf raise	3*	16-20
Donkey or leg press calf raise	3*	16-20

WORKOUT 6: BACK, TRAPS, BICEPS

Exercise	Sets	Reps
Lat pulldown	4*	16-20
Behind-the-neck pulldown	3*	16-20
Rope straight-arm pulldown	3*	16-20
Dumbbell shrug	4*	16-20
EZ-bar cable curl	3*	16-20
Incline dumbbell curl	3*	16-20
Dumbbell hammer curl	3*	16-20
Dumbbell reverse wrist curl	3*	16-20

WEEK 6
WORKOUT 1: CHEST, TRICEPS, ABS (MULTIJOINT)

Exercise	Sets	Reps
Bench press	4*	2-5
Incline bench press	3*	2-5
Decline dumbbell press	3*	2-5
Dips	4*	2-5
Close-grip bench press	4*	2-5
Smith machine crunch	3*	4-5
Hanging leg raise**	3*	4-5

WORKOUT 2: SHOULDERS, LEGS, CALVES

Exercise	Sets	Reps
Barbell shoulder press	4*	2-5
Dumbbell shoulder press (seated)	3*	2-5
Dumbbell upright row	3*	2-5
Squat	4*	2-5
Deadlift	3*	2-5

*On the last set do cardioaccelerated rest-pause/drop sets.

**Use ankle weights or hold dumbbell between feet if needed.

> continued

TABLE 13.2   Shortcut to Shred Program *(continued)*

WEEK 6 *(continued)*
WORKOUT 2: SHOULDERS, LEGS, CALVES *(continued)*

Exercise	Sets	Reps
Leg press	3*	2-5
Standing calf raise	3*	4-5
Seated calf raise	3*	4-5

WORKOUT 3: BACK, TRAPS, BICEPS

Exercise	Sets	Reps
Barbell bent-over row	4*	2-5
Incline dumbbell row	3*	2-5
Seated cable row	3*	2-5
Barbell shrug	4*	2-5
Barbell curl	3*	2-5
Seated barbell curl	3*	2-5
Reverse-grip barbell or EZ-bar curl	3*	4-5
Behind-the-back wrist curl	3*	4-5

WORKOUT 4: CHEST, TRICEPS, ABS (SINGLE JOINT)

Exercise	Sets	Reps
Cable crossover from low pulley	4*	21-30
Cable crossover	3*	21-30
Dumbbell fly	3*	21-30
Overhead cable triceps extension	3*	21-30
Lying triceps extension	3*	21-30

WORKOUT 4: CHEST, TRICEPS, ABS (SINGLE JOINT) *(cont.)*

Exercise	Sets	Reps
Rope triceps pressdown	3*	21-30
Crossover crunch	3*	21-30
Cable woodchopper	3*	21-30

WORKOUT 5: SHOULDERS, LEGS, CALVES

Exercise	Sets	Reps
Dumbbell lateral raise	4*	21-30
Cable front raise	3*	21-30
Lying cable rear delt fly	3*	21-30
Leg extension	4*	21-30
Leg curl	4*	21-30
Seated calf raise	3*	21-30
Donkey or leg press calf raise	3*	21-30

WORKOUT 6: BACK, TRAPS, BICEPS

Exercise	Sets	Reps
Lat pulldown	4*	21-30
Behind-the-neck pulldown	3*	21-30
Rope straight-arm pulldown	3*	21-30
Dumbbell shrug	4*	21-30
EZ-bar cable curl	3*	21-30
Incline dumbbell curl	3*	21-30
Dumbbell hammer curl	3*	21-30
Dumbbell reverse wrist curl	3*	21-30

*On the last set do cardioaccelerated rest-pause/drop sets.

**Use ankle weights or hold dumbbell between feet if needed.

Super Shredded 8 Program

This program, also known as SS8 (see table 13.3), incorporates numerous techniques to maximize fat burning while building muscle mass. The first is compound sets, which are supersets that pair exercises for the same muscle group. For each superset, one exercise is done with heavy weight for low reps and the other exercise is done with light weight for high reps. Typically the first exercise in the first superset pair is heavy weight for low reps. The first exercise for most muscle groups is typically a multijoint exercise, while the second one is a single-joint exercise. Then the second superset pair is typically done in the reverse order: light weight for high reps first and the heavy one second. For many muscle groups, this second exercise pair is done as a preexhaust superset; a single-joint (isolation) exercise is first with lighter weight and a multijoint exercise is next with heavy weight second.

Every two weeks the SS8 program progresses. The heavy exercises progress in a linear periodized fashion, so they get heavier and you complete fewer reps per set every two weeks. And every two weeks the light exercises progress in a reverse linear periodized fashion to get lighter and you perform more reps per set. This progression will help you get bigger and stronger as well as leaner, because it will further boost the calories burned during and after the workout.

Another change that occurs every two weeks on SS8 is rest between sets. Start off in weeks 1 and 2 allowing one minute of rest between supersets. But every two weeks the rest period drops by 15 seconds. So in weeks 3 and 4 you are allowed 45 seconds of rest, in weeks 5 and 6 you get only 30 seconds of rest, and in weeks 7 and 8 you get 15 seconds of rest, which is basically get no real rest period, between supersets. You go back and forth between the two exercises with no rest other than the time it takes to move into that next exercise, which is about 15 seconds. You do this until all three or four supersets are completed. Then you immediately move into the next superset.

The other addition to this program for maximal fat loss is the use of Tabata HIIT in between muscle groups. For example, on the chest, shoulders, and triceps workouts when you finish the last chest superset, do Tabata HIIT before you move on to supersets for shoulders. And after finishing shoulders, do Tabata HIIT before moving on to triceps. At the end of the workout, finish with more Tabata HIIT work. For info on Tabatas, see chapter 12.

Since the rest periods decrease every two weeks, you cannot use cardioacceleration (see chapter 12) properly with this program. So the next best thing, or maybe even the better thing, is Tabata HIIT in between muscle groups. In weeks 1 and 2 do just one Tabata exercise in between muscle groups for a total time of 12 minutes of Tabata per workout. But in week 3 that increases to two exercises done Tabata style between muscle groups for a total of six exercises and a total time of 24 minutes of Tabatas. If you are well conditioned and accustomed to HIIT, then you can consider starting in weeks 1 and 2 with two Tabata exercises between each muscle group trained.

TABLE 13.3 Super Shredded 8 Program

WEEKS 1, 2
WORKOUT 1 (MONDAY): CHEST, SHOULDERS, TRICEPS

Exercise	Sets/reps	Rest
Bench press	3/9-10	–
Superset with dumbbell fly	3/12-15	1 min
Incline dumbbell fly	3/12-15	–
Superset with incline dumbbell press	3/9-10	1 min
Push-up*	8/20 sec	10 sec
Dumbbell shoulder press	3/9-10	–
Superset with dumbbell lateral raise	3/12-15	1 min
Bent-over dumbbell lateral raise	3/12-15	–
Superset with dumbbell upright row	3/9-10	1 min
Kettlebell/dumbbell swing*	8/20 sec	10 sec
Close-grip bench press	2/9-10	–
Superset with lying triceps extension	2/12-15	1 min
Triceps pressdown	2/12-15	–
Superset with overhead cable triceps extension	2/9-10	1 min
Dead landmine*	8/20 sec	10 sec

WORKOUT 2 (TUESDAY): LEGS, CALVES, ABS

Exercise	Sets/reps	Rest
Squat jump	3/3-5	–
Superset with leg extension	3/12-15	1 min
Front squat	3/12-15	–
Superset with squat	3/9-10	1 min
Leg curl	3/12-15	–

WORKOUT 2 (TUESDAY): LEGS, CALVES, ABS (cont.)

Exercise	Sets/reps	Rest
Superset with dumbbell Romanian deadlift	3/9-10	1 min
Squat*	8/20 sec	10 sec
Leg press calf raise	3/12	–
Superset with body-weight standing calf raise	3/to failure	1 min
Lunge*	8/20 sec	10 sec
Hanging leg raise	3/to failure	–
Superset with oblique crunch	3/to failure	1 min
Crunch*	8/20 sec	10 sec

WORKOUT 3 (WEDNESDAY): BACK, TRAPS, BICEPS, FOREARMS

Exercise	Sets/reps	Rest
Barbell row	3/9-10	–
Superset with reverse-grip barbell row	3/12-15	30 sec
Straight-arm pulldown	3/12-15	–
Superset with wide-grip pulldown	3/9-10	30 sec
Kettlebell snatch*	8/20 sec	10 sec
Barbell shrug	3/9-10	–
Superset with behind-the-back barbell shrug	3/12-15	30 sec
Dumbbell clean*	8/20 sec	10 sec
Seated barbell curl	2/9-10	–
Superset with barbell curl	2/12-15	30 sec

*Do these exercises Tabata style.

> continued

TABLE 13.3   Super Shredded 8 Program *(continued)*

WEEKS 1, 2 *(continued)*
WORKOUT 3 (WEDNESDAY): BACK, TRAPS, BICEPS, FOREARMS *(continued)*

Exercise	Sets/reps	Rest
Prone incline dumbbell curl	2/12-15	–
Superset with dumbbell incline curl	2/9-10	30 sec
Barbell wrist curl	2/9-10	–
Superset with barbell reverse wrist curl	2/12-15	30 sec
Dead landmine*	8/20 sec	10 sec

WORKOUT 4 (THURSDAY): CHEST, SHOULDERS, TRICEPS

Exercise	Sets/reps	Rest
Incline bench press	3/9-10	–
Superset with incline dumbbell fly	3/12-15	1 min
Low cable crossover	3/12-15	–
Superset with cable crossover	3/9-10	1 min
Push-up*	8/20 sec	10 sec
Smith machine behind-the-neck shoulder press	4/9-10	–
Superset with Smith machine upright row	3/12-15	1 min
Cable rear delt fly	3/12-15	–
Superset with cable lateral raise	3/9-10	1 min
Kettlebell/dumbbell swing*	8/20 sec	10 sec
Lying triceps extension	2/9-10	–
Superset with bench dip	2/12-15	1 min
Reverse-grip triceps pressdown	2/12-15	–
Superset with triceps pressdown	2/9-10	1 min
Dead landmine*	8/20 sec	10 sec

WORKOUT 5 (FRIDAY): LEGS, CALVES, ABS

Exercise	Sets/reps	Rest
Squat	3/9-10	–
Superset with lunge	3/12-15	1 min
One-leg press (alternating legs)	3/12-15	–
Superset with leg press	3/9-10	1 min
Deadlift	3/9-10	–
Superset with Romanian deadlift	3/12-15	1 min
Squat*	8/20 sec	10 sec
Seated calf raise	3/12	–
Superset with body-weight standing calf raise	3/to failure	1 min
Lunge*	8/20 sec	10 sec
Cable crunch	3/12	–
Superset with oblique crunch	3/12	1 min
Reverse crunch*	8/20 sec	10 sec

*Do these exercises Tabata style.

WORKOUT 6 (SATURDAY): BACK, TRAPS, BICEPS, FOREARMS

Exercise	Sets/reps	Rest
Pulldown	3/9-10	–
Superset with reverse-grip pulldown	3/12-15	1 min
Straight-arm pulldown	3/12-15	–
Superset with standing pulldown	3/9-10	1 min
Kettlebell snatch*	8/20 sec	10 sec
Smith machine behind-the-back shrug	3/9-10	–
Superset with Smith machine shrug	3/12-15	1 min
Dumbbell clean*	8/20 sec	10 sec
EZ-bar curl	2/9-10	–
Superset with EZ-bar preacher curl	2/12-15	1 min
Dumbbell incline curl	2/12-15	–
Superset with standing dumbbell alternating curl	2/9-10	1 min
Dumbbell reverse wrist curl	2/9-10	–
Superset with dumbbell wrist curl	2/12-15	1 min
Dead landmine*	8/20 sec	10 sec

WEEKS 3, 4
WORKOUT 1 (MONDAY): CHEST, SHOULDERS, TRICEPS

Exercise	Sets/reps	Rest
Bench press	3/7-8	–
Superset with dumbbell fly	3/16-20	45 sec
Incline dumbbell fly	3/16-20	–
Superset with incline dumbbell press	3/7-8	45 sec
Push-up*	8/20 sec	10 sec
Jumping jack	8/20 sec	10 sec
Dumbbell shoulder press	3/7-8	–
Superset with dumbbell lateral raise	3/16-20	45 sec
Bent-over dumbbell lateral raise	3/16-20	–
Superset with dumbbell upright row	3/7-8	45 sec
Kettlebell/dumbbell swing*	8/20 sec	10 sec
Smith machine hang power clean*	8/20 sec	10 sec
Close-grip bench press	2/7-8	–
Superset with lying triceps extension	2/16-20	45 sec
Triceps pressdown	2/16-20	–
Superset with overhead cable triceps extension	2/7-8	45 sec
Dead landmine*	8/20 sec	10 sec
Burpee*	8/20 sec	10 sec

WORKOUT 2 (TUESDAY): LEGS, CALVES, ABS

Exercise	Sets/reps	Rest
Squat jump	3/5-6	–
Superset with leg extension	3/16-20	45 sec
Front squat	3/16-20	–
Superset with squat	3/7-8	45 sec
Leg curl	3/16-20	–
Superset with dumbbell Romanian deadlift	3/7-8	45 sec
Squat*	8/20 sec	10 sec
Kettlebell snatch*	8/20 sec	10 sec
Leg press calf raise	3/15	–
Superset with body-weight standing calf raise	3/to failure	45 sec
Lunge*	8/20 sec	10 sec
Mountain climber*	8/20 sec	10 sec
Hanging leg raise	3/to failure	–
Superset with oblique crunch	3/to failure	45 sec
Crunch*	8/20 sec	10 sec
Cable woodchopper*	8/20 sec	10 sec

WORKOUT 3 (WEDNESDAY): BACK, TRAPS, BICEPS, FOREARMS

Exercise	Sets/reps	Rest
Barbell row	3/7-8	–
Superset with reverse-grip barbell row	3/16-20	45 sec
Straight-arm pulldown	3/16-20	–
Superset with wide-grip pulldown	3/7-8	45 sec
Kettlebell snatch*	8/20 sec	10 sec
Bench step-up*	8/20 sec	10 sec
Barbell shrug	3/7-8	–
Superset with behind-the-back barbell shrug	3/16-20	45 sec
Dumbbell clean*	8/20 sec	10 sec
Bench hop-over*	8/20 sec	10 sec
Seated barbell curl	2/7-8	–
Superset with barbell curl	2/16-20	45 sec
Prone incline dumbbell curl	2/16-20	–
Superset with dumbbell incline curl	2/7-8	45 sec
Barbell wrist curl	2/7-8	–
Superset with barbell reverse wrist curl	2/16-20	45 sec
Dead landmine*	8/20 sec	10 sec
Jumping jack*	8/20 sec	10 sec

WORKOUT 4 (THURSDAY): CHEST, SHOULDERS, TRICEPS

Exercise	Sets/reps	Rest
Incline bench press	3/7-8	–
Superset with incline dumbbell fly	3/16-20	45 sec
Low cable crossover	3/15-20	–
Superset with cable crossover	3/7-8	45 sec
Push-up*	8/20 sec	10 sec
Jumping jack*	8/20 sec	10 sec
Smith machine behind-the-neck shoulder press	4/7-8	–
Superset with Smith machine upright row	3/16-20	45 sec
Cable rear delt fly	3/16-20	–
Superset with cable lateral raise	3/7-8	45 sec
Kettlebell/dumbbell swing*	8/20 sec	10 sec
Smith machine power clean*	8/20 sec	10 sec
Lying triceps extension	2/7-8	–
Superset with bench dip	2/16-20	45 sec
Reverse-grip triceps pressdown	2/16-20	–
Superset with triceps pressdown	2/7-8	45 sec
Dead landmine*	8/20 sec	10 sec
Burpees*	8/20 sec	10 sec

WORKOUT 5 (FRIDAY): LEGS, CALVES, ABS

Exercise	Sets/reps	Rest
Squat	3/7-8	–
Superset with lunge	3/15-20	45 sec
One-leg press (alternating legs)	3/16-20	–
Superset with leg press	3/7-8	45 sec
Deadlift	3/7-8	–
Superset with Romanian deadlift	3/16-20	45 sec
Squat*	8/20 sec	10 sec
Kettlebell snatch*	8/20 sec	10 sec
Seated calf raise	3/15	–
Superset with body-weight standing calf raise	3/to failure	45 sec
Lunge*	8/20 sec	10 sec
Mountain climber*	8/20 sec	10 sec
Cable crunch	3/10	–
Superset with oblique crunch	3/15	45 sec
Reverse crunch*	8/20 sec	10 sec
Barbell roll-out*	8/20 sec	10 sec

WORKOUT 6 (SATURDAY): BACK, TRAPS, BICEPS, FOREARMS

Exercise	Sets/reps	Rest
Pulldown	3/7-8	–
Superset with reverse-grip pulldown	3/16-20	45 sec

*Do these exercises Tabata style.

> *continued*

TABLE 13.3 Super Shredded 8 Program *(continued)*

WEEKS 3, 4 *(continued)*
WORKOUT 6 (SATURDAY): BACK, TRAPS, BICEPS, FOREARMS *(continued)*

Exercise	Sets/reps	Rest
Straight-arm pulldown	3/16-20	–
Superset with standing pulldown	3/7-8	45 sec
Kettlebell snatch*	8/20 sec	10 sec
Bench step-up*	8/20 sec	10 sec
Smith machine behind-the-back shrug	3/7-8	–
Superset with Smith machine shrug	3/16-20	45 sec
Dumbbell clean	8/20 sec	10 sec
Bench hop-over*	8/20 sec	10 sec
EZ-bar curl	2/7-8	–
Superset with EZ-bar preacher curl	2/16-20	45 sec
Dumbbell incline curl	2/16-20	–
Superset with standing dumbbell alternating curl	2/7-8	45 sec
Dumbbell reverse wrist curl	2/7-8	–
Superset with dumbbell wrist curl	2/16-20	45 sec
Dead landmine*	8/20 sec	10 sec
Jumping jack*	8/20 sec	10 sec

WEEKS 5, 6
WORKOUT 1 (MONDAY): CHEST, SHOULDERS, TRICEPS

Exercise	Sets/reps	Rest
Bench press	4/5-6	–
Superset with dumbbell fly	4/21-25	30 sec
Incline dumbbell fly	4/21-25	–
Superset with incline dumbbell press	4/5-6	30 sec
Push-up	8/20 sec	10 sec
Jumping jack	8/20 sec	10 sec
Dumbbell shoulder press	4/5-6	–
Superset with Dumbbell lateral raise	4/21-25	30 sec
Bent-over dumbbell lateral raise	4/21-25	–
Superset with dumbbell upright row	4/5-6	30 sec
Kettlebell/dumbbell swing*	8/20 sec	10 sec
Smith machine power clean*	8/20 sec	10 sec
Close-grip bench press	3/5-6	–
Superset with lying triceps extension	3/21-25	30 sec
Triceps pressdown	3/21-25	–
Superset with overhead cable triceps extension	3/5-6	30 sec
Dead landmine*	8/20 sec	10 sec
Burpee*	8/20 sec	10 sec

WORKOUT 2 (TUESDAY): LEGS, CALVES, ABS

Exercise	Sets/reps	Rest
Squat jump	4/7-8	–
Superset with leg extension	4/21-25	30 sec
Front squat	4/21-25	–
Superset with squat	4/5-6	30 sec
Leg curl	4/21-25	–
Superset with dumbbell Romanian deadlift	4/5-6	30 sec
Squat*	8/20 sec	10 sec
Kettlebell snatch*	8/20 sec	10 sec
Leg press calf raise	4/20	–
Superset with body-weight standing calf raise	4/to failure	30 sec
Lunge*	8/20 sec	10 sec
Mountain climber*	8/20 sec	10 sec
Hanging leg raise	4/to failure	–
Superset with oblique crunch	4/to failure	30 sec
Crunch*	8/20 sec	10 sec
Cable woodchopper*	8/20 sec	10 sec

WORKOUT 3 (WEDNESDAY): BACK, TRAPS, BICEPS, FOREARMS

Exercise	Sets/reps	Rest
Barbell row	4/5-6	–
Superset with reverse-grip barbell row	4/21-25	30 sec
Straight-arm pulldown	4/21-25	–
Superset with wide-grip pulldown	4/5-6	30 sec
Kettlebell snatch*	8/20 sec	10 sec
Bench step-up*	8/20 sec	10 sec
Barbell shrug	4/5-6	–
Superset with behind-the-back barbell shrug	4/21-25	30 sec
Dumbbell clean*	8/20 sec	10 sec
Bench hop-over*	8/20 sec	10 sec
Seated barbell curl	3/5-6	–
Superset with barbell curl	3/21-25	30 sec
Prone incline dumbbell curl	3/21-25	–
Superset with dumbbell incline curl	3/5-6	30 sec
Barbell wrist curl	3/5-6	–
Superset with barbell reverse wrist curl	3/21-25	30 sec
Dead landmine*	8/20 sec	10 sec
Jumping jack*	8/20 sec	10 sec

*Do these exercises Tabata style.

WORKOUT 4 (THURSDAY): CHEST, SHOULDERS, TRICEPS

Exercise	Sets/reps	Rest
Incline bench press	4/5-6	–
Superset with incline dumbbell fly	4/21-25	30 sec
Low cable crossover	4/21-25	–
Superset with cable crossover	4/5-6	30 sec
Push-up*	8/20 sec	10 sec
Jumping jack*	8/20 sec	10 sec
Smith machine behind-the-neck shoulder press	4/5-6	–
Superset with Smith machine upright row	4/21-25	30 sec
Cable rear delt fly	4/21-25	–
Superset with cable lateral raise	4/5-6	30 sec
Kettlebell/dumbbell swing*	8/20 sec	10 sec
Smith machine hang power clean*	8/20 sec	10 sec
Lying triceps extension	3/5-6	–
Superset with bench dip	3/21-25	30 sec
Reverse-grip triceps pressdown	3/21-25	–
Superset with triceps pressdown	3/5-6	30 sec
Dead landmine*	8/20 sec	10 sec
Burpee*	8/20 sec	10 sec

WORKOUT 5 (FRIDAY): LEGS, CALVES, ABS

Exercise	Sets/reps	Rest
Squat	4/5-6	–
Superset with lunge	4/21-25	30 sec
One-leg press (alternating legs)	4/21-25	–
Superset with leg press	4/5-6	30 sec
Deadlift	4/5-6	–
Superset with Romanian deadlift	4/21-25	30 sec
Squat*	8/20 sec	10 sec
Kettlebell snatch*	8/20 sec	10 sec
Seated calf raise	4/20	–
Superset with body-weight standing calf raise	4/to failure	30 sec
Lunges*	8/20 sec	10 sec
Mountain climber*	8/20 sec	10 sec
Cable crunch	4/8	–
Superset with oblique crunch	4/20	30 sec
Reverse crunch*	8/20 sec	10 sec
Barbell roll-out*	8/20 sec	10 sec

WORKOUT 6 (SATURDAY): BACK, TRAPS, BICEPS, FOREARMS

Exercise	Sets/reps	Rest
Pulldown	4/5-6	–
Superset with reverse-grip pulldown	4/21-25	30 sec

*Do these exercises Tabata style.

WORKOUT 6 (SATURDAY): BACK, TRAPS, BICEPS, FOREARMS *(continued)*

Exercise	Sets/reps	Rest
Straight-arm pulldown	4/21-25	–
Superset with standing pulldown	4/5-6	30 sec
Kettlebell snatch*	8/20 sec	10 sec
Bench step-up*	8/20 sec	10 sec
Smith machine behind-the-back shrug	4/5-6	–
Superset with Smith machine shrug	3/21-25	30 sec
Dumbbell clean*	8/20 sec	10 sec
Bench hop-over*	8/20 sec	10 sec
EZ-bar curl	3/5-6	–
Superset with EZ-bar preacher curl	3/21-25	30 sec
Dumbbell incline curl	3/21-25	–
Superset with Standing dumbbell alternating curl	3/5-6	30 sec
Dumbbell reverse wrist curl	3/5-6	–
Superset with Dumbbell wrist curl	3/21-25	30 sec
Dead landmine*	8/20 sec	10 sec
Jumping jack*	8/20 sec	10 sec

WEEKS 7, 8

WORKOUT 1 (MONDAY): CHEST, SHOULDERS, TRICEPS

Exercise	Sets/reps	Rest
Bench press	4/3-4	–
Superset with dumbbell fly	4/26-30	15 sec
Incline dumbbell fly	4/26-30	–
Superset with incline dumbbell press	4/3-4	15 sec
Push-up*	8/20 sec	10 sec
Jumping jack*	8/20 sec	10 sec
Dumbbell shoulder press	4/3-4	–
Superset with dumbbell lateral raise	4/26-30	15 sec
Bent-over dumbbell lateral raise	4/26-30	–
Superset with dumbbell upright row	4/3-4	15 sec
Kettlebell/dumbbell swing*	8/20 sec	10 sec
Smith machine power clean*	8/20 sec	10 sec
Close-grip bench press	3/3-4	–
Superset with lying triceps extension	3/26-30	15 sec
Triceps pressdown	3/26-30	–
Superset with overhead cable triceps extension	3/3-4	15 sec
Dead landmine*	8/20 sec	10 sec
Burpee*	8/20 sec	10 sec

> *continued*

TABLE 13.3 Super Shredded 8 Program *(continued)*

WEEKS 7, 8 *(continued)*
WORKOUT 2 (TUESDAY): LEGS, CALVES, ABS

Exercise	Sets/reps	Rest
Squat jump	4/9-10	–
Superset with leg extension	4/26-30	15 sec
Front squat	4/26-30	–
Superset with squat	4/3-4	15 sec
Leg curl	4/26-30	–
Superset with dumbbell Romanian deadlift	4/3-4	15 sec
Squat*	8/20 sec	10 sec
Kettlebell snatch*	8/20 sec	10 sec
Leg press calf raise	4/25	–
Superset with body-weight standing calf raise	4/to failure	15 sec
Lunges*	8/20 sec	10 sec
Mountain climber*	8/20 sec	10 sec
Hanging leg raise	4/to failure	–
Superset with oblique crunch	4/to failure	15 sec
Crunch*	8/20 sec	10 sec
Cable woodchopper*	8/20 sec	10 sec

WORKOUT 3 (WEDNESDAY): BACK, TRAPS, BICEPS, FOREARMS

Exercise	Sets/reps	Rest
Barbell row	4/3-4	–
Superset with reverse-grip barbell row	4/26-30	15 sec
Straight-arm pulldown	4/26-30	–
Superset with wide-grip pulldown	4/3-4	15 sec
Kettlebell snatch*	8/20 sec	10 sec
Bench step-up*	8/20 sec	10 sec
Barbell shrug	4/3-4	–
Superset with behind-the-back barbell shrug	4/26-30	15 sec
Dumbbell clean*	8/20 sec	10 sec
Bench hop-over*	8/20 sec	10 sec
Seated barbell curl	3/3-4	–
Superset with barbell curl	3/26-30	15 sec
Prone incline dumbbell curl	3/26-30	–
Superset with dumbbell incline curl	3/3-4	15 sec
Barbell wrist curl	3/3-4	–
Superset with barbell reverse wrist curl	3/26-30	15 sec
Dead landmine*	8/20 sec	10 sec
Jumping jack*	8/20 sec	10 sec

WORKOUT 4 (THURSDAY): CHEST, SHOULDERS, TRICEPS

Exercise	Sets/reps	Rest
Incline bench press	4/3-4	–
Superset with incline dumbbell fly	4/26-30	15 sec
Low cable crossover	4/26-30	–
Superset with cable crossover	4/3-4	15 sec
Push-up*	8/20 sec	10 sec
Jumping jack*	8/20 sec	10 sec
Smith machine behind-the-neck shoulder press	4/3-4	–
Superset with Smith machine upright row	4/26-30	15 sec
Cable rear delt fly	4/26-30	–
Superset with cable lateral raise	4/3-4	15 sec
Kettlebell/dumbbell swing*	8/20 sec	10 sec
Smith machine hang power clean*	8/20 sec	10 sec
Lying triceps extension	3/3-4	–
Superset with bench dip	3/26-30	15 sec
Reverse-grip triceps pressdown	3/26-30	–
Superset with triceps pressdown	3/3-4	15 sec
Dead landmine*	8/20 sec	10 sec
Burpee*	8/20 sec	10 sec

WORKOUT 5 (FRIDAY): LEGS, CALVES, ABS

Exercise	Sets/reps	Rest
Squat	4/3-4	–
Superset with lunge	4/26-30	15 sec
One-leg press (alternating legs)	4/26-30	–
Superset with leg press	4/3-4	15 sec
Deadlift	4/3-4	–
Superset with Romanian deadlift	4/25-30	15 sec
Squat*	8/20 sec	10 sec
Kettlebell snatch*	8/20 sec	10 sec
Seated calf raise	4/25	–
Superset with body-weight standing calf raise	4/to failure	15 sec
Lunge	8/20 sec	10 sec
Mountain climber*	8/20 sec	10 sec
Cable crunch	4/6	–
Superset with oblique crunch	4/25	15 sec
Reverse crunch*	8/20 sec	10 sec
Barbell roll-out*	8/20 sec	10 sec

WORKOUT 6 (SATURDAY): BACK, TRAPS, BICEPS, FOREARMS

Exercise	Sets/reps	Rest
Pulldown	4/3-4	–
Superset with reverse-grip pulldown	4/26-30	15 sec

*Do these exercises Tabata style.

WEEKS 7, 8 (*continued*)
**WORKOUT 6 (SATURDAY): BACK, TRAPS,
BICEPS, FOREARMS** (*continued*)

Exercise	Sets/reps	Rest
Straight-arm pulldown	4/26-30	–
Superset with standing pulldown	4/3-4	15 sec
Kettlebell snatch*	8/20 sec	10 sec
Bench step-up*	8/20 sec	10 sec
Smith machine behind-the-back shrug	4/3-4	–
Superset with Smith machine shrug	3/26-30	15 sec
Dumbbell clean*	8/20 sec	10 sec
Bench hop-over*	8/20 sec	10 sec

*Do these exercises Tabata style.

**WORKOUT 6 (SATURDAY): BACK, TRAPS,
BICEPS, FOREARMS** (*continued*)

Exercise	Sets/reps	Rest
EZ-bar curl	3/3-4	–
Superset with EZ-bar preacher curl	3/26-30	15 sec
Dumbbell incline curl	3/26-30	–
Superset with standing dumbbell alternating curl	3/3-4	15 sec
Dumbbell reverse wrist curl	3/3-4	–
Superset with dumbbell wrist curl	3/26-30	15 sec
Dead landmine*	8/20 sec	10 sec
Jumping jack*	8/20 sec	10 sec

HIIT 100s

In HIIT 100s, I have not just combined HIIT with weights, but I have combined HIIT with two very popular, very intense, and very effective weight training techniques: hundreds training and German volume training (GVT). German volume training is also known as 10 × 10 training. You do 10 sets of 10 reps. This technique is used in chapter 9 in the 5 × 10 program. As the name implies, hundreds training involves doing 100-rep sets.

With HIIT 100s you start each workout by doing 10 sets of 10 reps for one exercise per muscle group. The HIIT comes from the rest periods between those 10 sets. Start with just 60 seconds of rest between sets and progressively drop it down by 10 seconds over the 6 weeks, until you have no rest and you're doing 100 reps straight through. And that brings us to hundreds training. By the way, 10 sets of 10 reps is also 100 reps. And when you're resting only 10 or 20 seconds between sets in the last few weeks of the program, it feels just like you're doing 100 reps straight through. Most people are not able to complete all 100 reps straight through on HIIT 100s exercises in week 6. Don't worry. If you fail to reach 100 reps, simply rest as many seconds as you have reps left to complete until you hit 100 reps. For example, if you hit only 70 reps straight through, then rest 30 seconds and continue.

You start each workout doing one exercise per muscle group using HIIT 100s. Then follow that by doing three more sets of the same exercise using your 10-rep max (a weight that you can normally get for 10 reps). Of course, after doing 10 sets of 10

reps, you will no longer be able to complete 10 full reps with your 10-rep max weight. You will likely be able to complete only about 5 to 7 reps. On the third set, do a drop set by dropping down to the weight that you used for HIIT 100s and do as many reps as possible before you reach muscle failure. Then you do three sets of one or two more exercises for that same muscle group, depending on the muscle group. Rest between all sets after the HIIT 100s exercise will be only one minute to maximize fat burning.

Follow the muscle-group-specific weight training with a final HIIT 100s using a full-body weight exercise, such as barbell or dumbbell cleans, kettlebell swings, barbell or dumbbell deadlifts, barbell or dumbbell snatches, one-arm kettlebell or dumbbell snatch, or my unique lift known as the dead curl press.

On the HIIT 100s sets during weeks 1 through 3 when rest periods are 30 seconds or more, perform the first 3 sets of 10 as fast and explosively as possible. This will help to build more muscle power and strength, despite using such light weight. Then for sets 4 through 6, do them slowly and in control, focusing on the contraction with each rep and squeezing each rep at the top for 1 to 2 seconds. This helps to build the mind–muscle connection, which is critical for muscle size, shape, and separation. During weeks 4 through 6, when rest periods are down at 20 seconds and less, your goal is to just complete the hundred reps. So don't worry about rep speed or control. Just get the reps done with the best form possible while your muscles are on fire.

For each exercise, you will do HIIT 100s with select a weight that is equal to about 50 percent of what you normally could do on that exercise for 10 reps. Don't worry if you went too heavy. If you fail to complete all 10 sets of 10 reps during the program, you can adjust your weight either during that set or at the next workout. If you can't complete all 10 reps before hitting the eighth set of 10 reps, then immediately drop the weight by 5 or 10 pounds before the next set of 10 reps. If you can't complete 10 reps during or after the eighth set, finish all 10 sets doing as many reps as possible for those final sets. Then the next time you train that muscle group, lower the weight by 5 to 10 pounds.

If some of the exercises that you will do HIIT 100s with are new to you, then you'll need to spend some time figuring out how much weight you can do for 10 reps. The week before you start the actual HIIT 100s program, work these exercises into your training program to figure out an approximate weight that allows you to perform 10 reps but no more. Then when you start the program the next week, use half of that weight for your HIIT 100s sets.

When trying to estimate your 10-rep max on each exercise, be sure to do the HIIT exercise as the first exercise for that muscle group. For example, if you don't know what your 10-rep max is on the bench press, do bench press as the first exercise in your chest workout, aiming for a weight that allows you to complete just 10 reps. Then follow with your typical chest routine.

While the major benefit of this program (see table 13.4) is rapid fat loss, the fringe benefits are just as impressive. Even though weight is light, muscle growth will be a pleasant surprise, especially while you are simultaneously dropping body fat. You will have insane growth in muscle groups that you do not typically train with high volume, like traps, forearms, and calves. But you may also be surprised about the muscle growth you get in places like your arms and legs. One of the best ways to optimize muscle growth is by making a given weight more difficult. And HIIT 100s makes a very light weight difficult to move. The stress your muscle receives because of the difficulty in moving that weight repeatedly is what influences muscle growth. This pushes muscle fatigue to new levels, which stimulates the production and buildup of biochemical waste products. These waste products are not a complete waste, since they stimulate the release of hormones such as growth hormone (GH), which not only boosts muscle size but also encourages fat burning.

Of course, another obvious benefit to doing 100 reps with progressively shorter rest periods is an increase in muscle endurance. This will boost your conditioning for almost any sport. And even if you do not participate in any sport, this benefit will ring loud and clear in your workouts. When you go back to normal training, where you are resting a couple of minutes between sets, your muscle recovery will be quicker, which means you will be able to get more reps with the same weight than you normally would on successive sets. That's because progressively dropping your rest periods each week forces your muscles to gradually learn how to recover more quickly between sets.

Most people do not even need to add extra HIIT cardio when following this program. The HIIT 100s sets are adequate enough to stimulate fat burning. However, feel free to add some extra HIIT if you wish. You can add cardioacceleration to the non-HIIT 100s sets, or add HIIT in between muscle groups, or a HIIT workout after the HIIT 100s workout.

TABLE 13.4 HIIT 100s Workout

WEEK 1
WORKOUT 1 (MONDAY): CHEST, BACK, ABS

Exercise	Weight	Sets/reps	Rest
Bench press HIIT 100s	50% 10RM	10/10	60 sec
Bench press	10RM (from test)	3[1]/to failure	60 sec
Dumbbell incline press	10RM	3/to failure	60 sec
Cable crossover	15RM	3/to failure	60 sec
Wide-grip pulldown	50% 10RM	10/10	60 sec
Wide-grip pulldown	10RM (from test)	3[1]/to failure	60 sec
Barbell bent-over row	10RM	3/to failure	60 sec
Straight-arm pulldown	15RM	3/to failure	60 sec
Reverse crunch	Body weight[2]	10/10	60 sec
Crunch	Body weight[2]	10/10	60 sec
Dead curl press	Light dumbbells	10/10	60 sec

WORKOUT 2 (TUESDAY): LEGS, TRICEPS, CALVES

Exercise	Weight	Sets/reps	Rest
Squat HIIT 100s	50% 10RM	10/10	60 sec
Squat	10RM (from test)	3[1]/to failure	60 sec
Leg press	10RM	3/to failure	60 sec
Leg extension	15RM	3/to failure	60 sec
Leg curl	15RM	3/to failure	60 sec
Triceps pressdown	50% 10RM	10/10	60 sec
Triceps pressdown	10RM (from test)	3[1]/to failure	60 sec
Lying triceps extension	15RM	3/to failure	60 sec
Standing calf raise	50% 10RM	10/10	60 sec
Standing calf raise	10RM (from test)	3[1]/to failure	60 sec
Seated calf raise	15RM	3/to failure	60 sec
Kettlebell swing	Light kettlebell[3]	10/10	60 sec

WORKOUT 3 (WEDNESDAY): SHOULDERS, TRAPS, BICEPS, FOREARMS

Exercise	Weight	Sets/reps	Rest
Dumbbell shoulder press HIIT 100s	50% 10RM	10/10	60 sec
Dumbbell shoulder press	10RM (from test)	3[1]/to failure	60 sec
Dumbbell lateral raise	10RM	3/to failure	60 sec
Dumbbell rear delt raise	15RM	3/to failure	60 sec
Dumbbell shrug	50% 10RM	10/10	60 sec
Dumbbell shrug	10RM (from test)	3[1]/to failure	60 sec
Dumbbell curl	50% 10RM	10/10	60 sec
Dumbbell curl	10RM (from test)	3*/to failure	60 sec
Incline dumbbell curl	15RM	3/to failure	60 sec

[1] On the last set, do a drop set by reducing the weight to the same amount you used for HIIT 100s and do as many reps as possible to failure.

[2] Because this is a body-weight exercise, you cannot reduce the weight. So if you can't do 10 sets of 10 reps with 1 minute of rest on this exercise, do not reduce the rest each week. Instead, keep it at 1 minute until you are able to do all 10 sets for 10 reps. Then the next week start reducing the rest period each week.

[3] If you do not have access to kettlebells, you can use a dumbbell.

> continued

TABLE 13.4 HIIT 100s Workout *(continued)*

WEEK 1 *(continued)*
WORKOUT 3 (WEDNESDAY): SHOULDERS, TRAPS, BICEPS, FOREARMS *(continued)*

Exercise	Weight	Sets/reps	Rest
Barbell wrist curl	50% 10RM	10/10	60 sec
Barbell wrist curl	10RM (from test)	3*/to failure	60 sec
Dumbbell clean	50% 10RM	10/10	60 sec

WORKOUT 4 (THURSDAY): CHEST, BACK, ABS

Exercise	Weight	Sets/reps	Rest
Bench press HIIT 100s	50% 10RM	10/10	50 sec
Bench press	10RM (from test)	3[1]/to failure	60 sec
Reverse-grip incline bench press	10RM	3/to failure	60 sec
Incline dumbbell fly	15RM	3/to failure	60 sec
Wide-grip pulldown	50% 10RM	10/10	50 sec
Wide-grip pulldown	10RM (from test)	3[1]/to failure	60 sec
One-arm dumbbell bent-over row	10RM	3/to failure	[2]
Reverse-grip pulldown	15RM	3/to failure	60 sec
Reverse crunch	Body weight[3]	10/10	50 sec
Crunch	Body weight[3]	10/10	50 sec
Dead curl press	Light dumbbells	10/10	50 sec

WORKOUT 5 (FRIDAY): LEGS, TRICEPS, CALVES

Exercise	Weight	Sets/reps	Rest
Squat HIIT 100s	50% 10RM	10/10	50 sec
Squat	10RM (from test)	3[1]/to failure	60 sec
Dumbbell lunge	10RM	3/to failure	60 sec
Leg extension	15RM	3/to failure	60 sec
Romanian deadlift	15RM	3/to failure	60 sec
Triceps pressdown	50% 10RM	10/10	50 sec
Triceps pressdown	10RM (from test)	3[1]/to failure	60 sec
Cable overhead triceps extension	15RM	3/to failure	60 sec
Standing calf raise	50% 10RM	10/10	50 sec
Standing calf raise	10RM (from test)	3[1]/to failure	60 sec
Seated calf raise	15RM	3/to failure	60 sec
Kettlebell swing	Light kettlebell[2]	10/10	50 sec

WORKOUT 6 (SATURDAY): SHOULDERS, TRAPS, BICEPS, FOREARMS

Exercise	Weight	Sets/reps	Rest
Dumbbell shoulder press HIIT 100s	50% 10RM	10/10	50 sec
Dumbbell shoulder press	10RM (from test)	3[1]/to failure	60 sec
One-arm cable lateral raise	10RM	3/to failure	[2]
Machine rear delt fly	15RM	3/to failure	60 sec
Dumbbell shrug	50% 10RM	10/10	50 sec
Dumbbell shrug	10RM (from test)	3[1]/to failure	60 sec

[1] On the last set, do a drop set by reducing the weight to the same amount you used for HIIT 100s and do as many reps as possible to failure.

[2] Because this is a body-weight exercise, you cannot reduce the weight. So if you can't do 10 sets of 10 reps with 1 minute of rest on the exercises, do not reduce the rest each week. Instead, keep it at 1 minute until you are able to do all 10 sets for 10 reps. Then the next week start reducing the rest period each week.

WORKOUT 6 (SATURDAY): SHOULDERS, TRAPS, BICEPS, FOREARMS *(continued)*

Exercise	Weight	Sets/reps	Rest
Dumbbell curl	50% 10RM	10/10	50 sec
Dumbbell curl	10RM (from test)	3[1]/to failure	60 sec
Behind-the-back cable curl	15RM	3/to failure	[2]
Barbell wrist curl	50% 10RM	10/10	50 sec
Barbell wrist curl	10RM (from test)	3[1]/to failure	60 sec
Dumbbell clean	50% 10RM	10/10	50 sec

WEEK 2
WORKOUT 1 (MONDAY): CHEST, BACK, ABS

Exercise	Weight	Sets/reps	Rest
Bench press HIIT 100s	50% 10RM	10/10	40 sec
Bench press	10RM (from test)	3[1]/to failure	60 sec
Dumbbell incline press	10RM	3/to failure	60 sec
Cable crossover	15RM	3/to failure	60 sec
Wide-grip pulldown	50% 10RM	10/10	40 sec
Wide-grip pulldown	10RM (from test)	3[1]/to failure	60 sec
Barbell bent-over row	10RM	3/to failure	60 sec
Straight-arm pulldown	15RM	3/to failure	60 sec
Reverse crunch	Body weight[2]	10/10	40 sec
Crunch	Body weight[2]	10/10	40 sec
Dead curl press	Light dumbbells	10/10	40 sec

WORKOUT 2 (TUESDAY): LEGS, TRICEPS, CALVES

Exercise	Weight	Sets/reps	Rest
Squat HIIT 100s	50% 10RM	10/10	40 sec
Squat	10RM (from test)	3[1]/to failure	60 sec
Leg press	10RM	3/to failure	60 sec
Leg extension	15RM	3/to failure	60 sec
Leg curl	15RM	3/to failure	60 sec
Triceps pressdown	50% 10RM	10/10	40 sec
Triceps pressdown	10RM (from test)	3[1]/to failure	60 sec
Lying triceps extension	15RM	3/to failure	60 sec
Standing calf raise	50% 10RM	10/10	40 sec
Standing calf raise	10RM (from test)	3[1]/to failure	60 sec
Seated calf raise	15RM	3/to failure	60 sec
Kettlebell swing	Light kettlebell[3]	10/10	40 sec

WORKOUT 3 (WEDNESDAY): SHOULDERS, TRAPS, BICEPS, FOREARMS

Exercise	Weight	Sets/reps	Rest
Dumbbell shoulder press HIIT 100s	50% 10RM	10/10	40 sec
Dumbbell shoulder press	10RM (from test)	3[1]/to failure	60 sec

[3] If you do not have access to kettlebells, you can use a dumbbell.

[4] Take no rest and do each arm back-to-back until all 3 sets are completed for each arm.

> *continued*

TABLE 13.4 HIIT 100s Workout *(continued)*

WEEK 2 *(continued)*
WORKOUT 3 (WEDNESDAY): SHOULDERS, TRAPS, BICEPS, FOREARMS *(continued)*

Exercise	Weight	Sets/reps	Rest
Dumbbell lateral raise	10RM	3/to failure	60 sec
Dumbbell rear delt raise	15RM	3/to failure	60 sec
Dumbbell shrug	50% 10RM	10/10	40 sec
Dumbbell shrug	10RM (from test)	3[1]/to failure	60 sec
Dumbbell curl	50% 10RM	10/10	40 sec
Dumbbell curl	10RM (from test)	3[1]/to failure	60 sec
Incline dumbbell curl	15RM	3/to failure	60 sec
Barbell wrist curl	50% 10RM	10/10	40 sec
Barbell wrist curl	10RM (from test)	3[1]/to failure	60 sec
Dumbbell clean	50% 10RM	10/10	40 sec

WORKOUT 4 (THURSDAY): CHEST, BACK, ABS

Exercise	Weight	Sets/reps	Rest
Bench press HIIT 100s	50% 10RM	10/10	40 sec
Bench press	10RM (from test)	3[1]/to failure	60 sec
Reverse-grip incline bench press	10RM	3/to failure	60 sec
Incline dumbbell fly	15RM	3/to failure	60 sec
Wide-grip pulldown	50% 10RM	10/10	40 sec
Wide-grip pulldown	10RM (from test)	3[1]/to failure	60 sec
One-arm dumbbell bent-over row	10RM	3/to failure	[4]
Reverse-grip pulldown	15RM	3/to failure	60 sec
Reverse crunch	Body weight[2]	10/10	40 sec
Crunch	Body weight[2]	10/10	40 sec
Dead curl press	Light dumbbells	10/10	40 sec

WORKOUT 5 (FRIDAY): LEGS, TRICEPS, CALVES

Exercise	Weight	Sets/reps	Rest
Squat HIIT 100s	50% 10RM	10/10	40 sec
Squat	10RM (from test)	3[1]/to failure	60 sec
Dumbbell lunge	10RM	3/to failure	60 sec
Leg extension	15RM	3/to failure	60 sec
Romanian deadlift	15RM	3/to failure	60 sec
Triceps pressdown	50% 10RM	10/10	40 sec
Triceps pressdown	10RM (from test)	3[1]/to failure	60 sec
Cable overhead triceps extension	15RM	3/to failure	60 sec
Standing calf raise	50% 10RM	10/10	40 sec
Standing calf raise	10RM (from test)	3[1]/to failure	60 sec
Seated calf raise	15RM	3/to failure	60 sec
Kettlebell swing	Light kettlebell[3]	10/10	40 sec

[1] On the last set, do a drop set by reducing the weight to the same amount you used for HIIT 100s and do as many reps as possible to failure.

[2] Because this is a body-weight exercise, you cannot reduce the weight. So if you can't do 10 sets of 10 reps with 1 minute of rest on the exercises, do not reduce the rest each week. Instead, keep it at 1 minute until you are able to do all 10 sets for 10 reps. Then the next week start reducing the rest period each week.

WORKOUT 6 (SATURDAY): SHOULDERS, TRAPS, BICEPS, FOREARMS

Exercise	Weight	Sets/reps	Rest
Dumbbell shoulder press HIIT 100s	50% 10RM	10/10	40 sec
Dumbbell shoulder press	10RM (from test)	3[1]/to failure	60 sec
One-arm cable lateral raise	10RM	3/to failure	[4]
Machine rear delt fly	15RM	3/to failure	60 sec
Dumbbell shrug	50% 10RM	10/10	40 sec
Dumbbell shrug	10RM (from test)	3[1]/to failure	60 sec
Dumbbell curl	50% 10RM	10/10	40 sec
Dumbbell curl	10RM (from test)	3[1]/to failure	60 sec
Behind-the-back cable curl	15RM	3/to failure	[4]
Barbell wrist curl	50% 10RM	10/10	40 sec
Barbell wrist curl	10RM (from test)	3[1]/to failure	60 sec
Dumbbell clean	50% 10RM	10/10	40 sec

WEEK 3
WORKOUT 1 (MONDAY): CHEST, BACK, ABS

Exercise	Weight	Sets/reps	Rest
Bench press HIIT 100s	50% 10RM	10/10	30 sec
Bench press	10RM (from test)	3[1]/to failure	60 sec
Dumbbell incline press	12RM	3/to failure	60 sec
Cable crossover	20RM	3/to failure	60 sec
Wide-grip pulldown	50% 10RM	10/10	30 sec
Wide-grip pulldown	10RM (from test)	3[1]/to failure	60 sec
Barbell bent-over row	12RM	3/to failure	60 sec
Straight-arm pulldown	20RM	3/to failure	60 sec
Reverse crunch	Body weight[2]	10/10	30 sec
Crunch	Body weight[2]	10/10	30 sec
Dead curl press	Light dumbbells	10/10	30 sec

WORKOUT 2 (TUESDAY): LEGS, TRICEPS, CALVES

Exercise	Weight	Sets/reps	Rest
Squat HIIT 100s	50% 10RM	10/10	30 sec
Squat	10RM (from test)	3[1]/to failure	60 sec
Leg press	12RM	3/to failure	60 sec
Leg extension	20RM	3/to failure	60 sec
Leg curl	20RM	3/to failure	60 sec
Triceps pressdown	50% 10RM	10/10	30 sec
Triceps pressdown	10RM (from test)	3[1]/to failure	60 sec
Lying triceps extension	20RM	3/to failure	60 sec
Standing calf raise	50% 10RM	10/10	30 sec
Standing calf raise	10RM (from test)	3[1]/to failure	60 sec
Seated calf raise	20RM	3/to failure	60 sec
Kettlebell swing	Light kettlebell[3]	10/10	30 sec

[3] If you do not have access to kettlebells, you can use a dumbbell.

[4] Take no rest and do each arm back-to-back until all 3 sets are completed for each arm.

> *continued*

BISHOP BURTON COLLEGE

TABLE 13.4 HIIT 100s Workout *(continued)*

WEEK 3 *(continued)*
WORKOUT 3 (WEDNESDAY): SHOULDERS, TRAPS, BICEPS, FOREARMS

Exercise	Weight	Sets/reps	Rest
Dumbbell shoulder press HIIT 100s	50% 10RM	10/10	30 sec
Dumbbell shoulder press	10RM (from test)	3[1]/to failure	60 sec
Dumbbell lateral raise	12RM	3/to failure	60 sec
Dumbbell rear delt raise	20RM	3/to failure	60 sec
Dumbbell shrug	50% 10RM	10/10	30 sec
Dumbbell shrug	10RM (from test)	3[1]/to failure	60 sec
Dumbbell curl	50% 10RM	10/10	30 sec
Dumbbell curl	10RM (from test)	3[1]/to failure	60 sec
Incline dumbbell curl	20RM	3/to failure	60 sec
Barbell wrist curl	50% 10RM	10/10	30 sec
Barbell wrist curl	10RM (from test)	3[1]/to failure	60 sec
Dumbbell clean	50% 10RM	10/10	30 sec

WORKOUT 4 (THURSDAY): CHEST, BACK, ABS

Exercise	Weight	Sets/reps	Rest
Bench press HIIT 100s	50% 10RM	10/10	30 sec
Bench press	10RM (from test)	3[1]/to failure	60 sec
Reverse-grip incline bench press	12RM	3/to failure	60 sec
Incline dumbbell fly	20RM	3/to failure	60 sec
Wide-grip pulldown	50% 10RM	10/10	30 sec
Wide-grip pulldown	10RM (from test)	3[1]/to failure	30 sec
One-arm dumbbell bent-over row	12RM	3/to failure	[4]
Reverse-grip pulldown	20RM	3/to failure	60 sec
Reverse crunch	Body weight[2]	10/10	30 sec
Crunch	Body weight[2]	10/10	30 sec
Dead curl press	Light dumbbells	10/10	30 sec

WORKOUT 5 (FRIDAY): LEGS, TRICEPS, CALVES

Exercise	Weight	Sets/reps	Rest
Squat HIIT 100s	50% 10RM	10/10	30 sec
Squat	10RM (from test)	3[1]/to failure	60 sec
Dumbbell lunge	12RM	3/to failure	60 sec
Leg extension	20RM	3/to failure	60 sec
Romanian deadlift	20RM	3/to failure	60 sec
Triceps pressdown	50% 10RM	10/10	30 sec
Triceps pressdown	10RM (from test)	3[1]/to failure	60 sec
Cable overhead triceps extension	20RM	3/to failure	60 sec
Standing calf raise	50% 10RM	10/10	30 sec
Standing calf raise	10RM (from test)	3[1]/to failure	60 sec
Seated calf raise	20RM	3/to failure	30 sec
Kettlebell swing	Light kettlebell[3]	10/10	30 sec

[1] On the last set, do a drop set by reducing the weight to the same amount you used for HIIT 100s and do as many reps as possible to failure.

[2] Because this is a body-weight exercise, you cannot reduce the weight. So if you can't do 10 sets of 10 reps with 1 minute of rest on the exercises, do not reduce the rest each week. Instead, keep it at 1 minute until you are able to do all 10 sets for 10 reps. Then the next week start reducing the rest period each week.

WEEK 3 *(continued)*
WORKOUT 6 (SATURDAY): SHOULDERS, TRAPS, BICEPS, FOREARMS

Exercise	Weight	Sets/reps	Rest
Dumbbell shoulder press HIIT 100s	50% 10RM	10/10	30 sec
Dumbbell shoulder press	10RM (from test)	3[1]/to failure	60 sec
One-arm cable lateral raise	12RM	3/to failure	[4]
Machine rear delt fly	20RM	3/to failure	60 sec
Dumbbell shrug	50% 10RM	10/10	30 sec
Dumbbell shrug	10RM (from test)	3[1]/to failure	60 sec
Dumbbell curl	50% 10RM	10/10	30 sec
Dumbbell curl	10RM (from test)	3[1]/to failure	60 sec
Behind-the-back cable curl	20RM	3/to failure	[4]
Barbell wrist curl	50% 10RM	10/10	30 sec
Barbell wrist curl	10RM (from test)	3[1]/to failure	60 sec
Dumbbell clean	50% 10RM	10/10	30 sec

WEEK 4
WORKOUT 1 (MONDAY): CHEST, BACK, ABS

Exercise	Weight	Sets/reps	Rest
Bench press HIIT 100s	50% 10RM	10/10	20 sec
Bench press	10RM (from test)	3[1]/to failure	60 sec
Dumbbell incline press	12RM	3/to failure	60 sec
Cable crossover	20RM	3/to failure	60 sec
Wide-grip pulldown	50% 10RM	10/10	20 sec
Wide-grip pulldown	10RM (from test)	3[1]/to failure	60 sec
Barbell bent-over row	12RM	3/to failure	60 sec
Straight-arm pulldown	20RM	3/to failure	60 sec
Reverse crunch	Body weight[2]	10/10	20 sec
Crunch	Body weight[2]	10/10	20 sec
Dead curl press	Light dumbbells	10/10	20 sec

WORKOUT 2 (TUESDAY): LEGS, TRICEPS, CALVES

Exercise	Weight	Sets/reps	Rest
Squat HIIT 100s	50% 10RM	10/10	20 sec
Squat	10RM (from test)	3[1]/to failure	60 sec
Leg press	12RM	3/to failure	60 sec
Leg extension	20RM	3/to failure	60 sec
Leg curl	20RM	3/to failure	60 sec
Triceps pressdown	50% 10RM	10/10	20 sec
Triceps pressdown	10RM (from test)	3[1]/to failure	60 sec
Lying triceps extension	20RM	3/to failure	60 sec
Standing calf raise	50% 10RM	10/10	20 sec
Standing calf raise	10RM (from test)	3[1]/to failure	60 sec
Seated calf raise	20RM	3/to failure	60 sec
Kettlebell swing	Light kettlebell[3]	10/10	20 sec

[3] If you do not have access to kettlebells, you can use a dumbbell.

[4] Take no rest and do each arm back-to-back until all 3 sets are completed for each arm.

> *continued*

TABLE 13.4 HIIT 100s Workout *(continued)*

WEEK 4 *(continued)*
WORKOUT 3 (WEDNESDAY): SHOULDERS, TRAPS, BICEPS, FOREARMS

Exercise	Weight	Sets/reps	Rest
Dumbbell shoulder press HIIT 100s	50% 10RM	10/10	20 sec
Dumbbell shoulder press	10RM (from test)	3[1]/to failure	60 sec
Dumbbell lateral raise	12RM	3/to failure	60 sec
Dumbbell rear delt raise	20RM	3/to failure	60 sec
Dumbbell shrug	50% 10RM	10/10	20 sec
Dumbbell shrug	10RM (from test)	3[1]/to failure	60 sec
Dumbbell curl	50% 10RM	10/10	20 sec
Dumbbell curl	10RM (from test)	3[1]/to failure	60 sec
Incline dumbbell curl	20RM	3/to failure	60 sec
Barbell wrist curl	50% 10RM	10/10	20 sec
Barbell wrist curl	10RM (from test)	3[1]/to failure	60 sec
Dumbbell clean	50% 10RM	10/10	20 sec

WORKOUT 4 (THURSDAY): CHEST, BACK, ABS

Exercise	Weight	Sets/reps	Rest
Bench press HIIT 100s	50% 10RM	10/10	20 sec
Bench press	10RM (from test)	3[1]/to failure	60 sec
Reverse-grip incline bench press	12RM	3/to failure	60 sec
Incline dumbbell fly	20RM	3/to failure	60 sec
Wide-grip pulldown	50% 10RM	10/10	20 sec
Wide-grip pulldown	10RM (from test)	3[1]/to failure	30 sec
One-arm dumbbell bent-over row	12RM	3/to failure	[4]
Reverse-grip pulldown	20RM	3/to failure	60 sec
Reverse crunch	Body weight[2]	10/10	20 sec
Crunch	Body weight[2]	10/10	20 sec
Dead curl press	Light dumbbells	10/10	20 sec

WORKOUT 5 (FRIDAY): LEGS TRICEPS, CALVES

Exercise	Weight	Sets/reps	Rest
Squat HIIT 100s	50% 10RM	10/10	20 sec
Squat	10RM (from test)	3[1]/to failure	60 sec
Dumbbell lunge	12RM	3/to failure	60 sec
Leg extension	20RM	3/to failure	60 sec
Romanian deadlift	20RM	3/to failure	60 sec
Triceps pressdown	50% 10RM	10/10	20 sec
Triceps pressdown	10RM (from test)	3[1]/to failure	60 sec
Cable overhead triceps extension	20RM	3/to failure	60 sec
Standing calf raise	50% 10RM	10/10	20 sec
Standing calf raise	10RM (from test)	3[1]/to failure	60 sec
Seated calf raise	20RM	3/to failure	30 sec
Kettlebell swing	Light kettlebell[3]	10/10	20 sec

[1] On the last set, do a drop set by reducing the weight to the same amount you used for HIIT 100s and do as many reps as possible to failure.

[2] Because this is a body-weight exercise, you cannot reduce the weight. So if you can't do 10 sets of 10 reps with 1 minute of rest on the exercises, do not reduce the rest each week. Instead, keep it at 1 minute until you are able to do all 10 sets for 10 reps. Then the next week start reducing the rest period each week.

WORKOUT 6 (SATURDAY): SHOULDERS, TRAPS, BICEPS, FOREARMS

Exercise	Weight	Sets/reps	Rest
Dumbbell shoulder press HIIT 100s	50% 10RM	10/10	20 sec
Dumbbell shoulder press	10RM (from test)	3[1]/to failure	60 sec
One-arm cable lateral raise	12RM	3/to failure	[4]
Machine rear delt fly	20RM	3/to failure	60 sec
Dumbbell shrug	50% 10RM	10/10	20 sec
Dumbbell shrug	10RM (from test)	3[1]/to failure	60 sec
Dumbbell curl	50% 10RM	10/10	20 sec
Dumbbell curl	10RM (from test)	3[1]/to failure	60 sec
Behind-the-back cable curl	20RM	3/to failure	[4]
Barbell wrist curl	50% 10RM	10/10	20 sec
Barbell wrist curl	10RM (from test)	3[1]/to failure	60 sec
Dumbbell clean	50% 10RM	10/10	20 sec

WEEK 5
WORKOUT 1 (MONDAY): CHEST, BACK, ABS

Exercise	Weight	Sets/reps	Rest
Bench press HIIT 100s	50% 10RM	10/10	10 sec
Bench press	10RM (from test)	3[1]/to failure	60 sec
Dumbbell incline press	15RM	3/to failure	60 sec
Cable crossover	30RM	3/to failure	60 sec
Wide-grip pulldown	50% 10RM	10/10	10 sec
Wide-grip pulldown	10RM (from test)	3[1]/to failure	60 sec
Barbell bent-over row	15RM	3/to failure	60 sec
Straight-arm pulldown	30RM	3/to failure	60 sec
Reverse crunch	Body weight[2]	10/10	10 sec
Crunch	Body weight[2]	10/10	10 sec
Dead curl press	Light dumbbells	10/10	10 sec

WORKOUT 2 (TUESDAY): LEGS, TRICEPS, CALVES

Exercise	Weight	Sets/reps	Rest
Squat HIIT 100s	50% 10RM	10/10	10 sec
Squat	10RM (from test)	3[1]/to failure	60 sec
Leg press	15RM	3/to failure	60 sec
Leg extension	30RM	3/to failure	60 sec
Leg curl	30RM	3/to failure	60 sec
Triceps pressdown	50% 10RM	10/10	10 sec
Triceps pressdown	10RM (from test)	3[1]/to failure	60 sec
Lying triceps extension	30RM	3/to failure	60 sec
Standing calf raise	50% 10RM	10/10	10 sec
Standing calf raise	10RM (from test)	3[1]/to failure	60 sec
Seated calf raise	30RM	3/to failure	60 sec
Kettlebell swing	Light kettlebell[3]	10/10	10 sec

[3] If you do not have access to kettlebells, you can use a dumbbell.

[4] Take no rest and do each arm back-to-back until all 3 sets are completed for each arm.

> *continued*

TABLE 13.4 HIIT 100s Workout *(continued)*

WEEK 5 *(continued)*
WORKOUT 3 (WEDNESDAY): SHOULDERS, TRAPS, BICEPS, FOREARMS

Exercise	Weight	Sets/reps	Rest
Dumbbell shoulder press HIIT 100s	50% 10RM	10/10	10 sec
Dumbbell shoulder press	10RM (from test)	3[1]/to failure	60 sec
Dumbbell lateral raise	15RM	3/to failure	60 sec
Dumbbell rear delt raise	30RM	3/to failure	60 sec
Dumbbell shrug	50% 10RM	10/10	10 sec
Dumbbell shrug	10RM (from test)	3[1]/to failure	60 sec
Dumbbell curl	50% 10RM	10/10	10 sec
Dumbbell curl	10RM (from test)	3[1]/to failure	60 sec
Incline dumbbell curl	30RM	3/to failure	60 sec
Barbell wrist curl	50% 10RM	10/10	10 sec
Barbell wrist curl	10RM (from test)	3[1]/to failure	60 sec
Dumbbell clean	50% 10RM	10/10	10 sec

WORKOUT 4 (THURSDAY): CHEST, BACK, ABS

Exercise	Weight	Sets/reps	Rest
Bench press HIIT 100s	50% 10RM	10/10	10 sec
Bench press	10RM (from test)	3[1]/to failure	60 sec
Reverse-grip incline bench press	15RM	3/to failure	60 sec
Incline dumbbell fly	30RM	3/to failure	60 sec
Wide-grip pulldown	50% 10RM	10/10	10 sec
Wide-grip pulldown	10RM (from test)	3[1]/to failure	30 sec
One-arm dumbbell bent-over row	15RM	3/to failure	[4]
Reverse-grip pulldown	30RM	3/to failure	60 sec
Reverse crunch	Body weight[2]	10/10	10 sec
Crunch	Body weight[2]	10/10	10 sec
Dead curl press	Light dumbbells	10/10	10 sec

WORKOUT 5 (FRIDAY): LEGS, TRICEPS, CALVES

Exercise	Weight	Sets/reps	Rest
Squat HIIT 100s	50% 10RM	10/10	10 sec
Squat	10RM (from test)	3[1]/to failure	60 sec
Dumbbell lunge	15RM	3/to failure	60 sec
Leg extension	30RM	3/to failure	60 sec
Romanian deadlift	30RM	3/to failure	60 sec
Triceps pressdown	50% 10RM	10/10	10 sec
Triceps pressdown	10RM (from test)	3[1]/to failure	60 sec
Cable overhead triceps extension	30RM	3/to failure	60 sec
Standing calf raise	50% 10RM	10/10	10 sec
Standing calf raise	10RM (from test)	3[1]/to failure	60 sec
Seated calf raise	30RM	3/to failure	30 sec
Kettlebell swing	Light kettlebell[3]	10/10	10 sec

[1] On the last set, do a drop set by reducing the weight to the same amount you used for HIIT 100s and do as many reps as possible to failure.

[2] Because this is a body-weight exercise, you cannot reduce the weight. So if you can't do 10 sets of 10 reps with 1 minute of rest on the exercises, do not reduce the rest each week. Instead, keep it at 1 minute until you are able to do all 10 sets for 10 reps. Then the next week start reducing the rest period each week.

WORKOUT 6 (SATURDAY): SHOULDERS, TRAPS, BICEPS, FOREARMS

Exercise	Weight	Sets/reps	Rest
Dumbbell shoulder press HIIT 100s	50% 10RM	10/10	10 sec
Dumbbell shoulder press	10RM (from test)	3[1]/to failure	60 sec
One-arm cable lateral raise	15RM	3/to failure	[4]
Machine rear delt fly	30RM	3/to failure	60 sec
Dumbbell shrug	50% 10RM	10/10	10 sec
Dumbbell shrug	10RM (from test)	3[1]/to failure	60 sec
Dumbbell curl	50% 10RM	10/10	10 sec
Dumbbell curl	10RM (from test)	3[1]/to failure	60 sec
Behind-the-back cable curl	30RM	3/to failure	[4]
Barbell wrist curl	50% 10RM	10/10	10 sec
Barbell wrist curl	10RM (from test)	3[1]/to failure	60 sec
Dumbbell clean	50% 10RM	10/10	10 sec

WEEK 6
WORKOUT 1 (MONDAY): CHEST, BACK, ABS

Exercise	Weight	Sets/reps	Rest
Bench press HIIT 100s	50% 10RM	10/10	0 sec
Bench press	10RM (from test)	3[1]/to failure	60 sec
Dumbbell incline press	15RM	3/to failure	60 sec
Cable crossover	30RM	3/to failure	60 sec
Wide-grip pulldown	50% 10RM	10/10	0 sec
Wide-grip pulldown	10RM (from test)	3[1]/to failure	60 sec
Barbell bent-over row	15RM	3/to failure	60 sec
Straight-arm pulldown	30RM	3/to failure	60 sec
Reverse crunch	Body weight[2]	10/10	0 sec
Crunch	Body weight[2]	10/10	0 sec
Dead curl press	Light dumbbells	10/10	0 sec

WORKOUT 2 (TUESDAY): LEGS, TRICEPS, CALVES

Exercise	Weight	Sets/reps	Rest
Squat HIIT 100s	50% 10RM	10/10	0 sec
Squat	10RM (from test)	3[1]/to failure	60 sec
Leg press	15RM	3/to failure	60 sec
Leg extension	30RM	3/to failure	60 sec
Leg curl	30RM	3/to failure	60 sec
Triceps pressdown	50% 10RM	10/10	0 sec
Triceps pressdown	10RM (from test)	3[1]/to failure	60 sec
Lying triceps extension	30RM	3/to failure	60 sec
Standing calf raise	50% 10RM	10/10	0 sec
Standing calf raise	10RM (from test)	3[1]/to failure	60 sec
Seated calf raise	30RM	3/to failure	60 sec
Kettlebell swing	Light kettlebell[3]	10/10	0 sec

[3] If you do not have access to kettlebells, you can use a dumbbell.

[4] Take no rest and do each arm back-to-back until all 3 sets are completed for each arm.

> *continued*

TABLE 13.4 HIIT 100s Workout *(continued)*

WEEK 6 *(continued)*
WORKOUT 3 (WEDNESDAY): SHOULDERS, TRAPS, BICEPS, FOREARMS

Exercise	Weight	Sets/reps	Rest
Dumbbell shoulder press HIIT 100s	50% 10RM	10/10	0 sec
Dumbbell shoulder press	10RM (from test)	3[1]/to failure	60 sec
Dumbbell lateral raise	15RM	3/to failure	60 sec
Dumbbell rear delt raise	30RM	3/to failure	60 sec
Dumbbell shrug	50% 10RM	10/10	0 sec
Dumbbell shrug	10RM (from test)	3[1]/to failure	60 sec
Dumbbell curl	50% 10RM	10/10	0 sec
Dumbbell curl	10RM (from test)	3[1]/to failure	60 sec
Incline dumbbell curl	30RM	3/to failure	60 sec
Barbell wrist curl	50% 10RM	10/10	0 sec
Barbell wrist curl	10RM (from test)	3[1]/to failure	60 sec
Dumbbell clean	50% 10RM	10/10	0 sec

WORKOUT 4 (THURSDAY): CHEST, BACK, ABS

Exercise	Weight	Sets/reps	Rest
Bench press HIIT 100s	50% 10RM	10/10	0 sec
Bench press	10RM (from test)	3[1]/to failure	60 sec
Reverse-grip incline bench press	15RM	3/to failure	60 sec
Incline dumbbell fly	30RM	3/to failure	60 sec
Wide-grip pulldown	50% 10RM	10/10	0 sec
Wide-grip pulldown	10RM (from test)	3[1]/to failure	30 sec
One-arm dumbbell bent-over row	15RM	3/to failure	[4]
Reverse-grip pulldown	30RM	3/to failure	60 sec
Reverse crunch	Body weight[2]	10/10	0 sec
Crunch	Body weight[2]	10/10	0 sec
Dead curl press	Light dumbbells	10/10	0 sec

WORKOUT 5 (FRIDAY): LEGS, TRICEPS, CALVES

Exercise	Weight	Sets/reps	Rest
Squat HIIT 100s	50% 10RM	10/10	0 sec
Squat	10RM (from test)	3[1]/to failure	60 sec
Dumbbell lunge	15RM	3/to failure	60 sec
Leg extension	30RM	3/to failure	60 sec
Romanian deadlift	30RM	3/to failure	60 sec
Triceps pressdown	50% 10RM	10/10	0 sec
Triceps pressdown	10RM (from test)	3[1]/to failure	60 sec
Cable overhead triceps extension	30RM	3/to failure	60 sec
Standing calf raise	50% 10RM	10/10	0 sec
Standing calf raise	10RM (from test)	3[1]/to failure	60 sec
Seated calf raise	30RM	3/to failure	30 sec
Kettlebell swing	Light kettlebell[3]	10/10	0 sec

[1] On the last set, do a drop set by reducing the weight to the same amount you used for HIIT 100s and do as many reps as possible to failure.

[2] Because this is a body-weight exercise, you cannot reduce the weight. So if you can't do 10 sets of 10 reps with 1 minute of rest on the exercises, do not reduce the rest each week. Instead, keep it at 1 minute until you are able to do all 10 sets for 10 reps. Then the next week start reducing the rest period each week.

[3] If you do not have access to kettlebells, you can use a dumbbell.

[4] Take no rest and do each arm back-to-back until all 3 sets are completed for each arm.

WEEK 5 *(continued)*
WORKOUT 6 (SATURDAY): SHOULDERS, TRAPS, BICEPS, FOREARMS

Exercise	Weight	Sets/reps	Rest
Dumbbell shoulder press HIIT 100s	50% 10RM	10/10	0 sec
Dumbbell shoulder press	10RM (from test)	3[1]/to failure	60 sec
One-arm cable lateral raise	15RM	3/to failure	4
Machine rear delt fly	30RM	3/to failure	60 sec
Dumbbell shrug	50% 10RM	10/10	0 sec
Dumbbell shrug	10RM (from test)	3[1]/to failure	60 sec
Dumbbell curl	50% 10RM	10/10	0 sec
Dumbbell curl	10RM (from test)	3[1]/to failure	60 sec
Behind-the-back cable curl	30RM	3/to failure	4
Barbell wrist curl	50% 10RM	10/10	0 sec
Barbell wrist curl	10RM (from test)	3[1]/to failure	60 sec
Dumbbell clean	50% 10RM	10/10	0 sec

[1] On the last set, do a drop set by reducing the weight to the same amount you used for HIIT 100s and do as many reps as possible to failure.

[2] Because this is a body-weight exercise, you cannot reduce the weight. So if you can't do 10 sets of 10 reps with 1 minute of rest on the exercises, do not reduce the rest each week. Instead, keep it at 1 minute until you are able to do all 10 sets for 10 reps. Then the next week start reducing the rest period each week.

[3] If you do not have access to kettlebells, you can use a dumbbell.

[4] Take no rest and do each arm back-to-back until all 3 sets are completed for each arm.

Tabata Weight Blast Program

Tabata Weight Blast takes the Tabata that you think of only as cardio and turns it into a full weight-training program. This way you get the combined benefit of fat loss while actually building some muscle. Doing very high reps with light weight for short periods can help you blow past plateaus and add some serious lean muscle.

Because Tabata enhances endurance, it boosts your body's ability to burn more fat. And because it enhances explosive energy, the kind you use in a typical set of bench presses, it can help you get more reps with a given weight, or use more weight to get a given number of reps. And that crosses over to more strength as well as more muscle growth, since a greater overload on the muscle results in greater growth.

And the benefits won't end there. Because you do fairly high reps and take very short rest periods between sets, you'll increase the amount of blood vessels that feed your muscle fibers. This will help to get more nutrients, oxygen, and anabolic hormones to your muscles, which means they'll have more energy during workouts and better recovery and growth after the workout.

This Tabata program will have you doing several exercises per muscle group in Tabata fashion. Do 2 to 4 exercises per muscle group. Each exercise consists of 8 sets of 20 seconds, getting as many reps as possible in those 20 seconds. Rest only 10 seconds between the 20-second sets. Once you've completed 8 sets, rest 1 to 2 minutes and then do the same on the next exercise.

Finish each workout with four full-body or calisthenic exercises done in Tabata fashion for even more fat burning. When you do these four exercises, take no scheduled rest between the exercises. Once you have completed all eight cycles of one exercise, move into the next one as quickly as possible.

It will take some trial and error to select the proper weight for each exercise. I suggest you start very light because you can work up in weight each week. If you find a weight that allows you to complete 20 seconds of reps for the first five or six sets but you cannot do the full 20 seconds on the last two or three sets, stick with that weight. This way you can set a goal to complete the 20 seconds of reps for all eight sets before you move on to a heavier weight. Each week that you follow the Tabata Weight Blast program, your goal should be to increase the weight you use or the number of reps you complete in those 4 minutes. I suggest you follow the Tabata Weight Blast program in table 13.5 for about three to six weeks before returning to a more normal style of straight-set training.

TABLE 13.5 Tabata Weight Blast

WORKOUT 1 (MONDAY): CHEST/ABS

Exercise	Sets/time	Rest
Bench press*	8/20 sec	10 sec
Incline bench press*	8/20 sec	10 sec
Dumbbell fly*	8/20 sec	10 sec
Cable crossover*	8/20 sec	10 sec
Reverse crunch*	8/20 sec	10 sec
Crunch*	8/20 sec	10 sec
Push-up**	8/20 sec	10 sec
Dumbbell clean**	8/20 sec	10 sec
Dumbbell walking lunge**	8/20 sec	10 sec
Kettlebell swing	8/20 sec	10 sec

WORKOUT 2 (TUESDAY): LEGS/CALVES

Exercise	Sets/time	Rest
Squat*	8/20 sec	10 sec
Deadlift*	8/20 sec	10 sec
Leg extension*	8/20 sec	10 sec
Leg curl*	8/20 sec	10 sec
Standing calf raise*	8/20 sec	10 sec
Seated calf raise*	8/20 sec	10 sec
Dumbbell walking lunge**	8/20 sec	10 sec
Dead landmine**	8/20 sec	10 sec
Kettlebell snatch**	8/20 sec	10 sec
Band woodchopper	8/20 sec	10 sec

WORKOUT 3 (WEDNESDAY): SHOULDERS/TRAPS

Exercise	Sets/time	Rest
Smith machine shoulder press*	8/20 sec	10 sec
Smith machine upright row*	8/20 sec	10 sec
Dumbbell lateral raise*	8/20 sec	10 sec
Standing cable rear delt fly*	8/20 sec	10 sec
Barbell shrug*	8/20 sec	10 sec
Smith machine behind-the-back shrug*	8/20 sec	10 sec

WORKOUT 3 (WEDNESDAY): SHOULDERS/TRAPS (cont.)

Exercise	Sets/time	Rest
Medicine ball overhead throw**	8/20 sec	10 sec
Burpee**	8/20 sec	10 sec
Kettlebell swing**	8/20 sec	10 sec
Medicine ball slam	8/20 sec	10 sec

WORKOUT 4 (THURSDAY): BACK/ABS

Exercise	Sets/time	Rest
Bent-over barbell row*	8/20 sec	10 sec
Pulldown*	8/20 sec	10 sec
Seated cable row*	8/20 sec	10 sec
Straight-arm pulldown*	8/20 sec	10 sec
Crossover crunch*	8/20 sec	10 sec
Cable crunch*	8/20 sec	10 sec
Push-up**	8/20 sec	10 sec
Dead curl press**	8/20 sec	10 sec
Heavy bag work**	8/20 sec	10 sec
Dumbbell clean	8/20 sec	10 sec

WORKOUT 5 (FRIDAY): TRICEPS/BICEPS/FOREARMS

Exercise	Sets/time	Rest
Lying triceps extension*	8/20 sec	10 sec
Triceps pressdown*	8/20 sec	10 sec
Cable overhead extension*	8/20 sec	10 sec
Barbell curl*	8/20 sec	10 sec
Incline dumbbell curl*	8/20 sec	10 sec
Dumbbell hammer curl*	8/20 sec	10 sec
Barbell wrist curl*	8/20 sec	10 sec
Barbell reverse wrist curl*	8/20 sec	10 sec
Burpee**	8/20 sec	10 sec
Dumbbell walking lunge**	8/20 sec	10 sec
Dead landmine**	8/20 sec	10 sec
Band roundhouse elbow	8/20 sec	10 sec

* Rest 1-2 minutes between exercises.

**Take no rest between exercises.

Band Whole-Body Workout

This is a great exercise-bands-only workout for when you travel and don't have access to free weights or when you just want to switch things up (see table 13.6). It involves several high-intensity training techniques such as supersets and giant sets to increase calorie burn during and after the workout. It also is a whole-body training split, which means that all your major muscle groups will need to recover after the workout, which will boost metabolic rate after the workout. It also includes cardioacceleration to help burn the fat.

Do this workout three times per week. Or you can even use it as a cardio conditioning workout on your off days from weight training. Either way, it's a great way to increase your conditioning and decrease body fat.

TABLE 13.6 Band Whole-Body Workout

Exercise	Sets/reps	Exercise	Sets/reps
Power push-up	1/5-8	Giant set with band lateral raise	1/10
Superset with band straight-arm pullback	1/10	Giant set with band upright row	1/10
Cardioacceleration: Squat jump	1/5-8	Giant set with band shoulder press	1/10
Superset with body-weight squat	1/40 sec	Cardioacceleration: Body-weight lunge	1/60 sec
Power push-up	1/5-8	Band rear delt pull	1/10
Superset with band straight-arm pullback	1/10	Giant set with band lateral raise	1/10
Cardioacceleration: Squat jump	1/5-8	Giant set with band upright row	1/10
Superset with body-weight squat	1/40 sec	Giant set with band shoulder press	1/10
Power push-up	1/5-8	Cardioacceleration: Body-weight lunge	1/60 sec
Superset with band straight-arm pullback	1/10	Band triceps overhead extension	1/10
Cardioacceleration: Squat jump	1/5-8	Superset with band biceps curl	1/10
Superset with body-weight squat	1/40 sec	Cardioacceleration: Lateral hop	1/60 sec
Incline band press	1/15	Band triceps overhead extension	1/10
Superset with band bent-over row	1/15	Superset with band biceps curl	1/10
Cardioacceleration: Jumping jack	1/60 sec	Cardioacceleration: Lateral hop	1/60 sec
Incline band press	1/15	Band triceps overhead extension	1/10
Superset with band bent-over row	1/15	Superset with band biceps curl	1/10
Cardioacceleration: Jumping jack	1/60 sec	Cardioacceleration: Lateral hop	1/60 sec
Incline band press	1/15	Band triceps overhead extension	1/10
Superset with band bent-over row	1/15	Superset with band biceps curl	1/10
Cardioacceleration: Jumping jack	1/60 sec	Cardioacceleration: Lateral hop	1/60 sec
Band rear delt pull	1/10	Reverse crunch	1/20
Giant set with band lateral raise	1/10	Superset with twisting crunch	1/20
Giant set with band upright row	1/10	Cardioacceleration: Calf jump	1/60 sec
Giant set with band shoulder press	1/10	Reverse crunch	1/20
Cardioacceleration: Body-weight lunge	1/60 sec	Superset with twisting crunch	1/20
Band rear delt pull	1/10	Cardioacceleration: Calf jump	1/60 sec
		Reverse crunch	1/20
		Superset with twisting crunch	1/20
		Cardioacceleration: Calf jump	1/60 sec

PART V

TRAINING EXERCISES

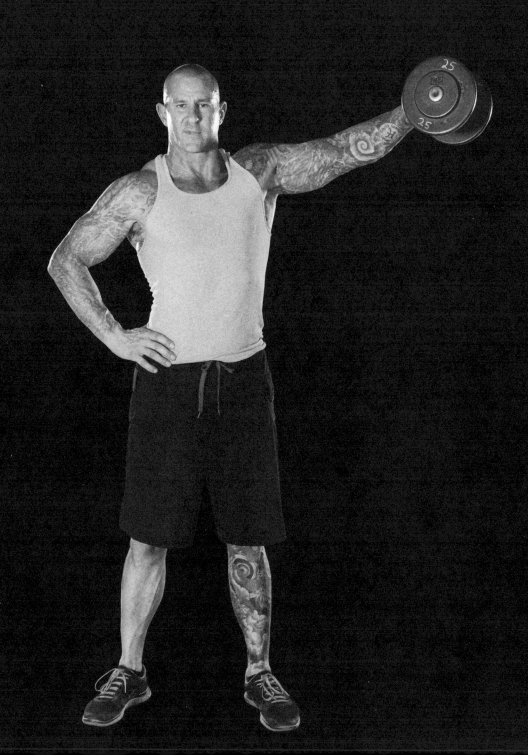

No matter how sound an exercise program is, it won't be effective without the proper execution of the exercises that make up that program. Contained in this section are the descriptions for proper form of every exercise covered in the previous chapters, in addition to many others not covered. This is a total of 381 exercises. Accompanying each exercise description is a photo or two of that exercise to help you visualize the proper execution of each exercise.

Each chapter covers the exercises that train one specific muscle group. These chapters organize the exercises into similar movements that train that muscle group in a similar manner. This is to encourage you to frequently substitute exercises in a program with other exercises that are similar in the effect they will have on a particular muscle. This not only will help to prevent stagnation of muscle adaptations and overall boredom but will also encourage the greatest gains in muscle growth and strength. This is because the slightest variation of an exercise can target different muscle fibers within a muscle group.

Regardless of your goals, having such an arsenal of exercises to choose from will help to maximize your results. Whatever program you are following, you can use this section to change the exercise selections. To do this for any exercise, simply choose from the list of exercises that accompany that exercise in the same category. For example, to find an alternative exercise for the bench press, just choose one of the other exercises from the barbell pressing exercises category, such as incline bench press, decline bench press, Smith machine flat bench press, Smith machine incline bench press, or Smith machine decline bench press. Just be sure to follow the guidelines discussed in chapters 5, 8, and 11 for exercise selection and order. Making the slightest alterations to a program while staying within the suggested guidelines is the best way to individualize a program for best results.

CHAPTER 14

Chest

This chapter contains detailed descriptions of all major exercises that focus on the chest (pectoral) muscles. The pectoralis major muscles are divided into the upper and lower sections (see diagram). Although many of these exercises are pressing movements (such as the bench press) that are multijoint exercises, requiring the use of the deltoids and triceps as well as the pectorals, they are considered primarily chest exercises because of the movement of the upper arms. The chest exercises are divided into barbell pressing exercises; dumbbell pressing exercises; machine, cable, or band pressing exercises; fly-type exercises; and push-up, dip, and pullover exercises. Wherever a certain type of exercise is used in a workout, any one of the same type can be substituted (for example, if the incline bench press is called for, any barbell press exercise can be substituted).

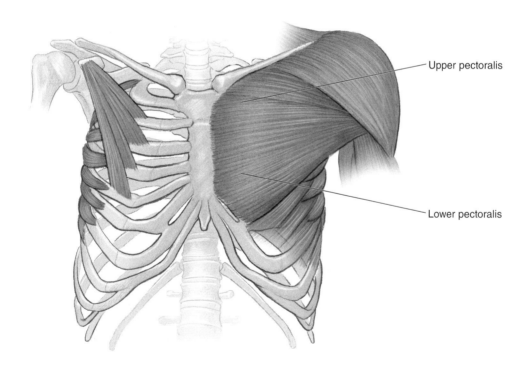

Upper pectoralis

Lower pectoralis

BENCH PRESS

START

Lie faceup on a bench-press bench with your feet flat on the floor. Grasp the barbell with an overhand grip, hands slightly wider than shoulder-width apart.

MOVE

Unrack the bar and slowly lower it toward your chest. Keep your wrists aligned with your elbows and your elbows pointed out to your sides so that your upper arms form a 30- to 60-degree angle with your torso. When the bar just touches your chest, press back up explosively, driving the weight away from you until you almost lock it out.

Note: For details on performing the bench press to maximize strength, see chapter 8.

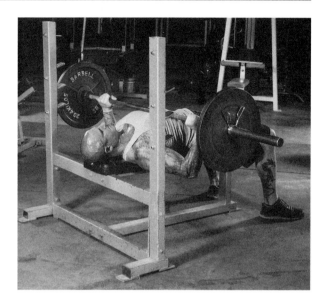

INCLINE BENCH PRESS

START

Lie on an incline bench-press bench and grasp the racked barbell with a grip that's slightly wider than shoulder width, palms facing toward the ceiling. Lift the bar off the rack and raise it until your arms are fully extended.

MOVE

Bend your elbows to lower the bar to your upper chest. At the bottom, your elbows should be out and away from your body but slightly in front of your shoulders. Contract your chest muscles and extend your elbows to press the bar up until your elbows are almost locked out.

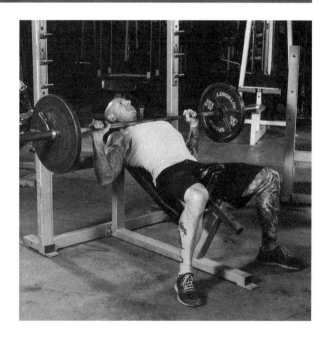

DECLINE BENCH PRESS

START

Lie back on a decline bench-press bench set to a 30- to 40-degree decline. Grasp the barbell with an overhand grip with both hands slightly wider than shoulder-width apart. Lift the bar off the supports and hold it over your lower chest with your arms extended.

MOVE

Lower the barbell to your lower chest. Immediately push the bar back up to full extension without locking your elbows out at the top.

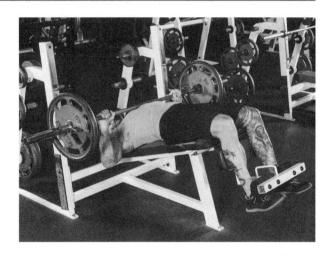

BARBELL BENCH PRESS WITH BANDS

START

Place an exercise band securely under the bench and secure each barbell cuff onto either side of the barbell. An easy way to secure the ends of the bands on the bar is by placing them between two weight plates. If you cannot place the band under the bench, then use one band on each end of the bar and secure it to a heavy dumbbell on each side under the bar.

MOVE

Perform the bench press as you normally would as described earlier in this chapter. You can also use the bands in a similar manner on the incline bench press and decline bench press.

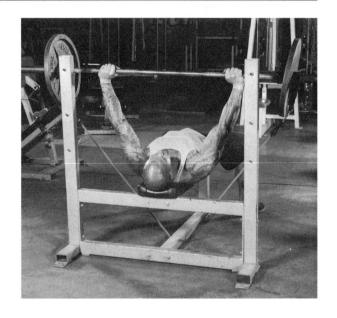

BARBELL FLOOR PRESS

START

Although this is a bench press done on the floor, unless you are very thin, you will not be able to fit under the bar even when it is loaded with 45-pound plates. So you will need to set the bar on the lower rack of a power rack. Once the barbell is set in the power rack, lie faceup on the floor in the middle of the power rack so that the bar is above your head. Keep your back flat on the floor and your knees bent with feet flat on the floor. Unrack the barbell and hold it over your chest.

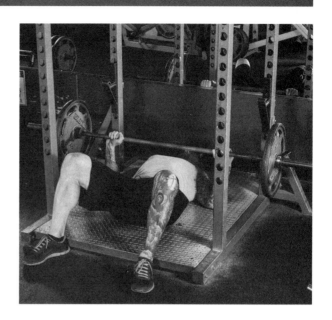

MOVE

Lower the bar toward your lower chest until the back of your upper arms touch the floor. The bar will be several inches above your chest and will not touch your chest. This is the point of doing the floor press because it lessens the range of motion, which allows you to use more weight. Press the bar up and toward your head so that the bar is above your upper chest in the top position.

REVERSE-GRIP BENCH PRESS

START

Grasp the barbell with an underhand grip with your hands spaced wider than shoulder-width apart.

MOVE

Have a spotter help you unrack the bar because it is difficult to do so alone with the underhand grip. Once the bar is positioned over your chest, lower the bar to your lower chest or upper abs and then press the bar back up toward your head. If you must do this exercise alone, unrack the bar with an overhand grip and lower it to your chest. With the bar on your chest, carefully swap your grip from overhand to underhand and perform the exercise. Research shows that this exercise recruits a greater number of muscle fibers in the upper pecs than the overhand grip. You can also use the reverse grip on the incline bench press to further hit the upper pecs.

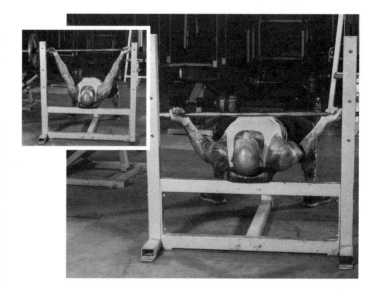

SMITH MACHINE FLAT BENCH PRESS

START

Position yourself on a flat bench that is positioned in a Smith machine so that the bar lines up with your lower chest (where your nipples are). Grasp the bar with an overhand grip spaced slightly wider than shoulder-width apart. Release the safety hooks.

MOVE

Lower the bar to your chest. Press the bar back up to full arm extension, stopping just short of elbow lockout. Pause at the top and lower the bar under control to your upper chest.

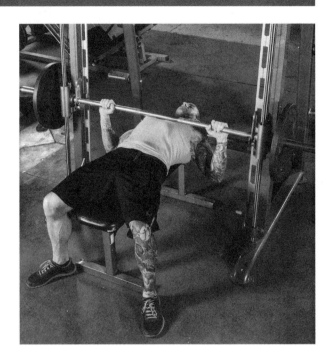

SMITH MACHINE INCLINE BENCH PRESS

START

Position yourself on an incline bench (set to about 30 to 40 degrees) that is positioned in a Smith machine so that the bar lines up with the top of your chest. Grasp the bar with an overhand grip spaced slightly wider than shoulder-width apart. Release the safety hooks.

MOVE

Lower the bar to your chest. Press the bar up to full arm extension, stopping just short of elbow lockout.

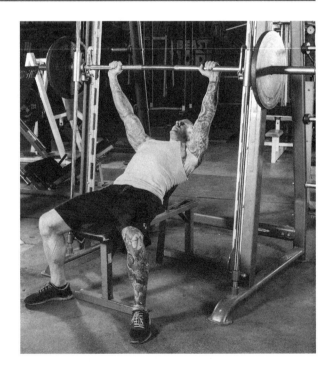

SMITH MACHINE DECLINE BENCH PRESS

START

Position yourself on a decline bench (set to about 30 to 45 degrees) that is positioned in a Smith machine so that the bar lines up with the lower part of your chest. Grasp the bar with an overhand grip that is slightly wider than shoulder-width apart. Release the safety hooks.

MOVE

Lower the bar to your chest. Press the bar up to full arm extension, stopping just short of elbow lockout.

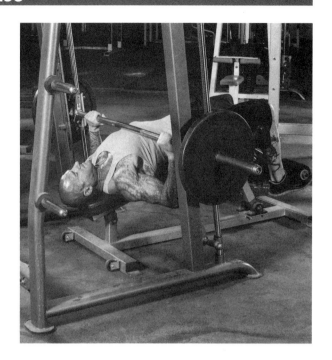

ONE-ARM SMITH MACHINE BENCH PRESS

START

Position yourself on a flat bench that is positioned in a Smith machine so that the bar lines up with your lower chest (where your nipples are). Grasp the bar with a one-hand overhand grip that is spaced slightly wider than shoulder-width apart.

MOVE

Release the safety hooks and then slowly lower the bar to your chest. Press the bar back up to full arm extension, stopping just short of elbow lockout. Complete all reps on one arm and then repeat with the other arm.

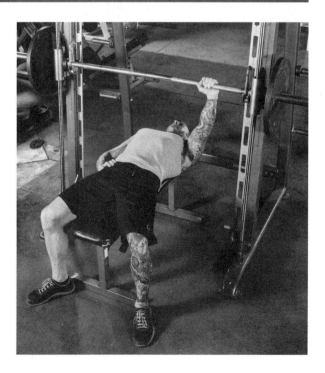

ONE-ARM SMITH MACHINE NEGATIVE BENCH PRESS

START

For those who train alone, doing negative reps is almost impossible. Yet the Smith machine allows you to train with negative reps one arm at a time. Position yourself on a flat bench that is in a Smith machine so that the bar lines up with your lower chest (where your nipples are). Grasp the bar with a one-hand overhand grip that is spaced slightly wider than shoulder-width apart.

MOVE

Release the safety hooks and then slowly lower the bar about a quarter of the way down. From there, resist the bar as long as you can to prevent the bar from lowering to your chest. It should take you no less than 3 seconds and no more than 8 seconds for the weight to reach your chest. If it's shorter than this, decrease the weight. If it's longer, increase the weight. Press the bar up using both arms and then repeat on the opposite arm. Alternate arms each rep.

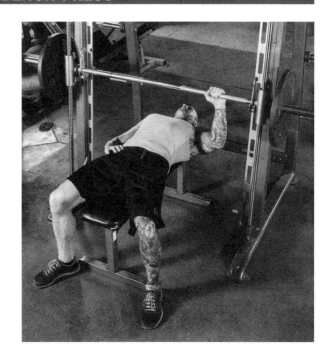

SMITH MACHINE BENCH PRESS THROW

START

Position yourself on a flat bench that is in a Smith machine so that the bar lines up with your lower chest (where your nipples are). Grasp the bar with an overhand grip that is spaced slightly wider than shoulder-width apart. Release the safety hooks.

MOVE

Slowly lower the bar to your chest and explode the bar off of your chest by pressing the bar back up to full arm extension with as much speed and power as possible. Allow the bar to leave your hands in the top position. Catch the bar on the return with slightly bent elbows without stopping the bar and guide it down to your chest and then immediately perform the next rep.

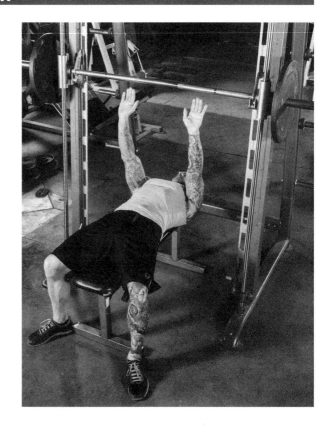

SMITH MACHINE REVERSE-GRIP BENCH PRESS

START

Position yourself on a flat bench that is in a Smith machine so that the bar lines up with your lower chest or upper abs. Grasp the bar with an underhand grip that is spaced slightly wider than shoulder-width apart. Release the safety hooks.

MOVE

Slowly lower the bar to your chest and then press the bar back up to full arm extension, stopping just short of elbow lockout. You can also do this on an incline bench.

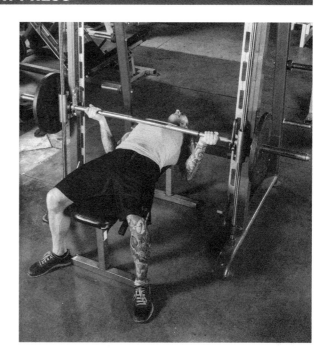

DUMBBELL BENCH PRESS

START

Lie faceup on a flat bench with your feet planted flat on the floor. Hold the dumbbells just outside your chest with your elbows out to your sides, so your upper arms form a 30- to 60-degree angle with your torso.

MOVE

Forcefully press the weights up in an arc (coming toward each other at the top) until your arms are fully extended above your chest. Reverse the motion, being sure not to lower the dumbbells below chest level.

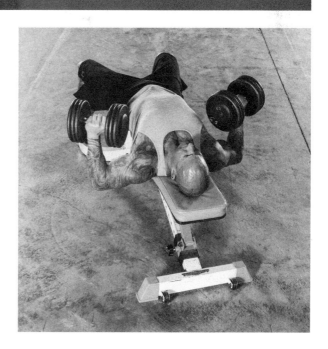

INCLINE DUMBBELL PRESS

START

Lie squarely on an incline bench, which should be set at a fairly low angle (less than 45 degrees). Hold the dumbbells just outside your shoulders with your elbows out to your sides and your feet planted flat on the floor.

MOVE

Forcefully press the weights up in an arc (coming toward each other at the top) until your arms are fully extended above your chest. Reverse the motion, being sure not to lower the dumbbells below chest level.

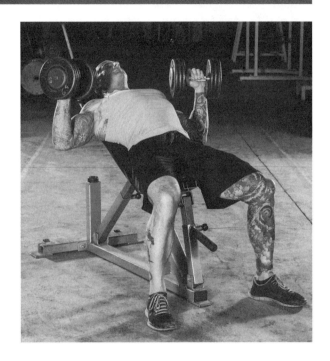

DECLINE DUMBBELL PRESS

START

Lie back on a decline bench set to 30 to 40 degrees with your feet secured under the foot pads. Hold the dumbbells just outside your lower chest with your elbows out to your sides.

MOVE

Forcefully press the weights up in an arc (coming toward each other at the top) until your arms are fully extended above your lower chest or upper abs.

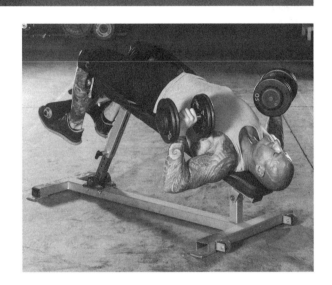

ONE-ARM DUMBBELL BENCH PRESS

START

Grasp a dumbbell and lie faceup on the bench. Hold the dumbbell just outside your shoulder with your elbow out to your sides. With your other arm, grasp the side of the bench down by your hip.

MOVE

Press the dumbbell up until your arm is fully extended above your chest. Reverse the motion, being sure not to lower the dumbbells below lower chest level. Complete the desired number of reps and repeat with your other arm.

Note: You can also do this exercise on the incline or decline bench in a similar manner.

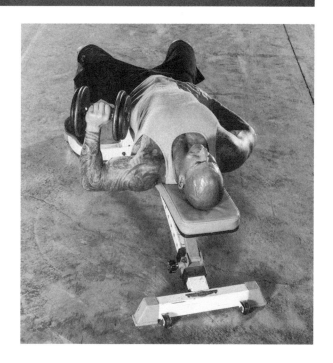

EXERCISE-BALL DUMBBELL PRESS

START

Grasping two dumbbells, lie with your upper back on an exercise ball with your feet planted firmly on the floor. Hold the dumbbells just outside your shoulders with your palms facing forward and your elbows out to your sides.

MOVE

Forcefully press the weights up in an arc (coming toward each other at the top) until your arms are fully extended above your chest. Reverse the motion, being sure not to lower the dumbbells below chest level.

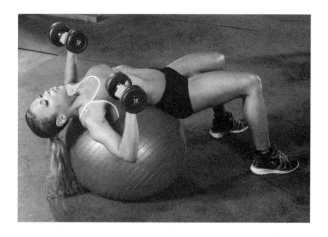

NEUTRAL-GRIP FLAT BENCH DUMBBELL PRESS

START

Grasping two dumbbells, lie on a flat bench and turn your wrists so that they are toward each other, hands at each side of your torso with the dumbbells above your body.

MOVE

Press the dumbbells upward, allowing them to naturally move toward each other at the top (without touching). Then reverse the move back to the starting position.

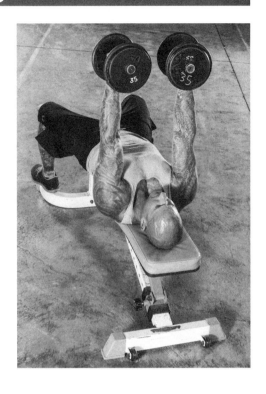

REVERSE-GRIP DUMBBELL PRESS

START

Lie on a flat bench while holding one dumbbell in each hand outside your chest. Turn your wrists outward so that your palms are pointed toward your face for the position known as the reverse grip.

MOVE

Press the dumbbells up and together in an arc over your chest while maintaining the reverse grip. Then slowly lower the dumbbells back to the start position and repeat for reps.

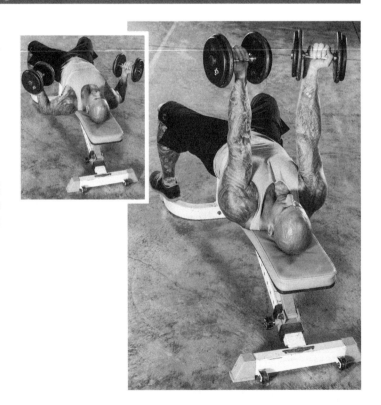

SEATED CHEST PRESS MACHINE

START

Position the handles of the machine so that they line up with your mid- to lower chest. Sit back in the seat and grab the handles with an overhand grip.

MOVE

Press the handles out in front of you until your arms are fully extended but not locked, then slowly bring the handles back toward your chest without letting the weights touch the stack. Some machines also offer an incline chest press version that allows you to mimic the incline bench press to focus more on the upper chest.

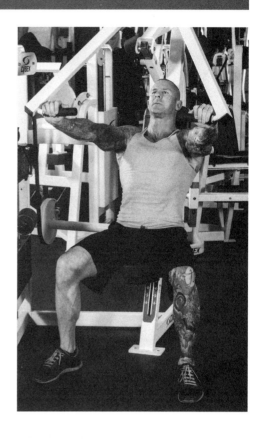

ONE-ARM CABLE CHEST PRESS

START

Stand facing away from a pulley cable apparatus with your feet shoulder-width apart or wider; maintain a slight bend in your knees. If the pulley height is adjustable, bring it to just above shoulder height. Grasp the single-handle D-grip with an overhand grip and hold it just outside your shoulder with your elbow out to your side so that your upper arm forms a 30- to 60-degree angle with your torso.

MOVE

Forcefully press the handle out in front of you until your arm is fully extended in front of your chest but your elbow is not locked out. Reverse the motion, being sure not to return the handle behind the level of your chest.

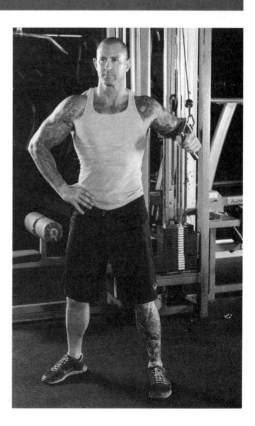

CABLE CROSSOVER CHEST PRESS

START

Attach single-handle D-grip handles to the high pulleys on a cable crossover apparatus. Stand in the direct center of the machine with one foot in front of the other and with your knees slightly bent. Grasp the handles with your palms facing down and keep your elbows slightly bent and facing up toward the ceiling. Lean slightly forward at the waist.

MOVE

In a simultaneous downward and inward motion, bring the handles to a point in front of your mid-section, keeping your arms slightly bent. Pause a moment and squeeze your pec muscles before slowly allowing the handles to return to the start position.

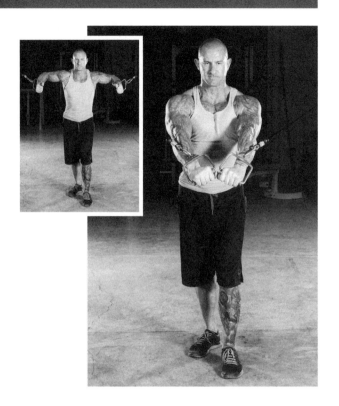

CABLE CROSSOVER CHEST PRESS (FROM LOW PULLEYS)

START

Attach single-handle D-grip handles to the lower pulleys on a cable crossover apparatus. Stand in the direct center of the apparatus with one foot in front of the other with your knees slightly bent. Grasp the handles with your palms facing up and keep your elbows bent and facing down toward the floor and behind you. Maintain the arch in your lower back and keep your chest up.

MOVE

In a simultaneous upward and inward motion, bring the handles to a point straight out in front of you so your hands are level with your chin or higher. Pause a moment and squeeze your pec muscles before slowly allowing the handles to return to the start position.

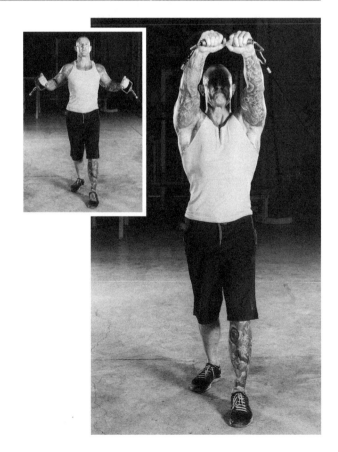

CABLE BENCH PRESS

START

Place a flat bench in the center of a cable cross-over apparatus. Lower the cable pulleys on the lowest setting. Grasp the D-handles in both hands and lie down onto the bench. Start with your elbows bent and hands evenly placed on the sides of the chest.

MOVE

With both hands, press firmly upward, squeezing the pecs and bringing the handles toward the center line of the body. Slowly lower down and repeat for reps. You can cross your hands in the top position for better recruitment of the inner-pec muscles. You can also do this exercise on an incline or decline bench.

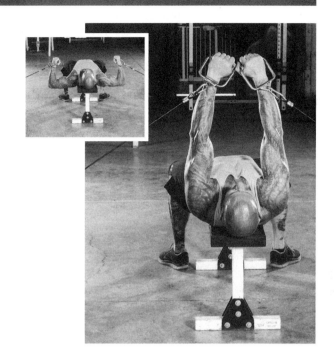

STANDING BAND CHEST PRESS

START

Secure the band at about shoulder height around an immobile object, or use the door attachment and face away from the door. Make sure that both lengths of the band on either side are equal. Either place both feet shoulder-width apart or stagger step with one foot forward and the other back.

MOVE

Press the bands out in front of the chest with both arms and bring the band handles together, squeezing the pecs as you press out, then return to the start and repeat until you complete the set. This targets more of the middle and lower pecs. To target more of the upper pecs, attach the band to a position close to the floor and press the bands up and together in front of your face.

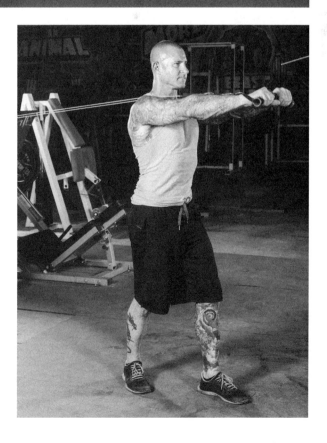

DUMBBELL FLY

START

Lie on a flat bench with your feet flat on the floor and your back pressed against the pad. Begin by holding the dumbbells with your arms straight up from your shoulders and the weights directly over your chest. Your palms should face each other and your elbows should be slightly bent. Maintain this angle of your elbows throughout the entire exercise.

MOVE

Slowly lower your arms out to your sides until your wrists come to about shoulder level or slightly above. Bring your arms back toward the midline of your body, focusing on using your pec muscles to draw them back together.

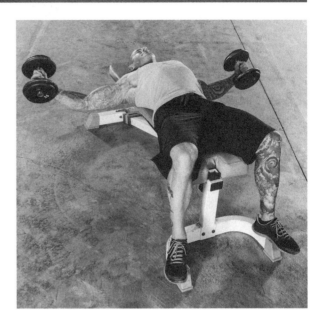

INCLINE DUMBBELL FLY

START

Set an incline bench at a 30- to 45-degree angle. Lie on the bench with your feet flat on the floor and your back pressed against the pad. Begin by holding the dumbbells with your arms straight up from your shoulders and the dumbbells directly over your upper chest. Your palms should face each other and your elbows should be slightly bent. Maintain this angle of your elbows through-out the entire exercise.

MOVE

Slowly lower your arms out to your sides until your wrists come to about shoulder level or slightly above. Bring your arms back toward the midline of your body, focusing on using your pec muscles to draw them back together.

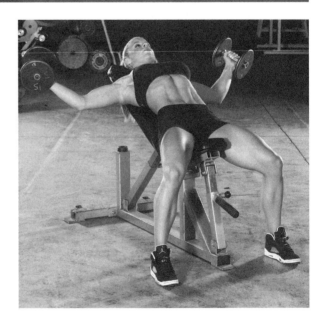

DECLINE DUMBBELL FLY

START

Set an decline bench at a 30- to 40-degree angle. Lie on the bench with your feet secured under the ankle pads and your back pressed against the pad. Begin by holding the dumbbells with your arms straight up from your shoulders and the dumbbells directly over your lower chest. Your palms should face each other and your elbows should be slightly bent. Maintain this angle of your elbows throughout the entire exercise.

MOVE

Slowly lower your arms out to your sides until your wrists come to about shoulder level or slightly above. Bring your arms back toward the midline of your body, focusing on using your pec muscles to draw them back together.

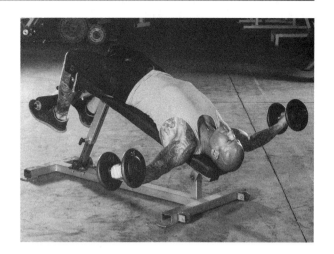

EXERCISE-BALL DUMBBELL FLY

START

This exercise is similar to the fly on the flat bench except that here your body works harder to keep you stabilized. Grab two dumbbells and lie back on a ball so that you face the ceiling. Your feet should be firmly planted on the floor about shoulder-width apart. Begin by holding the dumbbells with your arms straight up from your shoulders and the weights directly over your chest. Your palms should face each other and your elbows should be slightly bent. Maintain this angle of your elbows throughout the entire exercise.

MOVE

Slowly lower your arms out to your sides until your wrists come to about shoulder level or slightly above. Bring your arms back toward the midline of your body, focusing on using your pec muscles to draw them back together.

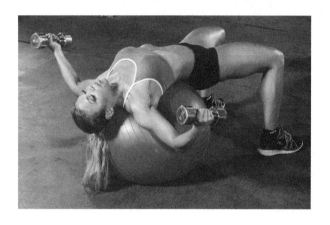

LEANING ONE-ARM DUMBBELL FLY

START

Take a dumbbell in one hand; with the opposite hand, grasp a secure post such as that on a power rack or cable apparatus. Lean out at about a 45-degree angle away from the rack and let the hand with the dumbbell hang to the floor.

MOVE

Keep the working arm straight with just a slight bend in the elbow. Raise the dumbbell in an upward fashion toward the opposite shoulder, squeezing the pecs at the top of the movement and then slowly lowering the dumbbell back to the start position. Repeat for reps on one arm and then on the other arm.

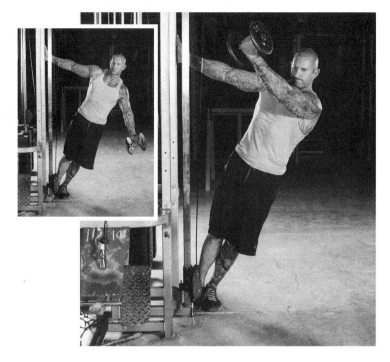

CABLE FLY

START

Connect two of the single-handle D-grips to the low pulleys of a cable crossover apparatus. Position the bench in the middle of the cable crossover apparatus so that the cables are in line with your chest. Lie on the bench with your feet flat on the floor and your back pressed against the pad. Begin by holding the handles with your arms straight out at your sides and your palms facing up while maintaining a slight bend in your elbows.

MOVE

Use your pecs to bring the arms up and together over your chest until your hands meet, maintaining the slight bend in your elbows as you do. Slowly return to the starting position by lowering your arms back out to your sides until your wrists come to about shoulder level or slightly above.

Note: You can also do this exercise on an incline bench, decline bench, or exercise ball in a similar manner.

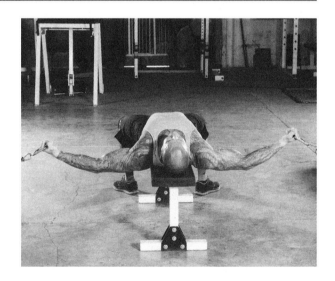

CABLE CROSSOVER

START

Attach single-handle D-grip handles to the upper pulleys on a cable crossover apparatus. Stand in the direct center of the machine with one foot in front of the other and your knees slightly bent. Grasp the handles with your palms facing down, and keep your elbows slightly bent and pointing up toward the ceiling. Lean slightly forward at the waist.

MOVE

In a simultaneous downward and inward motion, bring the handles to a point in the front of your midsection, keeping your arms slightly bent. Pause a moment and squeeze your pec muscles before slowly allowing the handles to return to the starting position.

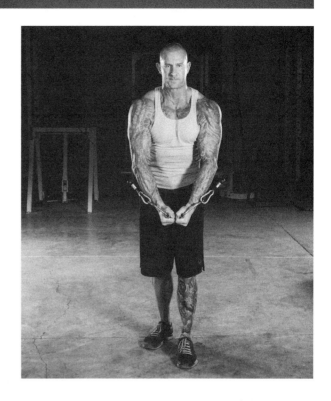

LOW-PULLEY CABLE CROSSOVER

START

Attach single-handle D-grip handles to the lower pulleys on a cable crossover apparatus. Stand in the direct center of the apparatus with one foot in front of the other and your knees slightly bent. Grasp the handles with your palms facing up, and keep your elbows slightly bent and pointing down toward the floor and behind you. Maintain the arch in your low back and keep your chest up.

MOVE

In a simultaneous upward and inward motion, bring the handles to a point straight out in front of you so that your hands are level with your forehead. Pause a moment and squeeze your pec muscles before slowly allowing the handles to return to the starting position.

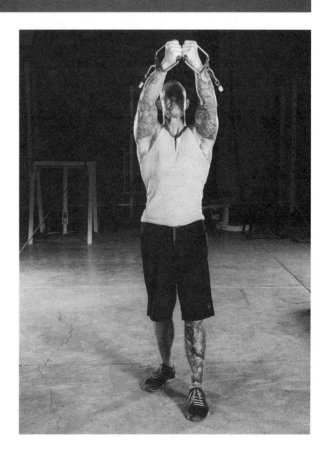

FLY MACHINE

START

Adjust the seat so that your shoulders, elbows, and hands are all in line and your arms are parallel to the floor when you grab the handles. Your elbows should be slightly bent and pointing behind you and your back should be flat against the back pad.

MOVE

Forcefully bring the handles all the way together, making sure to keep your elbows bent. Squeeze your pecs for a second before reversing the motion to allow the handles to go back to a point where your hands are even with your chest.

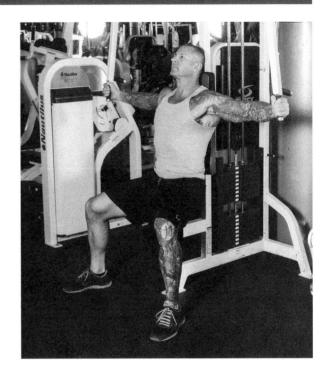

ONE-ARM STANDING BAND FLY

START

Although you could do this exercise with both arms, it's often tough to find enough space or area to attach two bands at the same height, so the one-arm version is easier to set up and allows you to focus on each side better. Attach the band to a secure spot or use a door anchor. Place the band at about shoulder height. Stand far enough away from the band so that you have adequate tension at the start of the movement. Hold the band with your arm extended to the side with a slight bend in your elbow.

MOVE

Contract your pec to bring your arm across the front of your body before returning your arm to the start position. Repeat all reps on one arm and then perform on the other arm. With the band in this position, the focus is on the middle pec. To target more of the upper pec, lower the attachment point of the band toward the floor and bring your arm up toward your face as it crosses your body. To target more of the lower pec, attach the band higher than shoulder height and bring your arm down toward your opposite hip as it crosses your body.

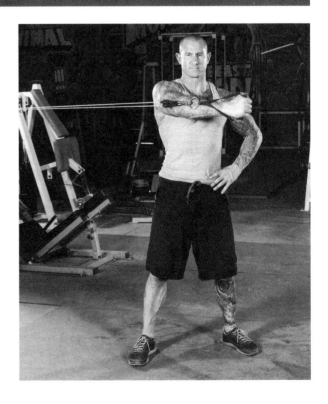

TRX FLY

START

Set the TRX at a height that reduces your body weight enough to perform this tough exercise. Get in the push-up position with your hands in the TRX handles, palms facing each other, and toes only on the floor.

MOVE

Maintaining a slight bend in your elbows, extend your arms out to your sides as wide as you can to stretch the pecs, and lower your body toward the floor. Then reverse the motion by contracting your pecs to bring your arms back together, lifting your body weight. Start with a short range of motion and gradually increase it as you get stronger on this exercise.

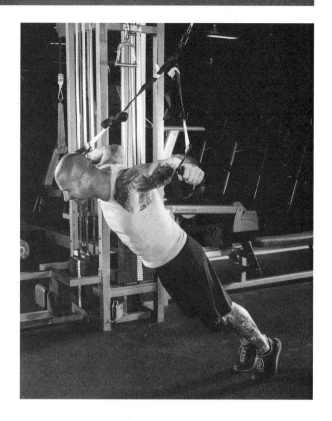

PUSH-UP

START

Lie facedown on the floor with your hands slightly wider than shoulder width. Your palms should be flat on the floor and your elbows out to your sides, so your upper arms form a 30- to 60-degree angle with your torso. Your body should be straight with just your palms and toes touching the floor.

MOVE

Raise your body up by pushing your palms into the floor to fully extend your arms without locking out the elbows at the top. Reverse the movement to return your body toward the floor.

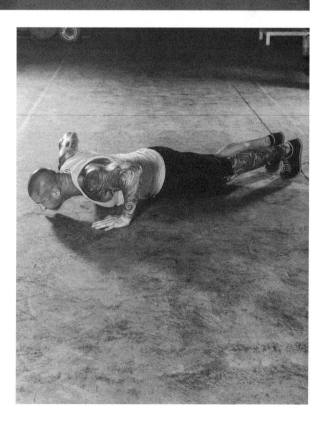

INCLINE PUSH-UP

START

This is similar to the push-up but with your hands on a bench. Although this is called the incline push-up, it focuses more on the lower pecs. Also, because your upper body is raised from the floor, the resistance your body provides is decreased compared to doing the push-up on the floor. This makes the incline push-up easier than the standard push-up. Your hands should be placed firmly on the bench and spaced slightly wider than shoulder-width apart. Elbows are bent and upper arms are out to your sides, so your upper arms form a 30- to 60-degree angle with your torso. Your body should be extended behind you with just your toes touching the floor.

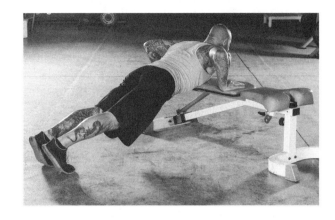

MOVE

Raise your body up by pushing your palms into the bench to fully extend your arms without locking out the elbows at the top. Reverse the movement to return your upper body toward the bench.

DECLINE PUSH-UP

START

This is similar to the incline push-up, but your body position is reversed. Although this is called the decline push-up, it focuses more on the upper pecs. Also, because your lower body is raised from the floor, the resistance your body provides is increased compared to doing the push-up on the floor. This makes the decline push-up harder than the standard push-up. Your hands are placed firmly on the floor and spaced slightly wider than shoulder-width apart. Elbows are bent and upper arms are out to your sides, so your upper arms form a 30- to 60-degree angle with your torso. Your body should be extended behind you with just your feet up on the bench and just your toes touching the bench.

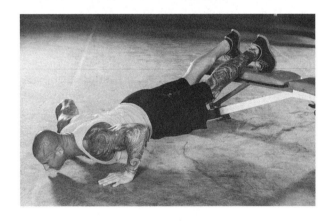

MOVE

Raise your body up by pushing your palms into the floor to fully extend your arms without locking out the elbows at the top. Reverse the movement to return your upper body toward the floor.

EXERCISE-BALL PUSH-UP

START

This exercise is similar to the incline push-up but uses a ball instead of a bench. The instability of the exercise ball makes the exercise far more difficult to perform than the standard push-up and helps to work the shoulder girdle stabilizer muscles and core. Make sure the ball is fairly secure and get into push-up position with your hands on the ball and feet on the floor. Your elbows should be bent with your upper arms out to your sides.

MOVE

Keeping your body straight, raise your body up by pushing your palms into the ball to fully extend your arms without locking out the elbows at the top. Reverse the movement to return your upper body toward the ball.

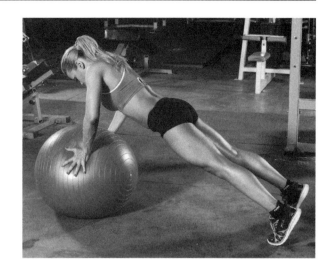

POWER PUSH-UP

START

Lie facedown on the floor with your hands slightly wider than shoulder-width apart. Palms are flat on the floor and elbows are out to your sides, so your upper arms form a 30- to 60-degree angle with your torso. Your body should be straight with just your palms and toes touching the floor.

MOVE

Raise your body up from the floor by explosively pushing your palms into the floor to fully extend your arms so that your palms leave the floor. As you land, allow your elbows to bend and immediately lower your body back to the floor.

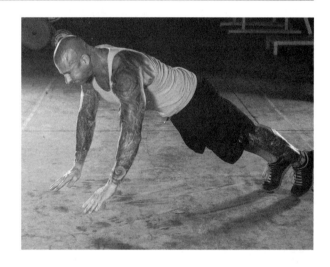

PUSH-UP LADDER

START

Get in push-up position on the floor near a Smith machine.

MOVE

Perform push-ups on the floor as described previously until you reach muscle failure. Immediately move to the bar of the Smith machine set on the lowest setting and continue doing push-ups with your hands on the bar and feet on the floor, similar to incline push-ups described previously. Once you reach muscle failure, raise the bar one notch on the Smith machine and continue doing push-ups. Continue in this manner doing push-ups to failure and raising the bar height on the Smith machine by one notch until the bar is just above waist height.

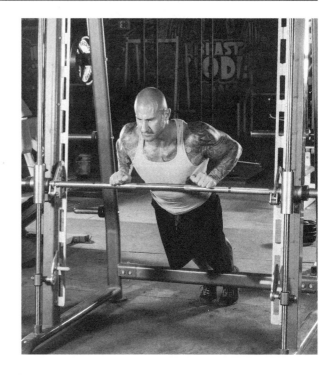

TRX PUSH-UP

START

Set the TRX at a height that reduces your body weight enough to perform this exercise. Get in the push-up position with your hands in the TRX handles and your feet firmly on the floor.

MOVE

Bend your elbows like in a normal push-up to lower your body until your chest is level with the handles. Keep your elbows tucked in slightly so that your upper arms form a 30- to 60-degree angle with your torso during this exercise. Reverse the motion by pressing your arms down to lift your body weight until your arms are fully extended.

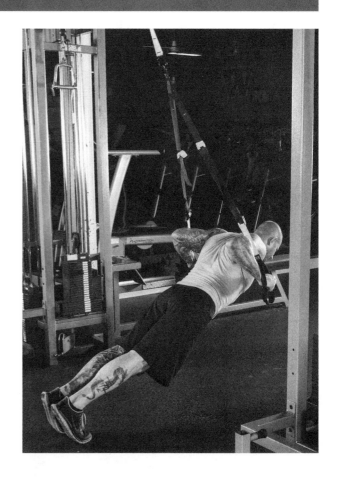

CHEST DIP

START

Grasp the dip bars with your arms extended and locked. Lean forward and bend your knees while keeping your legs crossed.

MOVE

Keep your elbows out to your sides as you bend them to lower your body down until your upper arms are about parallel to the floor. Press your hands into the bars to extend your arms and raise your body back up.

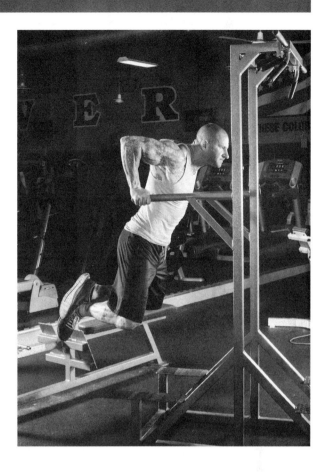

DUMBBELL PULLOVER

START

Lie across a flat bench with your upper back supported by the bench and your feet flat on the floor about shoulder-width apart or wider. Hold the inside edge of a dumbbell at arm's length directly over your chest and drop your hips slightly toward the floor.

MOVE

Bring your arms back behind your head as far as possible while keeping a slight bend in your elbows. Reverse the direction and pull the weight back up over your chest.

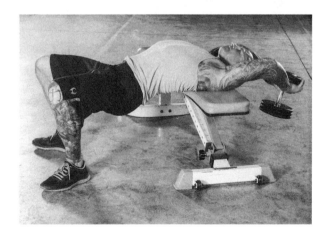

CHAPTER 15

Shoulders

This chapter contains detailed descriptions of all major exercises that focus on the shoulders, or deltoid muscles. The deltoid muscles are divided into the front (anterior) head, middle (lateral) head, and rear (posterior) head. (See the diagram.) Although many of these exercises are pressing movements (such as the barbell overhead press) that are multijoint exercises, requiring the use of the trapezius and the triceps as well as the deltoids, they are considered primarily shoulder exercises because of the movement of the upper arms overhead. The shoulder exercises are divided into pressing exercises, upright row exercises, and raises. There are also rotator cuff exercises at the end for keeping your shoulder stabilizers strong and preventing injury, which is an all-too-common problem among weightlifters with weak rotator cuff muscles. The pressing exercises are further divided into barbell overhead pressing exercises; dumbbell overhead pressing exercises; and machine, band, and body-weight overhead pressing exercises. The upright row exercises are further divided into barbell upright row exercises, Smith machine upright row exercises, dumbbell upright row exercises, cable upright row exercises, and band upright row exercises. The raises are further divided into front raise exercises, lateral raise exercises, and rear deltoid exercises. Wherever a certain type of exercise is used in a workout, any one of the same type can be substituted.

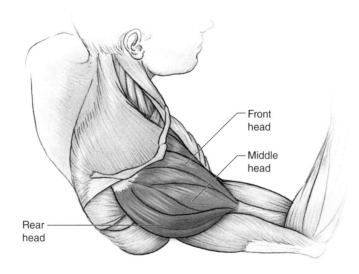

Front head

Middle head

Rear head

Barbell Overhead Pressing Exercises

Dumbbell Overhead Pressing Exercises

Machine, Band, and Body-Weight Overhead Pressing Exercise

Upright Rowing Exercises

Front Raise Exercises

Lateral Raise Exercises

Rear Deltoid Exercises

Rotator Cuff Exercises

SEATED BARBELL OVERHEAD PRESS

START

Sit on a bench with a vertical back, such as a shoulder press bench, or an adjustable bench that adjusts to 90 degrees. Plant your feet flat on the floor and unrack the bar using an overhand grip with your hands slightly wider than shoulder width on the bar. Bring the bar over and in front of your head to the starting position—under your chin and just above your upper chest.

MOVE

Press the bar straight up overhead until your arms are fully extended but not locked out. Slowly lower the bar back to the starting position.

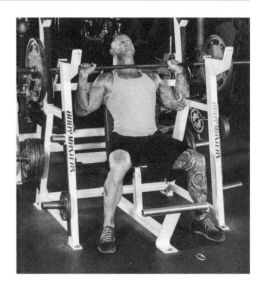

BARBELL OVERHEAD PRESS WITH BANDS

START

Depending on your setup, either place the bands underneath the bench and the cuffs around either side of the barbell, or use the straps and place bands on both sides of the base of the rack and up around either end of the barbell. Sit on a bench with a vertical back such as a shoulder press bench or an adjustable bench that adjusts to 90 degrees. Plant your feet flat on the floor and unrack the bar using an overhand grip with your hands slightly wider than shoulder width on the bar. Bring the bar over and in front of your head to the start position—under your chin and just above your upper chest.

MOVE

Press the bar straight overhead until your arms are fully extended but not locked out. Slowly lower the bar to the start position.

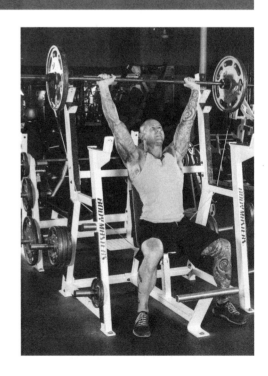

SEATED BARBELL BEHIND-THE-NECK PRESS

START

Sit on a bench with a vertical back, such as a shoulder press bench or an adjustable bench that adjusts to 90 degrees. Plant your feet flat on the floor and unrack the bar using an overhand grip with your hands slightly wider than shoulder width on the bar. Bring the bar behind your head to a level that is even with the lower part of your ears.

MOVE

Press the bar straight up overhead and slightly back until your arms are fully extended but not locked out. Slowly lower the bar back to the starting position.

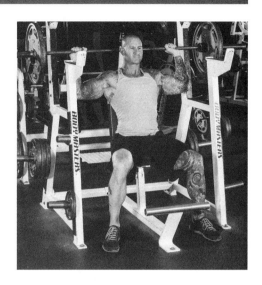

STANDING BARBELL OVERHEAD PRESS

START

Stand holding a barbell with an overhand grip with your hands spaced just outside shoulder width. Hold the bar just over your upper chest and below your chin. Your feet should be spaced just slightly wider than shoulder width and your knees should have a slight bend.

MOVE

Press the bar straight overhead, stopping just short of elbow lockout. Then slowly lower the bar back to the starting position.

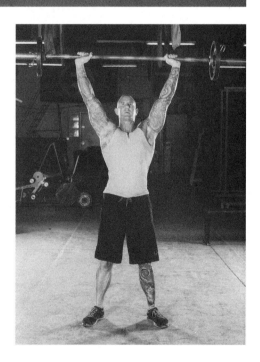

SMITH MACHINE SEATED OVERHEAD PRESS

START

Position an adjustable bench to 90 degrees or use a low-back bench, and place it within the Smith machine so that the bar lowers just in front of your face. Sit on the bench with your feet flat on the floor and your back flat against the bench. Grasp the bar just outside shoulder width and unlatch it from the safety supports. Lower the bar to just below your chin.

MOVE

Contract your shoulders and extend your arms to press the weight up until your arms are fully extended but not locked out. Slowly lower the bar back to the starting position.

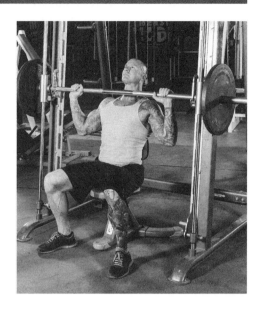

SMITH MACHINE SEATED BEHIND-THE-NECK PRESS

START

Position a low-back bench or an adjustable bench to 90 degrees, and place it within the Smith machine so that the bar lowers just behind your head. Sit on the bench with your feet flat on the floor and your back flat against the bench. Grasp the bar just outside shoulder width and unlatch it from the safety supports. Lower the bar behind the head to lower-ear level.

MOVE

Press the bar straight up overhead until your arms are fully extended but not locked out. Slowly lower the bar back to the starting position.

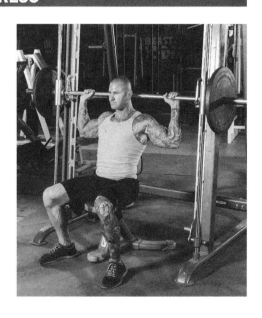

SMITH MACHINE SHOULDER PRESS THROW

START

Position a low-back bench in the Smith machine so that the bar lowers just in front of your face. Sit in the bench with your feet flat on the floor and your back flat against the bench. Grasp the bar just outside shoulder width and unlatch it from the safety supports. Lower the bar to just below your chin.

MOVE

Explosively contract your shoulders and extend your arms as fast as possible to press the weight up until your arms are fully extended and throw the bar upward, letting go with both arms. As the bar returns, catch it and slowly lower the bar back to the start position.

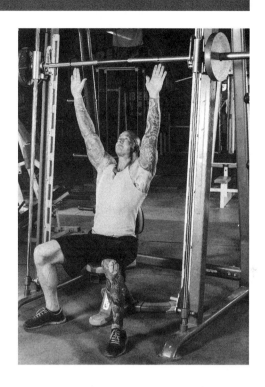

SEATED DUMBBELL OVERHEAD PRESS

START

Sit on a low-back bench with your feet firmly planted on the floor. Hold a pair of dumbbells at shoulder height. Begin with your palms facing forward and your elbows just below shoulder level but slightly forward. Forearms are angled in slightly so that the inner plates of the dumbbells are directly above your shoulders.

MOVE

Push the weights straight up, stopping just short of locking out your elbows. Then control the dumbbells all the way down until your upper arms are parallel with the floor or slightly lower and the weights are at approximately ear level.

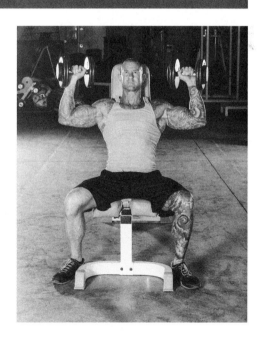

SEATED NEUTRAL-GRIP OVERHEAD DUMBBELL PRESS

START

Sit on a low-back bench with your feet firmly planted on the floor. Hold a pair of dumbbells at shoulder height. Begin with your palms facing toward each other and your elbows just below shoulder level and directed forward.

MOVE

Push the weights straight up, stopping just short of locking out your elbows. Then control the dumbbells all the way down until your upper arms are parallel with the floor or slightly lower and your elbows are pointed forward and the weights are at approximately ear level.

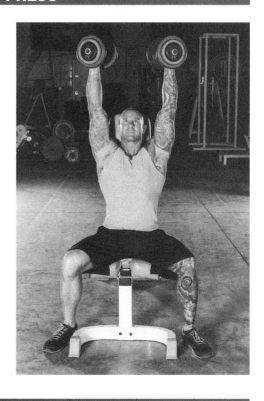

ARNOLD PRESS

START

Sit on a low-back bench with your feet firmly planted on the floor. Hold a pair of dumbbells at shoulder height. Begin with your palms facing toward your shoulders and your elbows down and forward.

MOVE

Push the weights straight up, pronating your hands once the dumbbells reach eye level so that your palms are facing forward at full arm extension. Control the dumbbells all the way back down in the reverse motion to the starting position.

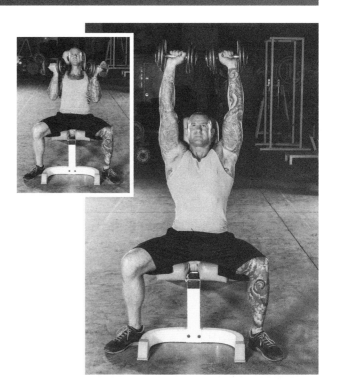

STANDING DUMBBELL OVERHEAD PRESS

START

Stand holding a pair of dumbbells at shoulder height with your feet about shoulder-width apart and knees slightly bent. Begin with your palms facing forward and your elbows just below shoulder level but slightly forward. Forearms are angled in slightly so that the inner plates of the dumbbells are directly above your shoulders.

MOVE

Push the weights straight up, stopping just short of locking out your elbows. Then control the dumbbells all the way down until your upper arms are parallel with the floor or slightly lower and the weights are at approximately ear level.

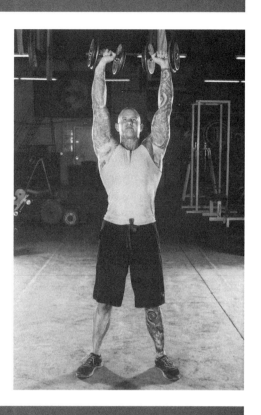

SEATED MACHINE OVERHEAD PRESS

START

Sit in a seated machine overhead press station with your feet firmly planted on the floor and your back flat against the seat back. Hold the machine handles with your palms facing forward and your hands slightly wider than shoulder-width apart.

MOVE

Push the handle up overhead to full arm extension, stopping just short of locking out your elbows. Then control the weight all the way down until your upper arms are parallel with the floor or slightly lower and the handle is at approximately ear level.

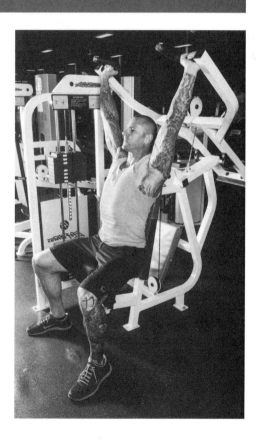

BAND SHOULDER PRESS

START

Stand in a staggered stance with the band placed securely under your back foot. Make sure that the band has equal lengths on either side. Step forward with your right foot. Bring the handles up and around behind the shoulders.

MOVE

Press straight up until your arms are completely extended but not locked out at the elbows. Return your arms to the start position and repeat for reps.

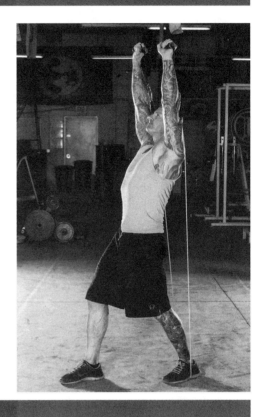

PIKE PUSH-UP

START

Place your hands on the floor in a push-up position with your feet up on something such as a bench or an exercise ball. Flex your hips to lift your glutes up and place your torso in a perpendicular position with the floor.

MOVE

Maintaining the bend in your hips, lower your body to the floor until the top of your head touches the floor and then contract your shoulders to extend your arms to full extension to lift your body back up.

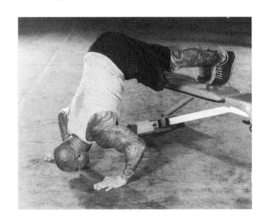

TRX PIKE PUSH-UP

START

Get in the push-up position with your hands on the floor and your feet in the TRX stirrups. Flex your hips to lift your glutes up and place your torso perpendicular with the floor.

MOVE

Maintaining the bend in your hips, lower your body to the floor until the top of your head touches the floor and then contract your shoulders to extend your arms to full extension to lift your body back up.

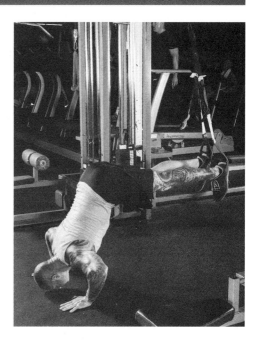

BARBELL UPRIGHT ROW

START

Stand holding a barbell across the front of your thighs with your feet shoulder-width apart and knees slightly bent. Place your hands wider than shoulder-width apart.

MOVE

Lift the bar straight up to chest height, keeping the bar close to your body and keeping your elbows higher than your wrists at all times. Pause for a moment at the top when the upper arms are parallel with the floor, and then slowly lower the bar back to the starting position.

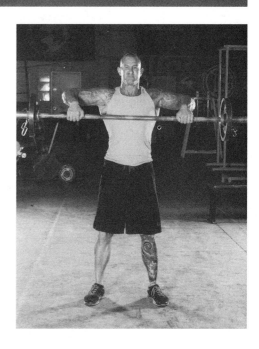

341

DUMBBELL UPRIGHT ROW

START

Stand with your feet shoulder-width apart, holding a pair of dumbbells in front of your thighs. Palms are facing toward your legs and elbows are slightly bent.

MOVE

Bring your elbows up and out to your sides as you lift the dumbbells, keeping your wrists straight and the dumbbells close to your body. When your elbows reach shoulder level, hold for a second in the top position before slowly lowering the dumbbells to the starting position.

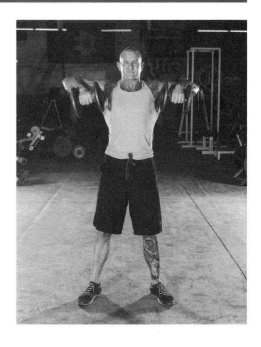

SMITH MACHINE UPRIGHT ROW

START

Stand in the middle of a Smith machine, holding the bar with an overhand grip across the front of your thighs. Your feet are shoulder-width apart and knees are slightly bent. Place your hands wider than shoulder-width apart.

MOVE

Lift the bar up to chest height while keeping your elbows higher than your wrists at all times. Pause for a moment at the top when the upper arms are parallel with the floor, and then slowly lower the bar back to the starting position.

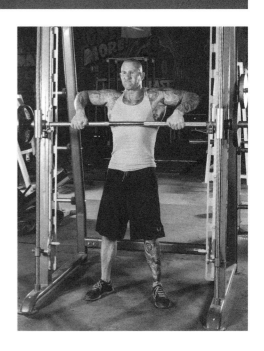

ONE-ARM SMITH MACHINE UPRIGHT ROW

START

Stand in the middle of a Smith machine with the bar set at about midthigh height. Grab the bar with your left hand using an overhand grip with your hand about 4 inches (10 centimeters) to the side of your thigh and unrack the bar

MOVE

Pull the bar up to chest height, leading with the elbow that you allow to flair out to the side as much as possible. This variation places the majority of the focus on the middle head of the deltoid and is a more natural movement for the shoulder, which prevents shoulder pain and risk of injury as can occur when upright rows are performed incorrectly. Another benefit of this exercise is that because you are using only one arm, you can focus more on each deltoid working. After finishing all reps on the left side, repeat on the right side.

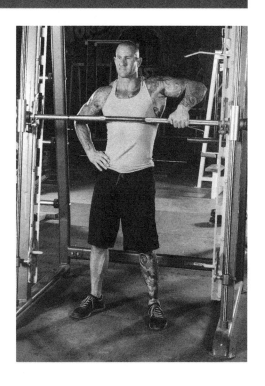

CABLE UPRIGHT ROW

START

Stand in front of a pulley cable apparatus holding a straight bar attached to a low pulley with an overhand grip that is about hip-width to shoulder-width apart or wider. Your feet should be shoulder-width apart and your knees are slightly bent. The bar is across the front of your thighs.

MOVE

Lift the bar up to chest height while keeping your elbows higher than your wrists at all times. Pause for a moment at the top and then slowly lower the bar back to the starting position.

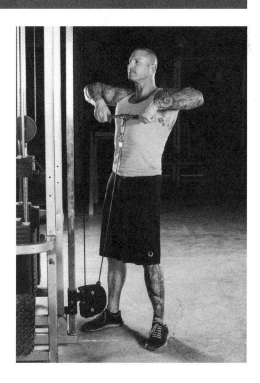

BAND UPRIGHT ROW

START

Stand lengthwise on an exercise band with a hip- to shoulder-width stance. Hold the handles of the bands with an overhand grip and your hands about shoulder-width apart in front of your legs.

MOVE

Keeping the band close to your body, pull the handles up to chest level, or until your upper arms are about parallel with the floor. Hold this top position for a second and then slowly lower the handles back to the start position and repeat for reps.

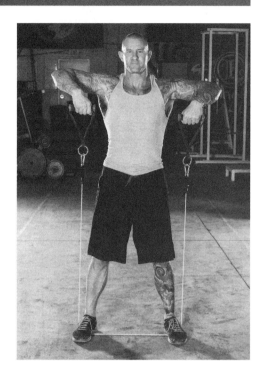

BARBELL FRONT RAISE

START

Stand holding a barbell across the front of your thighs. Your feet are shoulder-width apart and knees are slightly bent. You should have an overhand grip with your hands about shoulder-width apart.

MOVE

Lift the bar straight up and out in front of your body until your arms are just past parallel with the floor. Pause for a moment at the top before slowly lowering the bar back to the starting position.

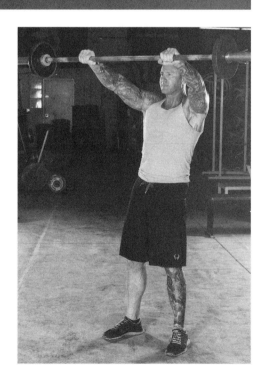

DUMBBELL FRONT RAISE

START

Stand holding a pair of dumbbells across the front of your thighs. Your feet are shoulder-width apart and knees are slightly bent. You should have an overhand grip.

MOVE

Lift the dumbbells straight up and out in front of your body until your arms are just past parallel with the floor. Pause for a moment at the top before slowly lowering the bar back to the starting position. To do alternating front dumbbell raise, lift one dumbbell up and down at a time, alternating sides.

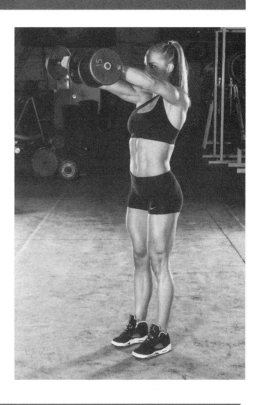

ONE-ARM DUMBBELL FRONT RAISE

START

Stand holding a dumbbell with one hand across the front of your thigh. Feet are shoulder-width apart and knees are slightly bent. You should have an overhand grip.

MOVE

Lift the dumbbell straight up and out in front of your body until your arm is just past parallel with the floor. Pause for a moment at the top before slowly lowering the dumbbell back to the starting position. Perform all reps on one side and then repeat with the other arm.

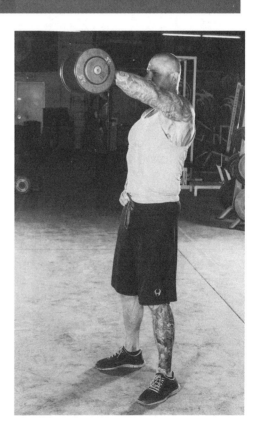

WEIGHT PLATE FRONT RAISE

START

Stand holding a weight plate by its edges in front of your thighs. Keep your feet shoulder-width apart and knees slightly bent.

MOVE

Lift the weight plate straight up and out in front of your body until your arms are just past parallel with the floor. Pause for a moment at the top before slowly lowering the plate back to the start position.

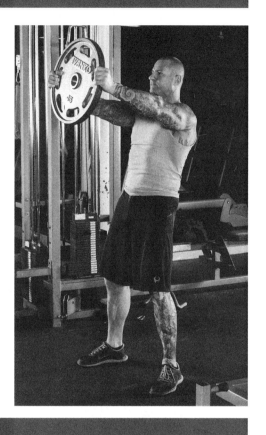

CABLE FRONT RAISE

START

Stand with your back toward a low-pulley cable apparatus. With an overhand grip, grab onto the straight-bar attachment connected to the low pulley. The bar should be in front of your thighs with the cable running through your legs. This can also be done with a rope attachment using a neutral grip.

MOVE

In a smooth motion, lift the handle up and straight out in front of you until your arms are just past parallel with the floor, keeping your arms straight throughout. Hold for a second and then slowly lower the attachment back to the starting position.

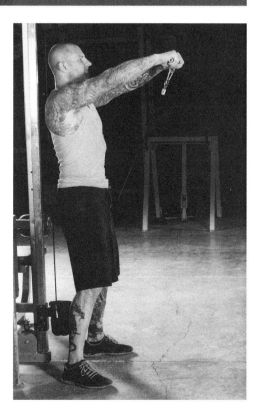

ONE-ARM CABLE FRONT RAISE

START

Stand with your back toward a low-pulley cable apparatus. With one hand in an overhand grip, grab onto the single-handle D-grip attachment connected to the low pulley. The handle should be on the side of your thighs.

MOVE

In a smooth motion, lift the handle up and straight out in front of you until your arm is just past parallel with the floor, keeping your arm straight throughout. Hold for a second and then slowly lower the attachment back to the starting position.

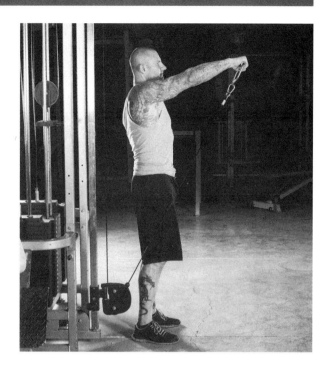

SEATED INCLINE FRONT RAISE

START

Sit on an incline bench set to 45 degrees while holding a barbell across your thighs. You should have an overhand grip on the bar using a shoulder-width grip.

MOVE

Lift the bar up in front of you until your arms are past parallel with the floor, keeping your arms straight throughout. Hold for a second and then slowly lower the bar back to the starting position.

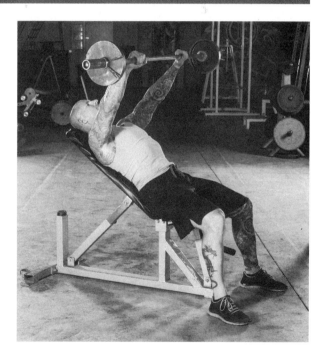

PRONE INCLINE FRONT RAISE

START

Sit in reverse direction straddling an incline bench set to 45 degrees while holding a barbell with an overhand grip. Your feet should be as flat as possible on the floor with your chest pressed into the bench and your chin above the top of the bench. With an overhand grip, hold the barbell with your hands shoulder-width apart. The barbell should hang straight down from your shoulders.

MOVE

Lift the bar up in front of you until your arms are parallel with the floor, keeping your arms straight throughout. Hold for a second and then slowly lower the bar back to the starting position.

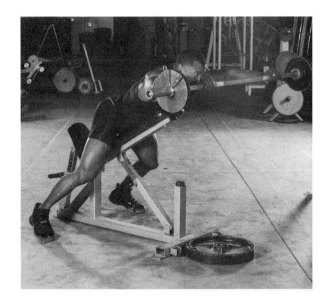

BAND FRONT RAISE

START

Standing upright, place the exercise band underneath both feet and grab the handles with an overhand grip. Be sure that the band heights on both sides are fairly even so that you have even resistance on both sides.

MOVE

Maintaining a slight bend in your elbows, slowly raise both arms up and out in front of you until your arms are parallel with the floor or higher. Hold this position for a second as you contract your shoulders as hard as you can and then slowly lower your arms back to the start position. Repeat for reps.

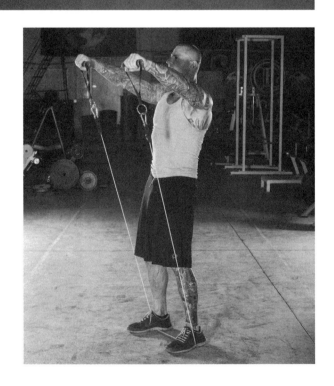

DUMBBELL LATERAL RAISE

START

Stand with your feet about shoulder-width apart while holding two dumbbells with neutral grips at your sides.

MOVE

Slowly raise the dumbbells up and out to your sides. Keep your arms straight with a very slight bend in your elbows. When your arms reach just above parallel with the floor, pause in this position for a second before slowly lowering the dumbbells back to the starting position.

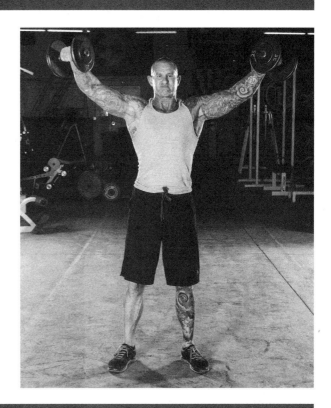

ONE-ARM DUMBBELL LATERAL RAISE

START

Stand with your feet about shoulder-width apart while holding one dumbbell with a neutral grip at your side.

MOVE

Slowly raise the dumbbell up and out to your side. Keep your arm straight with a very slight bend in your elbow. When your arm reaches just above parallel with the floor, pause in this position for a second before slowly lowering the dumbbell back to the starting position. Repeat with the other arm.

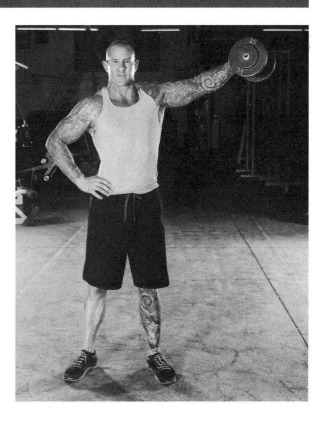

SEATED DUMBBELL LATERAL RAISE

START

Sit on a flat bench with your feet firmly planted on the floor while holding two dumbbells with neutral grips at your sides.

MOVE

Slowly raise the dumbbells up and out to your sides. Keep your arms straight with a very slight bend in your elbows. When your arms reach just above parallel with the floor, pause in this position for a second before slowly lowering the dumbbells back to the starting position.

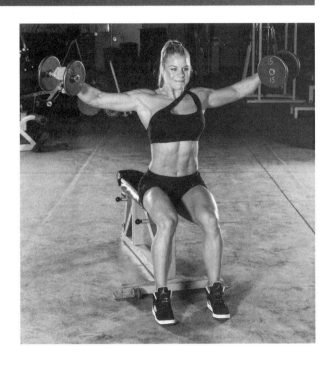

ONE-ARM CABLE LATERAL RAISE (FRONT OF BODY OR BEHIND)

START

Stand with your right shoulder toward a low-pulley cable apparatus. Your feet should be about shoulder-width apart. Hold a single-handle D-grip attachment that is attached to the low pulley in your left hand in front of your left thigh or behind your left thigh.

MOVE

Slowly raise the handle up and out to your side, keeping your arm straight with a very slight bend in your elbow. When your arm reaches just above parallel with the floor, pause in this position for a second before slowly lowering the handle back to the starting position.

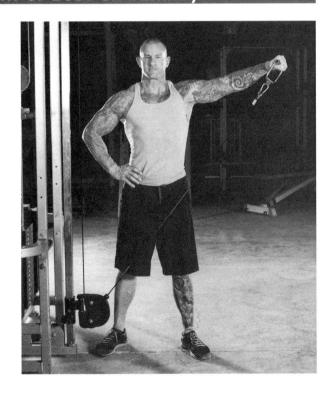

MACHINE LATERAL RAISE

START

Sit in a lateral raise machine with your upper arms pressed against the arm pads of the machine.

MOVE

Lift your upper arms up and out to your sides until your arms are parallel with the floor. Pause for a second and then slowly return your arms to the starting position.

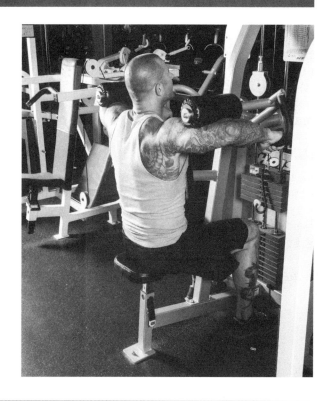

SMITH MACHINE LATERAL RAISE

START

Place light weight on the bar of a Smith machine and set the bar just above waist height. Stand in the middle of the Smith machine with your right arm touching the bar. Bend your right arm at the elbow 90 degrees so that your forearm is parallel with the bar. Unlatch the bar with your left hand and support the bar with your forearm.

MOVE

Maintaining the bend at your elbow, raise your arm to lift the bar to about shoulder height. Hold this position for a second, contracting your deltoid as hard as possible, then slowly lower the bar back to just above waist height, keeping the bar in contact with your forearm. Complete all reps with your right arm and then repeat in the same manner on the left side.

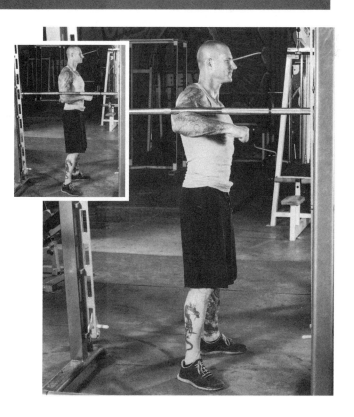

BAND LATERAL RAISE

START

Standing upright, place the exercise band underneath both feet and grab the handles with a neutral grip. Be sure that the band heights on both sides are fairly even so that you have even resistance on both sides.

MOVE

Maintaining a slight bend in your elbows, slowly raise both arms up and out to your sides until your arms are parallel with the floor or higher. Hold this position for a second as you contract your shoulders as hard as you can, and then slowly lower your arms to the start position. Repeat for reps.

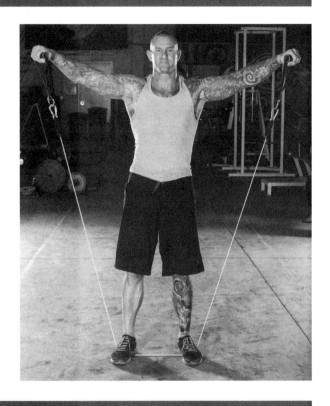

BENT-OVER LATERAL RAISE

START

Stand with your knees slightly bent. Holding a pair of dumbbells in front of you with your palms facing toward each other, bend forward from the hips, keeping your back flat and your head in line with your spine. Allow your arms to hang straight down from your shoulders and bend your elbows slightly.

MOVE

Slowly lift the dumbbells up and out to the sides of your body, pulling through the rear delts and middle traps. Pause a moment at the top of the motion before slowly lowering the weights back down to the starting position.

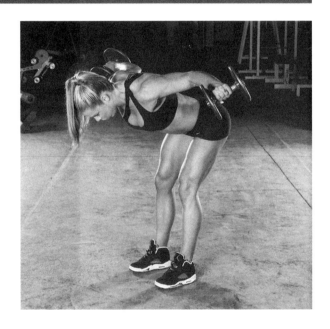

ONE-ARM BENT-OVER LATERAL RAISE

START

Lean forward at the hips, place your right hand on your thigh or a bench for support, and hold a dumbbell in your left hand with your arm extended straight down.

MOVE

Raise the weight straight out to the side until your arm is parallel with the floor. Pause a moment at the top of the motion before slowly lowering the weight back down to the starting position. Repeat with the right arm.

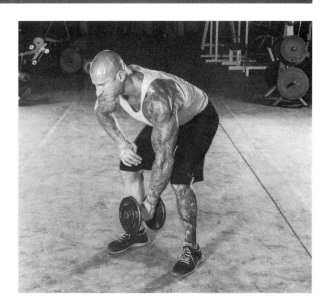

INCLINE BENCH REAR LATERAL RAISE

START

Sit in reverse direction straddling an incline bench set below 45 degrees while holding dumbbells with neutral grips. Your feet should be flat on the floor or positioned on the frame of the bench to secure your position with your chest pressed into the bench and your chin above the top of the bench. Hold the dumbbells so that they hang straight down from your shoulders.

MOVE

Slowly lift the dumbbells up and out to the sides of your body, pulling through the rear delts and middle traps. Pause a moment at the top of the motion before slowly lowering the weights back down to the starting position.

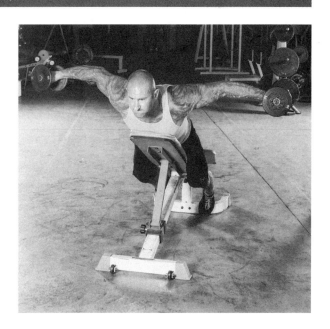

STANDING CABLE REVERSE FLY

START

Stand in the center of a cable crossover apparatus. Start with hands crossed in front of you at shoulder height with the left high cable in your right hand and the right in your left hand.

MOVE

Using your rear delts, pull your elbows out and back as far as possible, then return to the starting position.

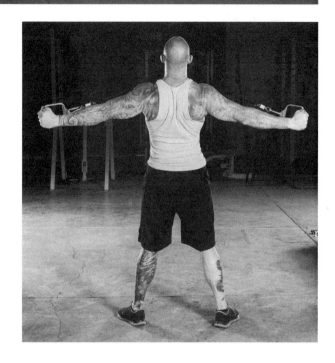

LYING CABLE REVERSE FLY

START

Lie faceup on a flat bench placed in the middle of a cable crossover apparatus. Hold D-handles attached to the high cable pulleys from opposite sides of the cable apparatus with a neutral grip. Hold your arms straight out above your chest with a slight bend in your elbows.

MOVE

Maintain the slight bend in your elbows as you extend at your shoulders to pull your arms out to your sides until your hands are parallel with your shoulders. Return the handles to the start position and repeat for reps.

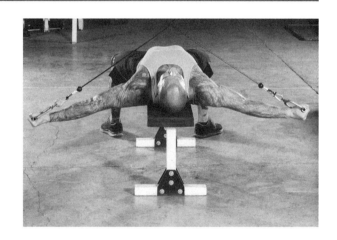

CROSS-BODY REAR DELTOID RAISE

START

Lie on a flat bench so that one side of your body is flush against it. Position your nonworking arm under your body on the bench. Position your working arm, dumbbell in hand, to hang across your body. Your elbow is slightly bent and your palm is down.

MOVE

Contract your shoulder to lift the dumbbell upward. Retrace the movement back to the starting position.

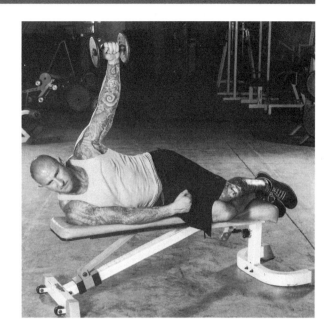

BAND BENT-OVER LATERAL RAISE

START

Place an exercise band on the floor in front of your feet. Stand on the middle of the band with both feet and bend forward from the hips to reach down and grab the handles with opposite-side hands. In other words, your right hand should grab the handle extending from your left foot and your left hand should grab the handle extending from your right foot. Keep your torso parallel with the floor or slightly higher and maintain a slight bend in your elbows.

MOVE

Squeeze your shoulder blades together as you contract your rear deltoids to extend your arms at the shoulders until your arms are parallel with the floor or higher. Hold this position for a second as you contract your rear delts and middle traps as hard as possible and then return your arms to the start position. Repeat for reps.

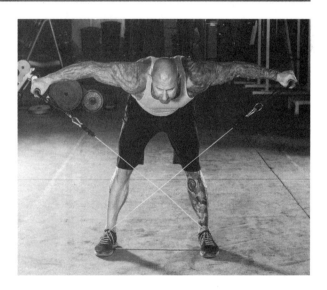

BAND PULL

START

Hold an exercise band with a shoulder-width grip and arms extended straight out in front of you.

MOVE

Contract your rear deltoids and middle traps to pull the band apart until your arms are out to your sides. Slowly return your hands to the start position.

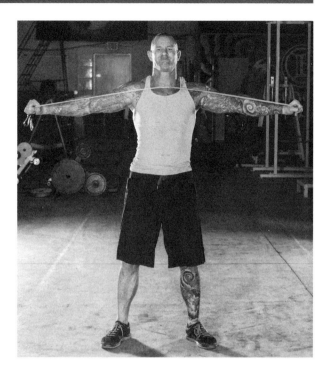

ONE-ARM BAND REAR DELT FLY

START

Attach the band to a stable post or door attachment at about shoulder height. Hold the band with a neutral grip and your arm extended straight out in front of you.

MOVE

Contract your rear deltoid and middle trap to extend your arm back until it is out to your side. Return your hand to the start position and repeat all reps on one side before performing on the other side.

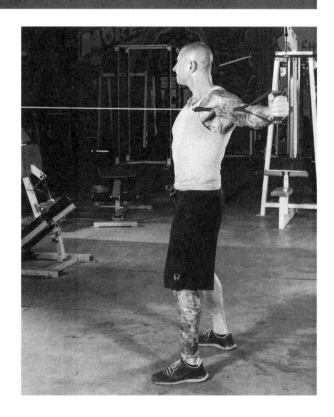

FACE PULL

START

Attach a rope to the cable pulley of a lat pulldown station. Grab the ends of the rope attachment using a neutral grip (palms facing each other) and place one foot up on the knee-pad post and lean back at about 45 degrees.

MOVE

Pull the rope toward your face as you spread the ends of the rope so they end up on the sides of your ears just above your shoulders in the finish position. Your upper arms should be straight out to your sides with elbows bent. Hold this position for a second as you squeeze your shoulder blades together, contracting rear delts and middle traps as hard as possible. Then slowly return the rope to the start position and repeat for reps. While this move somewhat mimics a cable row for the lats, because you are pulling the rope high to your shoulders, it places less focus on the lats and more focus on the rear delts and middle traps.

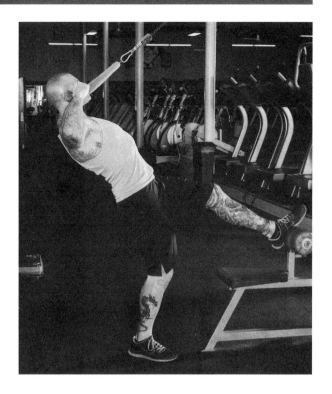

SMITH MACHINE FACE PULL

START

Stand in the Smith machine with a shoulder-width stance and bend forward from the hips so that your torso is just above parallel with the floor and your neck is lined up over the bar. Using a wider than shoulder-width grip, grab the bar.

MOVE

Slowly pull the bar up toward your neck. Hold this position for a second and then slowly lower the bar to the start and repeat for reps.

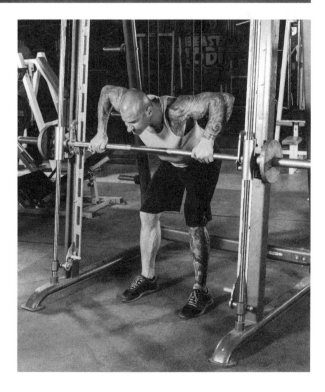

CABLE EXTERNAL ROTATION

START

This exercise is a great way to strengthen the rotator cuff muscles, particularly the infraspinatus and teres minor muscles. Position a cable pulley with a D-handle attached to it at waist height. Stand sideways to the cable so that the working arm is farthest from the pulley. Hold the cable while keeping a 90-degree bend in your elbow and with your hand reaching across to the opposite side of your waist.

MOVE

While maintaining the bend in your elbow, rotate your arm at the shoulder until you can no longer rotate it. Slowly return the handle to the start position. Complete all reps with that arm, then switch arms, facing the opposite direction. You can also do this with bands in the same manner.

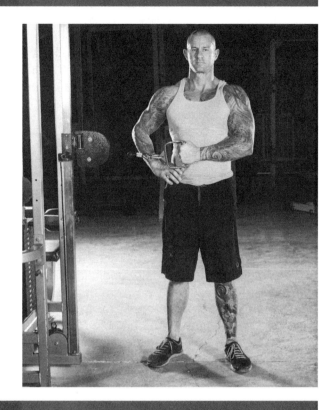

DUMBBELL EXTERNAL ROTATION

START

Lie on your side on a flat bench with your non-working arm lying on the bench. Your working arm should be bent at 90 degrees and your biceps should be pressed against your side while you hold a dumbbell directly in front of your torso.

MOVE

Keeping your upper arm pressed against your side and your elbow bent, lift the dumbbell until it is directly above your torso. Return to the start and repeat for reps. After completing all the reps with one arm, switch to the other arm.

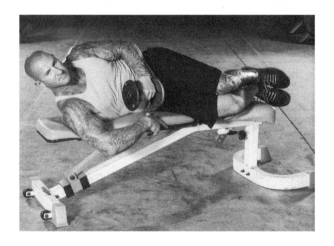

CABLE INTERNAL ROTATION

START

This exercise is a good rotator cuff exercise and specifically strengthens the subscapularis muscle. Position a cable pulley with a D-handle attached to it at waist height. Stand sideways with the working arm facing the pulley. Hold the handle in the hand closer to the pulley with your forearm in line with your abdomen and your arm bent 90 degrees and elbow in tight to your side.

MOVE

Keeping your arm bent and your elbow in at your side, slowly pull the handle across your body until your hand reaches the opposite side of your waist. Slowly return the handle to the start position. Complete all reps with that arm, then switch arms, facing the opposite direction. You can also do this with bands in the same manner.

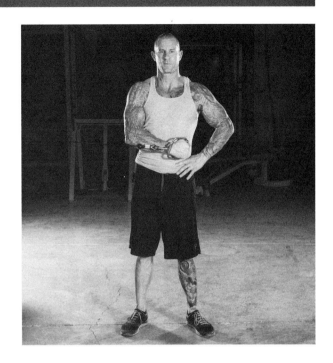

DUMBBELL INTERNAL ROTATION

START

Lie on your side on a flat bench with your working arm on the bench in front of you with your upper arm parallel to your torso and your elbow bent at 90 degrees and pressed against your side while you hold a dumbbell directly in front of your torso.

MOVE

Keeping your upper arm pressed against your side and your elbow bent, lift the dumbbell until it is directly above your torso. Return to the start and repeat for reps. After completing all the reps with one arm, switch to the other arm.

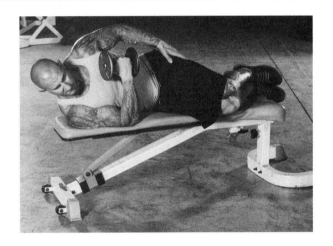

EMPTY CAN LIFT

START

Standing upright, hold a pair of light dumbbells or weight plates in your hands in front of your thighs with an overhand grip so that your palms face your thighs.

MOVE

Lift your arms up and out to your sides until your arms are parallel with the floor. In the top position your pinky fingers should be on top and your thumbs on the bottom.

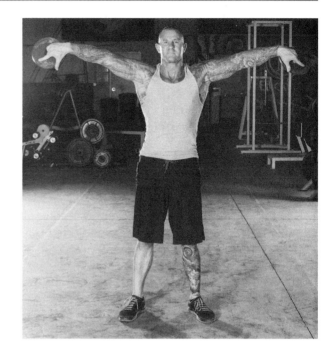

CHAPTER 16

Back

This chapter contains detailed descriptions of all major exercises that focus on the back muscles, including the latissimus dorsi (lat), teres major, rhomboids (just below the trapezius), and the deep spinal erectors. See the diagram for the location of each muscle. The back exercises are divided into barbell rowing exercises, dumbbell rowing exercises, cable or band and machine rowing exercises, body-weight rowing exercises, pull-up and pulldown exercises, pullover exercises, and low-back exercises. Wherever a certain type of exercise is used in a workout, any one of the same type can be substituted.

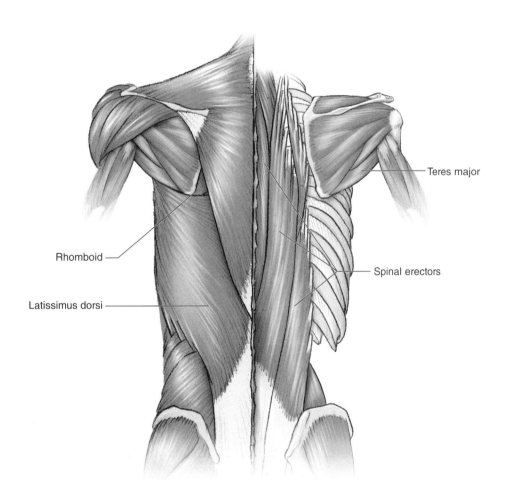

Rhomboid

Latissimus dorsi

Teres major

Spinal erectors

BARBELL ROW

START

Stand with your feet about shoulder-width apart with a slight bend in your knees. Bend forward from the hips, keeping your torso just above parallel to the floor and your chest lifted to maintain the natural arch in your back. Take an overhand grip on the bar, hands just outside shoulder width.

MOVE

Pull the bar into your lower abs, contract your lats and middle-back muscles hard, then slowly lower the bar all the way down to full arm extension.

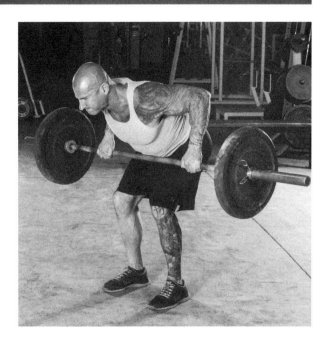

UNDERHAND-GRIP BARBELL ROW

START

Stand with your feet about shoulder-width apart with a slight bend in your knees. Bend forward from the hips, keeping your torso just above parallel to the floor and your chest lifted to maintain the natural arch in your back. Take an underhand grip on the bar, hands shoulder-width apart.

MOVE

Pull the bar into your lower abs, contract your lats and middle-back muscles hard, then slowly lower the bar all the way down to full arm extension.

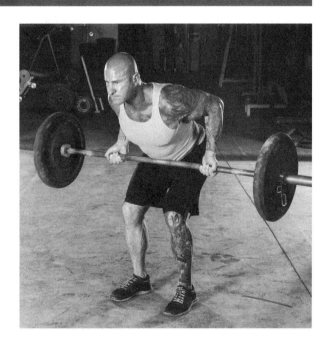

PENDLAY ROW

START

With your feet shoulder-width apart, bend over from the hips and grasp a barbell on the floor with an overhand grip. Bend your knees slightly and make sure that your back is perfectly straight and parallel to the floor.

MOVE

Maintaining the position of your legs and back, pull the bar up to your lower chest or upper abs. Hold this position for a second as you squeeze your lats hard at the top. Lower the bar with control to the floor. Relax your grip, reset, and repeat.

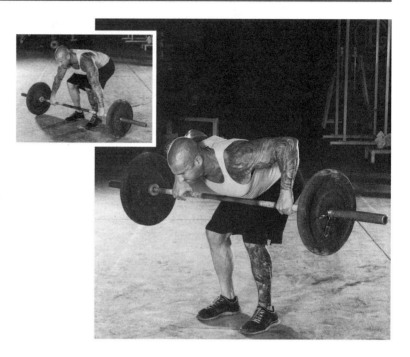

SUPPORTED BARBELL ROW

START

Adjust an incline bench so that the top of the back pad is about waist high. Stand behind the bench holding a barbell with an overhand grip just outside shoulder width. Bend forward from the hips and rest your chest on the top of the bench and let the barbell hang straight down below your shoulders. Your feet should be about shoulder-width apart and your knees should be slightly bent.

MOVE

Pull the bar in to your lower abs, contract your lats and middle-back muscles hard, then slowly lower the bar all the way down to full arm extension.

Note: You can also do this exercise with an underhand grip, as well as with dumbbells.

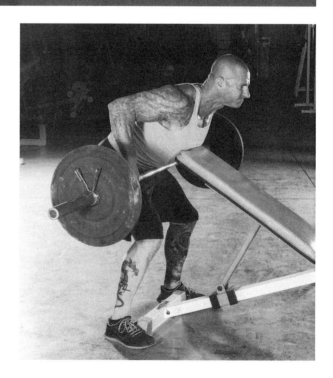

BARBELL ROW WITH BANDS

START

Place the ends of a band onto the ends of a loaded barbell as shown. Stand on the middle of the band with your feet about shoulder-width apart with a slight bend in your knees. Bend forward from the hips, keeping your torso just above parallel to the floor and your chest lifted to maintain the natural arch in your back. Take an overhand grip on the bar, hands just outside shoulder width.

MOVE

Pull the bar into your lower abs, contract your lats and middle-back muscles hard, then slowly lower the bar all the way down to full arm extension.

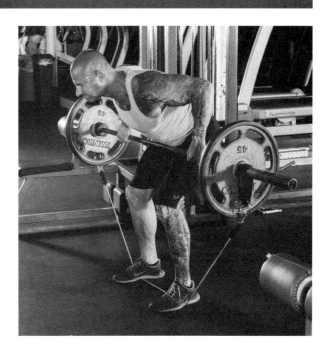

SMITH MACHINE BENT-OVER ROW

START

Stand in a Smith machine with the bar set on the lowest setting. Keep your feet about shoulder-width apart with a slight bend in your knees. Bend forward from the hips, keeping your torso just above parallel to the floor and your chest lifted to maintain the natural arch in your back. Take an overhand grip on the bar, hands just outside shoulder width.

MOVE

Pull the bar in to your lower abs, contract your lats and middle-back muscles hard, then slowly lower the bar all the way down to full arm extension.

Note: You can also do this exercise with an underhand grip.

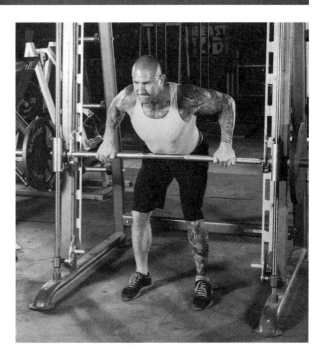

SMITH MACHINE ONE-ARM BENT-OVER ROW

START

Stand sideways in the middle of the Smith machine with the bar set on the lowest setting and on the side of your right leg. Stand in a staggered stance with your left leg in front of your right and a slight bend in your knees. Bend forward from the hips, keeping your torso just above parallel to the floor and your chest lifted to maintain the natural arch in your back. Rest your left hand on your lower thigh for support. Grab the bar in the middle with your right hand.

MOVE

Pull the bar up as high as possible as you contract your lats and middle-back muscles hard, then slowly lower the bar all the way down to full arm extension. Complete all reps with the right arm, then repeat on the left side.

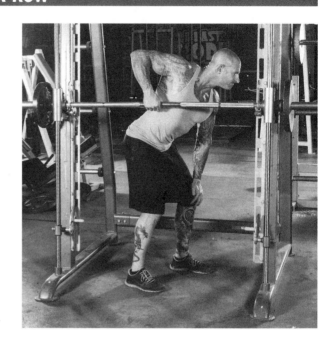

SMITH MACHINE POWER ROW

START

Stand sideways in the middle of the Smith machine so that the outside of your right leg is almost touching the bar. Bend forward from the hips so that your torso is at about a 45-degree angle with the floor. Grab the middle of the bar with your right hand using an open grip (thumb on same side as fingers).

MOVE

Use your legs, hips, and lower back to generate the initial power that will transfer to your lats and arm to pull the bar up as high as possible. Let go of the bar in the top position and then grab it as it starts its descent back to the start position. Repeat for reps, completing all reps on the right side and then switching your position to repeat on the left side.

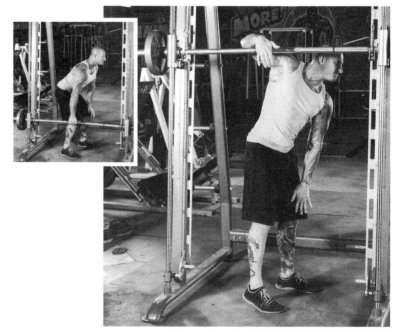

BARBELL POWER ROW

START

Stand in a power rack with a barbell resting on the safety pins set just above knee height. Keep your feet about shoulder-width apart with a slight bend in your knees. Bend forward from the hips, keeping your torso just above parallel to the floor and your chest lifted to maintain the natural arch in your back. Take an overhand grip on the bar, hands just outside shoulder width.

MOVE

With a fast and powerful move, pull the bar up to your waist and lower it back to the pins. Pause for several seconds with the bar on the pins before doing another rep.

Note: You can also do this exercise with an underhand grip.

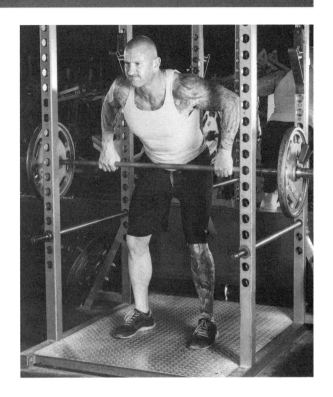

T-BAR ROW

START

With your feet shoulder-width apart and your knees slightly bent, grab the handles with an open grip. Bend at the hips and keep your back arched throughout the movement.

MOVE

Pull the bar all the way to your chest and pause at the top before lowering to a full stretch at the bottom.

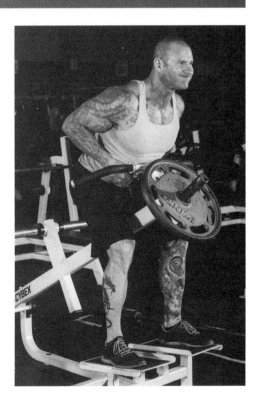

SUPPORTED T-BAR ROW

START

Lie on the pad of the T-bar row machine with your chest supported and your feet firmly planted on the foot platform. Take a wide, overhand grip on the handles and unhook the bar from the rack and support it with your arms hanging down at full extension.

MOVE

Pull the bar as high as the apparatus will allow and pause at the top before lowering to a full stretch at the bottom.

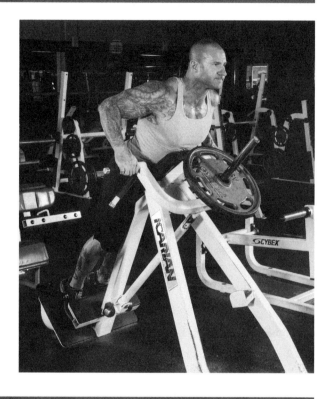

DUMBBELL ROW

START

Holding two dumbbells with a neutral grip, stand with your feet about shoulder-width apart while maintaining a slight bend in your knees. Bend forward from the hips, keeping your torso just above parallel to the floor and your chest lifted to maintain the natural arch in your back. Allow the dumbbells to hang straight down below your shoulders.

MOVE

Pull the dumbbells to your sides as high as possible while contracting your lats and middle-back muscles hard. Then slowly lower the dumbbells all the way down to full arm extension.

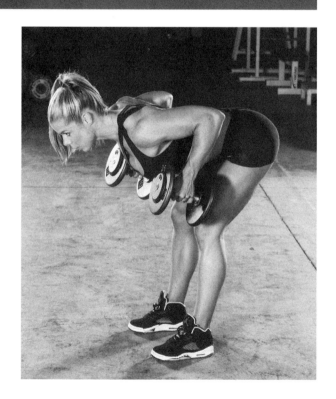

ONE-ARM DUMBBELL ROW

START

Grasp a dumbbell in one hand and rest your free hand and same side leg on a bench. Keep your chest slightly lifted as you bend forward from the hips. Keep the other foot flat on the ground for balance.

MOVE

Keeping your torso stable throughout the movement, pull the dumbbell all the way up to your side, lifting your elbow as high as possible. Then lower the dumbbell straight down to the starting position.

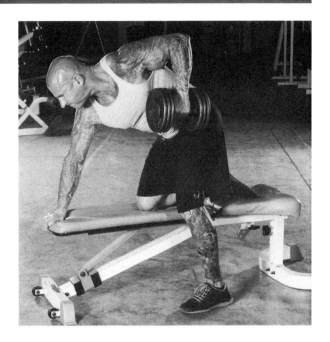

INCLINE DUMBBELL ROW

START

Grasp a dumbbell in each hand and straddle an incline bench set below 45 degrees. Your chest should be supported by the bench with your chin above the top. Let the dumbbells hang directly below your shoulders.

MOVE

With your palms facing each other and your elbows close to your body, pull the weights as high as possible, squeezing your shoulder blades together at the top. Hold this position for a second before returning the dumbbells to the start position.

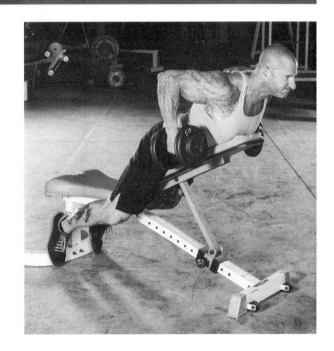

BISHOP BURTON COLLEGE

DUMBBELL POWER ROW

START

Place a dumbbell on the floor between your feet. Your legs should be about shoulder-width apart and your knees should be bent so that your thighs are just above parallel with the floor. With your left hand, grasp the dumbbell with an overhand grip and place your right hand firmly above your right knee to brace your upper body.

MOVE

Start the movement by forcefully extending your knees and hips to lift the dumbbell from the floor, and then pull the dumbbell up toward your left hip by pulling your elbow as high as possible. Your grip should turn so that when the dumbbell is at the top your palm is facing your torso (neutral grip). Slowly lower the dumbbell back to the floor in the opposite manner you lifted it. After finishing the desired number of reps, repeat on the right side.

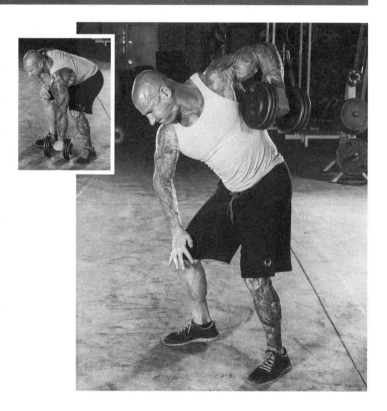

SEATED CABLE ROW

START

Sit on the cable row bench with your feet firmly planted on the foot plate. Grab a low row bar attached to the cable pulley. Keep your knees slightly bent and your back straight. Maintain a slight arch in your low back and keep your chest out.

MOVE

Pull the handle toward your midsection, focusing on driving your elbows back until the handle touches your lower abdomen. After squeezing your shoulder blades together at the peak of contraction, slowly return to the starting position.

Note: You can do this exercise with an overhand or underhand grip on a lat bar.

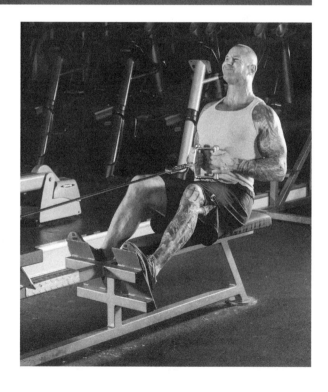

ONE-ARM SEATED CABLE ROW

START

Sit on the cable row bench so that your right leg is supported on the bench and your right foot is firmly planted on the foot platform. Your left leg should be bent and firmly planted on the floor. Grab a single-handle D-grip attached to the cable pulley. Keep your right knee slightly bent and your back straight. Maintain a slight arch in your lower back and keep your chest out.

MOVE

Pull the handle toward your side, focusing on driving your elbow back as far as possible. Slowly return to the starting position. After completing the desired number of reps, repeat on the left side.

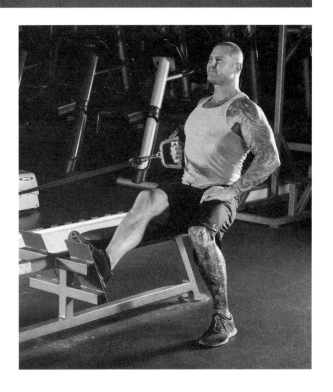

ONE-ARM BENT-OVER CABLE ROW

START

Grasp a single-handle D-grip attached to a low pulley with your left palm facing your body. Lean forward about 45 degrees. Use a split stance: The left foot should be back while the right is forward. Or use a shoulder-width stance if it feels more stable. Keep your chest up and shoulders squared. Maintain a slight arch in your back.

MOVE

Pull the handle in to the left side of your waist until your elbow is past your body. When you return to the starting position, go for a deep stretch. Complete the desired number of reps and repeat on the right side.

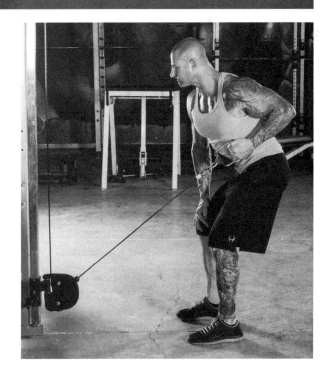

REVERSE INCLINE BENCH ONE-ARM CABLE ROW

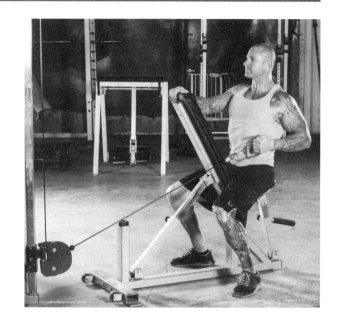

START

Place an incline bench next to a pulley apparatus so that the higher end is near the low pulley and to the right. Set the angle at about 45 to 60 degrees. Grasp the single-handle D-grip attachment attached to the low pulley with your left hand. Sit straddling the bench and facing the weight stack. Place your right hand on top of the bench to support your upper body while extending your left arm straight out in front of you.

MOVE

Pull on the handle, moving your elbow straight back as far as possible. Squeeze your shoulder blades together as you contract your lats briefly before returning to the starting position.

INCLINE BENCH CABLE ROW FROM HIGH PULLEY

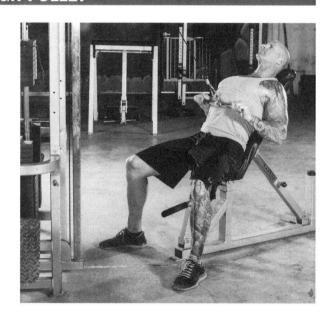

START

Place an incline bench (set to 45 degrees) about a foot from a high-pulley cable apparatus. Grab a straight bar attached to the high pulley and sit down on the bench. Your feet are flat on the floor and your back is flat against the bench. Extend your arms in front of you so that they follow the line of the cable.

MOVE

Pull the handle to your abdomen as you squeeze your shoulder blades together. Contract your lats briefly before returning the bar to the starting position.

Note: You can do this exercise with a low row bar or a rope attachment, and you can do it unilaterally using a single-handle D-grip attachment.

MACHINE ROW

START

Adjust the seat of the machine row so that your arms are parallel to the floor when you grab the handles. Adjust the chest pad so that the weight plates do not touch the bottom of the stack when you hold the handles with full arm extension. With your feet flat on the floor, keep your chest pressed against the chest pad while keeping your back straight.

MOVE

Pull the handles toward your ribs, bringing your elbows back as far as possible as you squeeze your shoulder blades together and you contract your lats briefly. Slowly return the handle to the starting position with your arms fully extended.

Note: You can also do this exercise unilaterally.

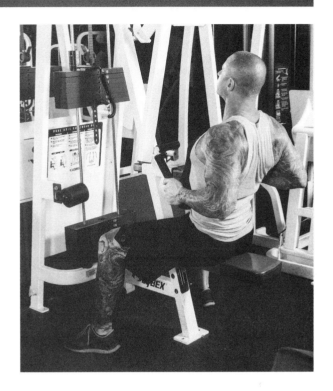

BAND BENT-OVER ROW

START

Stand on an exercise band with your right foot. Get in a staggered stance with your right leg in front of your left and hold the handle of the band with a neutral grip and your right arm extended straight down. You can hold the other end of the band with your left hand to stabilize the band. Bend forward slightly at the hips.

MOVE

Pull the band up as high as possible with your right arm. Hold the top position for a second while contracting your lats as hard as possible before slowly returning the handle to the start position. Complete all reps on the right side and then repeat on the left.

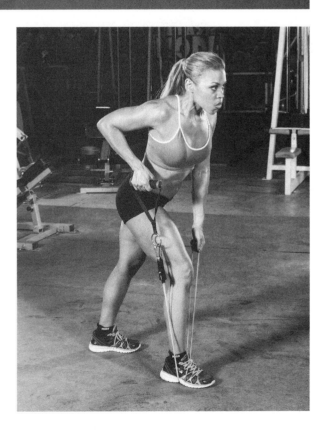

PULL-UP

START

Using an overhand grip, grab on to a chin-up bar with your hands spaced wider than shoulder-width apart. Hang from the bar with your arms fully extended and your chest high while exaggerating the arch in your lower back.

MOVE

Pull yourself up by squeezing your shoulder blades together and contracting your lats until your chin passes the bar. Hold the contraction at the top for a second before slowly lowering yourself back to the starting position.

Note: You can do this exercise with the hands closer together on the bar.

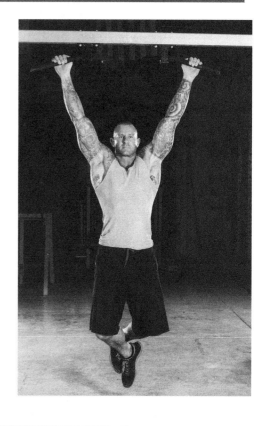

CHIN-UP

START

Using an underhand grip, grab on to a chin-up bar with your hands spaced shoulder-width apart. Hang from the bar with your arms fully extended and your chest high while exaggerating the arch in your low back.

MOVE

Pull yourself up by squeezing your shoulder blades together and contracting your lats until your chin passes the bar. Hold the contraction at the top for a second before slowly lowering yourself back to the starting position.

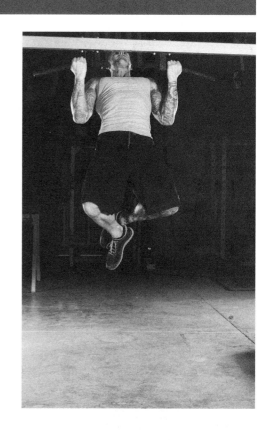

LAT PULLDOWN

START

Take an overhand grip that is wider than shoulder width on a lat bar attached to the pulley on the lat pulldown apparatus. Position yourself with your feet flat on the floor, chest up, and low-back arch exaggerated.

MOVE

Pull your shoulder blades together as you squeeze your lats to initiate the movement, pulling the bar down in a smooth motion to your midsection. Hold the contraction for a moment, then slowly return the bar all the way back to the starting position.

Note: You can do this exercise with the hands closer together on the bar.

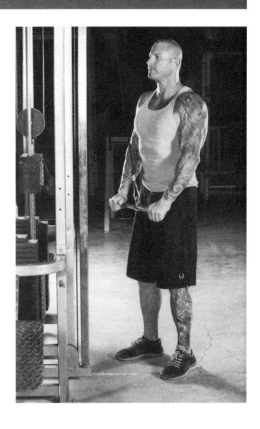

REVERSE-GRIP PULLDOWN

START

Take an underhand grip with your hands spaced about shoulder-width on a lat bar or straight bar attached to the pulley on the lat pulldown apparatus. Position yourself on the seat with your feet flat on the floor, arms extended overhead, chest up, and low-back arch exaggerated.

MOVE

Pull your shoulder blades together as you squeeze your lats to initiate the movement, pulling the bar down in a smooth motion to your chest. Hold the contraction for a moment, then slowly return the bar all the way back to the starting position.

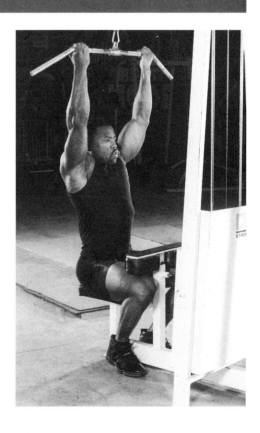

BEHIND-THE-NECK PULLDOWN

START

Take an overhand grip that is wider than shoulder width on a lat bar attached to the pulley on the lat pulldown apparatus. Position yourself on the seat with your feet flat on the floor, arms extended overhead, and back leaning slightly forward.

MOVE

Pull your shoulder blades together as you squeeze your lats to initiate the movement, pulling the bar down in a smooth motion to the back of your neck. Hold the contraction for a moment, then slowly return the bar all the way back to the starting position.

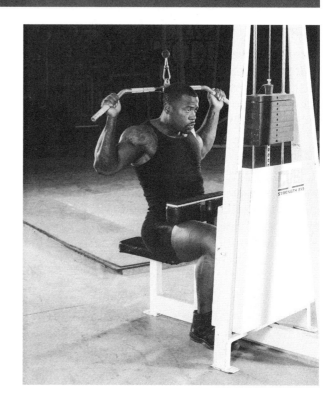

ONE-ARM PULLDOWN

START

Sit side saddle on the pulldown seat with your left arm closest to the pulley station. Grab a D-handle with your left hand using an overhand or neutral grip.

MOVE

Pull the handle down to the outside of your left shoulder, bringing your elbow down toward your hip. Hold the contraction for a second before returning the handle to the starting position. Repeat all reps on the left side and then perform on the right side.

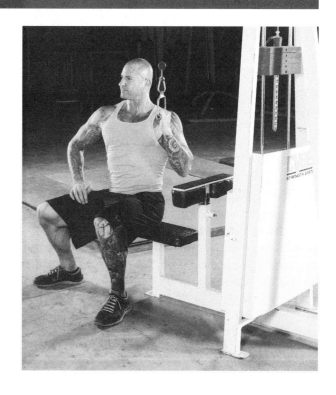

STANDING PULLDOWN

START

Stand at a pulldown station and place one foot up on the seat or on the knee pad as you hold on to the bar attachment with an overhand grip and lean back slightly while keeping your back arched and your chest up.

MOVE

Use your lats to pull the bar down to your chest and hold this position as you squeeze your shoulder blades together and flex your lats. Then return the bar to the start position and repeat for reps.

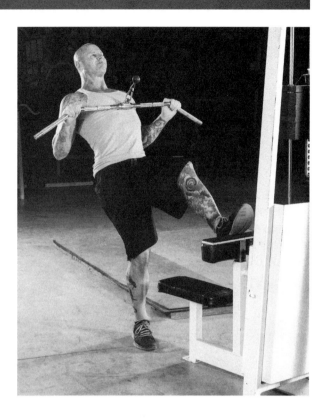

INVERTED ROW

START

Set the bar of a Smith machine or a power rack, just below hip height. Hold on to the bar using a shoulder-width, overhand grip and allow your body to hang below the bar with your body straight and your heels supported on the floor. This will look like an upside-down push-up position.

MOVE

Perform inverted rows by pulling your chest to the bar and then slowly lowering your body to the start position. To add resistance, wear a weight vest or place a weight plate on your chest.

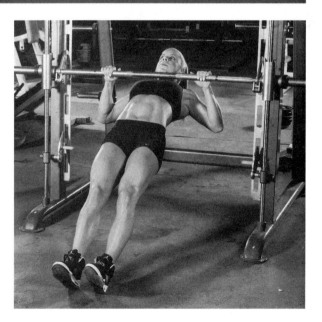

TRX INVERTED ROW

START

Set the handles of the TRX just below hip height. Hold on to the handles using a neutral grip and allow your body to hang below the bar with your body straight and heels supported on the floor. This will look like an upside-down push-up position.

MOVE

Perform inverted rows by using your lats to pull your elbows down past your sides, lifting your body up and then slowly lowering your body to the start position. To add resistance, wear a weight vest or place a weight plate on your chest.

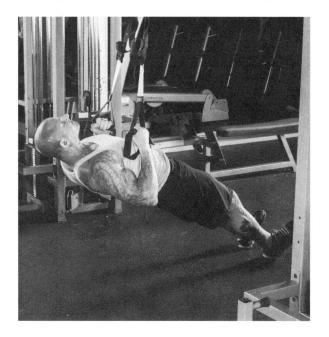

BAND PULLDOWN

START

Attach a band to a high stable crossbar or the top of the door attachment. Kneel down so that there is adequate tension on the bands when you hold the handles with your arms directly overhead. Alternatively, you can hold the bands directly without attaching handles to minimize the length of the bands, as seen in the photo.

MOVE

Pull the handles down to the outsides of your shoulders and hold this position for a second while focusing on contracting the lats. Slowly return the handles to the start position.

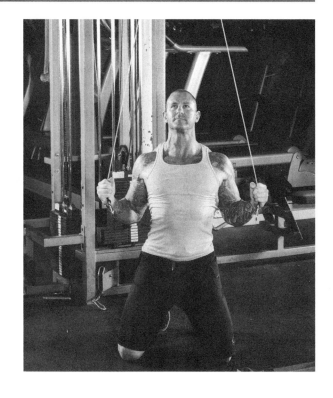

BAND STRAIGHT-ARM PULLDOWN

START

Attach a band to a high stable crossbar or the top of the door attachment. If you need to, kneel down so there is adequate tension on the bands when you hold the handles with your arms extended directly out in front of your chest.

MOVE

Keeping your arms straight, pull the handles down past your hips and hold this position for a second while focusing on contracting the lats. Slowly return the handles to the start position.

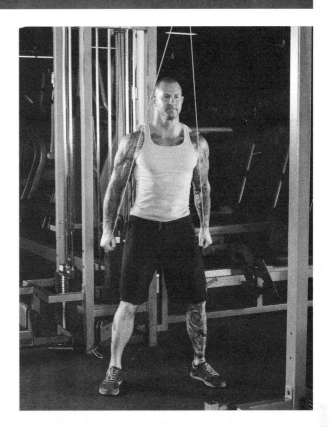

LYING STRAIGHT-ARM PULLDOWN

START

Lie on your back either on the floor or on a bench set lengthwise in a cable crossover apparatus with the pulley stationed above your head. If the pulley height is adjustable, lower it so that it is just above arm's reach. Grab a straight bar attached to the pulley with an overhand grip and your arms extended directly above you.

MOVE

Contract your lats as you keep your arms straight with a slight bend in your elbows to pull the bar down to your thighs. Hold this position for a second as you contract your lats as hard as possible before returning the bar to the start position.

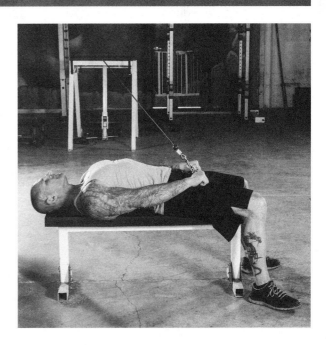

STRAIGHT-ARM PULLOVER

START

Lie on a flat bench with your feet flat on the floor and your head close to the end of the bench. Hold a straight bar or EZ curl bar with an overhand grip spaced shoulder-width apart and arms extended straight over your chest. Maintain a slight bend in your elbows throughout the entire exercise.

MOVE

Lower your arms back and down over your head until they are just below parallel to the floor. Pull the bar back up with straight arms until the bar is back over your chest.

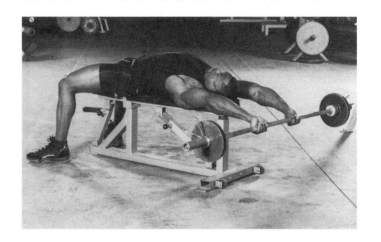

STRAIGHT-ARM DECLINE BENCH PULLOVER

START

Lie on a decline bench with your feet secured under the foot pads and your head close to the end of the bench. Hold a straight bar or EZ curl bar with an overhand grip spaced shoulder-width apart and arms extended straight up over your abs. Maintain a slight bend in your elbows throughout the entire exercise.

MOVE

Lower your arms back and down over your head as far as possible, then pull the bar back up with straight arms until the bar is back over your abs.

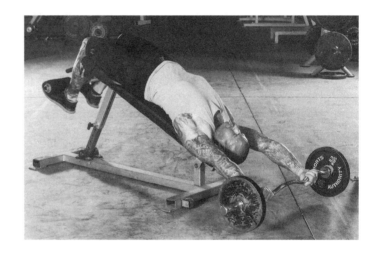

STRAIGHT-ARM PULLDOWN

START

Stand behind the bench of a lat pulldown apparatus with your feet hip-width to shoulder-width apart and knees slightly bent. Grab the lat bar with an overhand grip and your arms shoulder-width apart. In this position your arms should be extended straight out in front of you, forming about a 45-degree angle to the floor.

MOVE

Pull your arms down to bring the bar to your upper thighs while maintaining a slight bend in your elbows. Squeeze your lats hard in this position and slowly return the bar back to the starting position.

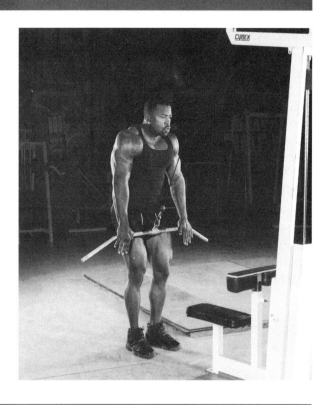

ONE-ARM STRAIGHT-ARM PULLDOWN

START

Stand about a foot (30.5 to 61 centimeters) or two away from a high-pulley cable so that your right arm is lined up with the pulley. Your feet should be hip-width to shoulder-width apart and your knees slightly bent. Grab a single-handle D-grip with an overhand grip. In this position your arm should be extended straight out in front of you, forming about a 45-degree angle to the floor.

MOVE

Pull your arm down to bring the handle to the side of your thigh while maintaining a slight bend in your elbow. Hold the contraction for a second before slowly returning the handle back to the starting position. Perform the desired number of reps and repeat on the left side.

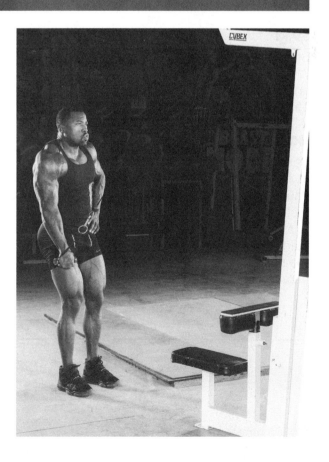

DUMBBELL STRAIGHT-ARM PULLBACK

START

Stand with your knees slightly bent and shoulder-width apart. Hold a dumbbell in your left hand with an overhand grip. Bend over from the hips until your back is just above parallel with the floor. Place your right hand on your lower thigh for support. Let the dumbbell hang straight down below your shoulder.

MOVE

Maintaining a straight arm, pull your arm back and up to your side until it is parallel with the floor. Then slowly return your arm to the starting position. Complete all reps with the left arm, then repeat with the right arm.

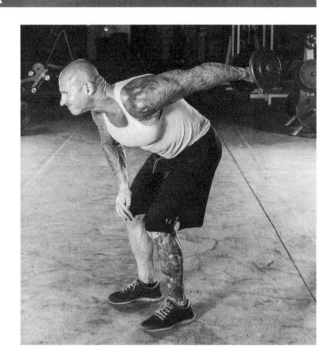

STIFF-LEG DEADLIFT

START

Stand with feet hip-width to shoulder-width apart. With hands in an overhand or staggered grip and spaced shoulder-width apart, hold a loaded barbell in front of your thighs.

MOVE

Bend over at the waist as you lower the bar in front of your legs down toward your ankles. Pause briefly before lifting your torso back up to a standing position.

Note: This exercise is different from the Romanian deadlift, which uses more movement at the hips than at the lower back and involves the hamstrings and glutes as the primary movers.

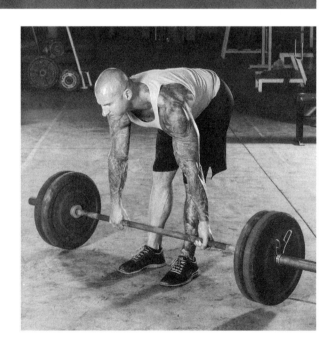

BARBELL GOOD MORNING

START

Stand with a barbell resting across your traps in a shoulder-width grip.

MOVE

Keeping your knees slightly bent, lean forward at the hips until your torso is almost parallel to the ground. Return to the starting position.

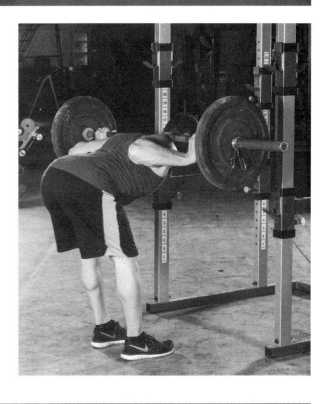

BACK EXTENSION

START

Lie facedown on a back extension bench with your heels under the footpads and your hips resting on the bench. Keep your body straight and your hands crossed over your chest.

MOVE

Lower your torso by bending at the waist to form an angle at your hips that approaches about 90 degrees. Use a smooth motion to rise back up to the starting position.

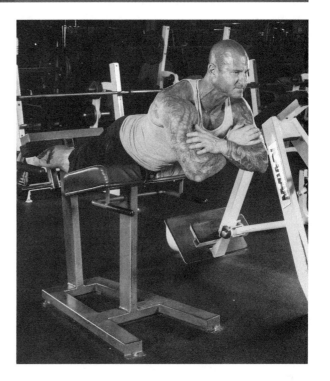

LYING BACK EXTENSION

START

Lie facedown on the floor with your arms extended in front of you.

MOVE

Raise your chest, shoulders, and arms off the floor as high as possible and hold for the desired amount of time.

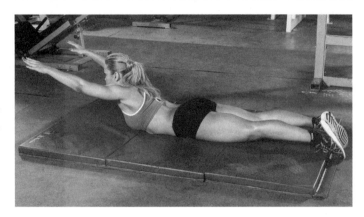

SUPERMAN BACK EXTENSION

START

Lie facedown on the floor with your arms extended in front of you.

MOVE

Simultaneously raise your chest, shoulders, arms, and legs off the floor as high as possible and hold for the desired amount of time.

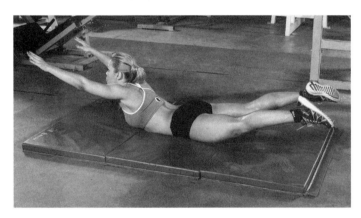

CHAPTER 17

Trapezius

This chapter contains detailed descriptions of all major exercises that focus on the trapezius (trap) muscles, including the upper-, middle-, and lower-trapezius muscle fibers. See the diagram for a detailed location of each of these areas of the trapezius muscle. The traps exercises are divided into barbell and Smith machine shrugging exercises; dumbbell shrugging exercises; cable, band, and machine shrugging exercises; and lower-trapezius exercises. Wherever a certain type of exercise is used in a workout, any one of the same type can be substituted.

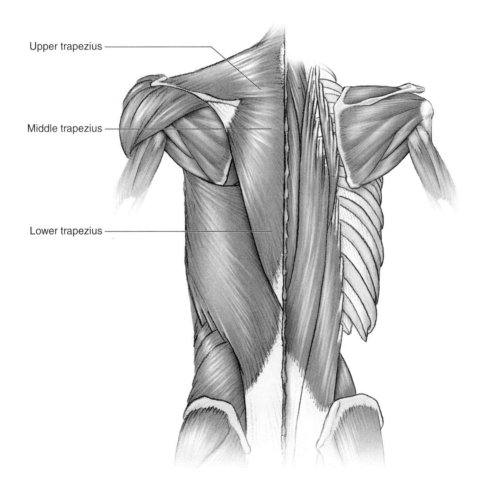

Upper trapezius

Middle trapezius

Lower trapezius

BARBELL SHRUG

START

Stand while holding a barbell with an overhand grip in front of your thighs. Both your hands and your feet should be shoulder-width apart.

MOVE

Lift your shoulders up toward your ears as high as possible while keeping your arms straight. Hold the contraction for a second before lowering the bar back to the starting position.

Note: You can do this exercise with a staggered grip (one hand using an overhand grip and the other using an underhand grip).

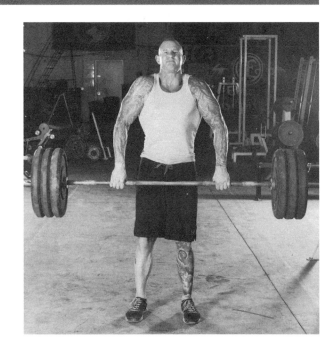

BEHIND-THE-BACK BARBELL SHRUG

START

Stand while holding a barbell with an overhand grip behind your thighs. Both your hands and your feet should be shoulder-width apart.

MOVE

Lift your shoulders up toward your ears as high as possible while keeping your arms straight. Hold the contraction for a second before lowering the bar back to the starting position.

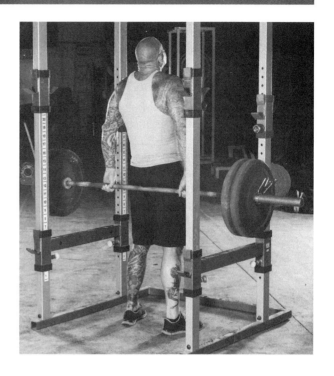

BARBELL SHRUG WITH BANDS

START

Attach the ends of an exercise band to the ends of a loaded barbell. Stand on the middle of the band with a wide stance to provide ample resistance from the bands. Grab the barbell with an overhand, shoulder-width grip and lift the barbell off the floor to get in a normal barbell shrug start position.

MOVE

Use your traps to pull your shoulders up as high as possible and lower your shoulders to the start position.

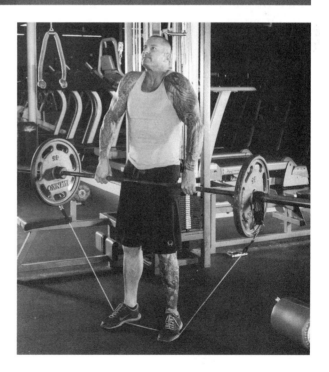

SMITH MACHINE SHRUG

START

Stand in a Smith machine holding the unlatched bar with an overhand grip in front of your thighs. Both your hands and your feet should be shoulder-width apart.

MOVE

Lift your shoulders up toward your ears as high as possible while keeping your arms straight. Hold the contraction for a second before lowering the bar back to the starting position.

Note: You can do this exercise with a staggered grip (one hand using an overhand grip and the other using an underhand grip).

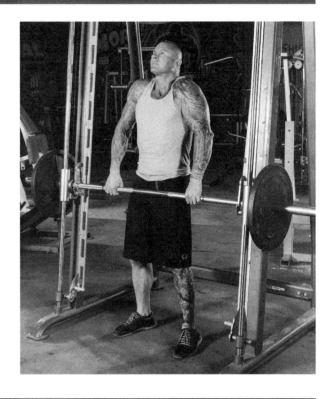

SMITH MACHINE BEHIND-THE-BACK SHRUG

START

Stand in a Smith machine holding the unlatched bar with an overhand grip in back of your thighs. Both your hands and your feet should be shoulder-width apart.

MOVE

Lift your shoulders up toward your ears as high as possible while keeping your arms straight. Hold the contraction for a second before lowering the bar back to the starting position.

Note: You can do this exercise with a staggered grip (one hand using an overhand grip and the other using an underhand grip).

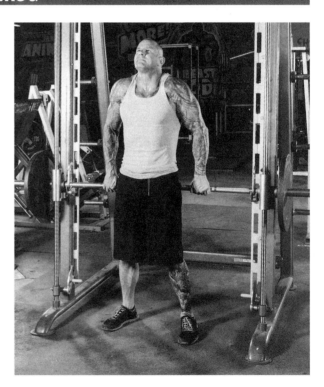

SMITH MACHINE ONE-ARM SHRUG

START

Stand in a Smith machine with your right side toward the bar. With your feet shoulder-width apart and your knees slightly bent, grab the bar in the middle with your right hand and unlatch it.

MOVE

Lift your shoulder up toward your ear as high as possible while keeping your arm straight. Hold the contraction for a second before lowering the bar back to the starting position. Complete the desired number of reps and repeat on the left side.

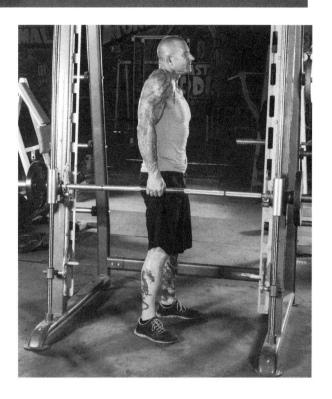

BARBELL POWER SHRUG

START

Stand while holding a barbell with an overhand grip in front of your thighs. Both your hands and your feet should be shoulder-width apart.

MOVE

Quickly bend down a little at the knees and immediately reverse that motion, exploding up with your thighs and calves while simultaneously shrugging your shoulders up toward your ears as high as possible while keeping your arms straight. Immediately lower the weight back to the starting position.

Note: You can do this exercise with a staggered grip (one hand using an overhand grip and the other using an underhand grip).

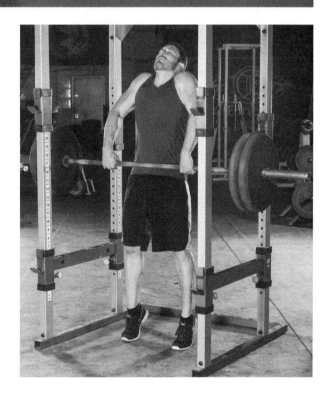

DUMBBELL SHRUG

START

Stand with feet shoulder-width apart while holding a pair of dumbbells at your sides.

MOVE

Slowly shrug your shoulders up toward your ears. At the top, pause for a moment and contract hard through your traps before slowly lowering the weights back to the starting position.

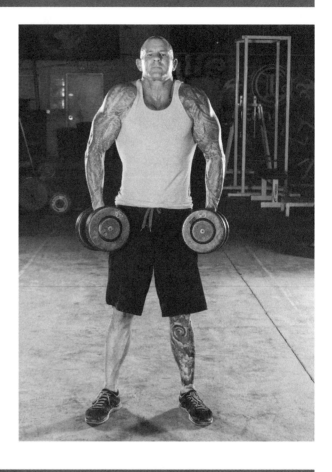

SEATED DUMBBELL SHRUG

START

Sit on a flat bench with your feet flat on the floor in front of you. Hold a pair of dumbbells with a neutral grip at your sides.

MOVE

Slowly shrug your shoulders up toward your ears. At the top, pause for a moment and contract hard through your traps and rhomboids before slowly lowering the weights back to the starting position.

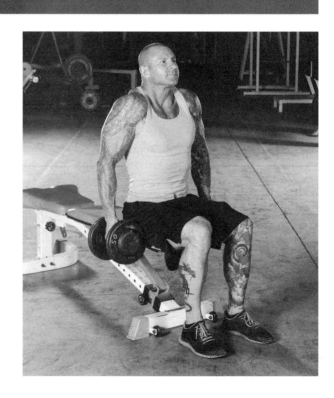

ONE-ARM DUMBBELL SHRUG

START

Stand with your feet shoulder-width apart. Hold a dumbbell in your left hand at your side.

MOVE

Slowly shrug your left shoulder up toward your ear. At the top, pause for a moment and contract the muscles hard before slowly lowering the weight back to the starting position. After completing all reps on the left side, repeat on the right side.

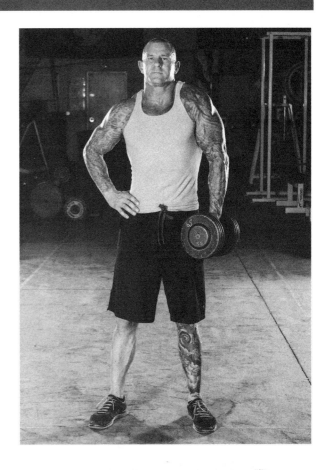

PRONE INCLINE BENCH DUMBBELL SHRUG

START

Grab a pair of dumbbells and straddle an adjustable-incline bench with your feet flat on the floor, or position them on the bench frame to support your body. Hold the dumbbells with a neutral grip at your sides.

MOVE

Slowly shrug your shoulders up toward your ears. At the top, pause for a moment and contract hard through your traps and rhomboids before slowly lowering the weights back to the starting position.

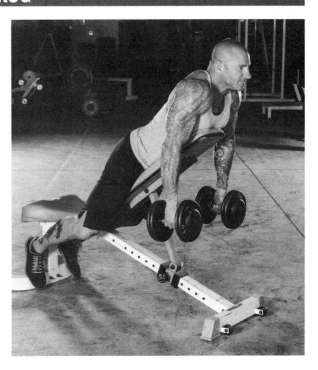

CABLE SHRUG

START

With feet shoulder-width apart, stand in front of a low-pulley cable while holding a straight bar attached to the low pulley.

MOVE

Slowly shrug your shoulders up toward your ears. At the top, pause for a moment and contract hard through your traps before slowly lowering the bar back to the starting position.

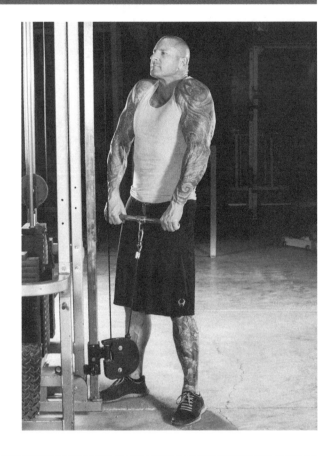

ONE-ARM CABLE SHRUG

START

Stand with your right side toward a low-pulley cable and maintain a shoulder-width stance while holding a single-handle D-grip in your right hand.

MOVE

Shrug your right shoulder up toward your ear. At the top, pause for a moment and contract the muscles hard before slowly lowering the handle back to the starting position.

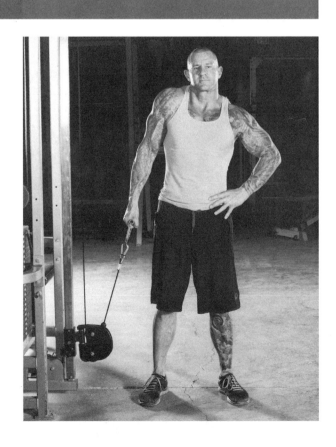

PRONE INCLINE CABLE SHRUG

START

Place an incline bench next to a pulley apparatus so that the higher end is near the low pulley and to the right. Set the angle at about 45 degrees or higher. With your left hand, grasp the single-handle D-grip attached to the low pulley. Sit straddling the bench and facing the weight stack. Lean against the bench to support your chest while extending your arm forward and down with a neutral grip.

MOVE

Slowly shrug your left shoulder up and back. At the top, pause for a moment and contract the muscles hard before slowly lowering the handle back to the starting position. Complete the desired number of reps and then repeat with the right arm.

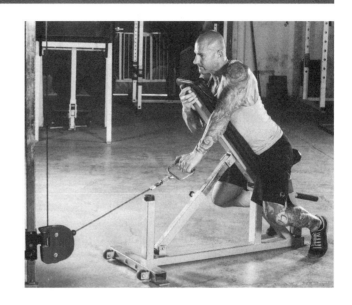

STANDING CALF MACHINE SHRUG

START

Stand in the standing calf machine with the pads on your shoulders and a slight bend in your knees. Allow the weight of the stack to drop your shoulders as low as possible to stretch the traps.

MOVE

Use your traps to shrug your shoulders up as high as possible. Hold this position for a second and then slowly lower your shoulders and repeat for reps.

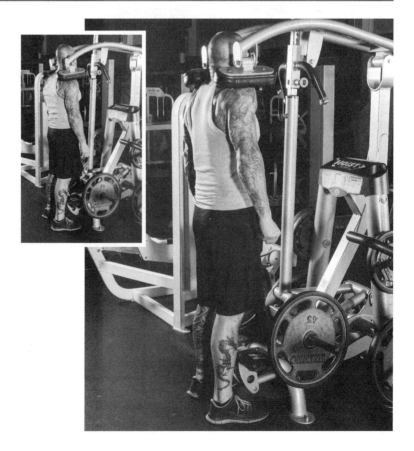

BAND SHRUG

START

Stand on top of an exercise band with both feet using a shoulder-width stance or wider to provide adequate resistance from the bands. Hold the handles of the band with a neutral grip with your arms extended down at the sides of your thighs.

MOVE

Contract your traps to shrug your shoulders up as high as possible. Hold the top position for a second as you contract your traps. Slowly lower your shoulders and repeat for reps

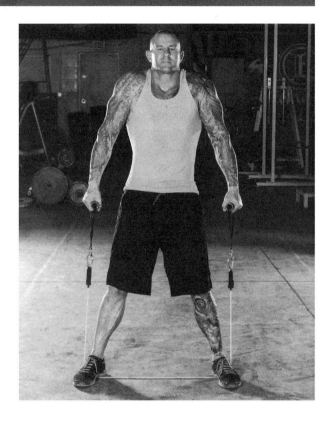

STRAIGHT-ARM DIP

START

Support your body on the dip bars with your arms straight and almost locked out.

MOVE

Without bending your elbows, allow your body to sink as low as you can and then use your lower traps to pull your scapulae down, which will raise your body up. Try to raise your body as high as possible and then lower it and repeat.

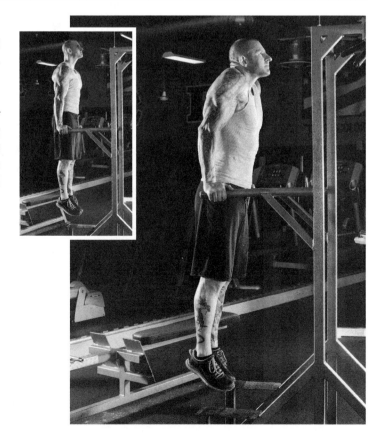

BEHIND-THE-BACK SMITH MACHINE STRAIGHT-ARM DIP

START

Set the bar of the Smith machine at a height so that when you sit back on the bar with your feet on the floor and place your hands on the bar your arms are straight and your shoulders are as high as possible.

MOVE

Keep your arms straight, contract your lower traps to depress your scapulae, and lift your body as high as possible, leaning the back of your legs against the bar for balance. Hold the top position for a second as you focus on contracting your lower traps and then lower your feet to the floor and repeat for reps. To increase the resistance, wear a weight vest or chain belt with weight plates attached.

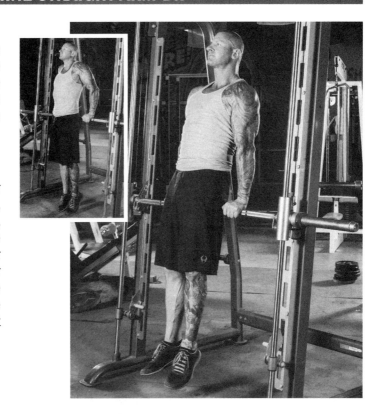

STRAIGHT-ARM PRESSDOWN

START

Attach a wide straight bar to a cable pulley and set the bar just below waist height. Stand with the bar behind your back and place your hands on the bar with an overhand, shoulder-width grip. Extend your arms so that your elbows are locked out. Without bending your elbows, allow the weight from the pulley station to raise your shoulders as high as possible. This is the start position.

MOVE

Use your lower traps to pull your shoulder blades down and together to lower your shoulders as much as possible. Hold this position for a second, focusing on contracting your lower traps as hard as possible before relaxing them and allowing your shoulders to rise to the start position.

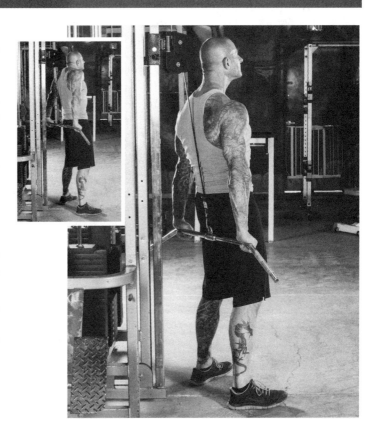

Y-RAISE

START

Lie facedown on a flat bench with your chin past the end of the bench. Hold two light dumbbells or weight plates with a neutral grip down toward the floor.

MOVE

Lift both dumbbells up as high as you can while forming a letter Y with your arms and torso. Hold this position for two seconds before returning the dumbbells to the starting position.

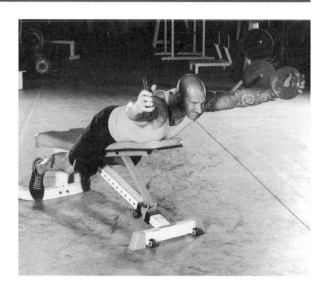

ONE-ARM CABLE Y-RAISE

START

Attach a rope handle to a low cable pulley. Stand facing the cable pulley as you hold the rope handle with a hammer grip and your arm extended straight out in front of you. Alternatively, you can just hold onto the end of the cable without an attachment, as shown in the photo.

MOVE

Keeping your arm straight, but allowing a slight bend in your elbow, raise the handle above your head. Your arm should make about a 30-degree angle with your head in the top position. Hold the top position for a second and then slowly return the handle to the start position. Perform all reps on one side and then repeat with the other arm.

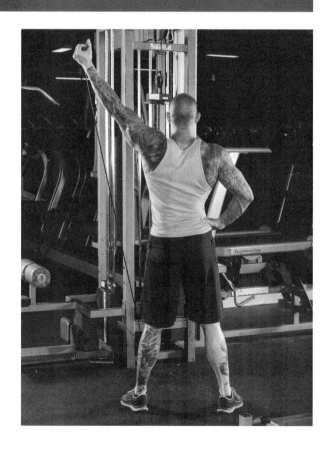

STANDING BAND Y-RAISE

START

Wrap a band around a stable structure so that both ends of the band are at about shoulder height. Hold the handles with a neutral grip (palms facing each other). Alternatively, you can hold the ends of the bands without attachments, as shown in the photo.

MOVE

While keeping your arms straight at the elbows, extend your arms straight up as high as possible so that they form about a 30-degree angle with your head. Slowly return your arms to the start position and repeat for reps.

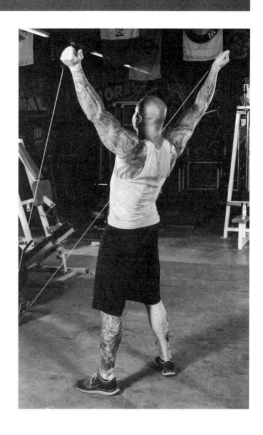

CHAPTER 18

Triceps

This chapter contains detailed descriptions of all major exercises that focus on the triceps muscles, including the lateral head, long head, and medial head. See the diagram for the location of each of theses triceps heads. The triceps exercises are divided into pressing, dip, and push-up exercises; pressdown and kickback exercises; lying and machine triceps extension exercises; and overhead triceps extension exercises. Wherever a certain type of exercise is used in a workout, any one of the same type can be substituted.

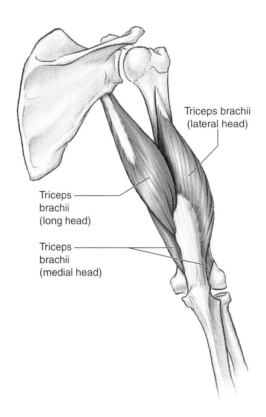

Triceps brachii (lateral head)

Triceps brachii (long head)

Triceps brachii (medial head)

Pressing, Dip, and Push-Up Exercises

Pressdown and Kickback Exercises

Lying and Machine Triceps Extension Exercises

Overhead Triceps Extension Exercises

CLOSE-GRIP BENCH PRESS

START

Lie faceup on a bench-press bench with your feet flat on the floor. With your hands shoulder-width apart, grasp the barbell with an overhand grip.

Note: Using anything closer than a shoulder-width grip does not increase triceps' involvement but may increase stress on the wrists.

MOVE

Unrack the bar and slowly lower it to your lower chest, keeping your elbows as close to your sides as possible. At the bottom of the movement, your elbows should be a little lower than your shoulders. Press the bar back up to the start position.

Note: You can do this exercise with an EZ bar.

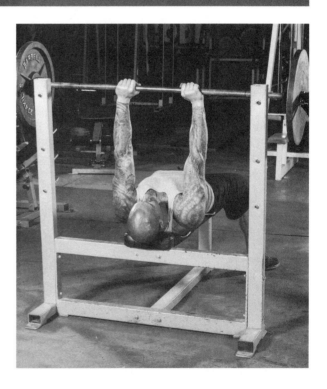

REVERSE-GRIP CLOSE-GRIP BENCH PRESS

START

Lie faceup on a bench-press bench with your feet flat on the floor. With your hands shoulder-width apart, grasp the barbell with an underhand grip.

MOVE

Have a spotter help you unrack the bar and slowly lower it to your lower chest, keeping your elbows as close to your sides as possible. At the bottom of the movement, your elbows should be a little lower than your shoulders. Press the bar back up to the starting position.

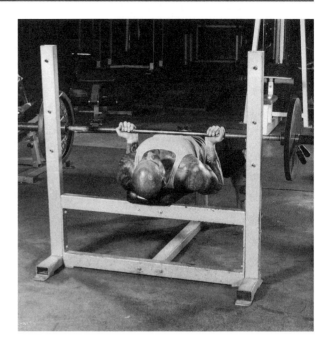

CLOSE-GRIP DUMBBELL PRESS

START

Lie back on a flat bench, holding two dumbbells at your chest with a neutral grip.

MOVE

Press the dumbbells straight overhead until your arms are fully extended. Flex your triceps hard at the top for a second before bringing the weights back down toward your chest.

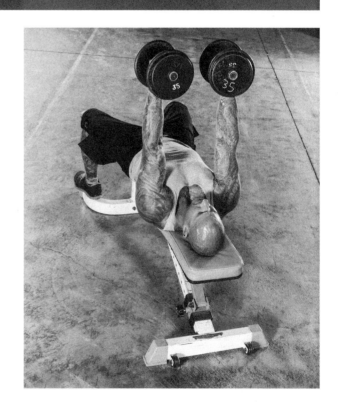

TRICEPS DIP

START

Grasp the dip bars with your arms extended and locked. Keep your body as vertical as possible to keep emphasis on the triceps and away from the chest. If the dip bars are high enough, keep your legs straight below you.

MOVE

Keep your elbows as close to your sides as possible as you bend them to lower your body down until your upper arms are about parallel to the floor. Press your hands forcefully into the bars to extend your arms and raise your body back up.

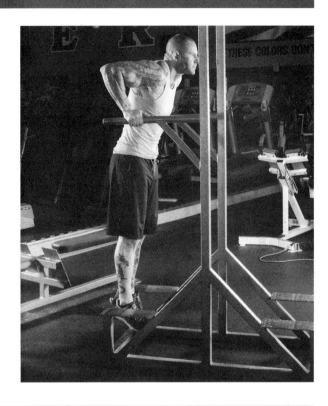

BENCH DIP

START

Place your hands on the side of a flat bench so that your body is perpendicular to the bench when you place your feet out in front of you. Only your heels should be on the floor and your legs should be straight. Or keep your knees and hips bent to support a weight plate on your thighs to add resistance. Your arms should be fully extended with just your palms on the bench.

MOVE

Bend your elbows to lower your body down until your elbows reach 90 degrees. Extend your arms to lift your body back to the starting position, flexing your triceps hard at the top.

Note: You can also do this exercise with your heels up on a bench that is parallel to the other bench. Have a partner load weight plates on your lap to make it even more difficult.

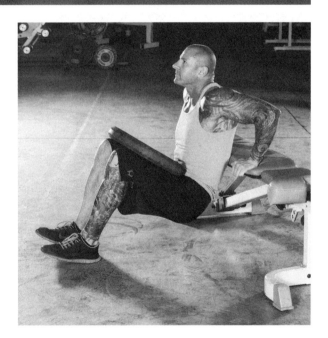

MACHINE DIP

START

Sit on the seat of a machine dip with your feet flat on the floor and your back pressed firmly against the pad. Grasp the handles with an overhand grip.

MOVE

With your arms close to your sides throughout (elbows pointed straight back behind you), press the handles down to full arm extension. Flex your triceps hard for a second and then slowly bring the handles back up until your elbows form a 90-degree angle.

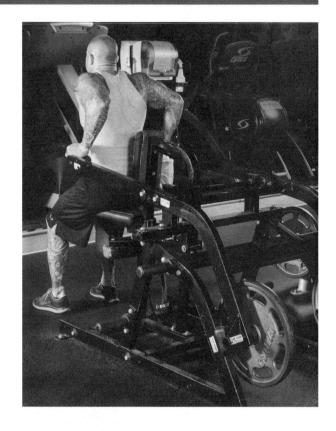

CLOSE-GRIP PUSH-UP

START

Lie facedown on the floor in a push-up position, placing your hands a few inches apart. Raise your body by extending your arms and coming up on your toes.

MOVE

With your forehead facing the floor and your abs pulled in, lower your body by bending your elbows. Stop the motion when your upper arms are about parallel to the floor, and reverse the movement to the starting position.

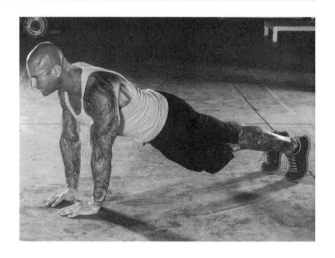

CLOSE-GRIP PUSH-UP LADDER

START

Get in the close-grip push-up position, as described earlier, next to a Smith machine.

MOVE

After reaching muscle failure, perform close-grip push-up ladders on the Smith machine bar as described for push-up ladders in chapter 14.

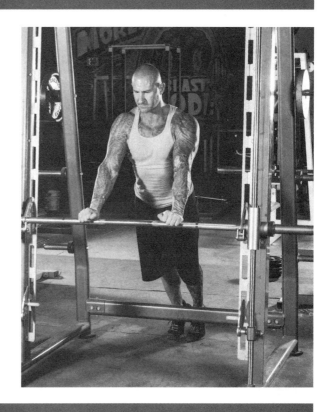

TRICEPS PRESSDOWN

START

With a slight bend in your knees, stand facing a high-pulley cable with a pressdown bar attached to it. Your feet should be about shoulder-width apart. Grasp the pressdown bar with an overhand grip and hold the bar at chest level with your elbows tight against your sides.

MOVE

Keeping your elbows stationary, straighten your arms until they are fully extended. Pause at full arm extension and flex your triceps, then slowly return the bar to the starting position.

Note: You can do this exercise with a rope, short straight bar, or EZ bar attachment.

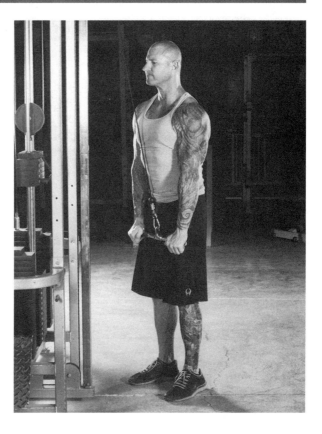

ONE-ARM CABLE PRESSDOWN

START

Stand facing a high-pulley cable with a single-handle D-grip attached to it. Your feet should be about shoulder-width apart and your knees should be slightly bent. Using an overhand grip, grasp the handle with your left hand and hold it at chest level with your elbow tight against your side.

MOVE

Keeping your elbow stationary, straighten your left arm until it is fully extended. Pause at full arm extension and flex your triceps, then slowly return the handle to the starting position. Complete as many reps as desired and then repeat with the right arm.

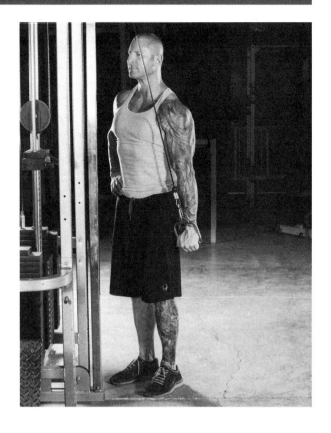

REVERSE-GRIP CABLE PRESSDOWN

START

With a slight bend in your knees, stand facing a high-pulley cable with a short straight bar attached to it. Your feet should be about shoulder-width apart. With an underhand grip, grasp the pressdown bar and hold the bar at chest level with your elbows tight against your sides.

MOVE

Keeping your elbows stationary, straighten your arms until they are fully extended. Pause at full arm extension and flex your triceps, then slowly return the bar to the starting position.

Note: You can do this exercise with an EZ bar attachment.

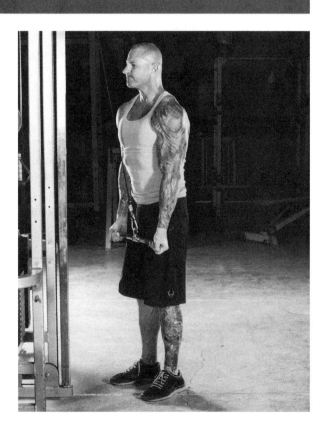

ONE-ARM REVERSE-GRIP CABLE PRESSDOWN

START

Stand facing a high-pulley cable with a single-handle D-grip attached to it. Your feet should be about hip-width to shoulder-width apart and your knees should be slightly bent. Using an underhand grip, grasp the handle with your left hand and hold it at chest level with your elbow tight against your side.

MOVE

Keeping your elbow stationary, straighten your left arm until it is fully extended. Pause at full arm extension and flex your triceps, then slowly return the handle to the starting position. Complete as many reps as desired, then repeat with the right arm.

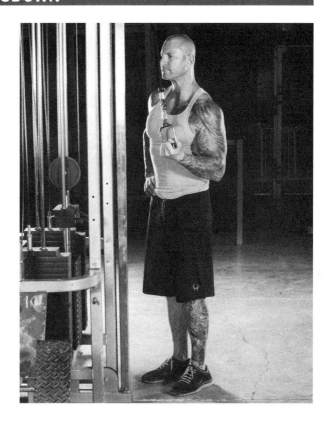

CROSS-BODY CABLE TRICEPS PRESSDOWN

START

Stand in the middle of a cable crossover apparatus holding in one hand a rope handle attached to the high pulley or to a pulley set slightly higher than shoulder height. Start with your upper arm extended to your side and almost parallel to the floor and your elbow bent so that your hand is in front of your chest.

MOVE

Keeping your upper arm stationary, extend your arm at the elbow until it is fully extended out to your side. Contract the triceps in this final position before returning your hand to the start. The upper-arm position this exercise requires takes the shoulder and chest completely out of the picture and forces you to use just your triceps for better isolation of the lateral head.

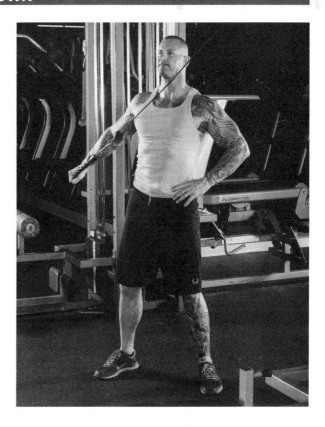

BAND TRICEPS PRESSDOWN

START

Attach a band to a high crossbar or the door attachment set at the top of the door. Stand back far enough to allow enough resistance from the bands with your upper arms parallel with your torso and pressed at your sides and your elbows bent at 90 degrees while holding the handles with an overhand grip. Alternatively, you can grab onto the bands directly without handles attached using a neutral grip. If there is not enough tension on the bands, do these in a kneeling position.

MOVE

Contract your triceps to extend your arms at the elbow. Bring the handles down to the sides of your legs. Hold this position for a second while forcefully contracting your triceps. Then slowly return the handles to the start position.

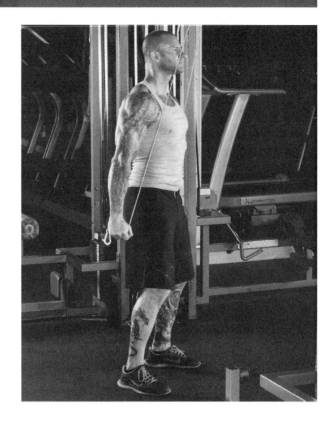

DUMBBELL KICKBACK

START

Place your right knee and palm on a flat bench so that your torso is parallel with the floor. While holding a dumbbell in the left hand and keeping the left foot flat on the floor, press your left arm tight against your side with the upper arm parallel to the floor.

MOVE

Extend at the elbow until your arm is straight back and fully extended. Flex the triceps hard for a second, then reverse to the starting position. Complete all reps on the left arm and then repeat on the right.

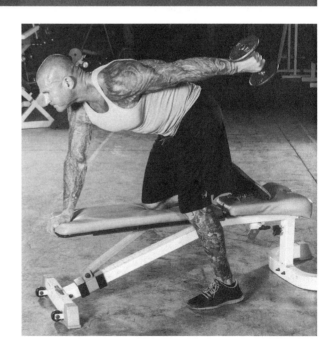

CABLE KICKBACK

START

Face the weight stack and bend from the waist so that your torso is about parallel to the floor. With an underhand grip, grasp a single-handle D-grip attached to a low pulley. Alternatively, you can grab onto the cable directly without a handle attached using a neutral grip. Raise your elbow so that your upper arm is parallel to the floor and your elbow is bent 90 degrees and tucked at your side. Brace your right arm on your thigh or on the pulley cable apparatus.

MOVE

Extend your arm back and up until your arm is fully extended. Flex the triceps hard for a second, then reverse to the starting position. Complete as many reps as desired, then repeat with the right arm.

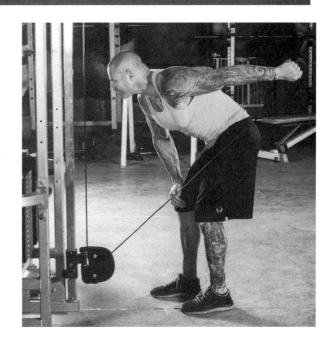

BAND TRICEPS KICKBACK

START

Stand in a staggered stance (one foot forward and one back). Stand on the middle of a band with the back foot. Grab the ends of the band with your left hand using a neutral grip. Bend forward from the hips and keep your upper arm parallel with your torso and pressed to your side. Allow your forearm to hang straight down at a 90-degree angle to your upper arm.

MOVE

Use your triceps to extend your forearm back until your arm is completely straight with your elbow locked out. Contract your triceps as hard as possible in this position, then return the band to the start position. Complete all reps with your left arm and then repeat with your right arm.

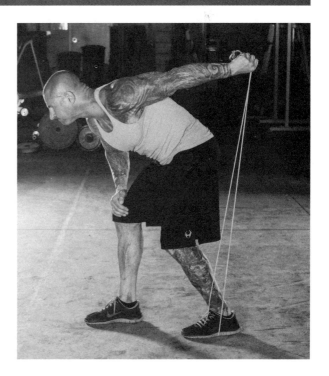

LYING TRICEPS EXTENSION

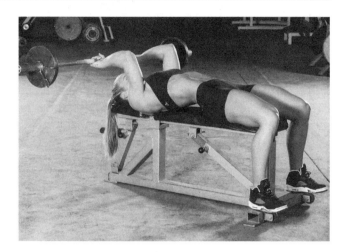

START

Lie faceup on a flat bench with your feet flat on the floor or up on the bench frame for those with shorter legs. Hold a barbell at full arm extension over your chest.

MOVE

Keeping your upper arms stationary, lower your lower arms to bring the bar down to your forehead, then push it back up.

Note: You can do this exercise with an EZ bar.

DECLINE TRICEPS EXTENSION

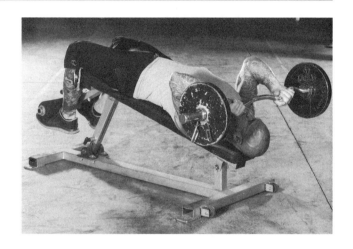

START

Lie faceup on an adjustable-decline bench with your feet secured under the foot pads. Take a shoulder-width, overhand grip on a barbell and lift it into position over your chest, keeping your arms straight.

MOVE

Bend your elbows and lower the weight to your forehead, then extend your arms to return the bar to the starting position.

DUMBBELL LYING TRICEPS EXTENSION

START

Lie faceup on a flat bench with your feet flat on the floor. With a neutral grip, hold a pair of dumbbells at full arm extension over your chest.

MOVE

Keeping your upper arms stationary, lower your lower arms to bring the dumbbells to the sides of your head, then push them back up.

Note: You can do this exercise on a decline bench.

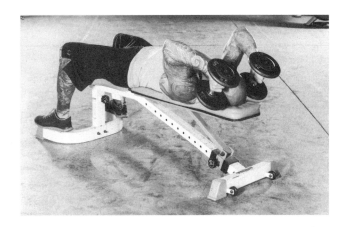

ONE-ARM DUMBBELL LYING TRICEPS EXTENSION

START

Lie on a flat bench and hold a dumbbell in your left hand with an overhand grip. Extend your arm so that the dumbbell is straight up from your left shoulder.

MOVE

Without letting your upper arm move, bend at the elbow to bring the dumbbell down to the side of your head across your body toward the right shoulder. Either way, stop when your elbow reaches 90 degrees and reverse the motion to bring the dumbbell back up to full arm extension. Complete as many reps as desired, then repeat with the right arm.

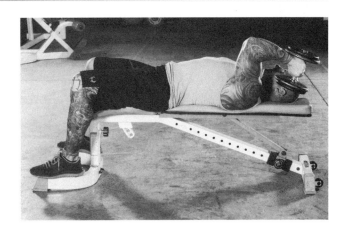

CABLE LYING TRICEPS EXTENSION

START

Lie faceup on the floor or on a bench lengthwise in the middle of a cable crossover apparatus. Your head is closest to the low-pulley cable. With an overhand grip, grab a straight bar handle attached to the low pulley and extend your arms straight over your head.

MOVE

Keeping your upper arms perpendicular to your torso, lower the bar to the top of your head. Extend your arms to lift the bar back up to full extension.

Note: You can do this exercise with an EZ bar attachment.

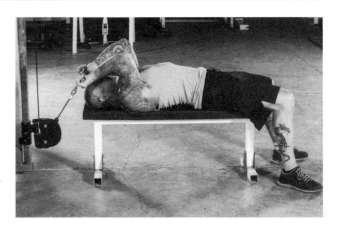

MACHINE TRICEPS EXTENSION

START

Sit in the seat of a triceps extension machine and place your upper arms on the arm pads while grasping the handles with your hands.

MOVE

Use your triceps to extend your arms at just the elbows while keeping your upper arms in the arm pads. Once your arms have reached full extension, slowly return the handles to the start position.

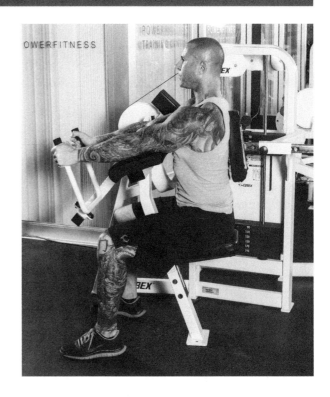

OVERHEAD BARBELL TRICEPS EXTENSION

START

Sit on a low-back bench and extend a barbell overhead, holding it with a shoulder-width grip.

MOVE

Keeping your upper arms right beside your head, lower the bar behind your head until your elbows form 90-degree angles, then lift it back to full arm extension.

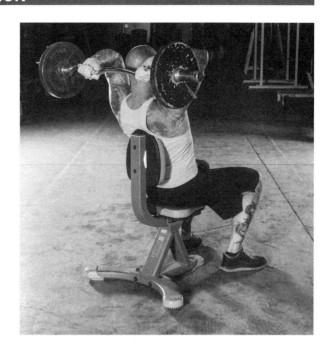

OVERHEAD DUMBBELL TRICEPS EXTENSION

START

Sit on a low-back bench and hoist a dumbbell overhead, holding it with both hands, palms cupped against the upper inside plates.

MOVE

Keeping your upper arms right beside your head, lower the dumbbell behind your head until your elbows form 90-degree angles, then lift it back to full arm extension.

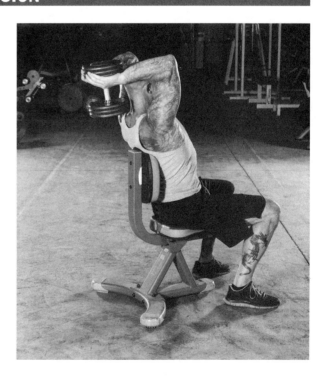

411

ONE-ARM OVERHEAD DUMBBELL TRICEPS EXTENSION

START

Sit on a low-back bench and lift a dumbbell overhead with your right hand. Hold it straight overhead with an overhand grip (palm facing forward).

MOVE

Keeping your upper arm right beside your head, lower the dumbbell behind your head and toward your left shoulder until your elbow forms a 90-degree angle, then lift it back to full arm extension.

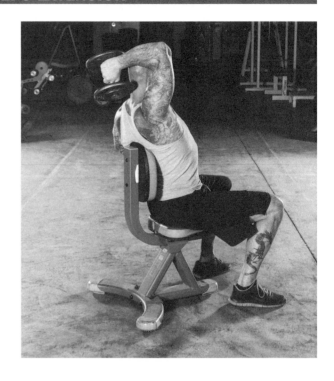

INCLINE OVERHEAD TRICEPS EXTENSION

START

Recline on an incline bench set to 45 degrees and raise a barbell overhead with an overhand grip.

MOVE

Bend your elbows to begin slowly lowering the bar until it is behind your head. Push the weights back up to full arm extension.

Note: You can do this exercise with a barbell, one dumbbell, or a pair of dumbbells.

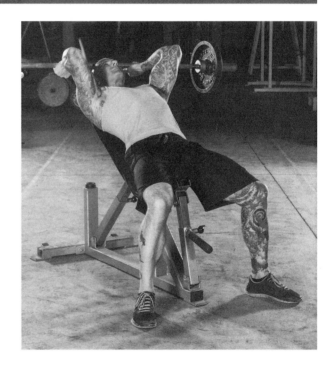

OVERHEAD CABLE TRICEPS EXTENSION

START

Stand with your back to a high pulley with a rope attached to it. With a neutral grip, grasp the rope just behind your head and stand with your torso leaning forward. Keep your elbows beside your ears and bring your forearms back to form a 90-degree angle.

MOVE

Keep your upper arms stationary as you move only from the elbows to press the weight to full arm extension.

Note: You can do this exercise with a short straight bar or EZ bar attachment.

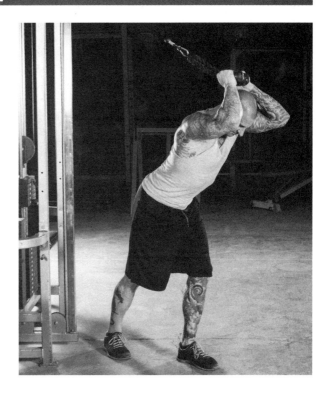

OVERHEAD CABLE TRICEPS EXTENSION (FROM LOW PULLEY)

START

Stand with your back to a cable pulley set below shoulder height with a rope attached to it. With a neutral grip, grasp the rope just behind your head and stand with your torso as upright as possible. Keep your elbows beside your ears with your upper arms as upright as possible.

MOVE

Keep your upper arms stationary as you move only from the elbows to extend the weight to full arm extension overhead.

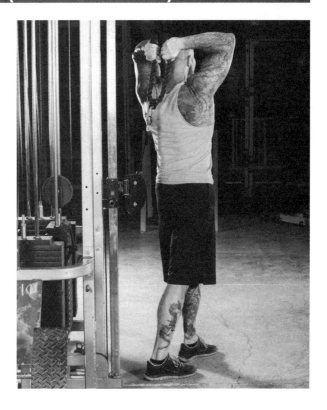

BAND OVERHEAD TRICEPS EXTENSION

START

Stand in a staggered stance (one foot in front and one in back). Stand on an exercise band with the back foot and hold the handles with an overhand grip. Bring your upper arms up so that your elbows are at the sides of your head and elbows are bent with your forearms flexed behind your head.

MOVE

Extend your arms just at the elbows, keeping your upper arms stationary to bring your arms straight overhead. Contract your triceps in this top position and then slowly return the handles to the start position.

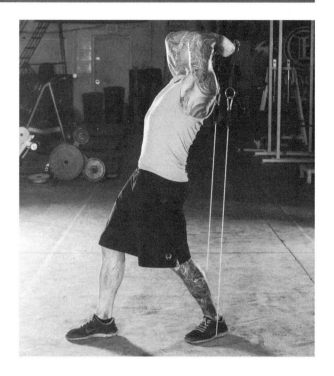

TRX TRICEPS EXTENSION

START

Hold the TRX handles with an overhand grip. Lean forward and bend your arms at the elbows so that your arms are bent less than 90 degrees. Only your toes should be touching the floor. The TRX length should be adjusted so that your body is leaning forward enough to provide enough resistance to limit you to the rep range you are shooting for.

MOVE

Extend your arms at the elbows to straighten your arms, lifting your body weight up. Hold this position with your arms fully extended, and contract your triceps as hard as possible. Resist your body weight as you return your arms to the start position. Continue performing reps in this manner.

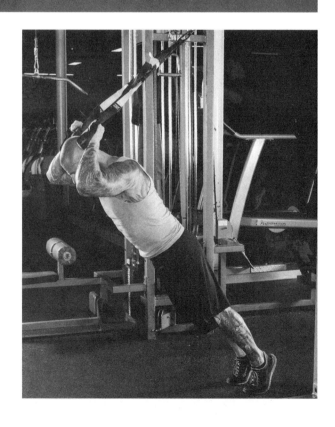

CHAPTER 19

Biceps

This chapter contains detailed descriptions of all major exercises that focus on the biceps muscles, including the biceps brachii and brachialis. The biceps muscles include the long head and short head, which can be seen in the diagram. The brachialis is located beneath the biceps. The biceps exercises are divided into standing curl exercises; seated curl exercises; cable curl exercises; preacher and concentration curl exercises; body-weight curl exercises; and hammer and reverse-grip curl exercises. Wherever a certain type of exercise is used in a workout, any one of the same type can be substituted.

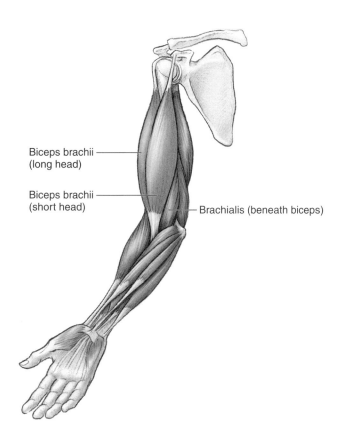

Biceps brachii (long head)

Biceps brachii (short head)

Brachialis (beneath biceps)

BARBELL CURL

START

With your knees slightly bent and your feet about shoulder-width apart, grasp a barbell with a shoulder-width, underhand grip. Let the bar hang to your thighs. Keep your abs pulled in and your elbows stationary.

MOVE

Without swaying, slowly curl the bar in an arc toward your shoulders. Pause at the top of the movement, squeeze your biceps, and slowly lower the bar to the starting position.

   Note: You can do this exercise with an EZ bar.

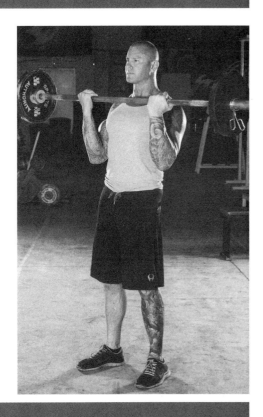

BARBELL CURL WITH BANDS

START

Attach both ends of a band to the ends of a barbell or EZ bar. Stand on the middle of the band and pick up the bar using an underhand grip.

MOVE

Perform curls as you normally would, focusing on the extra tension in the top position that the bands provide by concentrating on the biceps contractions. Slowly lower the bar to the start position.

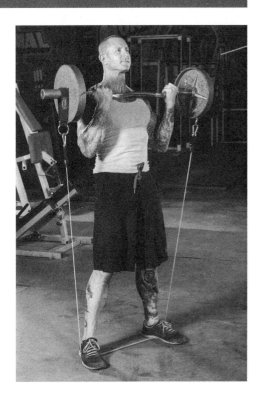

STANDING DUMBBELL CURL

START

Stand with your knees slightly bent and your feet about hip-width apart. Grasp a pair of dumbbells with an underhand grip. Let the dumbbells hang at the sides of your thighs.

MOVE

Without swaying, slowly curl the dumbbells in an arc toward your shoulders. Pause at the top of the movement, squeeze your biceps, and slowly lower the weights to the starting position.

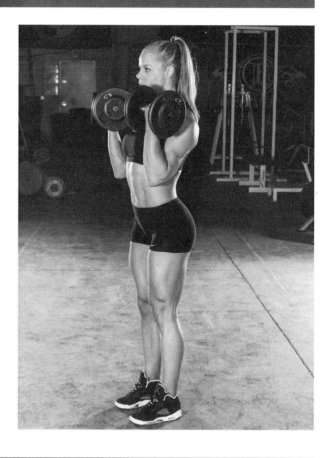

STANDING ALTERNATING DUMBBELL CURL

START

Stand with your knees slightly bent and your feet about hip-width apart. Grasp a pair of dumbbells with a neutral grip. Let the dumbbells hang at the sides of your thighs.

MOVE

Slowly curl the left arm in an arc toward your shoulder. As the dumbbell passes your hip, start to supinate your wrist (turn it out) until your palm is facing your shoulder at the top position. Pause at the top of the movement, squeeze your biceps, and slowly lower the weight in the reverse manner. Repeat the movement with the right arm. One curl with both arms equals one rep.

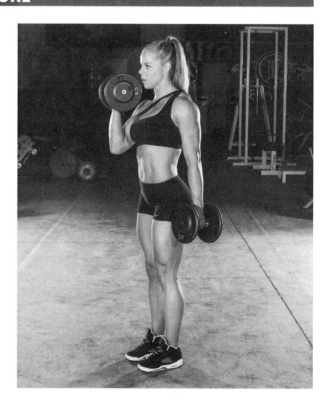

SMITH MACHINE DRAG CURL

START

Unlock the bar on the Smith machine and hold it in front of your thighs with an underhand grip, as you would holding a free-weight barbell.

MOVE

Slowly curl the bar upward, allowing your elbows to track behind your body as the barbell goes up. Stop at about chest height and slowly lower the bar to the start position. This exercise helps to minimize the involvement of the front delts, which come into play when the elbows move forward during curls. And with the biceps moving behind the body, this exercise further targets the long head of the biceps.

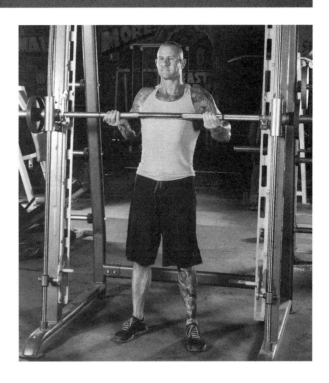

SMITH MACHINE CURL THROW

START

Unlock the bar on the Smith machine and hold it in front of your thighs with an underhand grip, as you would holding a free-weight barbell.

MOVE

As quickly and as explosively as possible, curl the bar upward, allowing it to leave your hands in the top position. Catch the bar with an underhand grip as it comes down, assisting it back into the start position. Reset your grip if you need to and repeat.

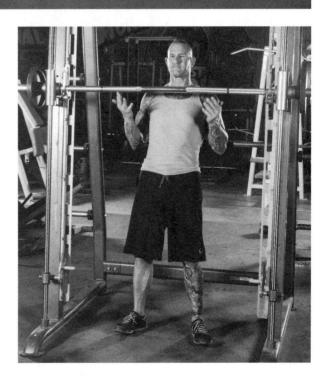

BAND CURL

START

Stand on the middle of an exercise band with a wide-enough stance to provide adequate resistance on the bands. Hold the handles with an underhand grip.

MOVE

Curl the handles up toward your shoulders and contract your biceps as hard as you can. Slowly lower the handles to the start position.

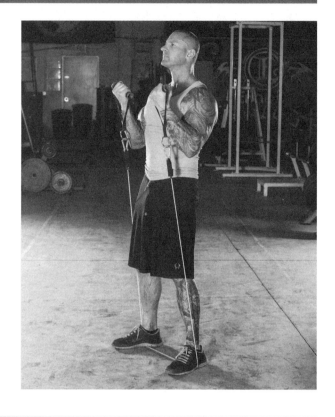

SEATED DUMBBELL CURL

START

Sit at the end of a flat bench or on a low-back bench with your feet planted firmly on the floor. Hold a pair of dumbbells with an underhand grip and let them hang at the sides of the bench.

MOVE

Curl the dumbbells up in an arc toward your shoulders. Pause at the top of the movement, squeeze your biceps, and slowly lower the weights to the starting position.

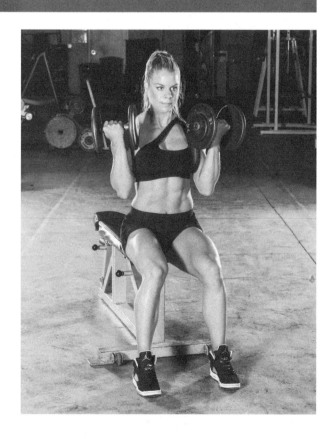

SEATED ALTERNATING DUMBBELL CURL

START

Sit at the end of a flat bench or on a low-back bench with your feet planted firmly on the floor. Hold a pair of dumbbells with a neutral grip and let them hang at the sides of the bench.

MOVE

Slowly curl the right arm in an arc toward your shoulder. As the dumbbell passes your hip, start to supinate your wrist (turn it out) until your palm is facing your shoulder at the top position. Pause at the top of the movement, squeeze your biceps, and slowly lower the weight in the reverse manner. Repeat the movement with the left arm. One curl with both arms equals one rep.

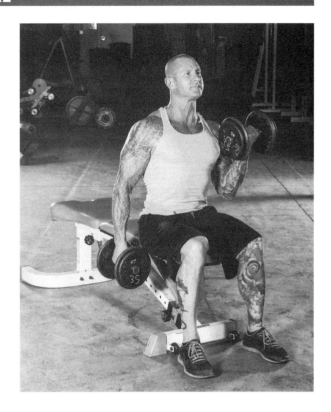

INCLINE DUMBBELL CURL

START

Grasp a pair of dumbbells and lie back on an incline bench set at about 45 to 60 degrees, allowing your arms to hang straight down toward the floor by your sides. Use an underhand grip, with your palms facing forward.

MOVE

Keeping your shoulders back and upper arms in a fixed position perpendicular to the floor, lock your elbows at your sides and curl both dumbbells toward your shoulders. Slowly return the dumbbell to the starting position.

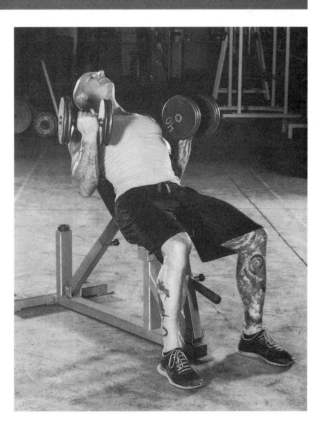

INCLINE ALTERNATING DUMBBELL CURL

START

Grasp a pair of dumbbells and lie back on an incline bench set at about 45 to 60 degrees, allowing your arms to hang straight down toward the floor by your sides. Use a neutral grip, with your palms facing in.

MOVE

Keeping your shoulders back and upper arms in a fixed position perpendicular to the floor, lock your elbows at your sides and curl one arm toward your shoulder. As you curl, supinate your wrist so that your palm faces your shoulder at the top of the movement. Slowly return the dumbbell to the starting position along the same path and repeat with the other arm.

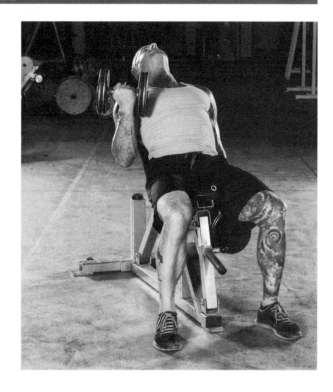

PRONE INCLINE DUMBBELL CURL

START

Lie facedown on an incline bench with a dumbbell in each hand. Let your arms hang straight down perpendicular to the floor. Your chest should be right at the top of the bench. Keep your head up and chest high to ensure easy breathing.

MOVE

Curl your right arm up and toward your left shoulder. Contract your biceps as hard as possible then slowly lower the dumbbell to the start position. Perform with the left arm and alternate arms in this manner.

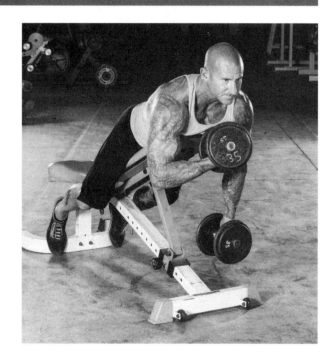

SEATED BARBELL CURL

START

Sit on a short-back bench or an adjustable bench set to 90 degrees and rest the bar on your thighs. Hold the bar with an underhand grip with your hands spaced shoulder-width apart.

MOVE

Curl the weight toward your shoulders. Contract your biceps as hard as possible in the top position for a second then slowly lower the weight and repeat.

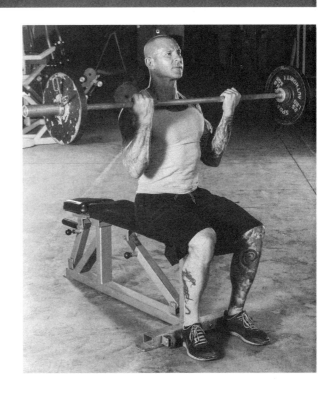

STANDING CABLE CURL

START

Stand in front of a low-pulley cable with your knees slightly bent and your feet about hip-width apart. With an underhand, shoulder-width grip, grab a straight bar attached to the low pulley. Hold the bar in front of your thighs and step back from the pulley enough to keep the weight plates from touching the bottom plate.

MOVE

Curl the bar up in an arc toward your shoulders. Pause at the top of the movement, squeeze your biceps, and slowly lower the bar to the starting position.

Note: You can do this exercise with an EZ bar attachment.

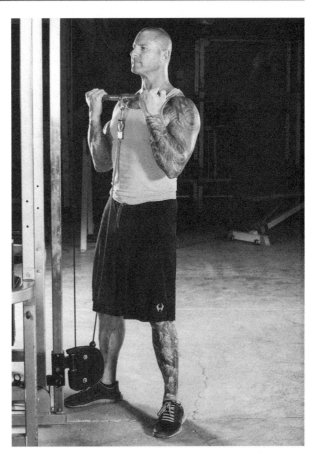

LYING CABLE CURL

START

Lie on the floor or on a bench in front of a low-pulley cable with the pulley in the middle of your feet. With an underhand, shoulder-width grip, grasp a straight bar attached to the low pulley and lean back until your back is flat against the floor.

MOVE

Curl the bar in an arc toward your shoulders. Pause at the top of the movement, squeeze your biceps, and slowly lower the bar to the starting position.

Note: You can do this exercise with an EZ bar attachment.

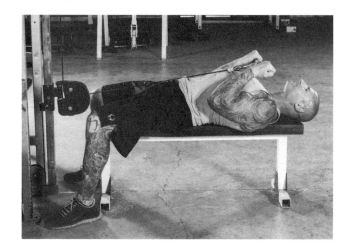

ONE-ARM CABLE CURL

START

With your feet shoulder-width apart, stand in front of a low-pulley cable apparatus. Using an underhand grip with your left hand, hold a single-handle D-grip attached to a low-pulley handle.

MOVE

Curl the handle up in an arc across your body toward your opposite shoulder. Hold the contraction at the top for a second before returning to the starting position. Complete the desired number of reps and repeat on the right side.

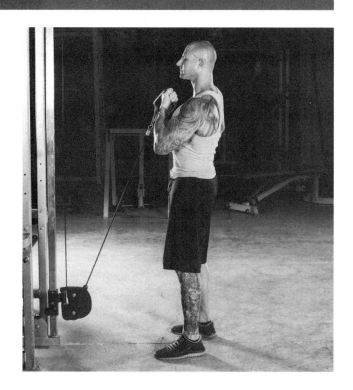

INCLINE CABLE CURL

START

Place an incline bench set at 45 to 60 degrees in the middle of a cable crossover apparatus. Grab the single-handle D-grips attached to the low pulleys and sit on the incline bench holding your arms down and out to your sides in line with the cables.

MOVE

Curl both arms toward your shoulders. Slowly return the handles to the starting position.

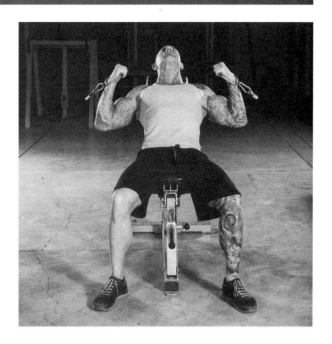

ONE-ARM HIGH-CABLE CURL

START

With an underhand grip, grasp the single-handle D-grip attached to the upper pulley. Your working arm should be extended out to your side and parallel with the floor or slightly higher. Hold on to the opposite side of the cable crossover apparatus.

MOVE

Curl the handle in toward your shoulder while keeping your upper arm stationary. Hold for a second in the flexed position while squeezing your biceps hard. This will look like a bodybuilder doing a biceps pose. Slowly return the handle to the starting position. You can also do this exercise two arms at a time.

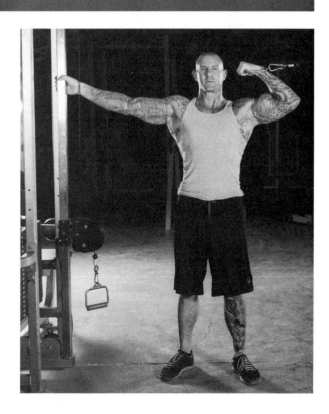

SEATED ONE-ARM CABLE CONCENTRATION CURL

START

Sit on the floor about two feet (61 centimeters) in front of a low-pulley cable with a single-handle D-grip attached to the pulley. Using an underhand grip, grasp the handle with your right hand and brace your arm against the inside of your right thigh.

MOVE

Curl the handle up toward your shoulder while keeping your upper arm stationary against your leg. Hold for a second in the flexed position while squeezing your biceps hard. Slowly return the handle to the starting position. Complete all reps with the right arm then repeat with the left arm.

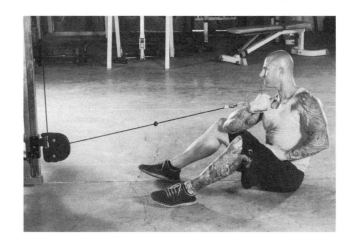

LYING CABLE CONCENTRATION CURL

START

Lie faceup on a flat bench set lengthwise in the middle of a cable crossover apparatus with your head closest to the pulley. With an underhand grip, grab a straight-bar handle attached to the high pulley and extend your arms straight over your chest.

MOVE

Keeping your upper arms perpendicular to your torso, curl the bar toward your forehead. Hold the contraction for a second, then slowly return the bar to the starting position.

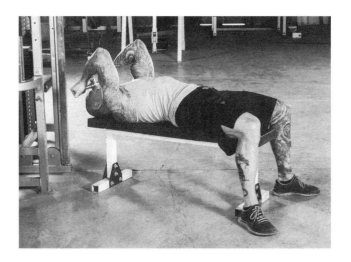

426

BEHIND-THE-BACK CABLE CURL

START

Attach a D-handle to a low cable and stand with your back to the pulley in a staggered stance (left foot forward and right foot back slightly to the left of the pulley). Hold the handle with an underhand grip in your right hand and keep your right arm straight and extended behind your body.

MOVE

Keeping your upper arm stationary, curl the handle by flexing your elbow until your hand is close to your shoulder. Contract your biceps as hard as possible and then return the handle to the start position. Perform all reps on the right arm and then repeat with the left arm.

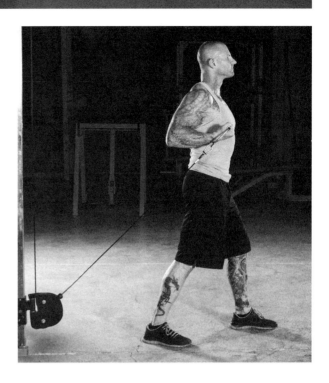

STANDING CABLE CONCENTRATION CURL

START

Attach a D-handle to a cable pulley on the cable station and adjust the cable pulley to about shoulder height. If your cable station does not adjust, do this from the top pulley in the same manner as described in this exercise's Move section. Hold the handle with a hammer grip with your arm extended out in front of you.

MOVE

Keeping your upper arm stationary, flex your arm at just the elbow to bring the handle toward your chest. Contract your biceps as hard as possible in this position and then slowly return the handle to the start position. Complete all reps on one arm before repeating on the other arm.

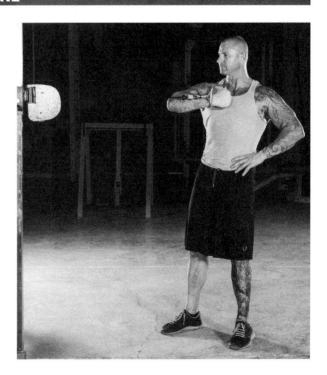

OVERHEAD CABLE CURL

START

Attach a straight or EZ bar attachment to the pulley of a lat pulldown station. Reach overhead and grab the bar with an underhand, shoulder-width grip. Your arms and shoulders should all be in a straight line overhead. Sit down on the lat pulldown seat with your legs secured under the support pads.

MOVE

Keeping your upper arms stationary, slowly curl the bar down behind your head. Focus on curling using the biceps and reaching a controlled contraction just behind the top of your head. You can also do this exercise kneeling in a cable crossover station. It is the same motion described earlier, but from a kneeling position on the floor using the high pulley on a cable crossover station.

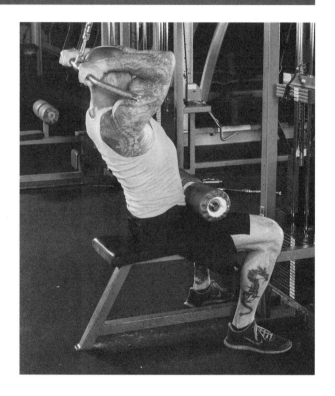

BARBELL PREACHER CURL

START

Set the seat height of the preacher curl bench so that when you sit down, the armrest is slightly below shoulder level. Place your upper arms over the armrest and grab a barbell with an underhand grip.

MOVE

With the backs of your upper arms pressed firmly against the pad, curl the bar up toward your shoulders until your elbows are just a bit beyond 90 degrees. Forcefully flex the biceps at the top of the movement, then slowly lower the weight.

Note: You can do this exercise with an EZ bar.

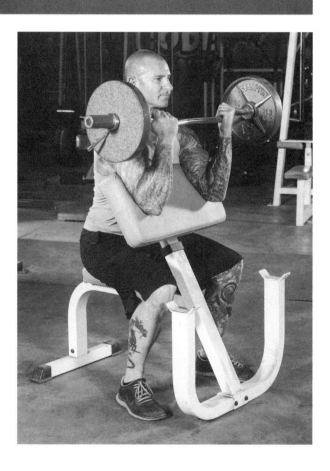

ONE-ARM DUMBBELL PREACHER CURL

START

Set the seat height of the preacher curl bench so that when you sit down or stand up in a standing preacher bench (as shown in photo), the armrest is slightly below shoulder level. Grasp a dumbbell in your left hand and place the back of your upper arm flush against the angled side of the preacher bench pad. Brace yourself with the right arm for stability.

MOVE

Curl the dumbbell up toward your shoulder until your elbow is just a bit beyond 90 degrees. Forcefully flex the biceps at the top of the movement, then slowly lower the weight to the starting position. Complete the desired number of reps and then repeat on the right side.

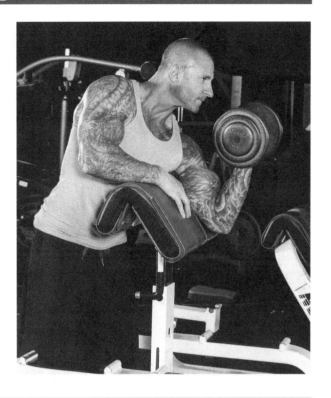

SCOTT CURL

START

Flip the pad on a preacher bench so that your chest and abs rest on the inclined side and your arms lie along the flat, vertical side. Lean into the pad so that your body weight is partially supported. Take an underhand, shoulder-width grip on a barbell or EZ bar and allow your arms to hang straight down from your shoulders along the flat side of the armrest.

MOVE

Slowly curl the bar up toward your shoulders, keeping your upper arms pressed into the pad and your upper body steady. Hold the contraction at the top for a second and flex the biceps as hard as possible. Slowly return the weight to the starting position.

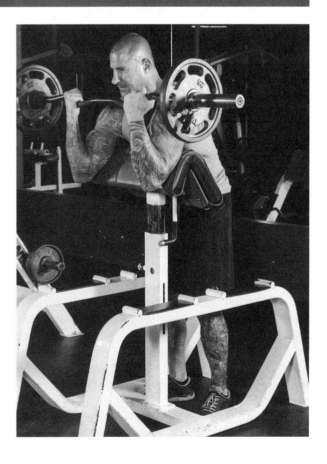

DUMBBELL CONCENTRATION CURL

START

Stand with a shoulder-width stance and bend forward from the hips. Bend over and let your arm hang straight down while holding a dumbbell with an underhand grip in your left hand.

MOVE

Contract your biceps to curl the dumbbell up toward your chest, then lower it under control all the way down to the starting position. Complete the desired number of reps and then repeat on the right side.

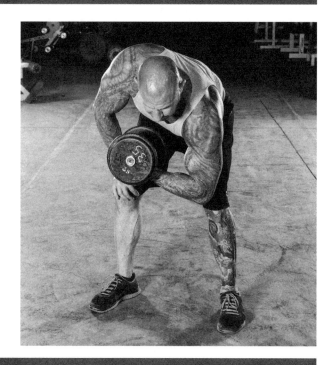

BICEPS LADDER

START

The easiest place to do this exercise is on a Smith machine, but you can also do it in a power rack. Set the bar in the Smith machine at a height that allows you to hang from the bar as when during an inverted row so that your back just clears the floor with only your heels making contact with the floor. Use an underhand and shoulder-width grip on the bar.

MOVE

Curl your body up toward the bar, bringing your face to the bar. Slowly lower your body to the start position. Do as many reps as you can until you reach muscle failure, then immediately raise the bar up one notch and continue doing body-weight curls. Each time you reach muscle failure, raise the bar up one notch until you have reached the very top notch. Each time you raise the bar up, it reduces the resistance that your body provides, making it easier to continue the set. In essence, this is one long, extended set. The novel movement of this exercise will stimulate muscle fibers that you likely have been ignoring. This exercise also places a high load on the negative part of the rep (especially on the lower rungs) on the biceps, which induces a lot of muscle damage for stimulating new muscle growth.

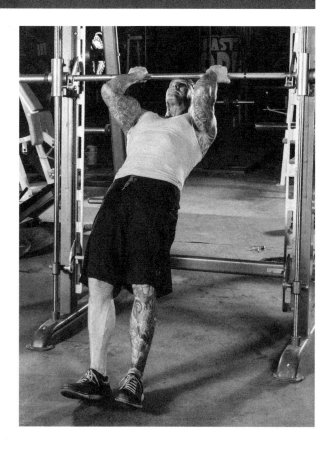

TRX BODY-WEIGHT CURL

START

Set the handles of the TRX at a height that decreases your body weight enough to allow for this tough exercise. Hold the handles with an underhand grip and start with just your heels touching the floor while your extended arms support your body weight.

MOVE

Trying to keep your arms as stationary as possible, curl your forearms toward your head to lift your body up to the handles. Slowly lower your body until your arms are fully extended again in the start position.

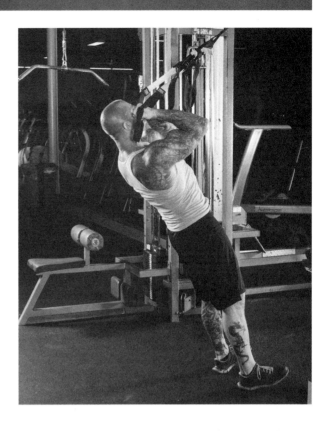

DUMBBELL HAMMER CURL

START

With your knees slightly bent and your feet about hip-width apart, grasp a pair of dumbbells with a neutral grip. Let the dumbbells hang at the sides of your thighs.

MOVE

Slowly curl the dumbbells up in an arc toward your shoulders while maintaining the neutral grip. Pause at the top of the movement, and slowly lower the weights back to the starting position.

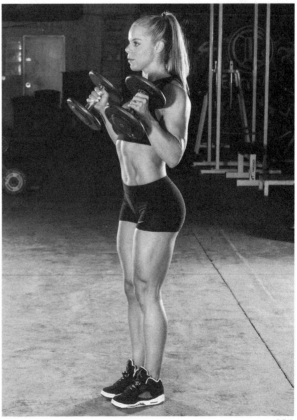

ALTERNATING DUMBBELL HAMMER CURL

START

With your knees slightly bent and your feet about hip-width apart, grasp a pair of dumbbells with a neutral grip. Let the dumbbells hang at the sides of your thighs.

MOVE

Slowly curl the left arm in an arc toward your shoulder while maintaining the neutral grip. Pause at the top of the movement and then slowly lower the weight in the reverse manner. Repeat the movement with the right arm. One curl with both arms equals one rep.

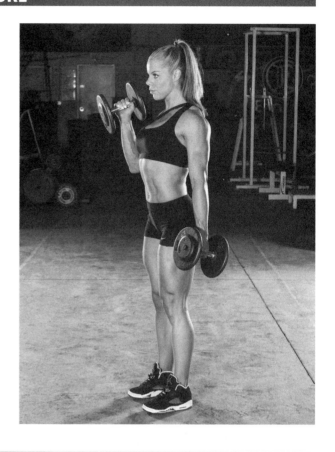

SEATED DUMBBELL HAMMER CURL

START

Sit at the end of a flat bench or on a low-back bench with your feet planted firmly on the floor. Hold a pair of dumbbells with a neutral grip and let them hang at the sides of the bench.

MOVE

Slowly curl the dumbbells in an arc toward your shoulders while maintaining the neutral grip. Pause at the top of the movement and slowly lower the weight in the reverse manner.

Note: You can do this exercise as a seated alternating dumbbell curl.

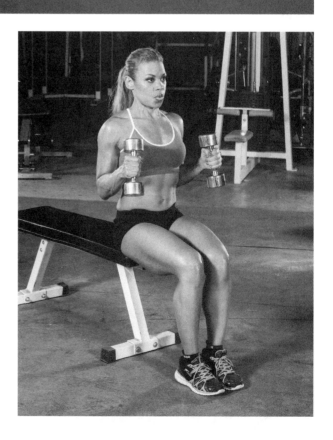

ROPE CABLE HAMMER CURL

START

With a neutral grip, grasp a rope handle attached to the low pulley of a cable apparatus. Knees are slightly bent and feet are shoulder-width apart.

MOVE

Curl your arms up, keeping them stationary at your sides as you do so. Bring your hands all the way up to your shoulders (as close as you can without shifting your elbows too far forward) and pause for a second at the top. Lower the rope to the starting position.

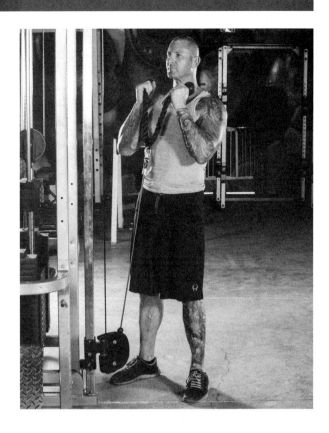

REVERSE-GRIP BARBELL CURL

START

With your knees slightly bent and your feet about shoulder-width apart, grasp a barbell with a shoulder-width, overhand grip. Let the bar hang to your thighs. Keep your abs pulled in and your elbows stationary.

MOVE

Without swaying, slowly curl the bar in an arc toward your shoulders. Pause at the top of the movement and slowly lower the bar to the starting position.

Note: You can do this exercise with an EZ bar.

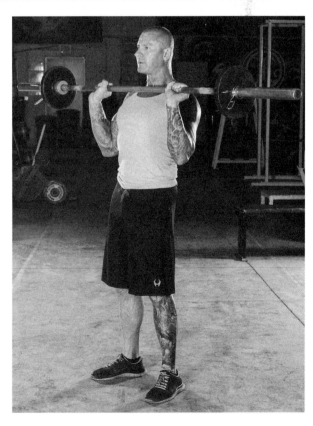

REVERSE-GRIP CABLE CURL

START

Stand in front of a low-pulley cable with your knees slightly bent and your feet about shoulder-width apart. With an overhand shoulder-width grip, grab a straight bar attached to the low pulley. Hold the bar in front of your thighs and step back from the pulley to keep the weight plates from touching the bottom plate.

MOVE

Curl the bar up in an arc toward your shoulders. Pause at the top of the movement and slowly lower the bar to the starting position.

Note: You can do this exercise with an EZ bar attachment.

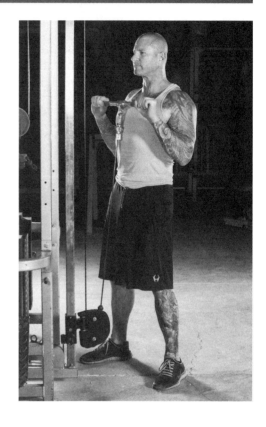

CHAPTER 20

Forearms

This chapter contains detailed descriptions of all major exercises that focus on the forearm muscles, including the wrist flexors and wrist extensors. The wrist flexors are located on the front of the forearms, while the wrist extensors are located on the back of the forearm. See the diagram for the location of each group. The forearm exercises are divided into wrist curl exercises, reverse wrist curl exercises, and grip exercises. Wherever a certain type of exercise is used in a workout, any one of the same type can be substituted.

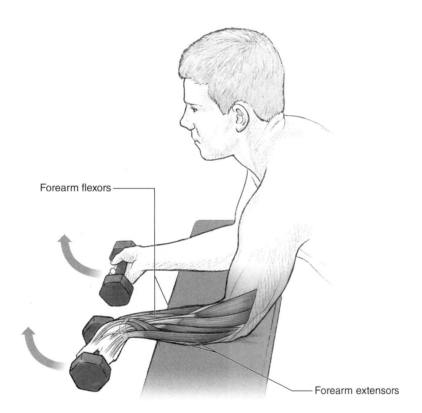

Forearm flexors

Forearm extensors

BARBELL WRIST CURL

START

Sit at the end of a flat bench with your legs in front of you and feet flat on the floor, hip-width apart. While holding a barbell with a shoulder-width, underhand grip, rest your forearms on the tops of your thighs so that your wrists and hands hang off your knees. Extend your wrists so that your hands hang down from your wrists at about a 90-degree angle. The bar should be supported with just your fingers.

MOVE

Curl the weight up, starting with your fingers and then your wrists, until your wrists are flexed and your hands are as much past parallel with the floor as possible. Hold this position for a second while forcefully contracting your forearm muscles, then slowly return the bar back to the start in the reverse manner.

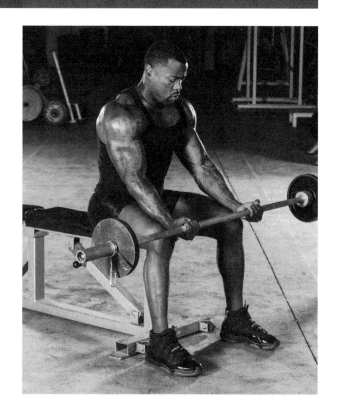

DUMBBELL WRIST CURL

START

Sit at the end of a flat bench with your legs in front of you and feet flat on the floor or bench base, or up on the bench frame depending on the height of the bench. While holding a dumbbell with an underhand grip in your right hand, rest your right forearm on top of your right thigh so that your wrist and hand hang off your knee. Extend your wrist so that your hand hangs down from your wrist at about a 90-degree angle. The dumbbell should be supported with just your fingers.

MOVE

Curl the weight up, starting with your fingers and then your wrist, until your wrist is flexed and your hand is as much past parallel with the floor as possible. Hold this position for a second while forcefully contracting your forearm muscles, then slowly return the dumbbell back to the start in the reverse manner. Complete the desired number of reps and repeat with the left arm.

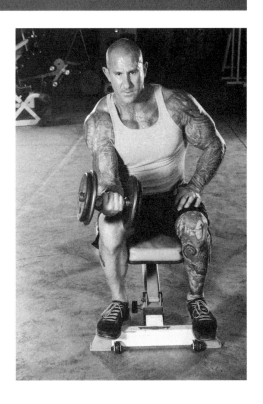

STANDING BEHIND-THE-BACK WRIST CURL

START

Stand while holding a barbell with an overhand grip behind your thighs. Both your hands and feet should be shoulder-width apart. The barbell should be supported with just your fingers.

MOVE

Curl the weight up, starting with your fingers and then your wrists, until your wrists are flexed and your hands are as close to parallel with the floor as possible. Hold this position for a second while forcefully contracting your forearm muscles, then slowly return the barbell back to the starting position.

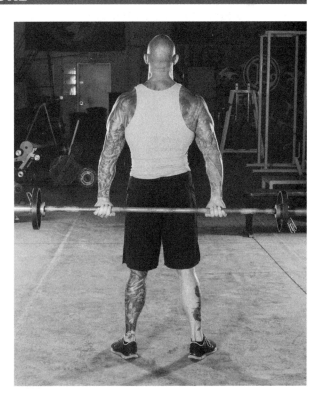

BARBELL REVERSE WRIST CURL

START

Sit at the end of a flat bench with your legs in front of you and feet flat on the floor, or on the bench frame depending on the height of the bench. While holding a barbell with a shoulder-width, overhand grip, rest your forearms on the tops of your thighs so that your wrists and hands hang off your knees. Flex your wrists so that your hands hang down from your wrists at about a 90-degree angle.

MOVE

Extend your wrists to lift the weight up as high as you can. Hold this position for a second while forcefully contracting your forearm muscles, then slowly return the bar back to the starting position.

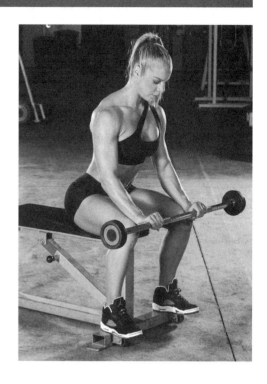

DUMBBELL REVERSE WRIST CURL

START

Sit at the end of a flat bench with your legs in front of you and feet flat on the floor, or on the bench frame depending on the height of the bench. Using an overhand grip to hold a dumbbell with your right hand, rest your forearm on the top of your right thigh so that your wrist and hand hang off your knee. Flex your wrist so that your hand hangs down from your wrist at about a 90-degree angle.

MOVE

Extend your wrist to lift the weight up as high as you can. Hold this position for a second while forcefully contracting your forearm muscles, then slowly return the dumbbell back to the starting position. Complete the desired number of reps and repeat with the left arm.

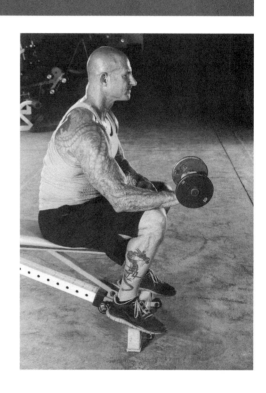

STANDING REVERSE WRIST CURL

START

While standing and using an overhand grip, hold a barbell about four to six inches (10 to 15 centimeters) in front of your thighs. Both your hands and feet should be shoulder-width apart.

MOVE

Extend your wrist to lift the weight up as high as you can. Hold this position for a second while forcefully contracting your forearm muscles, then slowly return the bar back to the starting position.

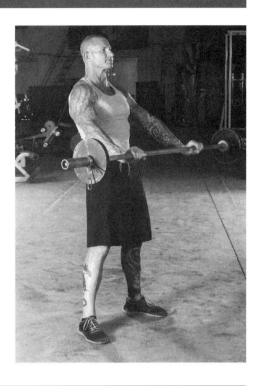

WRIST ROLLER

START

Hold the wrist roller out in front of you at arm's length and about shoulder height with the attached weight on the floor.

MOVE

To work the wrist extensors on the back of the forearm turn each wrist up in succession from left to right until the weight has reached the wrist roller bar. Then slowly lower the weight by resisting the flexion of the wrists in the same succession as used to lift the weight. Once the weight has reached the floor reverse the movement and keep going in this manner until reaching muscle failure. Once you can roll the weight up and back down 6-8 times, consider adding more weight. This unique exercise utilizes all concentric contractions to lift the weight and then all eccentric contractions to lower the weight. You can also work your wrist flexors on the front of the forearm by flexing your wrists to lift the weight up instead of extending them. Some wrist rollers are designed to go over the safety bars in a power rack. This way you do not need to support the weight with your shoulders and can better focus on the forearms.

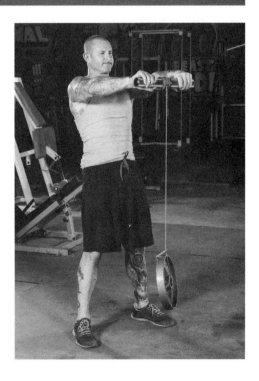

WEIGHT PLATE PINCH

START

Take two equal-sized weight plates and place them together on their sides with the smooth sides out by your left foot. Hold them together with your left hand fingertips, placing your thumb on one side and your fingers on the other.

MOVE

Pick up the plates and hold them at the side of your left thigh, similar to a unilateral deadlift. Hold the plates in this position for several seconds and then return the plates to the floor without letting go until you have performed as many reps as desired. Repeat with the right hand.

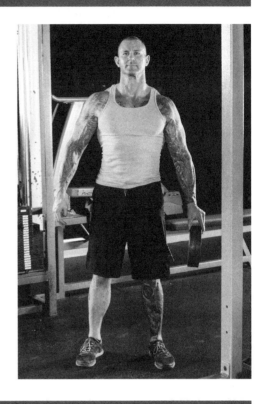

GORILLA HANG

START

Grab on to a pull-up bar with just your left hand.

MOVE

Lift your feet off the floor and hang for as long as possible with your left hand. Repeat with your right hand.

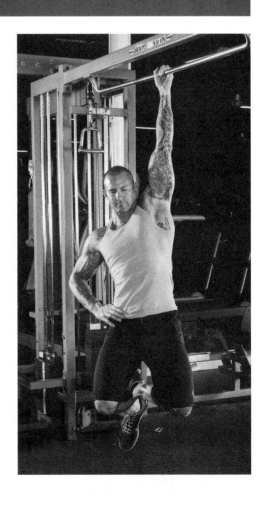

FARMER'S WALK

START

Using a neutral grip, hold on to two heavy dumbbells.

MOVE

Walk back and forth across the room as many times as you can while holding the dumbbells.

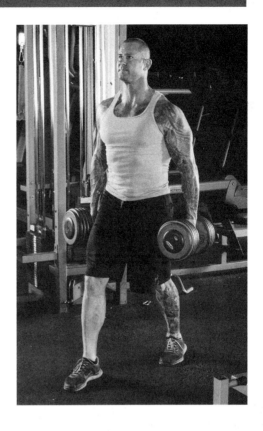

HAND GRIPPER

START

Hold a hand gripper in your hand with your upper arm straight by your side and your elbow bent about 90 degrees so that your forearm is parallel with the floor and out in front of you.

MOVE

Start with the gripper fully open and squeeze it closed as explosively as possible. Try to get the bottom of the handles to touch in the closed position. Hold this closed position for 1-2 seconds and then slowly open. Once you have completed all reps with one hand repeat with the other hand.

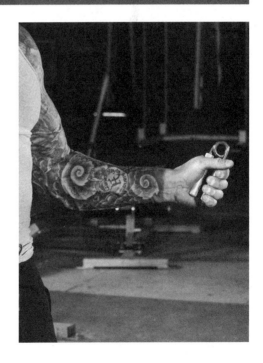

CHAPTER 21

Quadriceps

This chapter contains detailed descriptions of all major exercises that focus on the quadriceps muscles, including the vastus lateralis, vastus medialis, vastus intermedius, and rectus femoris. See the diagram for the location of each quadriceps muscle. The quadriceps exercises are divided into squat exercises, leg press and machine squat exercises, lunge and step exercises, and leg extension

exercises. Wherever a certain type of exercise is used in a workout, any one of the same type can be substituted. Although the squat, lunge, and step-up exercises involve the quadriceps, hamstrings, and glutes (as well as the adductor muscles in the inner thigh), I have categorized them as quadriceps exercises for the sake of simplicity.

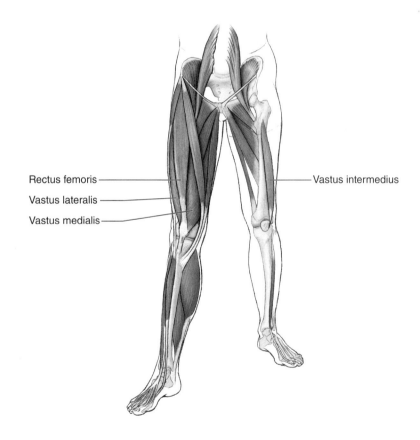

Rectus femoris

Vastus lateralis

Vastus medialis

Vastus intermedius

Squat Exercises

Leg Press and Machine Squat Exercises

Lunge and Step Exercises

Leg Extension Exercises

BARBELL SQUAT

START

Stand with a barbell rested on your shoulders and traps. Both your hands and your feet should be about shoulder-width apart. Maintain the natural arch in your lower back and keep your head directed forward.

MOVE

Bend at the knees and hips, letting your glutes track backward to lower yourself. At the point where your thighs are parallel to the floor or lower, reverse direction, driving up forcefully through your heels to a standing position.

Note: For a detailed description of using the squat for maximal strength, see chapter 8.

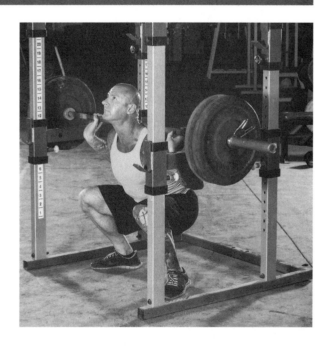

BARBELL FRONT SQUAT

START

Stand with a barbell rested on your shoulders and upper chest, holding with either an Olympic-style grip or cross-grip (as pictured). Maintain the natural arch in your lower back and keep your head directed forward.

MOVE

Perform a basic squat, bending your knees and driving your hips back to lower yourself until your thighs are parallel to the floor. Then forcefully extend your legs to stand back up to the starting position.

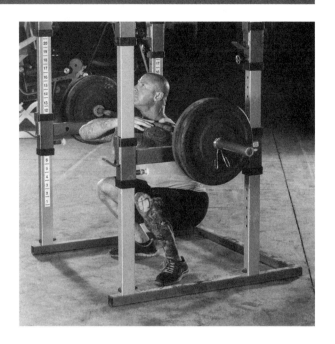

BOX SQUAT

START

Place a box or bench that is about knee height behind you in the power rack or squat rack. Unrack the bar and move back so that you're several inches in front of the box or bench.

MOVE

Squat back and down until your glutes make contact with the box, and immediately explode back up by pressing through your heels until you're back in the standing position. Do not "plop" or fully sit down on the box. The goal is to squat down slowly and softly on the box and then immediately explode up. This is a great exercise for learning how to squat because it reinforces the sitting-back portion of the squat. It is also a great exercise for increasing power in the squat, which can translate into stronger squats.

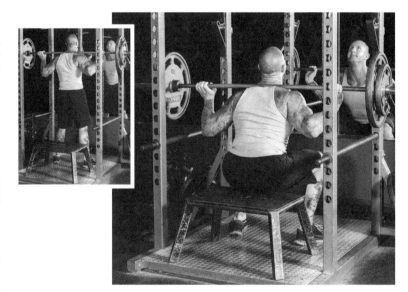

SISSY SQUAT

START

Stand with your feet hip-width to shoulder-width apart and hold on to something sturdy that can support you.

MOVE

Rise on your toes and lean back. Slowly descend, allowing your knees to go ahead of your toes. Go as low as you can and return to upright. The best way to make sure this exercise is executed correctly is to try to keep your hips and back straight. Act as if you were kneeling to the ground without moving your upper body. The only moving part of your body is the lower portion of the leg. To add resistance, hold a weight plate on your chest with the arm that is not stabilizing your body.

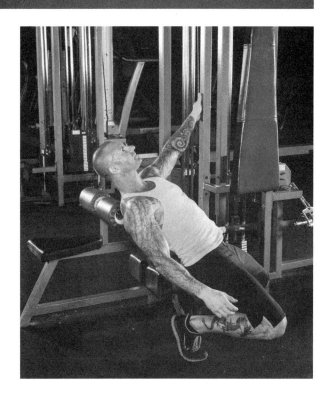

SMITH MACHINE SQUAT

START

Stand in a Smith machine with the bar across your shoulders and traps, grasping it just outside your shoulders. Twist the bar to unrack it.

MOVE

With your chest high, head forward, and back slightly arched, bend your knees and hips as if you're sitting back in a chair until your thighs are parallel to the floor. Reverse the motion by driving through your heels and pressing your hips forward to return to the starting position.

Note: You can also do this exercise as a front squat.

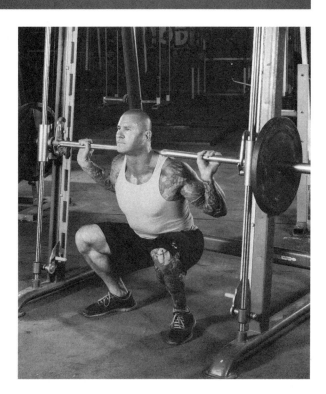

DUMBBELL SQUAT

START

Stand while holding two dumbbells in a shoulder-width, neutral grip by your sides. Maintain the natural arch in your lower back and keep your head directed forward.

MOVE

Bend at the knees and hips, letting your glutes track backward to lower yourself. At the point where your thighs are parallel to the floor, reverse direction, driving up forcefully through your heels to a standing position.

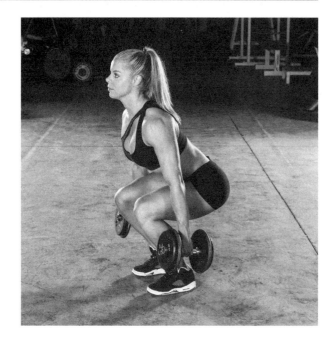

DUMBBELL FRONT SQUAT

START

Stand with your feet shoulder-width apart. Bring the dumbbells up and rest the ends on your shoulders, the same as in the catch with dumbbell cleans.

MOVE

Keeping your torso as upright as possible, squat until your thighs are parallel with the floor or lower and then explode back up by pressing through your heels.

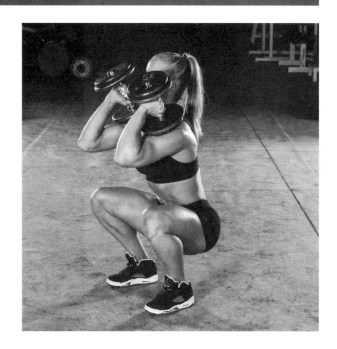

ONE-LEG SQUAT

START

Stand with a barbell rested on your shoulders and traps, holding it with a shoulder-width grip. Rest the top of your right foot on a flat bench placed two to three feet (half a meter to one meter) behind you. Maintain the natural arch in your lower back and keep your head directed forward.

MOVE

Bend your left knee and hip to lower your body until your left thigh is parallel to the floor. Reverse the direction, driving up forcefully through the left heel to the starting position. Perform the desired number of reps and then repeat with the right leg.

Note: You can do this exercise with dumbbells.

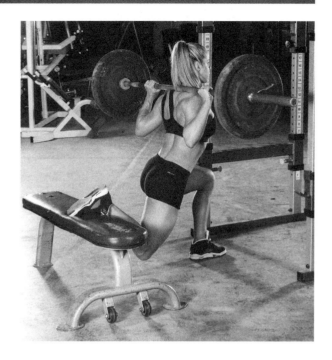

JUMP SQUAT

START

Stand with your feet about shoulder-width apart and your knees slightly bent.

MOVE

Quickly drop down by bending at the knees and hips, letting your glutes track backward to lower yourself into a squat. At the point where your thighs are parallel to the floor, quickly and explosively reverse direction, driving up through your heels and the balls of your feet to lift your body off the floor as high as possible. Land with soft knees and immediately lower into the next rep.

Note: Research shows that doing this exercise with just body weight and no added resistance produces the greatest amount of power.

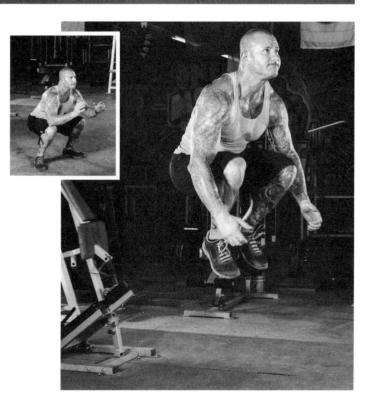

BARBELL HACK SQUAT

START

Stand with feet shoulder-width apart. Using a shoulder-width grip, hold a barbell behind your thighs. Maintain the natural arch in your lower back and keep your head directed forward.

MOVE

Bend at the knees and hips, letting your glutes track backward to lower yourself. At the point where your thighs are parallel to the floor or the bar touches the floor, reverse direction, driving up forcefully through your heels to a standing position.

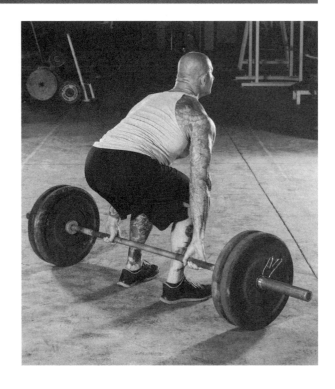

JEFFERSON SQUAT

START

Straddle a loaded barbell placed on the floor and running sideways between your feet. Squat down to pick up the bar, grabbing it with one hand facing palm backward and one hand facing palm forward. Hold the bar as you stand with a grip that's wider than shoulder width.

MOVE

Bend at the knees and hips, letting your glutes track backward to lower yourself. At the point where your thighs are parallel to the floor or the bar touches the floor, reverse direction, driving up forcefully through your heels to a standing position.

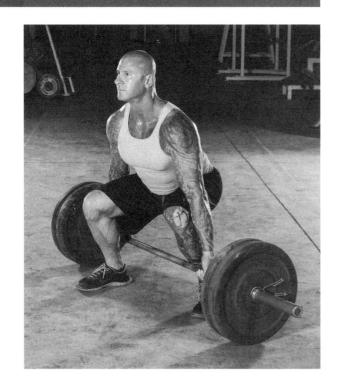

ZERCHER SQUAT

START

Stand with a shoulder-width grip while holding a barbell at waist height in the crook of your crossed arms.

MOVE

Bend at the knees and hips, letting your glutes track backward to lower yourself. At the point where your thighs are parallel to the floor, reverse direction, driving up forcefully through your heels to the standing position.

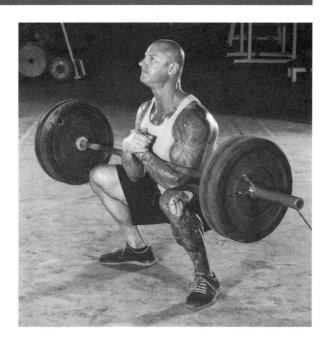

BARBELL SQUAT WITH BANDS

START

Attach a band to each side of the barbell. Attach the other end of each band to the bottom of the power rack or squat rack or to a heavy dumbbell. Stand with the barbell resting on your shoulders and traps. Both your hands and your feet should be about shoulder-width apart. Maintain the natural arch in your lower back and keep your head directed forward.

MOVE

Bend at the knees and hips, letting your glutes track backward to lower yourself. At the point where your thighs are parallel to the floor, reverse direction, driving up forcefully through your heels to a standing position.

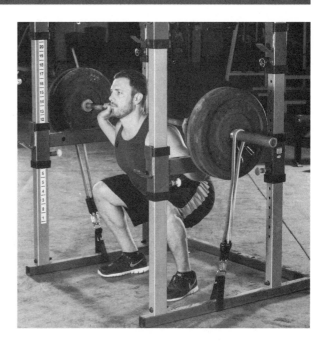

BAND SQUAT

START

Stand with your feet about shoulder-width apart on top of an exercise band. Be sure to keep your feet planted and straight throughout the exercise so that the band does not slip out. For light resistance, keep your arms at your sides. For maximal resistance, lift your arms so that the handles are near your shoulders with the bands running down behind your shoulders as if you were doing band shoulder presses.

MOVE

Squat by sitting back to bend at the hips and knees until your thighs are about parallel with the floor. Drive through your heels to stand back up into a fully upright position. Repeat for reps.

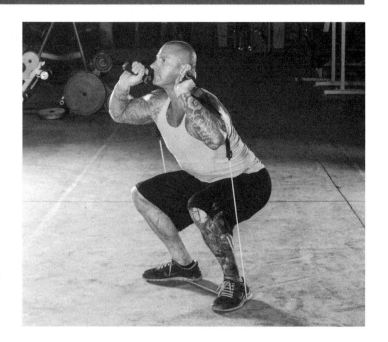

LEG PRESS

START

Sit in an angled leg press machine and place your feet shoulder-width apart in the center of the foot plate. Unhook the safety stoppers and support the weight with your legs.

MOVE

Slowly lower the weight, bringing your knees toward your chest but stopping when your knees are at a 90-degree angle. Pause a moment before pressing through your heels to return the weight to the starting position at full leg extension but without locking out at the knees.

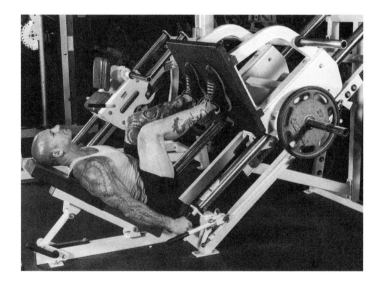

ONE-LEG LEG PRESS

START

Sit in a leg press machine and place your left foot in the middle of the platform, keeping the right foot flat on the floor for stability. Unhook the safety stoppers and support the weight with your left leg.

MOVE

Slowly lower the weight, bringing your left knee toward your chest but stopping when your knee is at a 90-degree angle. Pause a moment before pressing through your heel to return the weight to the starting position at full leg extension but without locking out at the knee. Perform the desired number of reps and then repeat with the right leg.

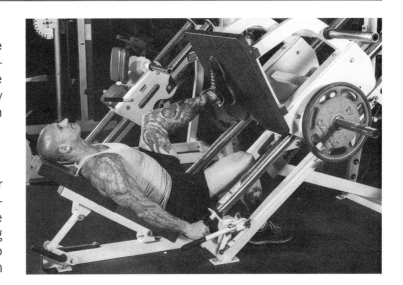

HORIZONTAL LEG PRESS

START

Lie in a horizontal leg press machine with your back flat against the pad. Place your feet shoulder-width apart in the center of the foot plate. Unhook the safety stopper and support the weight with your legs.

MOVE

Slowly lower yourself toward the foot plate, bringing your knees toward your chest but stopping when your knees are at a 90-degree angle. Pause a moment before pressing through your heels to return the weight to the starting position at full leg extension but without locking out the knees.

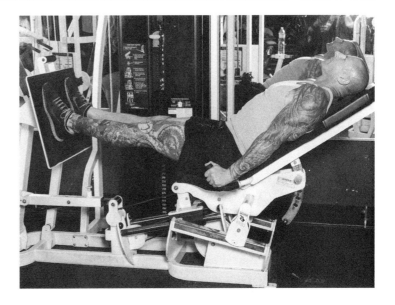

HACK SQUAT

START

Stand in a hack squat machine with your feet hip-width apart in the middle of the foot plate. Unhook the safety stopper and support the weight with your legs.

MOVE

Slowly squat down until your hips and knees are at or just below a 90-degree angle. From there, stand back up by pressing through your heels to lift the weight to an upright position. Come almost to a full extension at the top without locking out your knees.

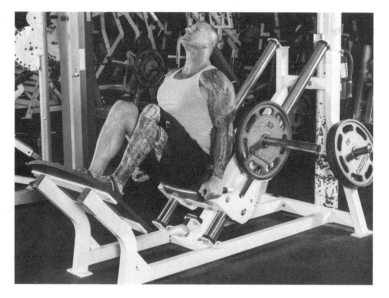

LUNGE

START

Support a barbell across your shoulders and traps and hold it with a shoulder-width grip while standing with your feet together. Keep your head directed forward and maintain the arch in your low back.

MOVE

Step forward with your right foot, leading with your heel, and lunge down toward the floor, maintaining control over the speed of your descent. Lower yourself until your left knee almost touches the floor. Push back off your right foot, returning to the starting position. Repeat with the left leg and alternate reps.

Note: You can do this exercise with dumbbells.

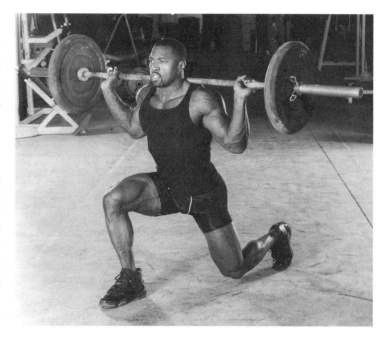

WALKING LUNGE

START

Support a barbell across your shoulders and traps and hold it with a shoulder-width grip while standing with your feet together. Keep your head directed forward and maintain the arch in your low back.

MOVE

Step forward with your right foot, leading with your heel, and lunge down toward the floor, maintaining control over the speed of your descent. Lower yourself until your left knee almost touches the floor. Lift yourself up and toward your right foot by pulling with your right leg. Come to a standing position with both feet together and repeat the motion with your left leg. Alternate legs with each rep.

Note: You can do this exercise with dumbbells.

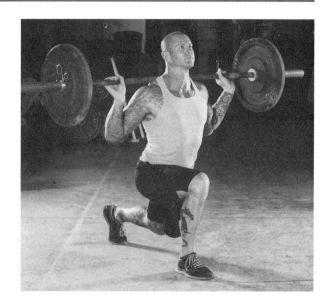

BACK LUNGE

START

Stand with your feet about hip-width apart while supporting a barbell on your shoulders, holding dumbbells in your hands, or using just your body weight.

MOVE

Step backward with your left leg and lower your body until your front leg is bent at the knee about 90 degrees. Push from the back leg to initiate the movement and continue lifting your body with the front leg until your back leg is back next to your front leg. Repeat by stepping back with the right leg and continue alternating legs until all reps are completed.

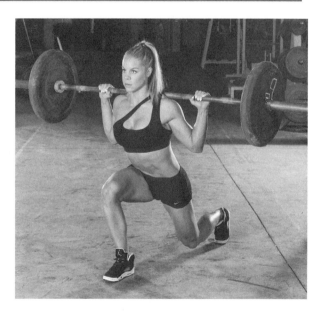

SIDE LUNGE

START

You can do this exercise by holding dumbbells or a barbell or by just using your body weight. In any case, stand with your feet about shoulder-width apart.

MOVE

Step out to your right as far as you can with your right foot. The forefoot should be turned out slightly as you plant it on the floor. Squat, shifting your weight to the right until your right leg is about parallel with the floor. Extend your right leg back up to lift your body up, and land with your right foot in a shoulder-width stance again. Repeat in the same manner with your left leg and continue alternating legs each rep until all reps are completed.

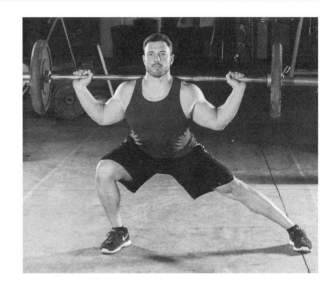

SPLIT SQUAT

START

Support a barbell across your shoulders and traps and hold it with a shoulder-width grip while standing with your feet together. Keep your head directed forward and maintain the arch in your low back. Take a large step forward with your right leg. Your left heel will lift off the floor.

MOVE

Drop your body downward by bending your right knee and lowering your left knee toward the floor. Reverse the motion and press back up into a standing split squat. Complete all reps for the right side, then switch to the left side.

Note: You can do this exercise with dumbbells.

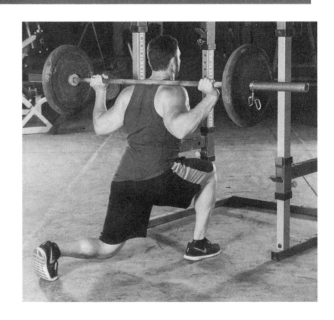

STEP-UP

START

Place a knee-high box or bench in front of you and grasp a dumbbell in each hand or use just your body weight. Stand with your feet in a comfortable hip-width stance.

MOVE

Step forward with one leg onto the step and drive through that thigh to bring your body upward. Bring the trailing leg to the top of the step and stand on the box, then step back with the opposite leg to the floor and lower yourself. Be sure to keep your low back in its natural arch and your upper body upright throughout the whole movement. Alternate legs with each rep.

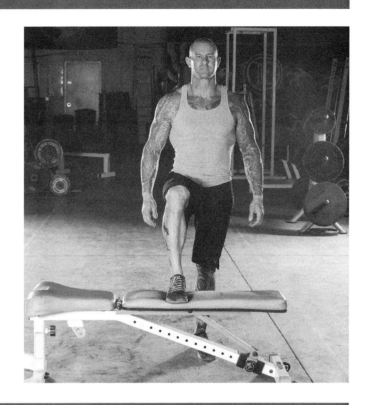

DIAGONAL STEP-UP

START

Place a box or a bench that's about knee-height in front of you.

MOVE

Step up on to the box or bench with the working leg at about a 45-degree angle to the back leg. Extend at the knees, hips, and ankles to lift your body so that both feet are on the box. Lower yourself to the floor using the same leg you stepped up with and switch legs once you have finished the descent. To add resistance, grasp dumbbells in each hand, or place a barbell on your back, or wear a weighted vest. Research shows that diagonal step-ups target the quadriceps better than standard step-ups, which better target the hamstrings and glutes.

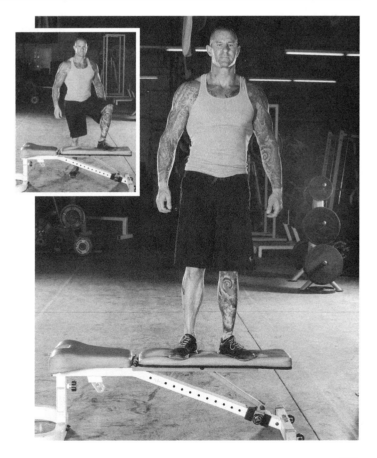

LEG EXTENSION

START

Adjust the seat back and footpad of a leg extension machine so that when you sit in it your knees are at the edge of the bench and your ankles are just below the footpad or rollers. Sit back with your back pressed firmly against the back pad.

MOVE

Grasp the handles or the seat edges behind your hips and keep your upper body stable as you extend your legs in a smooth movement until fully extended. Contract your quads at the top and slowly lower the weight under control to the starting position.

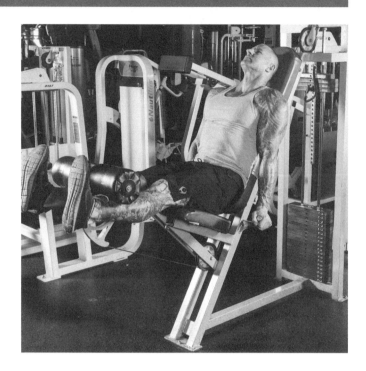

CABLE LEG EXTENSION

START

Attach an ankle cuff to your right ankle and connect it to a low-pulley cable. Your lower leg should form a 90-degree angle at the knee.

MOVE

Kick your lower leg forward and up until your leg is fully extended. Contract the quad muscles for a second and then return your foot to the starting position. Complete the desired number of reps and repeat with the left leg.

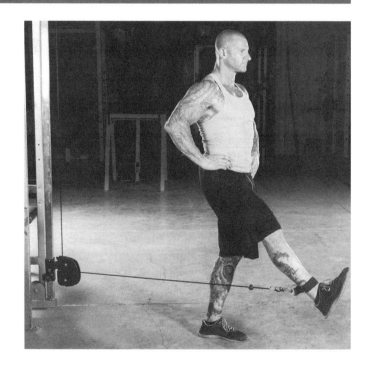

CHAPTER 22

Hamstrings and Glutes

This chapter contains detailed descriptions of all major exercises that focus on the hamstrings and gluteal (glute) muscles, including the biceps femoris, semitendinosus, semimembranosus, gluteus maximus, and gluteus medius. See the diagram for the location of each of these muscles. The hamstring and glute exercises are divided into hip extension exercises and leg curl exercises. Wherever a certain type of exercise is used in a workout, any one of the same type can be substituted.

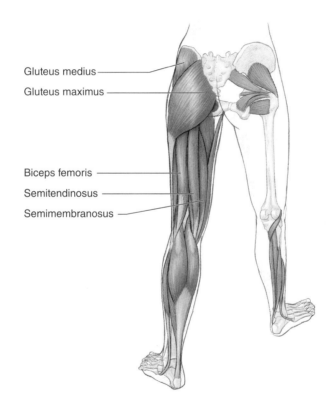

Gluteus medius

Gluteus maximus

Biceps femoris

Semitendinosus

Semimembranosus

BISHOP BURTON COLLEGE

ROMANIAN DEADLIFT

START

Stand with your feet shoulder-width apart and knees slightly bent. Using an overhand, shoulder-width grip or a staggered grip, hold a barbell in both hands in front of your thighs.

MOVE

Lean forward from your hips, pushing your hips back as you guide the bar down your legs until the bar is at mid-shin height. Slowly extend at the hips to raise the bar back to the starting position.

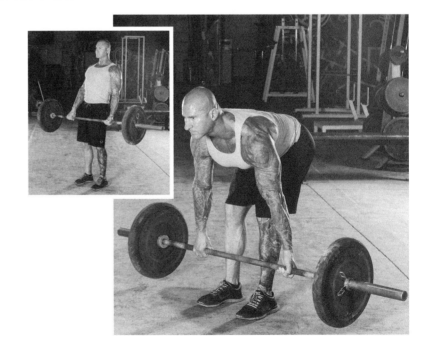

DUMBBELL ROMANIAN DEADLIFT

START

Stand with your feet shoulder-width apart and your knees slightly bent. Using an overhand grip, hold a pair of dumbbells in both hands in front of your thighs.

MOVE

Lean forward from your hips, pushing your hips back as you guide the dumbbells down your legs until they are mid-shin height. Slowly extend at the hips to raise the weights back to the starting position.

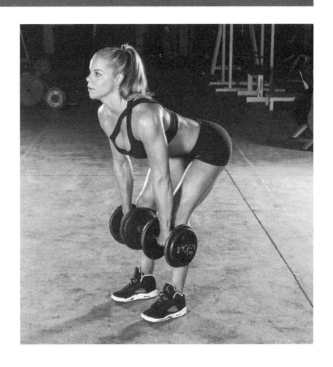

GLUTE AND HAM RAISE

START

Position yourself in a glute-ham raise bench with your thighs resting on the rounded pad and your ankles in the ankle pads and feet pressed firmly on the foot plate. Bend forward from the hips so that your torso hangs down toward the floor.

MOVE

Start the move by extending at the hips. Once your torso is in line with your thighs, immediately flex your hamstrings to curl your body up from the knees until your thighs and torso are upright.

Note: There is an apparatus known as a glute and ham raise that is designed specifically for this exercise as seen in the photos. However, very few gyms have this apparatus.

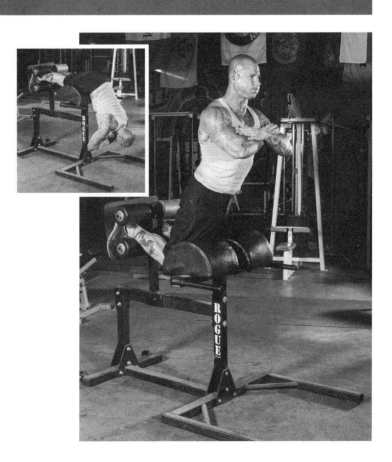

REVERSE HAMSTRING EXTENSION

START

Lie facedown on a horizontal back extension bench. Hold the footpads with your arms to support your torso on the pad. Your hips and legs should hang off the end of the pad at a 90-degree angle.

MOVE

Extend at the hips to raise your legs up to parallel with the floor. Hold this position for a second, then reverse the motion to lower your legs back to the starting position.

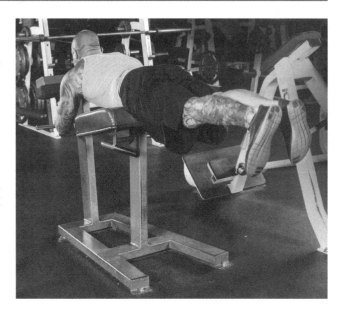

BENCH BRIDGE

START

Lie on the floor next to a bench with your back flat on the floor and your heels up on the bench. You can keep your arms at your sides on the floor or place them across your chest.

MOVE

Press through your heels to extend at the hips to lift your glutes up until your torso and upper legs are in a straight line with just your upper back touching the floor. Contract your hamstrings and glutes as hard as you can for a second before returning to the start position and repeating for reps. You can increase the resistance by holding a weight plate on your abs. To reduce the resistance, do this exercise with your feet on the floor instead of on the bench.

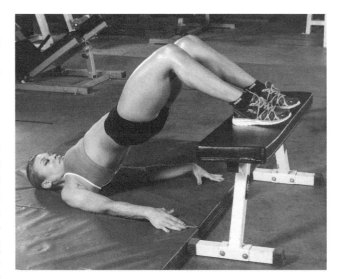

CABLE HAMSTRING RAISE

START

Stand facing a low-pulley cable with an ankle collar attached to your left ankle and connected to the low pulley. Hold the cable apparatus for support.

MOVE

Keeping your back straight, kick your left leg back behind you and as high up as possible. Hold it in the top position for a second before lowering the leg to the starting position. Complete the desired number of reps and repeat with the right leg.

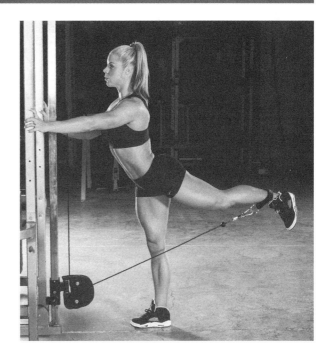

LYING LEG CURL

START

Lie facedown on a leg curl machine. Position your Achilles tendons below the padded lever and place your knees just off the edge of the bench. Grasp the bench or the handles for stability. Make sure your knees are slightly bent to protect them from overextension.

MOVE

Keeping your hips down on the bench, use your hamstrings to flex your knees and raise your feet toward your glutes. Squeeze the hamstrings at the top, then lower the lever arm to the starting position.

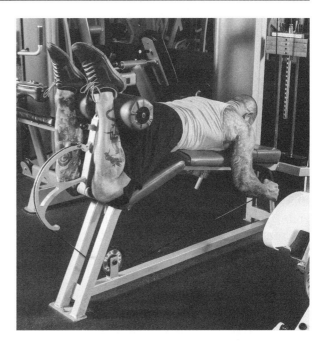

LYING DUMBBELL LEG CURL

START

Place a dumbbell between your feet and lie down on a flat bench with your legs extended. Hold on to the edge of the pad or the legs of the bench for stability.

MOVE

Slowly bring the weight up by flexing your knees until your lower legs are just short of vertical. Slowly lower the dumbbell back to the starting position.

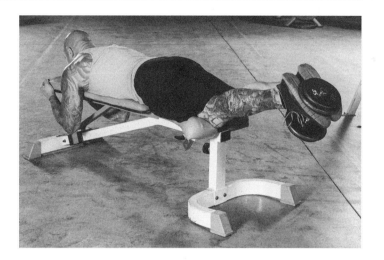

SEATED LEG CURL

START

Sit in a seated leg curl machine with your knees just past the bench and your ankles placed on the ankle pad. Hold the handles to support your body.

MOVE

Curl your lower legs under you by flexing at the knees to bring your feet as close to the bottom of the bench as possible. Hold this position for a second and squeeze your hamstrings hard. Return your feet to the starting position.

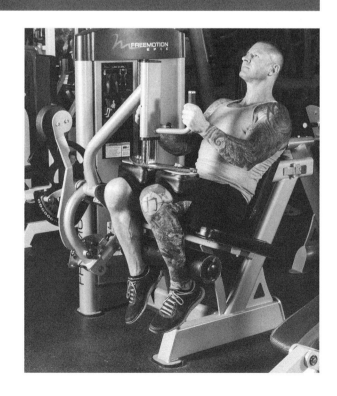

CABLE LEG CURL

START

Stand facing a low-pulley cable with an ankle collar attached to your left ankle and connected to the low pulley. Step back two to three feet (half a meter to one meter) from the pulley and lift your left leg out to form a 45-degree angle to your body.

MOVE

Slowly flex your knee to curl your lower leg down to form a 90-degree angle at your knee. Hold this position for a second and then return your foot to the start. Complete the desired number of reps and repeat with the right leg.

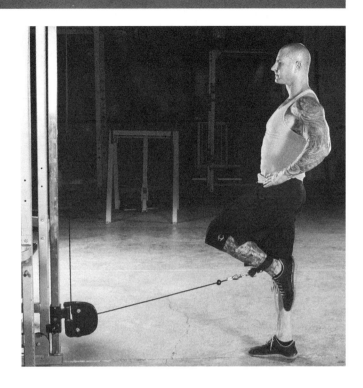

CHAPTER 23

Calves

This chapter contains detailed descriptions of all major exercises that focus on the calf muscles, including the gastrocnemius and soleus muscles. It also includes exercises for the major muscle on the front of the shin, the tibialis anterior. Keeping this muscle strengthened and in balance with the gastrocnemius and soleus can help to prevent lower-leg injuries, such as shinsplints. The gastrocnemius has a medial head and a lateral head. The soleus lies beneath the gastrocnemius. See the diagram for the location of these muscles. The calf exercises are divided into exercises that focus on the gastrocnemius and exercises that target the soleus, as well as exercises for the tibialis anterior. Wherever a certain type of exercise is used in a workout, any one of the same type can be substituted.

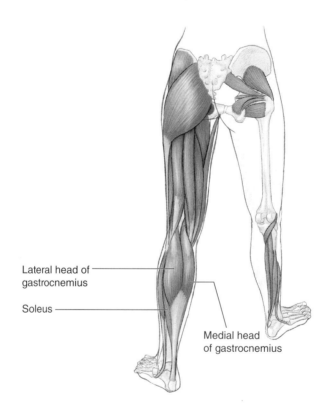

Lateral head of gastrocnemius

Soleus

Medial head of gastrocnemius

Gastrocnemius Exercises

Soleus Exercises

Tibialis Anterior Exercises

STANDING CALF RAISE

START

Stand beneath the shoulder pads of a standing calf raise machine with the balls of your feet at the edge of the foot rest. Keep your legs straight and your heels down to stretch the calves.

MOVE

Lift your heels by contracting the calf muscles to rise as high as you can on the balls of your feet. Hold this position for a second, flexing your calf muscles, then lower your heels back to the starting position.

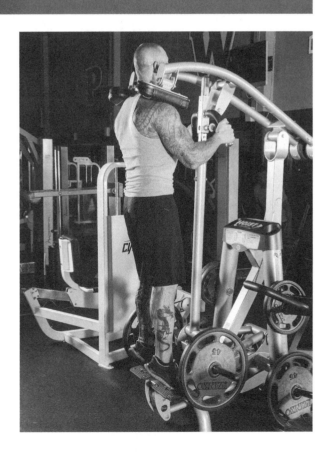

POWER RACK STANDING CALF RAISE

START

Stand underneath a barbell set in a power rack. You can stand on a block or weight plate, or simply just the floor (as pictured). The barbell should be set at a height lower than your shoulders. Rest the bar on your shoulders and traps and hold it with a shoulder-width, overhand grip.

MOVE

Lift your heels by contracting the calf muscles to rise as high as you can on the balls of your feet, raising the bar up along the sides of the power rack. Hold this position for a second, flexing your calf muscles, then lower your heels back to the starting position.

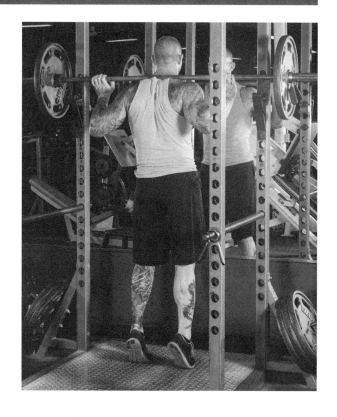

SMITH MACHINE STANDING CALF RAISE

START

Stand on a block or weight plate set underneath the bar of a Smith machine. You can also just use the floor. Rest the bar on your shoulders and traps. Hold it with a shoulder-width, overhand grip and unlatch the safety hooks.

MOVE

Lift your heels by contracting the calf muscles to rise as high as you can on the balls of your feet, raising the bar up along the guides of the Smith machine. Hold this position for a second, flexing your calf muscles, then lower your heels back to the starting position.

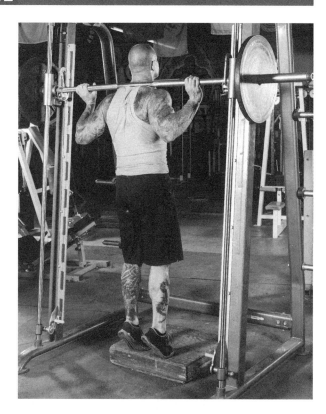

LEG PRESS CALF RAISE

START

Sit in a leg press machine and place your feet on the bottom of the foot plate so that your heels hang off the foot plate. Press the foot plate up from the safety hooks (but do not unlatch them) by straightening your legs. Drop your toes down toward your shins to stretch your calves.

MOVE

Press the weight up with your toes by contracting your calf muscles. Hold this position for a second, flexing your calf muscles, then lower your heels back to the starting position.

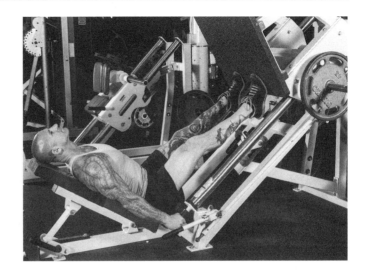

ONE-LEG PRESS CALF RAISE

START

Sit in a leg press machine and place your left foot on the bottom of the foot plate so that your heel hangs off the foot plate. Press the foot plate up from the safety hooks (but do not unlatch them) by straightening your leg. Drop your toes down toward your shin to stretch your calf.

MOVE

Press the weight up with your toes by contracting your calf muscles. Hold this position for a second, flexing your calf muscles, then lower your heel back to the start position. Perform all reps with the left leg and then repeat with the right leg.

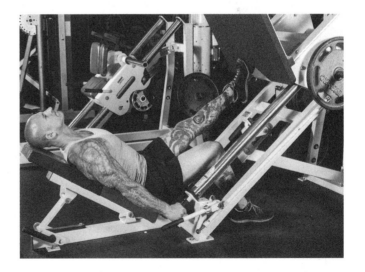

HACK SQUAT CALF RAISE

START

Stand in a hack squat machine with your back flat against the back pad. Place the balls of your feet on the end of the foot plate so that your heels hang off. Release the safety latches to support the weight with your body and lower your heels to get a good stretch on the calves.

MOVE

Extend at your ankles to lift your heels as high as possible and hold this position for a second as you contract your calves as hard as possible. Lower your heels back to the start and repeat for reps.

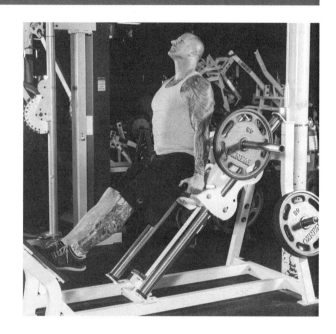

DONKEY CALF RAISE

START

Position yourself in a donkey calf raise machine so that your feet are on the foot plate. Your torso is bent at the hips and parallel to the ground. Your forearms rest on the forearm pad and your low back supports the back pad. Drop your heels as low as you can to get a good stretch in your calves.

MOVE

Lift your heels by contracting the calf muscles to rise as high as you can on the balls of your feet, raising the weight up by the pad placed on the low back. Hold this position for a second, flexing your calf muscles, then lower your heels back to the starting position.

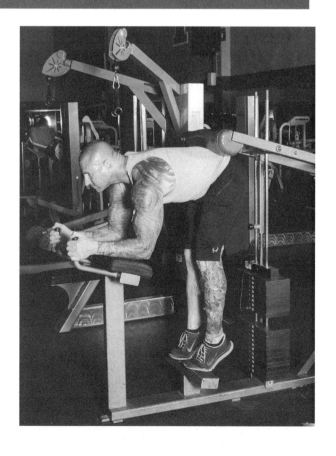

CALF JUMP

START

This exercise is much like a squat jump, but without squatting before the jump. To do this exercise, stand with your feet about hip-width apart.

MOVE

Bend only very slightly at the knees and then jump up as high as possible by extending your feet at the ankles. Be sure to land on the balls of your feet to take advantage of the negative force for inducing muscle damage. Repeat for reps.

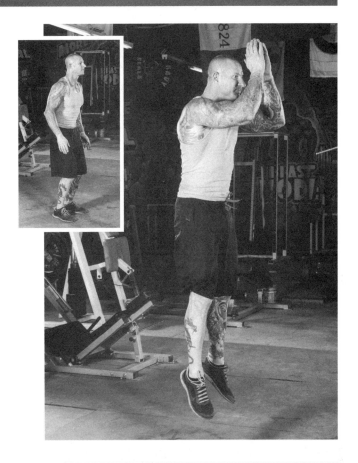

SEATED CALF RAISE

START

Sit in the seated calf machine and place the balls of your feet on the foot plate so that your heels hang off the edge. Place the knee pad on your knees and unrack the weight. Drop your heels as low as you can to get a good stretch in your calves.

MOVE

Lift your heels by contracting the calf muscles to raise the weight as high as you can on the balls of your feet. Hold this position for a second, flexing your calf muscles, then lower your heels back to the starting position.

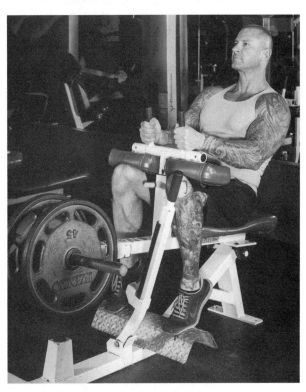

ONE-LEG SEATED CALF RAISE

START

Sit in the seated calf raise machine and place your right leg on the foot plate with your right knee under the knee pad. Keep your left leg on the floor. Unrack the weight supporting it with just your right leg.

MOVE

Lower your heel as low as possible to get a good stretch, then press the weight up on the ball of your foot to raise your heel as high as possible. Hold this position for a second as you flex your calf as hard as possible. Then lower your heel to repeat for reps. Once you have completed all reps with your right leg, perform in the same manner with the left leg.

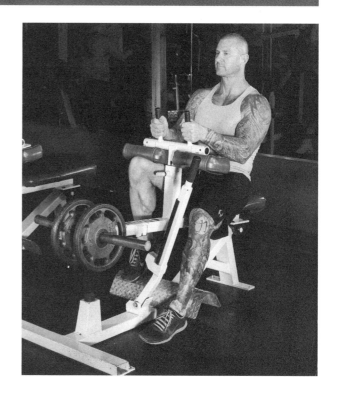

DUMBBELL SEATED CALF RAISE

START

Sit on the end of a flat bench with your legs hip-width apart and your feet on a block or foot plate set on the floor. Place a dumbbell on the top of each knee and secure them there with your hands. Drop your heels as low as you can to get a good stretch in your calves.

MOVE

Lift your heels by contracting the calf muscles to raise the weight as high as you can on the balls of your feet. Hold this position for a second, flexing your calf muscles, then lower your heels back to the starting position.

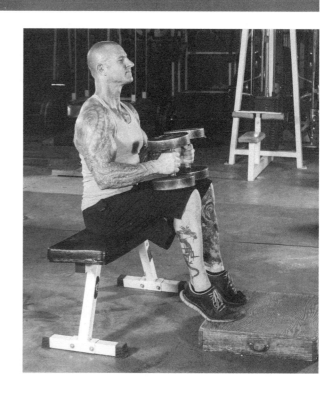

POWER RACK SEATED CALF RAISE

START

Place a flat bench or box in a power rack and set a block or foot plate (or if you have neither, try 25-pound plates) about one foot in front of the bench. You can also simply use the floor, as pictured. Set the safety pins so that when the bar rests on them, it is at the same height as your knees or slightly lower when you sit on the bench. Sit on the bench with the bar resting on your thighs (a few inches up from your knee caps). The balls of your feet are on the plates and your heels are on the floor.

MOVE

Lift your heels by contracting the calf muscles to raise the weight as high as you can on the balls of your feet. Hold this position for a second, flexing your calf muscles, then lower your heels back to the starting position.

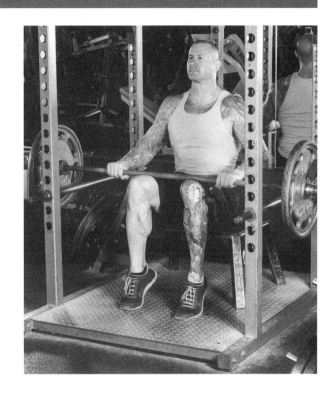

SMITH MACHINE SEATED CALF RAISE

START

Place a flat bench in a Smith machine and set a block or foot plate (or if you have neither, try 25-pound plates) about one foot in front of the bench. You can also use the floor or the frame of the bench, as pictured. Sit on the bench with the unlatched bar resting on your thighs (a few inches up from your knee caps). The balls of your feet are on the plates and your heels are on the floor.

MOVE

Lift your heels by contracting the calf muscles to raise the weight as high as you can on the balls of your feet. Hold this position for a second, flexing your calf muscles, then lower your heels back to the starting position.

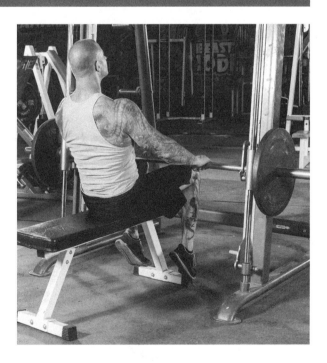

SEATED DUMBBELL TOE RAISE

START

Sit on the end of a bench with a light dumbbell placed on its end on the floor in front of you. Place your feet under the weight plates of the top end of the dumbbell and extend your legs out enough so that the dumbbell hangs freely. If you need to, use an adjustable bench with the bench raised up enough to allow clearance for the dumbbell to hang, as pictured.

MOVE

Raise your toes up toward your knees as high as possible and then reverse the motion to extend your toes as far as you can without dropping the dumbbell and repeat for reps.

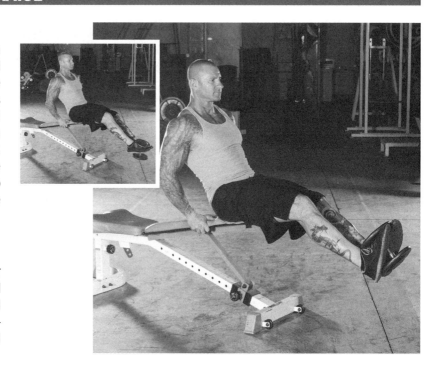

SEATED CABLE TOE RAISE

START

Place a flat bench next to a low-cable pulley with a D-handle or stirrup-handle attachment connected to it. Place your left foot through the attachment so that the handle is on the top of your foot. Sit on the bench and slide back so that your left leg is supported on the bench with your foot freely hanging off the end.

MOVE

Extend your ankle to point your toes forward as far as possible without the handle attachment slipping off of your foot, then reverse the motion to flex your ankle and lift your foot toward your shin as far back as you can. Extend your ankle again and repeat for reps. After you perform all reps on the left foot, repeat on the right.

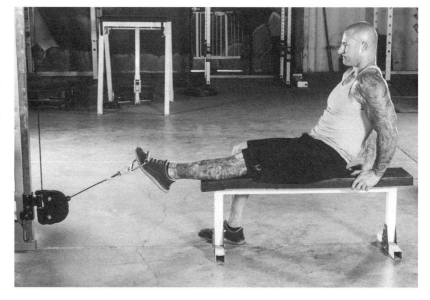

STANDING KETTLEBELL TOE RAISE

START

Stand on a block or box or a pile of 45-pound plates that are almost as high as the handle of the kettlebell you are using. Place one foot under the handle so that the handle is resting on the top of your foot.

MOVE

Pull your foot up as high as you can. Hold this position for a second and slowly lower the kettlebell back to the floor. Complete all reps for one leg and then repeat on the other leg.

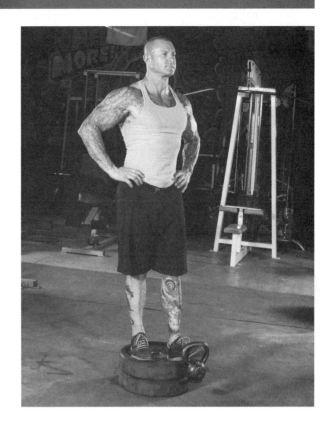

CHAPTER 24

Abdominals and Core

This chapter contains detailed descriptions of all major exercises that focus on the abdominal muscles, including the rectus abdominis, external obliques, internal obliques, and transverse abdominis. See the diagram below for the location of each. The abdominal exercises are divided into upper-abdominal exercises, lower-abdominal exercises, oblique exercises, and core exercise. Wherever a certain type of exercise is used in a workout, any one of the same type can be substituted.

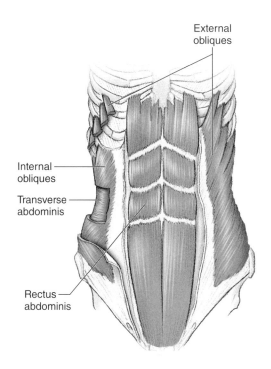

External obliques

Internal obliques

Transverse abdominis

Rectus abdominis

CRUNCH

START

Lie on the floor with your knees bent. Feet and low back are flat on the floor.

MOVE

With your hands cupped loosely behind your head, contract through your abs to lift your shoulders and upper back off the floor. Hold this position for a second before slowly lowering back to the starting position, making the negative portion of the rep as slow and deliberate as the positive portion.

Note: To make this exercise more difficult, hold a weight plate on your chest.

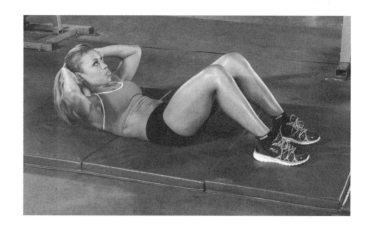

STRAIGHT-LEG CRUNCH

START

Lie faceup on the floor with your legs straight up in the air.

MOVE

Curl up as high as you can to bring your shoulders and upper back off the floor. Hold this position for a second before slowly lowering back to the starting position.

Note: To make this exercise more difficult, hold a weight plate on your chest.

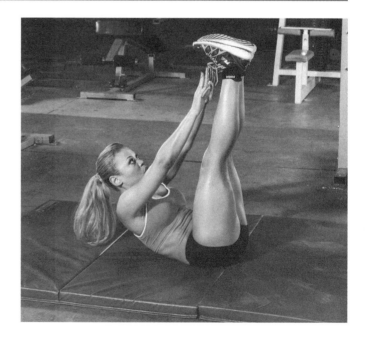

DECLINE CRUNCH

START

Lie back in a decline bench with your feet secured under the foot pad. Cup your hands behind your head, or place them by your ears as shown.

MOVE

Curl up as high as you can to bring your shoulders and upper back off the bench, simultaneously pressing your lower back into the bench. Hold this position for a second before slowly lowering back to the starting position.

Note: To make this exercise more difficult, hold a weight plate on your chest.

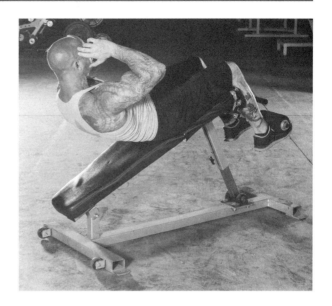

ROMAN CHAIR CRUNCH

START

Sit facing up on a back extension bench so that your shins are touching the ankle pads and your butt is on the bench.

MOVE

Extend back at the hips until your torso is below parallel with the floor and then crunch up as high as possible. Slowly lower down and repeat for reps. Focus on getting a good stretch in the abs in the start position, which will make for a stronger contraction of the abs. Add resistance by holding a weight plate on your chest.

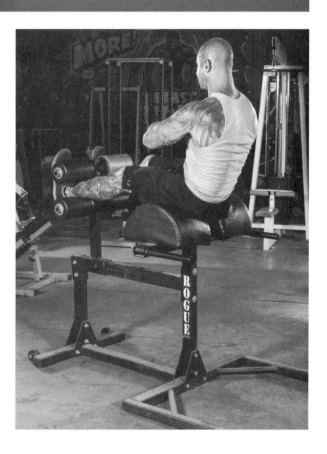

MACHINE CRUNCH

START

Sit in the machine crunch and select the proper weight.

MOVE

Keep your feet stationary and perform crunches as instructed in the machine directions, focusing on the contraction of your abs. This is a convenient way to add resistance to your ab work for better ab development.

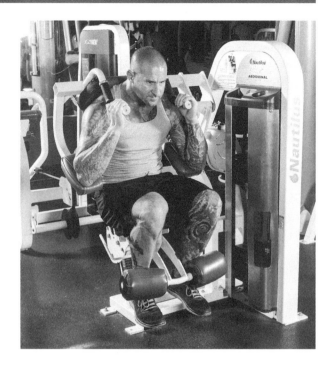

EXERCISE BALL CRUNCH

START

Lie on your back on a stability ball with your feet flat on the floor.

MOVE

Curl up as high as you can to bring your shoulders and upper back off the ball. Hold this position for a second before slowly lowering back to the starting position.

Note: To make this exercise more difficult, hold a weight plate on your chest.

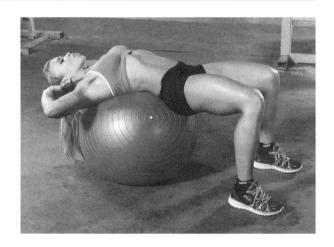

CRUNCH WITH MEDICINE BALL THROW

START

Get in a crunch position on the floor with your feet close to a sturdy wall or exercise ball net. Hold a medicine ball overhead with your knees bent and feet flat on the floor.

MOVE

Explosively crunch up as you simultaneously throw the medicine ball from overhead at the wall. Maintain the upright position to catch the ball on its return and allow it to take you down right into the next rep.

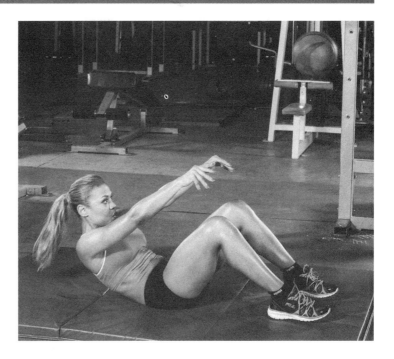

EXERCISE BALL CRUNCH WITH MEDICINE BALL THROW

START

Lie on your back on a stability ball with your feet flat on the floor. Hold a medicine ball with your arms extended back over your head.

MOVE

Curl up explosively to bring your shoulders and upper back as high as possible off the ball while throwing the medicine ball to a training partner. Hold the top position. Your partner then throws the ball back to you. Use your abs to resist the direction of the ball and return to the starting position.

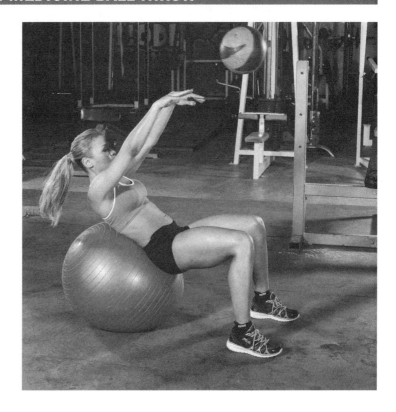

BICYCLE CRUNCH

START

Lie flat so that your lower back is pressed to the floor. Place your hands behind your head and lift your knees to about a 45-degree angle.

MOVE

Go through a bicycle pedaling motion with your legs as you alternately touch your elbows to the opposite knees, twisting back and forth.

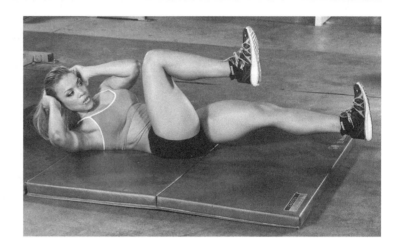

CABLE CRUNCH

START

Kneel facing a high-pulley cable with a rope attached to it. Grasp the ends of the rope and bring your hands down to the top of your head, where they remain fixed throughout the movement. Bend over at the waist so that your back is almost parallel with the floor.

MOVE

Curl your torso down to bring your elbows toward your knees. Hold this position and flex your abs for a second before slowly going back to the starting position.

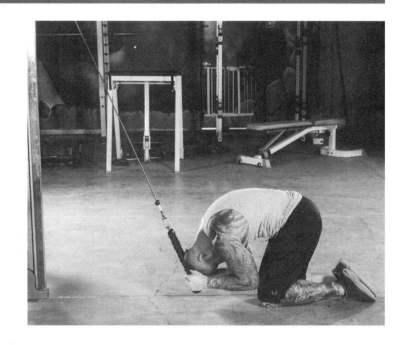

STANDING CABLE CRUNCH

START

Stand with your back toward a high-pulley cable with a rope attached to it. Grasp the end of the rope with a neutral grip and bring your hands down to your collarbone. Your feet are shoulder-width apart and your knees are slightly bent.

MOVE

Curl your torso down to bring your elbows toward your knees. Hold this position and flex your abs for a second before slowly going back to the starting position.

Note: This exercise can be done seated, as shown in the photo.

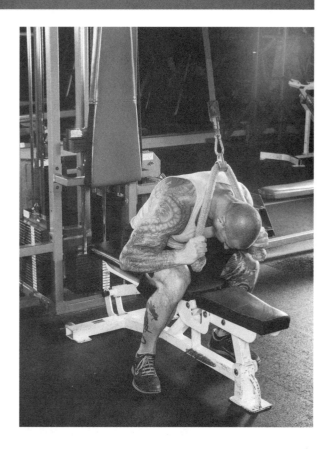

SMITH MACHINE CRUNCH

START

Place a bench in the middle of a Smith machine. Lie faceup on the bench with your knees bent and feet flat on the bench. The bar should line up over your upper abs as you hold the bar at arm's length above you with your back flat on the bench.

MOVE

Use your abs to explosively lift your torso up as high as you can, pushing the bar up as your body rises. Slowly lower your upper body to the bench and repeat for reps.

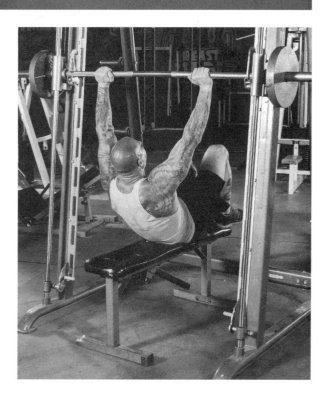

BELL TOWER CRUNCH

START

Attach a rope handle to a high cable pulley, or grab the end of the cable as shown. Grab the rope with your left hand above your right hand and stand in a staggered stance with your right leg in front of your left.

MOVE

Using your abs and obliques, pull the rope down in front of you and toward your right knee (flexing and rotating your spine). Hold this position for a second as you exhale and squeeze your abs as tight as possible. Slowly return to the start position and repeat for reps. When you have completed all reps on the right side, switch your foot and hand position and perform in a similar manner on the left.

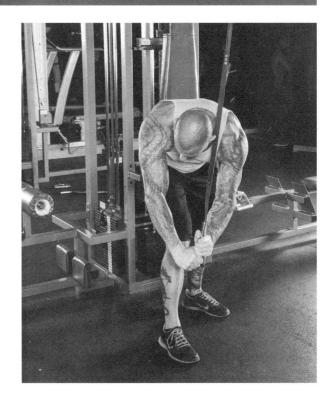

V-UP

START

Sit at the end of a flat bench with your hands grasping the edges and your feet off the floor. Lean back until your body is almost straight and parallel to the floor.

MOVE

Start with your legs straight, then bring your knees toward your chest while simultaneously curling your upper body toward your knees to form a V at the waist. Return your legs and torso to the starting position.

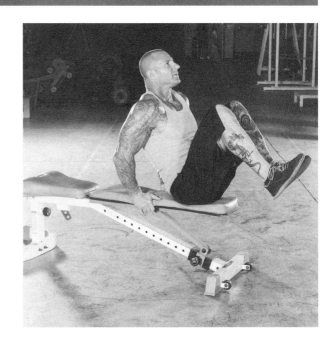

DUMBBELL V-SIT

START

Lie faceup on the floor. Arms are fully extended overhead and resting on the floor. Hold a dumbbell with both hands.

MOVE

Contract your abs to flex your spine, slowly drawing your legs and shoulders off the floor. Crunch hard until your feet and hands point at the ceiling and your body is in a V position. Slowly lower back to the starting position.

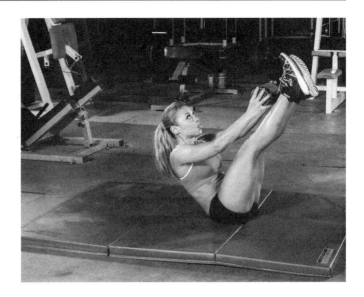

REVERSE CRUNCH

START

Lie faceup on the floor with your hands extended at your sides. Feet are up and thighs are perpendicular to the floor (your hips and knees should form a 90-degree angle).

MOVE

Slowly bring your knees toward your chest, lifting your hips and glutes off the floor. Try to maintain the bend in your knees throughout the movement. Return to the starting position under control.

Note: To make this exercise more difficult, perform it on a decline bench with your head on the high end.

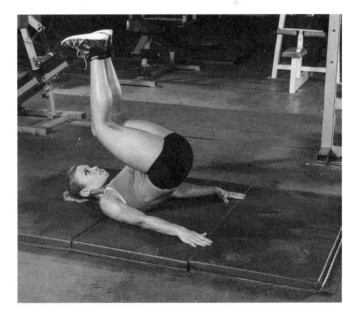

INCLINE REVERSE CRUNCH

START

Lie on an incline, such as on a decline bench or raised ab board, with your head where your feet normally go. Hold on to the leg pads to hold your torso in place on the bench. Bend your hips and knees to 90-degree angles for the start position of the reverse crunch.

MOVE

Maintain the bend in your knees and hips and flex your spine from the bottom to lift your hips up off the bench and curl your knees toward your head. Slowly reverse the motion to return your legs to the start position.

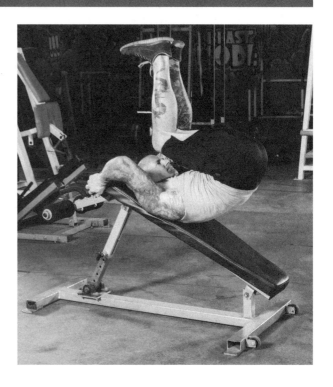

EXERCISE BALL REVERSE CRUNCH

START

Place an exercise ball next to an exercise machine or other apparatus that you can grab for stability. Lie on your back on the stability ball with your feet up and thighs perpendicular to the floor (your hips and knees should form a 90-degree angle). Reach back over your head and grab on to the apparatus for stability.

MOVE

Slowly bring your knees toward your chest, lifting your hips and glutes off the ball. Try to maintain the bend in your knees through-out the movement. Return to the starting position under control.

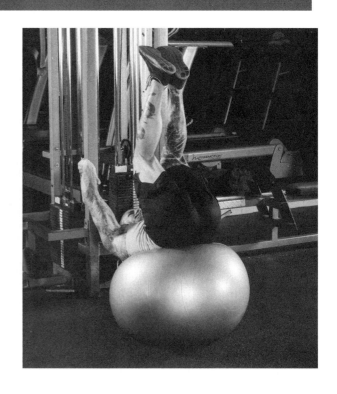

HIP THRUST

START

Lie faceup on the floor with your hands extended at your sides. Your legs are perpendicular to the floor.

MOVE

Raise your hips and glutes straight up off the floor by using your abdominals. Hold for a second in this position, then lower your hips back to the starting position.

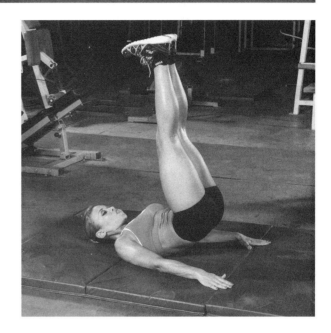

SMITH MACHINE HIP THRUST

START

Lie on your back on a bench or on the floor or on a flat bench in the middle of a Smith machine. Place your feet on the bottom of the bar and roll the bar with your feet to unlatch the safety hooks. Extend your legs straight up while supporting the bar with the soles of your feet. Your body should form an L in this position with your hips bent at about 90 degrees and your knees fairly straight. Hold on to the machine or place your hands firmly on the floor or on the bench at your sides.

MOVE

Use your lower abs to lift your legs straight up as high as you can go. Hold the top position for a second and then slowly lower your legs until your butt and lower back are on the floor.

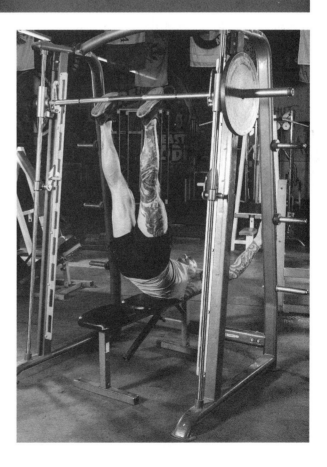

HANGING KNEE RAISE

START

Position yourself on a vertical bench and hang from it with your torso straight and your knees slightly bent.

MOVE

Lift your legs, bending your knees on the way up to pull your knees up toward your chest while rounding your lower back to bring your glutes forward and up. Pause in this position for a second, then slowly lower your legs to the starting position.

Note: This exercise can also be done hanging from a chin-up bar.

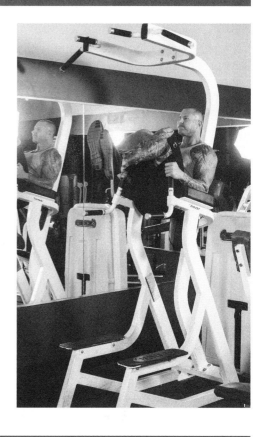

HANGING LEG RAISE

START

Position yourself on a vertical bench with your entire body completely straight.

MOVE

Keeping your legs straight, lift your legs up as high past parallel with the floor as possible by flexing at the waist while rounding your lower back to bring your glutes forward and up. Pause in this position for a second, then slowly lower your legs to the starting position.

Note: This exercise can also be done hanging from a chin-up bar.

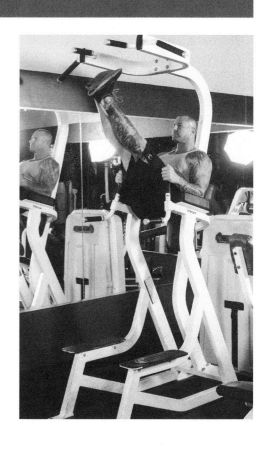

EXERCISE BALL TUCK

START

Lie on the floor in a push-up position with your feet resting on top of an exercise ball.

MOVE

Tuck your knees in toward your chest while rolling the ball forward. Hold the tucked position for a second, and then return to the starting position by extending your legs back.

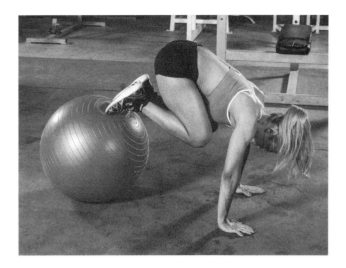

TRX KNEE TUCK

START

Get on the floor in a push-up position with your feet placed in the stirrups of a TRX. Adjust the TRX handles so that they are just above the floor

MOVE

Tuck your knees in toward your chest. Hold the tucked position for a second, and then return to the starting position by extending your legs back.

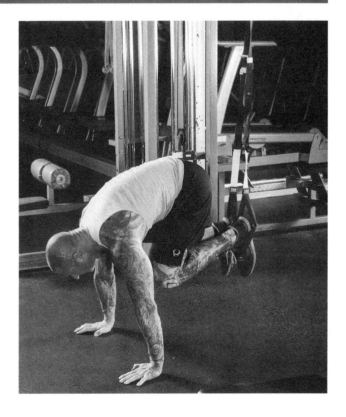

BAND RISING KNEE

START

Attach a band to a stable structure as low to the floor as possible and attach the other end of the band to your left ankle with an ankle cuff. Stand in a fighting stance with your right foot in front of your left.

MOVE

As quickly and as explosively as possible, drive your knee up toward your chest as high as possible and return your foot back to the start position. Complete all reps on the left leg and then perform in the same way with your right leg.

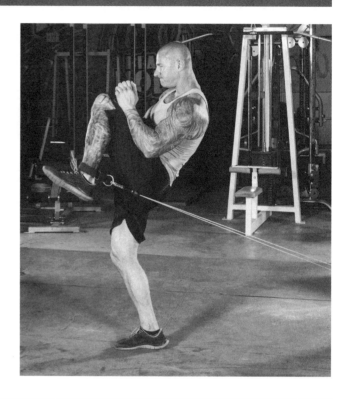

CROSSOVER CRUNCH

START

Lie faceup on the floor with your knees bent and feet flat on the floor. Cup your hands behind your head or place them at the sides of your head.

MOVE

Curl up as high as you can, bringing your left shoulder and upper back off the floor. Simultaneously bring your left elbow across your body toward your right knee. Hold at the top for a second, then slowly lower yourself back to the starting position. Repeat on the right side and continue alternating sides in this manner.

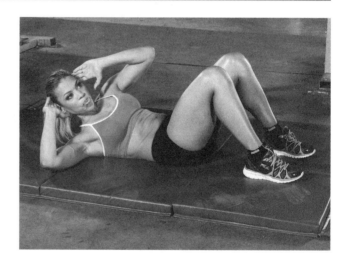

REACHING CROSSOVER CRUNCH

START

Lie on your back, knees bent and feet flat on the floor. Hold your arms extended a few inches off the floor alongside your hips.

MOVE

Raise your left shoulder and upper back off the floor as you reach with your left arm across your torso to your right knee. Return to the start and repeat on the right side.

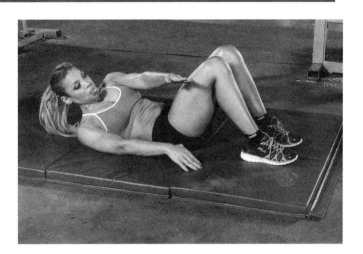

OBLIQUE CRUNCH

START

Lie on the floor on your right side with your hips and knees bent. Cup your left hand behind your head and place your right hand across your body. Placing your hand on your obliques can help you feel the muscles contract and enhance the mind–muscle connection.

MOVE

Contract your obliques to lift your shoulder off the floor. Hold this position for a second, contracting your obliques as hard as possible, then return to the start position. Complete all reps on the left side and then repeat on the right side.

Note: To make this exercise more difficult, hold a weight plate on your chest.

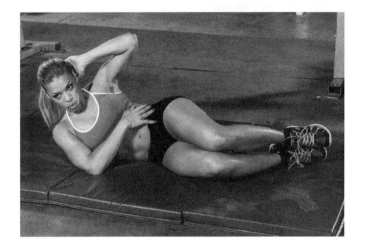

DUMBBELL SIDE BEND

START

Stand with your feet shoulder-width apart while holding a dumbbell with a neutral grip in your left hand with your arm hanging at your side.

MOVE

Bend sideways at the waist to the right as low as possible using your oblique muscles to pull your torso down. Hold for a second and return to the starting position. Complete the desired number of reps and repeat on the left side.

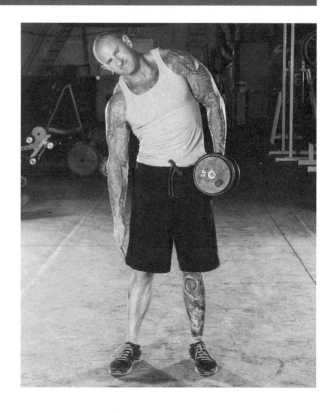

STANDING CABLE OBLIQUE CRUNCH

START

Stand with your right side toward a high-pulley cable with a single-handle D-grip attached to the pulley. Grip the handle with your right hand, palm up, and bring it toward your temple while keeping your elbow tucked tightly at your side.

MOVE

Contract though your obliques, pulling your torso down to the right. Pause a moment in this position before slowly returning to the starting position. Complete the desired number of reps and repeat on the left side.

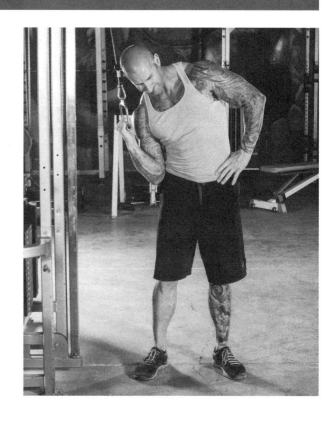

STANDING CABLE OBLIQUE PUSHDOWN

START

Attach a D-handle to a high cable pulley and, if possible, adjust it to just above hip height. Stand sideways to the pulley station with your right side closest to the pulley and right hand holding on to the handle attachment. Straighten your arm to create tension on the cable.

MOVE

Bend down on your right side, pushing the handle down toward the floor just outside your right foot. Focus on contracting your oblique muscle in this down position and then slowly return upright to the starting position. Perform all reps on the right side then repeat on the left.

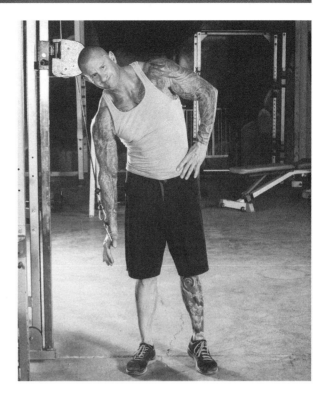

KNEELING OBLIQUE CABLE CRUNCH

START

Face a high cable pulley with a rope attached to it on your knees with your body angled about 45 degrees from the pulley. Grab the ends of the rope with your right hand and keep your arm out in front of you with your elbow bent about 90 degrees. Maintain this arm position throughout the movement.

MOVE

Use your obliques and abs to bend at the waist, bringing your right elbow down toward your right knee. Hold the bottom position for a second as you contract your obliques and abs and then slowly return to the start and repeat for reps. Once you have completed all reps on the right side, repeat on the left.

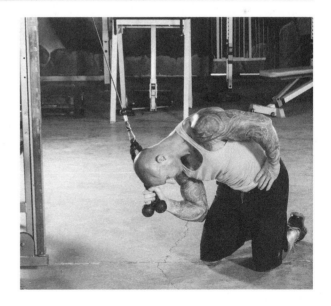

SIDE JACKKNIFE

START

Lie on the floor on your right side, keeping your left leg over your right one. Both legs are straight. Place your right hand in a comfortable position and cup your left hand behind your head.

MOVE

As you pull with your obliques, bring your torso and left leg toward each other. Hold the contraction briefly and lower slowly to the starting position. Complete the desired number of reps and repeat on the other side.

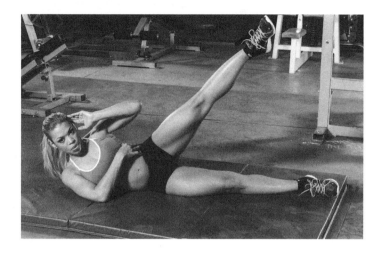

RUSSIAN TWIST

START

Lie faceup on the floor with your head about a foot (30.5 centimeters) from a stable object such as an exercise machine. Extend your arms overhead to grab the apparatus for stabilizing your torso. Lift your legs straight up so that they are perpendicular to the floor.

MOVE

Slowly lower your legs to the floor on your right side. Reverse the movement to bring them back up above you and then lower them to the left side.

Note: To make this exercise more difficult, add resistance by holding a medicine ball between your knees.

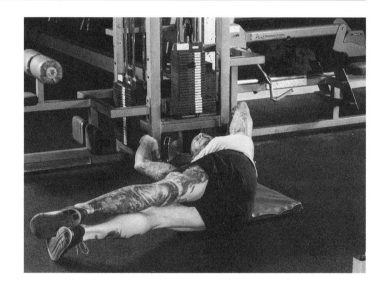

STANDING MEDICINE BALL ROTATION

START

Stand straight with knees slightly bent. Hold a medicine ball with both hands at shoulder level. Your training partner assumes the same position behind you but without a medicine ball.

MOVE

Keeping your lower body in place, rotate your torso to one side and pass the ball high to your partner, who has simultaneously rotated in that same direction. Then rotate in the other direction and receive the ball back from your partner, this time in a lower position (hands at your waist rather than at shoulder level). Continue passing and receiving the ball in this fashion for the desired number of reps. Then do the same number of reps beginning with the ball high on the other side.

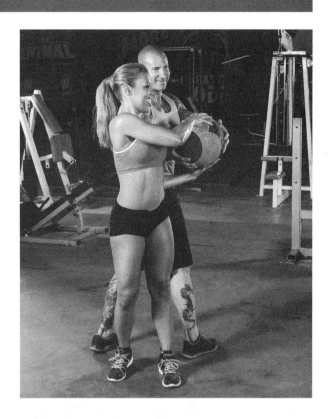

BAND ROUNDHOUSE ELBOW

START

Take a strength band and wrap it around a secure base such as a power rack, machine, or other suitable structure. The band should be a little below shoulder height. Attach a handle or ankle strap to the bands. Stand sideways to the attachment point of the bands with your left foot closest to it. Slide your left arm through the handle so that the handle sits on the inside of your elbow. Move your body far enough back from the band attachment so that there is adequate tension. Take a shoulder-width stance and hold your left arm out to the side with a full bend at the elbow. Your elbow should be pointing straight out to your side. Hold your left wrist with your right hand.

MOVE

Once in place, rotate about the waist in an explosive but controlled fashion, contracting the abs and obliques and pivoting on the back foot during the movement. Slowly return to the start position and repeat for reps. After completing all reps on the left side, repeat on the right side.

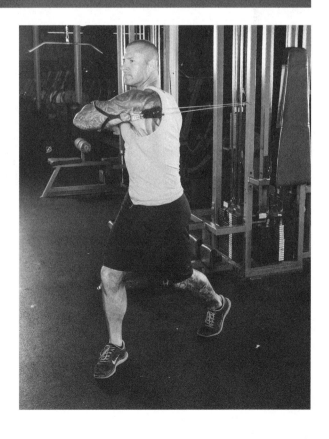

LYING LEG RAISE

START

Lie faceup on the floor with your entire body straight and your hands at your sides on the floor to stabilize your torso. Hold your legs a few inches off the floor.

MOVE

Raise your legs up toward the ceiling until they are just short of perpendicular to the floor. Slowly lower your legs back to the starting position.

Note: To make this exercise more difficult, perform it on a decline bench with your head on the higher end.

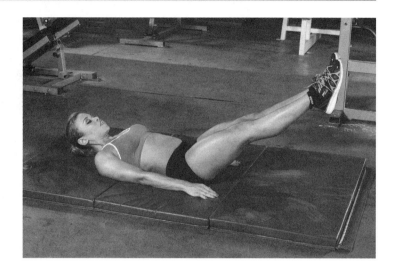

SCISSOR KICK

START

Lie faceup on the floor with your entire body straight and your hands at the sides of your head. Hold your legs a few inches off the floor.

MOVE

Make small, rapid, alternating up-and-down scissorlike motions as you lift each leg about 45 degrees into the air and lower each until your heel is a few inches off the floor.

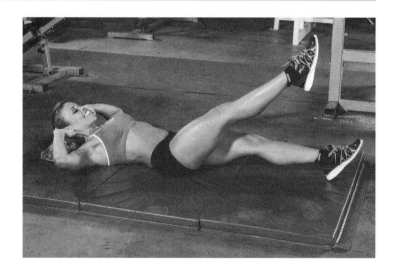

EXERCISE BALL PASS

START

Lie on your back with your legs and arms extended. Hold an exercise ball in your hands.

MOVE

Raise the ball overhead with your arms while simultaneously bringing your legs toward it. When your hands and feet meet, pass the ball from your hands to your feet. Without pausing, lower your arms and legs back down. Continue in alternating fashion.

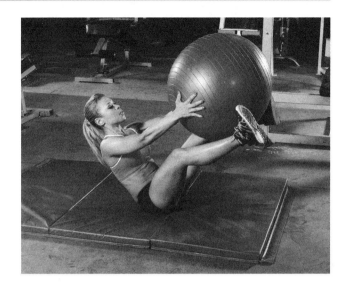

BARBELL ROLL-OUT

START

Kneel on the floor in front of a loaded barbell and grab the barbell with an overhand, shoulder-width group. Your arms should be straight and your torso fairly upright in the start position.

MOVE

Allow the bar to roll forward as far as possible with just your knees and toes touching the floor while you maintain your grip on the bar. The goal is to be as flat as possible in the finish position with your torso and upper legs parallel with floor and hovering just a couple inches above it. Then reverse the motion to pull the bar back toward your knees until your body is upright again. Repeat for as many reps as possible.

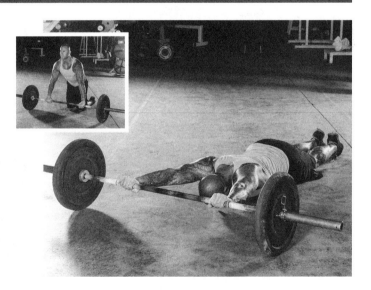

DUMBBELL WOODCHOPPER

START

Stand with your feet about shoulder-width apart and knees slightly bent. Grasp a light dumbbell in both hands, holding it outside and above your left shoulder.

MOVE

Slowly lower the dumbbell diagonally across your body until it is beside your right hip. Reverse the direction, returning to the starting position. Complete the desired number of reps, then repeat on the right side.

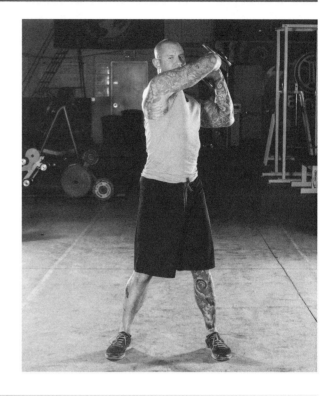

CABLE WOODCHOPPER

START

Stand with your right side toward a high-pulley cable with a rope handle attached to it. Grab the handle with both hands and hold it outside your right shoulder in a similar manner to the start of the dumbbell woodchopper exercise.

MOVE

Pull the handle across the front of your body to your left hip. Slowly resist the handle back to the starting position. Complete the desired number of reps and repeat on the left side.

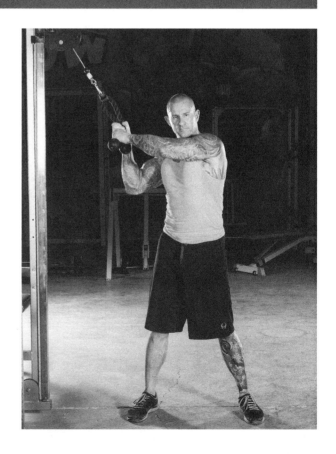

BAND WOODCHOPPER

START

Stand with your left side facing the attachment point of the band set above shoulder height. Grab the band with both hands, just like an ax, and hold it outside your left shoulder in a manner similar to the start of an actual swing with an ax.

MOVE

Explosively pull the band across the front of your body to the outside of your right hip as though really swinging an ax. Slowly resist the band back to the start position. Complete the desired number of reps on one side and then repeat on the other side.

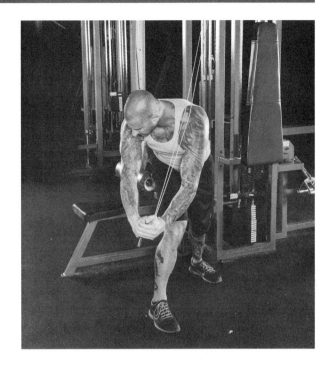

PLANK

START

Get into a modified push-up position by balancing your body on your forearms and toes with your body in a straight line from head to feet.

MOVE

Hold this position for the prescribed amount of time while pulling your abs in and keeping your hips from dropping toward the floor.

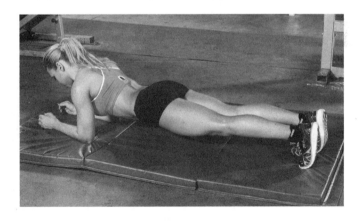

SIDE PLANK

START

Get in a side plank position by lying on your right side on the floor with your left foot rested on top of the inner side of your right foot and your left arm rested on top of your left side. Raise your body by placing your right forearm flat on the floor so that it's perpendicular to your torso. Lift your torso until your right upper arm is straight underneath you with your elbow bent 90 degrees and your forearm flat on the floor. In this position, only your right forearm and the outer side of your right foot are making contact with the floor and your body forms a diagonal line that is at about a 20-degree angle to the floor.

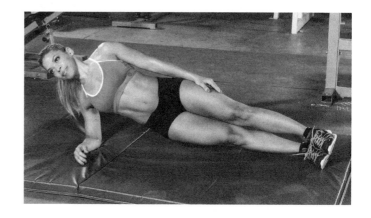

MOVE

Keep your abs pulled in tight and hold this position for as long as you can and then repeat on the left side.

SIDE PLANK WITH REACH-THROUGH

START

Get in a side plank position with your right arm as described in the side plank exercise.

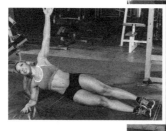

MOVE

Raise your left arm straight above you. Then lower your arm under the opposite armpit and through the other side as you turn your body from a sideways position to facing down toward the floor. Then reverse the motion to bring your arm back up above you. Focus on getting a good stretch in your rear delts and middle traps as your arm reaches the top position. When you have completed all reps on one side, repeat on the opposite side.

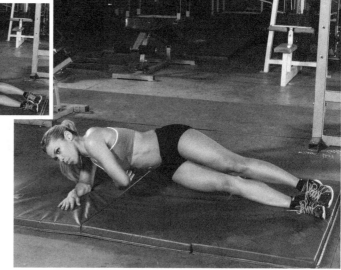

CHAPTER 25

Whole Body

This chapter contains detailed descriptions of the exercises that involve multiple joints and use multiple large muscle groups of the upper and lower body. Not only are these great exercises for building sheer power and strength, but they make great cardio alternatives, especially with techniques such as Power HIIT, Tabatas, and cardioacceleration as discussed in chapter 12. These exercises are divided into barbell whole-body exercises and dumbbell, kettlebell, and medicine ball whole-body exercises. Wherever a certain type of exercise is used in a workout, any one of the same type can be substituted.

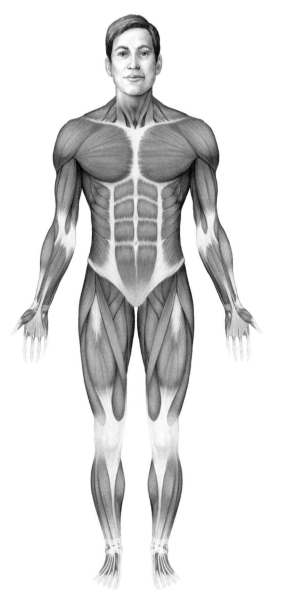
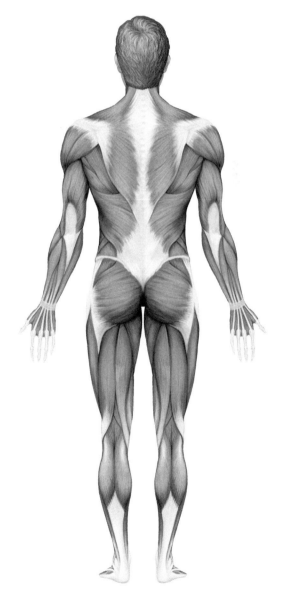

DEADLIFT

START

Stand over a loaded barbell resting on the floor with a hip-width stance. Your shins should touch the bar. Squat down to grab the bar using a staggered grip. Your hands should be about shoulder-width apart. Your torso should be bent at 45 degrees over the bar and your arms should be tensed and pulling on the bar. Your thighs are slightly higher than parallel with the floor.

MOVE

Keep your abs pulled in tight and tense your entire body. Drive through your heels to straighten your knees and bring your hips forward until you are in a standing position. Once standing, bring your shoulders back slightly and pause. Lower the barbell along the same path (close to your body all the way down) to the floor. Touch the plates lightly to the floor and begin your next rep.

Note: For a detailed description on using the deadlift for maximal strength, as well as doing the sumo deadlift, see chapter 8.

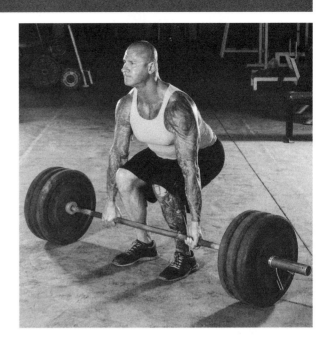

HEX BAR DEADLIFT

START

Stand in the middle of a loaded hex bar and squat to grab the handles. In the start position your thighs should be just above parallel with the floor with your torso bent forward at about a 45-degree angle with the floor.

MOVE

Drive your heels through the floor as you extend at the knees and hips to reach a fully upright position and then slowly lower the bar to the floor. You can lift significantly more weight in hex bar deadlifts than in traditional deadlifts, and hex bar deadlifts use more of the quadriceps and place less stress on the lower back.

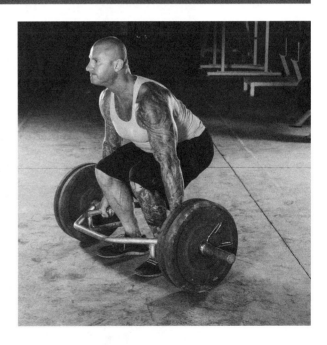

DEAD LANDMINE

START

Load one end of a barbell with weight and place the opposite and empty end of the barbell on the floor or in a landmine base. Stand facing the loaded end of the barbell with the weight plate in between your feet and your left foot closer to the end of the barbell. Squat and grab the barbell using an underhand grip with your left hand and an overhand grip with the right.

MOVE

Extend at the hips and knees to drive the weighted end of the barbell off the floor. As the weight passes your hips, use your arms to continue lifting the bar as you pivot your feet to swing the end of the bar across your chest and toward your right side. Continue pivoting your feet as you lower the bar to the floor on the right side. Once the barbell touches the floor, repeat on the right side to swing it over to the left side and repeat for the prescribed number of reps or time interval.

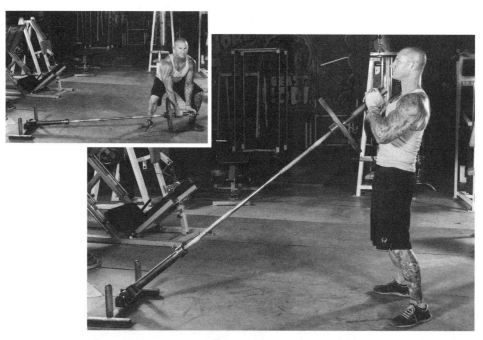

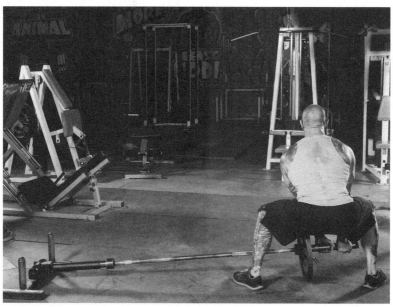

DEAD CURL PRESS

START

Place a barbell on the floor in front of you to assume a deadlift start with your hands reversed in an underhand grip so that the palms are facing forward.

MOVE

Deadlift the barbell to the midthigh and then immediately curl the barbell into a biceps curl to the shoulders; immediately complete the movement with a reverse barbell shoulder press. Reverse these movements to return the bar to the floor and repeat for reps.

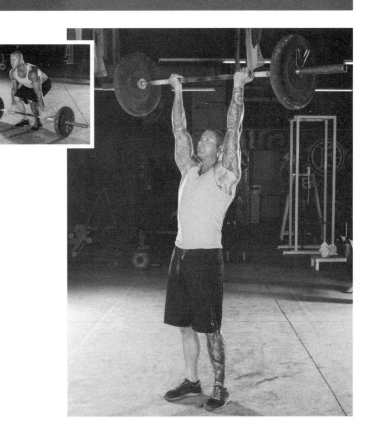

SNATCH

START

Stand over a barbell placed on the floor. Your legs are hip-width apart and your shins are about an inch (2.5 centimeters) from the bar. Squat down and grab the barbell with a very wide overhand grip. Your shoulders should be over the barbell and your back should be tightly arched.

MOVE

With one smooth motion, forcefully extend at the hips and knees as you swing the barbell forward and up with your arms. The extension at the hips and knees should be minimal—just enough to start the barbell moving from the floor. Immediately squat back down by flexing at the hips and knees as you extend the barbell straight overhead. With the barbell extended straight overhead, forcefully extend at the hips and knees to stand straight up. Return the barbell to the floor.

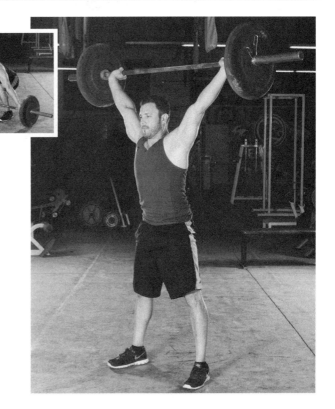

CLEAN AND JERK

START

Squat and grab a loaded barbell bar resting on the floor using an overhand grip with your feet spaced about hip-width apart. Your hands should be about shoulder-width apart with your shins about an inch from the bar. Your torso should be bent at 45 degrees over the bar, and your arms should be tensed and pulling on the bar. Your thighs will be slightly higher than parallel with the floor.

MOVE

Keep your abs pulled in tight as you drive explosively through your heels to straighten your knees and hips to lift the bar to hip height. Immediately pull the bar up to shoulder height as you squat under it to catch it on your upper chest and shoulders. Extend at the hips and knees to stand straight up with a slight bend in the knees. Extend forcefully at the knees and hips as you press the bar straight overhead. You can perform the press with your feet stationary. Or you can split your legs to drive one foot forward and the other back, then bring your legs together while keeping your arms extended overhead. Return the bar back to the starting position.

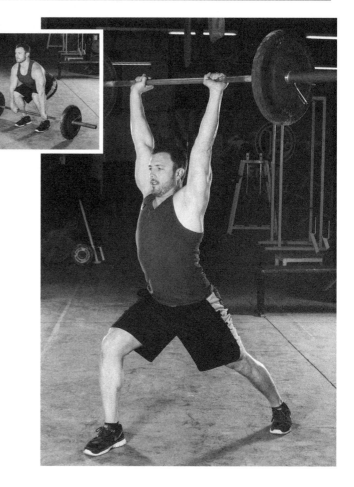

POWER CLEAN

START

Stand over a loaded barbell resting on the floor with your feet spaced hip-width apart. Your shins are about an inch (2.5 centimeters) from the bar. Squat to grab the bar using an overhand grip. Your hands should be spaced about shoulder-width apart. Your torso should be bent at 45 degrees over the bar with your arms tensed and pulling on the bar. Your thighs are slightly higher than parallel with the floor.

MOVE

Keep your abs pulled in tight and tense your entire body. Drive explosively through your heels to straighten your knees and bring your hips forward until the bar is at hip height. Pull the bar up to your shoulders and squat under the bar as you catch it on your shoulders and whip your arms around so that the elbows are pointing forward. Extend at the hips and knees so that you are standing straight up with a slight bend in the knees with the bar resting on your upper chest.

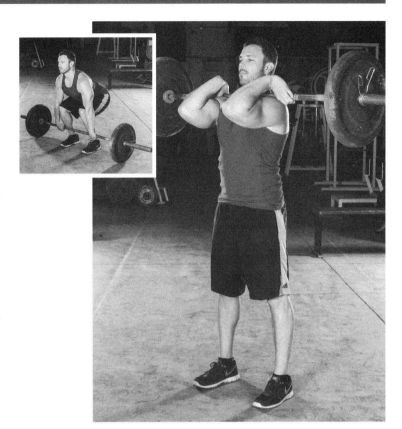

HANG POWER CLEAN

MOVE

This exercise is performed similar to a power clean but the bar starts just below the knees.

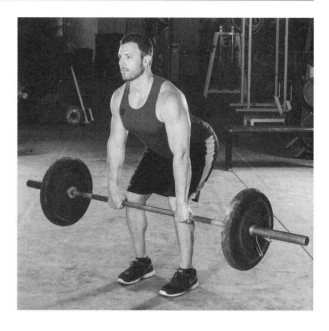

HIGH PULL

START

The first part of the movement is the same as for the clean and jerk.

MOVE

When the bar reaches thigh level, explosively move it upward by extending the hip, knee, and ankle joints in a jumping motion. When you reach full extension, shrug your shoulders. Then pull with your arms, bringing the bar as high as possible. Slowly lower the bar and reset.

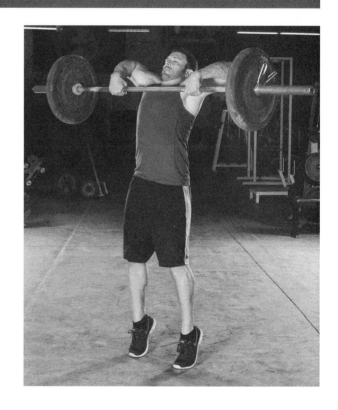

HANG PULL

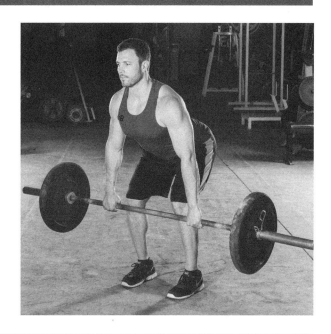

START

Stand while holding a barbell in front of your knees with an overhand grip. Both your hands and feet are shoulder-width apart. Your knees are slightly bent and your torso is leaned forward slightly.

MOVE

Pull the bar upward in an explosive manner by extending the hip, knee, and ankle joints in a jumping motion. Simultaneously shrug your shoulders, then pull with your arms, bringing the bar as high as possible. Slowly lower the bar to thigh level.

SMITH MACHINE HANG POWER CLEAN

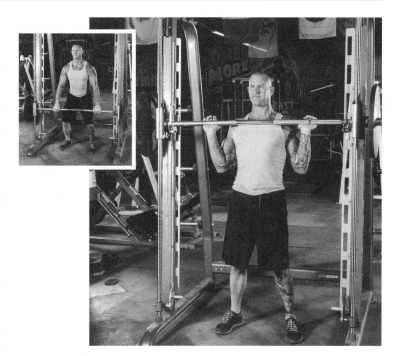

START

Stand in the middle of the Smith machine and position the bar at just above knee height. Take an overhand grip (I suggest a hook grip where the fingers wrap over the thumb) on the bar outside of shoulder width and unhook the bar from the machine. Your arms should be fully extended with your head and chest up. Your elbows should be pointed out with your shoulders back and down. Your hips should be back and knees should be slightly bent.

MOVE

Initiate the movement by forcefully extending the hips, knees, and ankles, accelerating into the bar. Use your traps to initiate pulling the bar up and transfer that motion into the shoulders to continue raising the bar. Once your lower body has reached full extension, bend the hips and knees again to lower your receiving position. Allow the arms to flex at this point, rotating the elbows around the bar to receive it on your shoulders. Extend through the hips and knees to come to a standing position with the bar racked on your shoulders to complete the movement. Lower the bar to the start position and repeat for reps.

DUMBBELL HIGH PULL

START

Stand while holding the dumbbells in front of your thighs with an overhand grip. Both your hands and feet are shoulder-width apart. Your knees are slightly bent and your torso is leaning forward slightly.

MOVE

Pull the dumbbells upward in an explosive manner by extending the hip, knee, and ankle joints in a jumping motion. Simultaneously shrug your shoulders, then pull with your arms, bringing the dumbbells as high as possible. Slowly lower the dumbbells to thigh level.

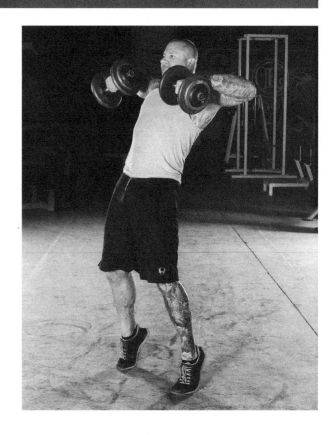

PUSH PRESS

START

Assume a front squat starting position.

MOVE

Bend slightly at the knees and then explode upward onto the balls of your feet, simultaneously pressing the bar overhead. Hold this position for a split second before returning to the bent-knee position.

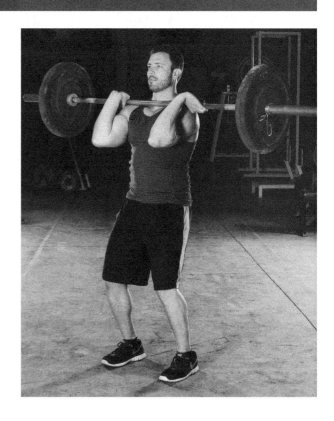

OVERHEAD SQUAT

START

Press a barbell straight overhead with a wider-than-shoulder-width grip. Lock out your arms and hold the bar overhead.

MOVE

Squat down into a full squat, pause at the bottom, and return to a standing position while holding the bar overhead.

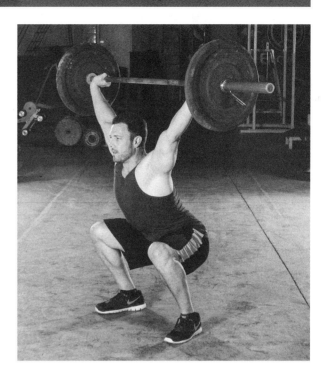

DUMBBELL DEADLIFT

START

Stand with your feet shoulder-width apart with a dumbbell on the floor outside of each foot. Squat down to grab the dumbbells using a neutral grip. Your torso is bent at 45 degrees over the floor with your arms tensed and pulling on the dumbbells. Your thighs are slightly higher than parallel with the floor.

MOVE

Keep your abs pulled in tight and tense your entire body, then drive through your heels to straighten your knees and bring your hips forward until you are in a standing position with the dumbbells at your sides. Once standing, bring your shoulders back slightly and pause. Lower the dumbbells along the same path to the floor. Touch the weights lightly to the floor and begin your next rep.

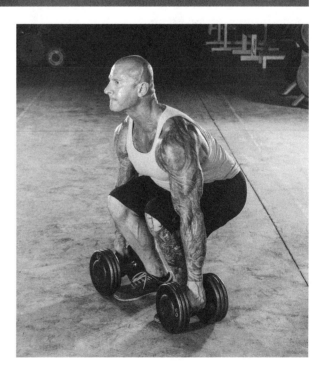

DUMBBELL CLEAN AND JERK

START

Stand with your feet shoulder-width apart with a dumbbell on the floor outside of each foot. Squat down to grab the dumbbells using a neutral grip. Your torso is bent at 45 degrees over the floor with your arms tensed and pulling on the dumbbells. Your thighs are slightly higher than parallel with the floor.

MOVE

Keep your abs pulled in tight, and tense your entire body. Drive explosively through your heels to straighten your knees and bring your hips forward until the dumbbells are at hip height. Pull the dumbbells up to your shoulders and squat under them as you catch them on your shoulders and whip your arms around so that the elbows are pointing forward. Extend at the hips and knees so that you are standing straight up with a slight bend in the knees and with the dumbbells resting on your shoulders. Extend forcefully at the knees and hips as you press the dumbbells straight overhead. You can also use a split stance as shown. Return the dumbbells back to the starting position.

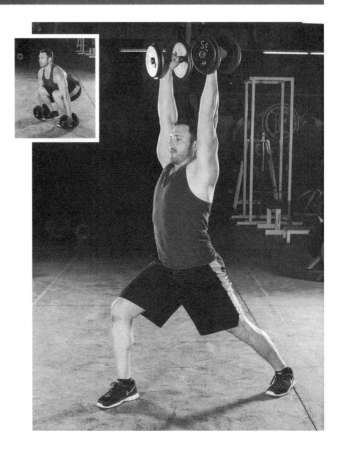

ONE-ARM DUMBBELL SNATCH

START

Stand with your feet shoulder-width apart with a dumbbell on the floor in the middle of your feet. Squat down to grab the dumbbell using an overhand grip with your right hand. Your torso is bent at 45 degrees over the floor with your arm tensed and pulling on the dumbbell. Your thighs are slightly higher than parallel with the floor.

MOVE

With one smooth motion, forcefully extend at the hips and knees as you pull the dumbbell up keeping it close to your body. The extension at the hips and knees should be minimal—just enough to start the dumbbells moving from the floor. Immediately squat back down by flexing at the hips and knees as you extend the dumbbell straight overhead. With the dumbbell extended straight overhead, forcefully extend at the hips and knees to stand straight up. Return the dumbbell back to the floor, and repeat on the left side.

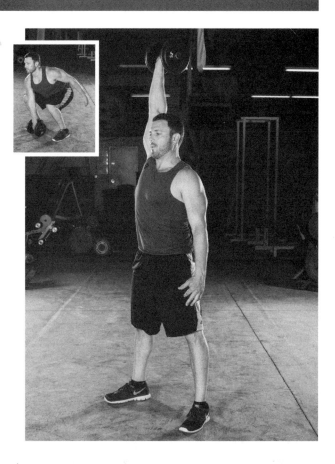

DUMBBELL POWER CLEAN

START

Stand with your feet hip-width apart with a dumbbell on the floor outside of each foot. Squat down to grab the dumbbells using a neutral grip. Your torso is bent at 45 degrees over the floor with your arms tensed and pulling on the dumbbells. Your thighs are slightly higher than parallel with the floor.

MOVE

Keep your abs pulled in tight, and tense your entire body. Drive explosively through your heels to straighten your knees and bring your hips forward until the dumbbells are at hip height. Pull the dumbbells up to your shoulders and squat under them as you catch them on your shoulders and whip your arms around so that the elbows are pointing forward. Extend at the hips and knees so that you are standing straight up with a slight bend in the knees and with the dumbbells resting on your shoulders. Carefully return the dumbbells to the floor.

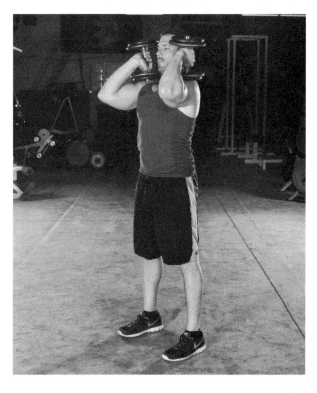

DUMBBELL HANG CLEAN

MOVE

This exercise is similar to the dumbbell power clean, but you start by holding the dumbbells at the sides of your thighs.

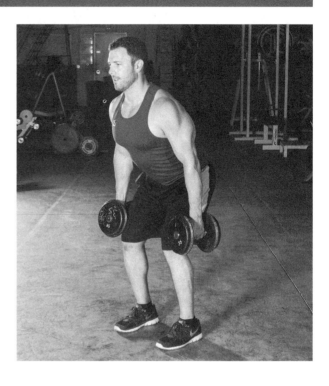

DUMBBELL PUSH PRESS

MOVE

This exercise is similar to the part of the dumbbell clean and jerk where the dumbbells rest on your shoulders.

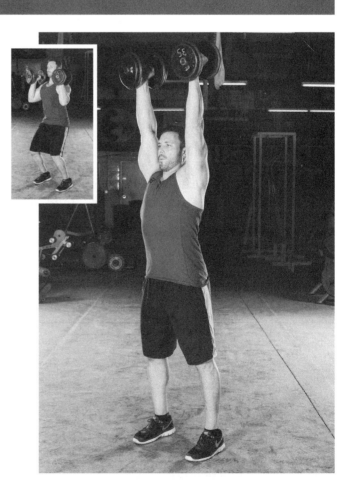

DUMBBELL OVERHEAD SQUAT

START

Stand with your feet shoulder-width apart and extend the dumbbells over your head and lock your wrists and elbows.

MOVE

Keeping your heels flat on the floor, squat down as close to parallel as you can, shifting the dumbbells back behind your head to counter-balance the movement. Come back up to the start position all the while keeping your abs tight and chest out.

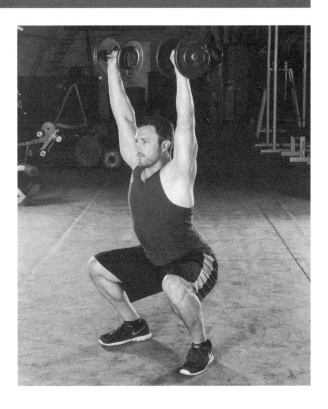

POWER DUMBBELL RAISE

START

Stand erect while holding a pair of dumbbells at your sides. Knees are slightly bent, feet are shoulder-width apart, and toes are slightly pointed out.

MOVE

Bend your knees slightly and then straighten them as you raise the dumbbells up toward your armpits. As the weights approach that position, push off the balls of your feet.

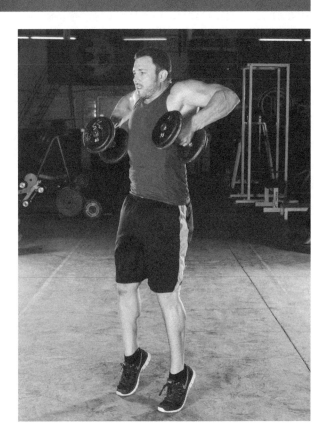

KETTLEBELL SNATCH

START

In a shoulder-width stance with a kettle-bell between your feet, squat to grasp the kettlebell with your left hand while keeping your torso at a 45-degree angle with the floor.

MOVE

Explode up by extending at the hips, knees, and ankles. Drive your heels into the floor as you pull the kettlebell up, keeping it close to your body. As the kettlebell reaches your head, allow the momentum it has gathered to swing over and end up on the top side of your forearm with your arm extended straight overhead. Reverse the motion to lower the kettlebell to the floor and then immediately perform in the same way with your right arm. Alternate arms each time until you have completed the desired number of reps or amount of time.

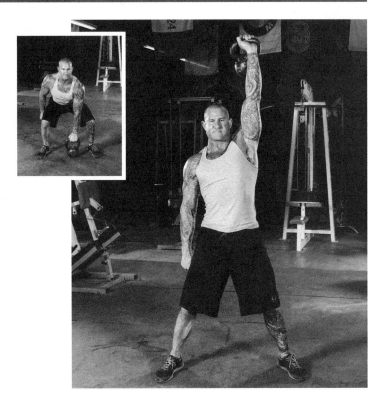

KETTLEBELL SWING

START

Stand with your feet shoulder-width apart holding the kettlebell with both arms in front of you.

MOVE

Drop your hips back and down just as you would sit in a chair, allowing the kettlebell to swing down in between your legs. Use your legs and hips to explosively extend at the knees and hips to swing the kettlebell up. The most important aspect of the lift is the hip thrust. As you swing the kettlebell up, you are not using your shoulders or your arms to help the kettlebell up; all you should use is your hips.

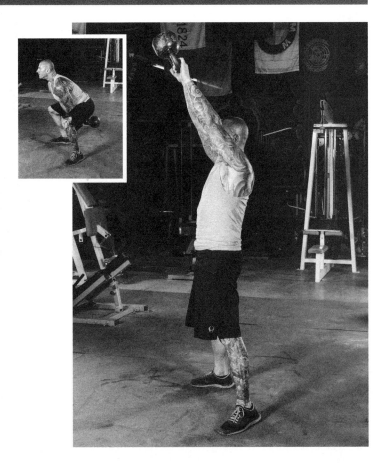

MEDICINE BALL OVERHEAD THROW

START

Hold a medicine ball with both hands in front of your upper chest.

MOVE

Squat and explode up as you launch the ball up overhead by explosively extending your arms. As the ball leaves your hands, your feet should be off the floor. Land on the ground with soft knees to absorb the force of the landing and allow the ball to land on the floor, but make sure that it doesn't land on you. Pick up the ball and repeat.

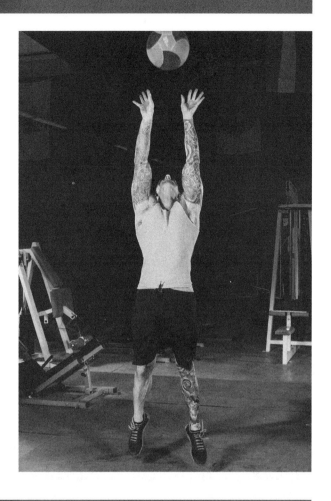

MEDICINE BALL SLAM

START

Hold a medicine ball with both hands in front of your chest.

MOVE

In an explosive manner, use your entire body to slam the medicine ball to the floor. If the medicine ball bounces high enough, catch it and repeat for the desired number of reps or time. If not, pick the medicine up and repeat.

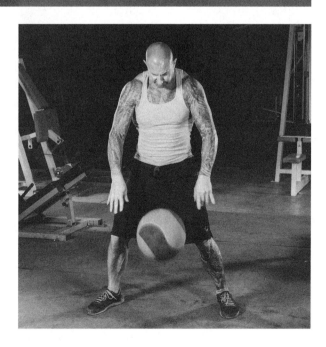

SQUAT-JUMP-PUSH-PRESS

START

In a shoulder-width stance, hold dumbbells at shoulder level so that your palms face each other.

MOVE

Descend into a full squat and then explode upward, jumping out of the squat as you press the weights to full extension so that your feet leave the floor. As you land, lower the weights back to your shoulders, making sure to bend your knees to "catch" them smoothly. Descend immediately into another rep.

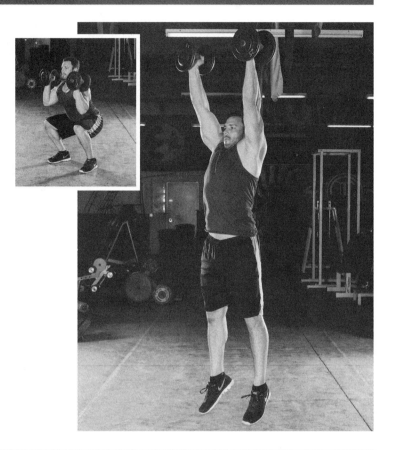

DUMBBELL SQUAT AND OVERHEAD PRESS

START

Hold two dumbbells at shoulder level with the ends of the dumbbell resting on the top of your shoulders. Keep your low back arched. Feet are slightly wider than shoulder width and toes are pointed out slightly.

MOVE

Squat down, holding the dumbbells in position at shoulder level. Pause for a second at the bottom when your thighs reach parallel with the ground, then drive back up to the starting position. When your knees are almost fully extended, press the dumbbells overhead. Finish with your arms fully extended overhead with your elbows straight but not locked. Slowly lower the dumbbells back to shoulder level and begin the next rep.

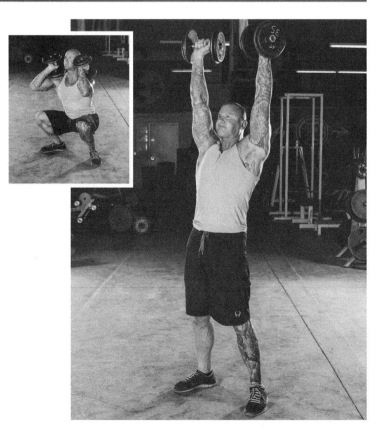

DUMBBELL PUSH-UP AND ROW

START

Place two dumbbells about shoulder-width apart on the floor. Get set in the bottom of a push-up position with your hands holding on to the weights. Place your feet about one to two feet (30.5 to 61 centimeters) apart for support and balance.

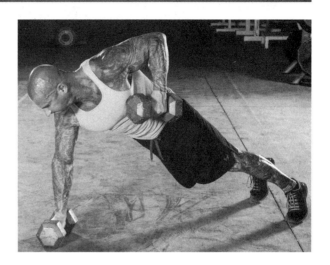

MOVE

Press yourself up by extending your elbows until your upper body is completely off the floor. When your elbows are fully extended, shift your body weight to your right arm and row the left dumbbell up to your left side, keeping your elbow as close to your body as possible. Lower the dumbbell back to the floor, shift your body weight over to your left side, and row the left dumbbell up to your right side. Lower the weight back to the floor and then lower your upper body back to the floor by bending your elbows. That completes one rep.

DUMBBELL DEADLIFT AND UPRIGHT ROW

START

The start is similar to the start of the dumbbell deadlift.

MOVE

Drive through your legs to lift the weights to a standing position. From there, go immediately into a dumbbell upright row, keeping the weights close to your body and pulling them to mid-chest level. Slowly reverse the movements to return the weights to the floor.

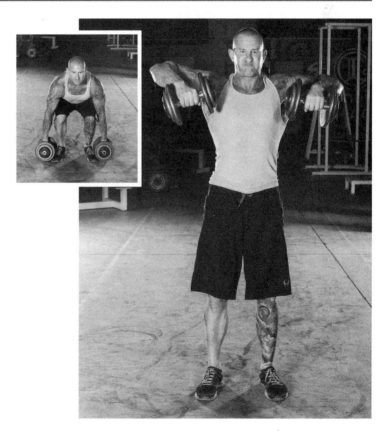

CHAPTER 26

Calisthenics

This chapter contains detailed descriptions of rhythmic calisthenic-type exercises that generally use many muscles. The exercises covered in this chapter typically make a great alternative to standard cardio, such as jogging, especially when employing HIIT cardio methods, including standard HIIT, Tabatas, Power HIIT, and cardioacceleration, as covered in chapter 12.

These exercises are not broken down into specific categories as the previous exercise chapters are, but they are grouped with exercises that are similar in nature. You can replace almost any one of these exercises with any other in this chapter.

BENCH HOP-OVER

START

Place your hands on the top of a flat weight bench with both feet on the left side of the bench toward the end of it.

MOVE

Hold the bench securely with both hands and hop your legs over the top of the bench and land them on the right side. Immediately hop back over to the left side. Keep hopping over the bench in this manner for the prescribed time.

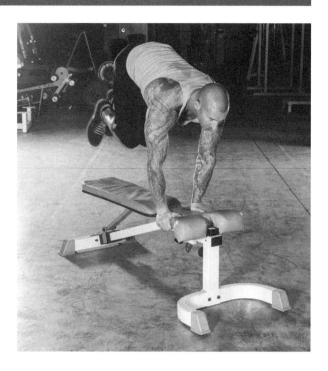

BOX JUMP

START

Stance facing a box or platform approximately a foot or so in front of you with your arms down at your sides and legs slightly bent.

MOVE

Using your arms to aid in the initial burst, jump upward and forward, landing with both feet simultaneously on top of the box. Immediately drop back to the start position and continue in this manner.

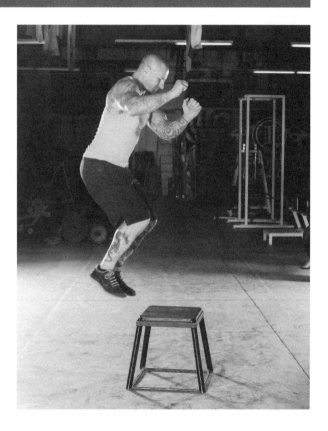

519

BURPEE

START

Start in a standing position.

MOVE

Crouch down, placing your hands on the floor in front of you. Kick your feet back into a solid plank push-up position and then bend your elbows and execute a full push-up. Hop your feet toward your hands into a crouch position. Use your legs to explode upward into a jump as high as you can with your arms extended overhead. Land on the floor and repeat for the desired number of reps or time.

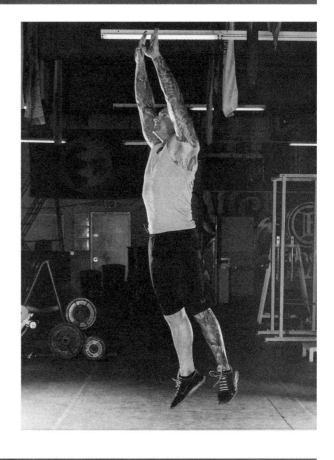

JUMPING JACK

START

Stand with your arms at your sides and your feet together.

MOVE

In one movement, jump up and separate your legs as you raise your arms to the sides and over your head. You should land with your arms over your head and your feet more than hip-width apart. Immediately jump up again and, in one movement, bring your legs together and your arms back to your sides. That completes one jumping jack. Continue in this manner.

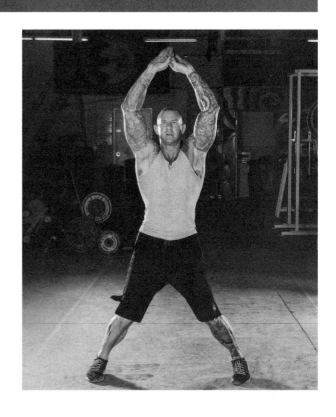

LATERAL BOUND

START

Stand in a half-squat position.

MOVE

Allow your left leg to do a countermovement inward as you shift your weight to the right leg. Immediately push off of your right foot to bound to the left side as far as possible. Land on your left leg. After absorbing the force by going down into a half squat, immediately push off your left leg in the opposite direction, returning to the start position. Continue back and forth in this manner.

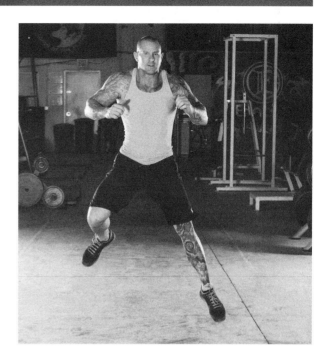

LATERAL BOX JUMP

START

Stand to the right of a box that is less than knee height.

MOVE

Drop into a half squat and explode up to jump up and over, landing on the top of the box. Absorb the impact by squatting slightly as you land. Immediately jump down to the left side of the box, landing with soft knees to absorb the force. Repeat in the other direction and continue this way for the prescribed amount of time.

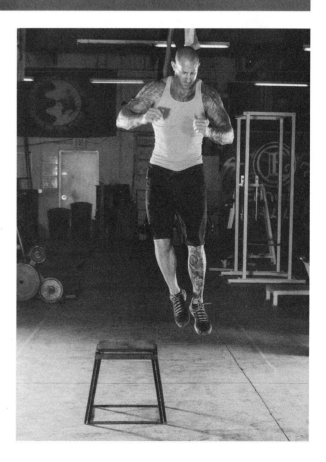

MOUNTAIN CLIMBER

START

Get in a push-up position with your weight supported by your hands and toes. Flexing your knee and hip, bring one leg up until the knee is under your chest.

MOVE

Explosively reverse the positions of your legs. Extend the bent leg until the leg is straight back and supported by the toe, and bring the other foot up with the hip and knee flexed until it is under your chest. Repeat in this alternating fashion for the prescribed amount of time.

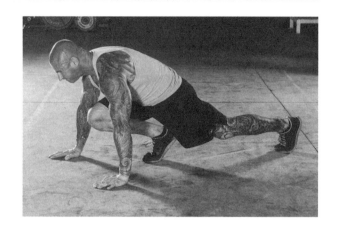

SIDE-TO-SIDE BOX SHUFFLE

START

Stand to one side of a box with your left foot resting on the middle of it.

MOVE

Jump up and over to the other side of the box, landing with your right foot on top of the box and your left foot on the floor. Swing your arms to aid your movement. Continue shuffling back and forth across the box in this manner.

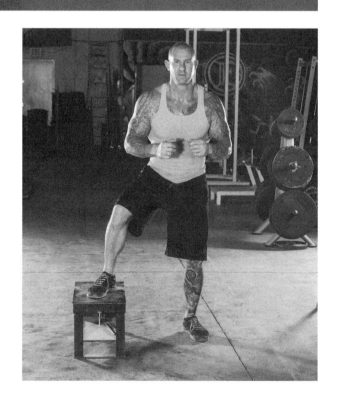

STEP-UP WITH RISING KNEE

START

Stand facing a box or bench that is anywhere from midshin to knee height with your feet together.

MOVE

Put your right foot on the top of the bench and extend your hip and knee to lift your body off of the floor. As your left leg passes the top of the bench, flex your left hip and knee to perform a rising knee, bringing your knee as high as you can. Reverse this motion to bring your left leg back to the floor and then lower your right foot back to the floor. Repeat this by stepping up with your left leg. Continue alternating legs like this for the desired amount of time. The higher the box or bench, the more intense the exercise will be. Perform the rising knee with explosive power as though you are performing a knee strike.

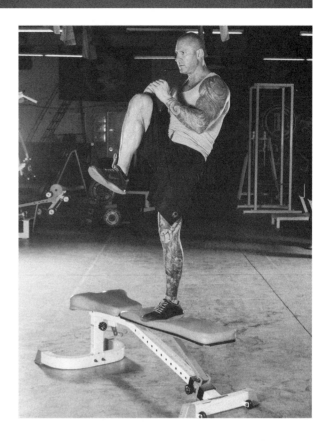

BAND SPRINT

START

Connect two resistance bands with handles to a stable structure. Hold the bands securely in front of your shoulders.

MOVE

Sprint as far forward as you can and as explosively as possible. Then quickly but carefully return to the start and repeat in this fashion for 20 seconds. This exercise is similar to running up a hill that gradually increases in steepness; the farther you sprint from the base, the more resistance the bands provide.

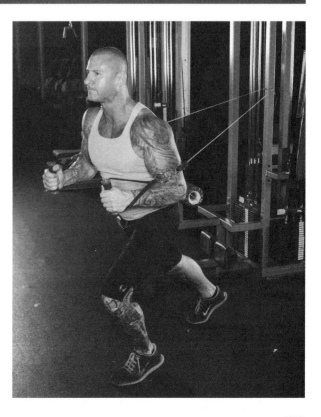

PART VI

NUTRITION FOR MAXIMIZING MUSCLE MASS, STRENGTH, AND FAT LOSS

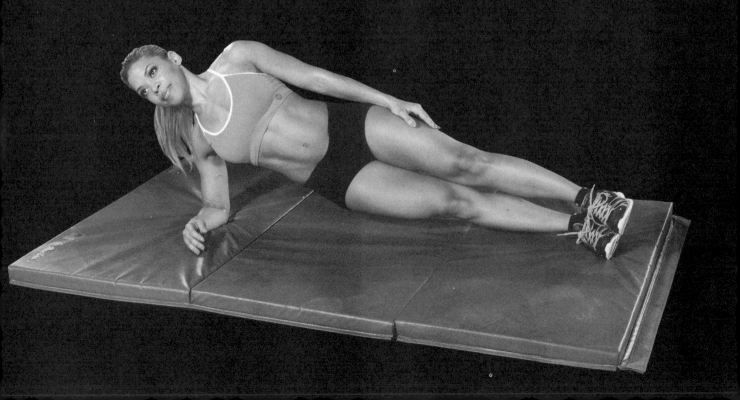

Even if you're following the proper training program, if you're not eating properly for your goals, then your results will be less than ideal. Having the proper diet will help to fuel your workouts so you have more energy and strength during the workout. And the proper diet will provide the right nutrients at the right time needed for recovery after the workout.

There's no doubt about it: Nutrition is a big part of the results you get from your training program. And it's a big part of maintaining health and general well-being.

Part VI is not an all-encompassing section on nutrition for weightlifting. That would make a book of its own. I've included this section to give you some general guidelines on nutrition and supplementation to support your goals.

Chapter 27 contains guidelines on nutrition for maximizing muscle mass and strength. This chapter includes ten nutrition goals and sample meal plans based on the times you typically work out during the day. These diet guidelines will work well with any of the programs in part IV of the book. This chapter also presents an overview of the most critical dietary supplements to take while following a weightlifting program. These are ingredients that enhance workout performance and recovery as well as promote gains in muscle mass, strength, and endurance and in some cases fat loss.

Chapter 28 presents nutrition guidelines for maximizing fat loss. It includes eight steps to achieving fat loss.

CHAPTER 27

Nutrition for Maximizing Muscle Mass and Strength

When it comes to maximizing muscle mass and strength gains, the general rules regarding nutrition are fairly the same. After all, building muscle mass and muscle strength go hand in hand to some degree. So nutrient requirements and timing are very similar whether you are trying to maximize muscle hypertrophy or muscle strength. And more often than not, you are trying to do both at the same time.

As mentioned in the introduction to this part, there is not enough room in this book to provide you with all the nutrition basics you will need to understand. However, the guidelines here will serve you well in meeting your goals.

These guidelines are what I have found to be most effective over decades of working with people to maximize muscle growth and strength naturally. They are backed by science done in the lab, but more important they are backed by real-world evidence in the gym on literally millions of people using them over the years. I've divided the guidelines into 10 goals to focus on with your diet. After the goals are sample meal plans based on the goals; you will discover how to incorporate these plans into your day based on when you work out.

GOAL 1: FOCUS ON PROTEIN

Muscle is made of protein. To build muscle, you need to boost muscle protein synthesis as well as decrease muscle breakdown. Research in the lab and the gym confirms that the best way to do this is with a diet that gets you a minimum of 1 gram per pound of body weight (a little over 2 grams of protein per kilogram of body weight) and even closer to about 1.5 grams of protein per pound of body weight (about 3 grams of protein per kilogram

of body weight) per day. This is especially true for those following more intense training programs.

Several studies support the notion that getting up to 1.5 grams of protein per pound of body weight is effective for producing better gains in muscle mass. Victoria University (Australia) researchers had weight-trained men consume about 1.5 grams of protein per pound of body weight per day or 0.75 gram of protein per pound during an 11-week weight training program (Cribb et al. 2007). The higher protein intake was achieved by supplementing with whey protein. The men who ingested the higher protein gained significantly greater strength and muscle fiber protein in the quadriceps than the control group did. In a 2006 study by Candow and colleagues, male and female participants supplemented with either whey protein or soy protein to bump up their daily protein intake to about 1.5 grams per pound of body weight per day during 6 weeks of weight training. The control group consumed about 0.75 gram of protein per pound. The participants getting the greater protein, regardless of the source, had significantly greater gains in muscle strength and growth. And in a study by Burke and colleagues (2001), participants' protein intake was increased to 1.5 grams per pound of body weight per day during 6 weeks of weight training with whey protein, while control participants consumed 0.5 gram of protein per pound. At the end of the six weeks the participants getting the extra protein gained significantly more strength and muscle mass. A 2011 study by Witard and colleagues has also shown that even in endurance athletes, when they double their protein intake to close to 1.5 grams per pound of body weight per day when training intensity is increased, they recover better and maintain better performance.

Despite these studies and the many others that confirm that higher protein intake produces better gains in muscle strength and mass, many misinformed dieticians, doctors, and scientists still believe that protein requirements for those who weight train are not that much different than for sedentary people who do little to no exercise. This is because there is also research showing that increasing protein intake during a weight-training program has little impact on muscle growth or strength gains.

A review study (Bosse and Dixon 2012) on protein intake and strength training finally gives us an answer to why some studies show that higher protein intakes produce better gains in muscle mass and strength and why others show that it doesn't. Many studies do not show a benefit of increased protein intake because protein intake was not increased enough from their baseline diets or protein intake was not increased enough compared to the lower-protein group. However, when you look at studies that increase protein intake by almost double the participants' baseline intake or increase protein intake by at least 50 percent of that consumed by the lower-protein group or control group, then high protein intake does lead to significant gains in lean muscle mass and muscle strength.

The bottom line is that eating a higher-protein diet is effective for gaining more muscle and increasing muscle strength. Shoot for 1 to 1.5 grams of protein per pound of body weight for optimal results.

GOAL 2: GET AMPLE FAT

Many people still are misguided when it comes to dietary fat. There is still a tendency to believe that you must keep fat low to be fit and healthy. Yet nothing could be further from the truth. Fat is an important macronutrient for anyone interested in building muscle and gaining strength as well as optimizing health.

One reason you need to take in adequate fat is that your body needs certain types of fat, such as omega-3 fat (from fatty fish like salmon). This type of fat has recently been found to be a critical player in muscle recovery and growth. It also keeps body fat at bay, aids joint health, protects from heart disease, and boosts brain function, among other benefits. A study by Smith and colleagues (2011)

suggests that those supplementing with fish oil have a higher anabolic response (higher rates of muscle protein synthesis) when consuming protein, which can lead to greater muscle growth in the long run.

Then there is monounsaturated fat. This is not an essential fat, but it is a healthy fat because it provides numerous health benefits and is readily burned for fuel rather than stored as body fat. On top of that, male athletes consuming more monounsaturated fat maintain higher testosterone levels (Hamalainen et al. 1983; Reed et al. 1987). Actually, male athletes consuming more monounsaturated fat *and* saturated fat maintain higher testosterone levels. So, yes, you actually should try to consume some saturated fat rather than try to avoid it at all costs. Good sources are beef, dairy (full fat or reduced fat, but not fat-free), and whole eggs. The only fat that you want to avoid is trans fat. The Malmo Diet and Cancer Study reported that individuals receiving more than 30 percent of their total daily energy from fat and more than 10 percent from saturated fat did not have increased mortality (Leosdottir et al. 2005).

A simple rule for fat intake is to consume half your body weight in pounds (or about your entire body weight in kilograms) in grams of fat. So, if you weigh 200 pounds (90 kg), you would consume about 100 grams of fat per day, 33 percent of it as monounsaturated fat, 33 percent as polyunsaturated fat (mainly omega-3 fat), and 33 percent as saturated fat each day. Also consider supplementing with 4 to 10 grams of fish oil per day. If you really want to fine-tune this recommendation, look to see how much DHA (docosahexaenoic acid) and EPA (eicosapentaenoic acid) your fish oil provides per capsule and try to get close to 1500 milligrams DHA and 1800 milligrams of EPA per day for maximal benefits.

GOAL 3: MANIPULATE CARBOHYDRATE

Because you want to make sure you're eating ample protein and ample fat for maximizing muscle growth, the amounts of these two critical macronutrients should stay about the same regardless of where you are in your diet or your goals. That means to gain more mass or to lose more fat you should change your carb intake. The body can make all the glucose (blood sugar) it needs from protein and fat. So there is no essential carbohydrate you need from your diet. Unlike with essential fat you need to consume, and with protein there are essential amino acids you need to consume because the body doesn't make them.

For maximizing muscle growth and strength gains while minimizing fat gains, start off somewhere around 1.5 to 2.0 grams of carbohydrate per pound of body weight. Then you can either increase this amount if you find that you are not gaining mass rapidly enough and are not gaining any body fat. Similarly, you can also gradually lower this amount if you find that you are gaining too much body fat. Everyone's body is different, and your body will respond to carbohydrate differently. So you need to experiment with carbohydrate intake.

GOAL 4: COUNT CALORIES

Calorie intake is important for building muscle and strength because you need to be in a positive energy balance (consuming more calories than you are burning) to truly maximize muscle growth. However, if you are hitting the proper amount of protein and fat and have your carb intake dialed in for your body, then how far over your energy needs or under you are doesn't really matter . . . to a point. As stated in rule 3, it is possible to gain muscle while losing body fat. That being said, to maximize muscle mass, you should be eating more calories than you are burning each day. And to maximize fat loss, you should be burning more calories than you are consuming. However, it is possible to burn slightly more calories than you are consuming yet gain muscle because you are eating ample amounts of protein and fat. We know that 1 gram of protein provides 4 calories, as does 1 gram of carbs. We also know that 1 gram of fat provides about 9 calories (8 to 10 calories, depending on the type of fat). If you build a diet from the macronutrients up and want to be sure to get in 1.5 grams of protein per pound of body weight and 0.5 gram of fat per pound of body weight, then that is about 11 calories per pound of body weight. If you shoot for about 1 to 2 grams of carbohydrate per pound of body weight, then you know that you should be eating at least 15 calories per pound of body weight to build muscle. If you find you need a good 3 grams of carbohydrate per pound of body weight, then you need about 23 calories per pound.

GOAL 5: EAT FREQUENTLY

It makes sense that if you're trying to eat ample amounts of protein, fat, carbohydrate, and total calories every day, then a smart strategy is to eat frequent meals throughout the day. Decades of experience show that bodybuilders who eat more frequent meals build more muscle. Just about every top-level professional bodybuilder consumes a meal every couple of hours. These are men who carry the most muscle mass in the world. And on the other end of the spectrum, newborn infants, the smallest humans in the world, eat every 2 to 3 hours during the first few months of life when it is absolutely critical that they rapidly gain mass.

All this anecdotal evidence is interesting; however, clinical research also supports this notion that more frequent meals better promote muscle growth. In a study by Moore and colleagues (2012), participants performed a leg workout and then ate a total of 80 grams of whey protein over the next 12 hours in three methods. They consumed eight 10-gram doses of whey protein every 1.5 hours, or consumed four 20-gram doses of whey every 3 hours, or consumed two 40-gram doses of whey every 6 hours. The researchers reported that protein net balance, which is essentially muscle protein synthesis minus muscle protein breakdown, was significantly greater when they consumed the four 20-gram doses of whey protein every 3 hours as compared to the other two dosing strategies. Greater protein net balance essentially means more muscle growth.

There are a couple of take-home points from this study. The first has to do with amounts of protein. That the 10-gram doses of whey every 1.5 hours did not lead to greater protein net balance than the 20-gram doses every 3 hours is more a message about protein quantity than frequency. So you need to get an adequate dose of protein at each meal, and the minimum appears to be 20 grams. They didn't look at higher doses taken more frequently, but I would suggest shooting for 20 to 40 grams of protein per meal depending on the source.

The second take-home point of the study is that, to maximize muscle growth, you should not go much longer than 3 hours between meals. Any longer than this appears to increase protein breakdown too much so that any major boost in protein synthesis you get is just making up for the breakdown and not maximizing the potential for muscle growth. So your meals should be spaced no more than 3 hours apart throughout the day, and each meal should have about 20 to 40 grams of protein.

GOAL 6: USE A MIXED PROTEIN POWDER

Using a protein powder can definitely help you get in your needed protein intake of 1 to 1.5 grams of protein per pound of body weight per day. But using a protein powder isn't just convenient; it also provides direct benefits for muscle growth, if you use the right kind.

For the best protein powder, you definitely want to have some form of whey protein. Whey protein is a milk protein. Milk contains two primary types of protein: whey and casein. Whey is the soluble portion of milk protein, making up 20 percent of the protein, while casein is the globular portion and makes up the remaining 80 percent. So whey starts out as whole milk from cows. The whey is separated from the casein in the cheese manufacturing process. It's literally drained off and sent on its way to processing for whey protein. It then undergoes a variety of filtering steps to remove a good deal of the carbohydrate (lactose) and fat and take the whey from being about 15 percent protein to 35 percent protein, then to 50 percent protein, and then to 80 percent protein concentrate. These are all considered whey protein concentrates; the 80 percent protein is the one most commonly used in protein powders using whey protein concentrate. The gentle filtration process that produces whey protein concentrate leaves the whey protein microfractions in place. These include beta-lactoglobulin (~50-55%), alpha-lactalbumin (~20-25%), glyco-macropeptide (~10-15%), immunoglobulins (~10-15%), serum albumin (~5-10%), lactoferrin (~1%), lactoperoxidase (<1%), and other minor proteins such as beta-microglobulin, lysozyme, insulin-like growth factors (IGFs), and gamma-globulins, which provide the major benefits of whey, such as anti-oxidant and immune-boosting benefits, as well as enhance muscle growth and strength.

To further purify the whey protein and create a whey protein isolate that is greater than 90 percent protein, the 80 percent whey protein concentrate undergoes a further process, often involving microfiltration or ion exchange chromatography to remove more of the carbohydrate and fat. Depending on the processing involved, creating an isolate

sometimes damages the microfractions of whey. So there can be a cost of a purer whey protein powder. This is the reason my whey protein isolate undergoes microfiltration and ultrafiltration, which preserves the important whey microfractions, is sought after. Some whey protein also undergoes the process of hydrolysis. This essentially breaks the long whey protein chains into much shorter chains, or peptides; some are just two or three amino acids in length. These hydrolyzed whey proteins are even quicker to digest than whey isolate. The whey protein concentrate, isolate, or hydrolysate is then spray-dried to form a powder. The powder is often instantized so that it mixes better in fluids and does not clump.

Whey is definitely the king of the protein powders. This is due to several factors. The first is that it is rich in the branched-chain amino acids (BCAAs), which are the most critical for muscle growth, as well as energy. For more on BCAAs, read goal 8 later in this chapter. No other protein is as fast as whey protein, meaning that it gets its amino acids into the bloodstream quite rapidly. Whey delivers the majority of its amino acids to the bloodstream in about 60 to 90 minutes (figure 27.1; Boirie 1997). This allows it to rapidly turn on muscle protein synthesis for instigating muscle growth. This is important around workouts to enhance recovery and aid muscle growth while the muscle is primed for it. Whey protein also provides special peptides and microfractions that other protein sources or straight-up amino acids don't. These peptides and microfractions provide numerous benefits to health, performance, and physique. For example, some peptides relax the blood vessels to cause vasodilation. Not only does this provide cardiovascular health benefits, but it helps to deliver whey's amino acids to the muscles in a more efficient manner. A study comparing whey protein to an amino acid mix that provided the same amino acids that whey provides showed that whey protein increased muscle protein synthesis better than the amino acids (Kanda et al. 2013).

Yet as good as whey is at rapidly spiking muscle protein synthesis, by itself, it may offer too transient a boost in protein synthesis. Combining casein protein (which is very slow digesting) with whey prolongs the length of time that muscle protein is spiked and leads to better long-term gains in muscle growth and strength, as compared to whey protein alone (Soop et al. 2012; Reidy et al. 2014; Reidy et al. 2013; Kerksick 2006).

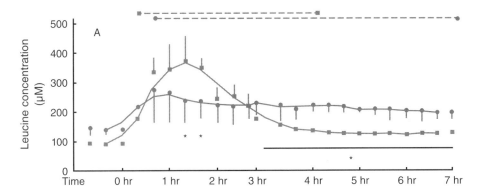

FIGURE 27.1 Plasma leucine concentrations after ingestion of whey or casein.

Reprinted, by permission, from Y. Boirie, M. Dangin, P. Gashon, et al., 1997, "Slow and fast dietary proteins differently modulate postprandial protein accretion," *Proceedings of the National Academy of Sciences of the United States of America* 94(26): 14930-14935. Copyright (1997) National Academy of Sciences, U.S.A.

Anytime you have a protein shake, you should consider having whey and some form of casein. Your best bet is a form of casein that provides micellar casein, the natural form of casein in milk, which digests the slowest. You can do this by buying a separate jug of whey protein and a separate jug of casein protein and mixing them at about 1:1 ratio. Or you can go for the more convenient method of buying a protein powder blend that already combines whey and casein. An even easier method is to mix whey protein in about 2 cups of low-fat milk or 1 cup of Greek yogurt. Both milk and Greek yogurt are good sources of micellar casein and can make the protein powder much tastier than mixing it in water.

The most critical times to take this protein blend are within 30 minutes before workouts and within 30 minutes after workouts. Shoot for about 20 to 40 grams of protein at each dose.

Another crucial time to take a mixed protein powder is as soon as you wake up in the morning. Because you have been fasting while you sleep, your muscle protein has been broken down for fuel. By drinking a mixed protein shake of whey and casein, you rebuild the broken-down protein and put your body back in an anabolic state.

You should also have a mixed protein powder containing whey and casein immediately before bed. Micellar casein can take up to 7 hours to fully digest. This is because casein literally forms a clot when it is in the stomach. To visualize this, consider when you mix a whey protein powder compared to when you mix a casein protein powder. The whey tends to mix very easily yet the casein tends to form clumps in the fluid. This is similar to what happens in your stomach when you consume casein. Although the clumps of casein may be

bad for palatability when drinking a casein shake, it provides benefits when these clumps form in your stomach. These clumps decrease the surface area of the casein that is available to digestive enzymes. The enzymes must digest the casein clumps one layer at a time, much like peeling the layers of an onion. This means that casein provides a slow and steady supply of amino acids for most of the night. That can help to prevent the breakdown of muscle protein while you sleep, helping you to gain more muscle mass in the long run.

GOAL 7: USE DIFFERENT TYPES OF CARBOHYDRATE BEFORE AND AFTER WORKOUTS

It should be obvious that before a workout you want to provide your body ample fuel to keep your muscles running as strong as possible for as long as possible throughout the workout. Having a protein shake, as discussed earlier, will help with those energy needs, as will the supplements discussed in goal 8. However, during your workouts one of the major fuel sources that your muscles use is glycogen. Glycogen is the storage form of carbohydrate. In simplified terms, when you consume carbohydrate, most is broken down into or converted into glucose, which is what blood sugar is. Glucose can either be used fairly immediately for fuel or it can be stored, mainly in muscle fibers and the liver. It is stored in the form of glycogen, which is just long branched chains of glucose connected together. The glycogen in your muscle cells and liver is broken down into glucose and used as one of the main fuels for your workouts.

Given all of this, you want to make sure that before workouts you provide your body a readily available source of glucose that will also last long into the workout. The best source of such a carb is a low-glycemic carb. Fruit works well because it is a low-glycemic carb and because most fruit is about half glucose and half fructose. *Low glycemic* means that it doesn't spike blood glucose levels, which then spikes insulin levels. Because when insulin levels are spiked, it rushes all of the glucose into the muscle cells and depletes the levels of glucose in the blood, which puts you in a state of hypoglycemia (low blood sugar). That leaves you lethargic, fatigued, slow, and weak. So when you consume fruit before a workout, the glucose component of fruit will give your body a small source of quick energy that it can use. But the fructose, on the other hand, is low glycemic despite being a sugar. This is because the body can't readily use the form of sugar that fructose is. So it has to go to the liver, where it gets converted to glycogen. Then the liver controls when the glycogen is released into the bloodstream as glucose. This allows fructose to provide longer-lasting energy. So with fruit you get a small dose of quick energy, but also longer lasting energy to prevent you from crashing. Within 30 minutes before workouts consume about 20 to 40 grams of carbohydrate from fruit or other low-glycemic carb source along with a protein shake.

After the workout, your best bet is to do the opposite of before the workout and consume a high-glycemic carb. At the end of a workout, your muscle glycogen levels are depleted. If your muscle glycogen levels are not restored, your performance in the next workout can suffer and muscle growth may be compromised.

One way that muscle growth can be compromised is because muscle glycogen levels serve as a barometer for how much energy the body has stored. If energy levels are low, as it seems when muscle glycogen is low, then the muscles may not want to expend energy-building muscle. Building muscle requires energy, and bigger muscles require more energy to maintain. If your body is unsure that you have adequate energy to fuel other, more critical processes and to maintain more muscle mass, it may choose not to go gangbusters in building muscle.

Another way that muscle growth may be compromised by not consuming adequate carbohydrate is because glycogen pulls water into the muscle fibers. The more glycogen, the more water in the muscle fibers. More water makes the muscles fuller. This makes your muscles appear significantly bigger. If your muscles are low in glycogen, then they are also low in water and that means that they look flatter and smaller than they could. Having muscles that are fuller due to more glycogen and water can also instigate muscle growth. There is evidence that having more water in the muscle fibers stretches the muscle membranes, and that stretch instigates chemical pathways that increase muscle protein synthesis, which can lead to greater muscle growth.

The best way to fully replenish muscle glycogen after workouts is with high-glycemic (fast-digesting) carbohydrate. These types of carbohydrate make it into the bloodstream and to your muscle fibers almost as quickly as you ingest them. The quicker you get carbohydrate to your muscles after workouts, the faster and better the muscle glycogen replenishment. One of the best sources of fast carbohydrate is dextrose, which is glucose. This form of sugar requires no digestion and is absorbed immediately into your bloodstream. You can use straight dextrose or glucose powder or Pixy Stix (100% dextrose) or gummy bears, which tend to be made out of dextrose and corn syrup. Corn syrup is essentially branched glucose molecules that are immediately broken down and absorbed. Corn syrup is completely different from high-fructose corn syrup. White bread and white potatoes are also good sources because they are mainly starch, which is branched glucose molecules bound together that break apart rapidly upon ingestion.

These fast carbs also spike insulin levels. After a workout is the one of the rare times of day when you want to spike the anabolic hormone insulin. Insulin is critical for pushing creatine into muscle fibers. Without a big spike in insulin, creatine uptake is not optimal. Insulin also helps amino acids, such as beta-alanine and BCAAs; the other critical ones from your protein shake get taken up by the muscle fibers. And let's not forget about the glucose from fast carbohydrate, which insulin helps to gain entry into the muscle fibers. For more information on these supplements, see goal 8.

Having fast carbohydrate after workouts is a sweet treat that doesn't damage your diet. Whether you are trying to maximize gains in mass or lose fat and gain muscle, you should be following a fairly "clean" diet. That is, doughnuts, French fries, and ice cream should not be staples in your nutrition plan. Having a dose of sweets in the form of dextrose, gummy bears, Pixy Stix, or white bread with jelly is a great way to get your sweet fix in for the day and actually have it enhance your results. Why would you ever want to skip that?

Some research shows that consuming a protein shake after workouts with or without fast carbs spikes muscle protein synthesis to an equivalent level. In other words, adding carbohydrate to a protein shake postworkout does not increase muscle protein synthesis any more than the protein shake did alone without carbohydrate. This has caused some experts to claim that you do not need carbohydrate after workouts. Well, that's a bit extreme. It's true that you can still build muscle without having carbohydrate after workouts. But I wouldn't recommend that unless you are on a very low-carb diet and you have removed carbohydrate from every other meal of your diet. In fact, it makes no sense to eat carbohydrate at other meals but avoid eating carbohydrate postworkout. If you are eating carbohydrate at any meals, the most critical meal to eat it is the postworkout meal when it will aid in recovery.

Some people worry that eating carbohydrate postworkout will blunt growth hormone and testosterone levels after the workout. Here's what they don't understand. Growth hormone and testosterone levels rise during the workout and peak toward the end of the workout, depending on the workout. After the workout, the levels of theses hormones begin to drop sharply so that they are back to resting levels about 60 to 90 minutes after the workout is over. The release of these hormones has already peaked before you consume the carbohydrate. After the workout it is too late for the carbohydrate to have a negative effect on hormone levels.

Some people worry that consuming fast carbohydrate after workouts will lead to diabetes. This is due to the media's demonization of all sugar. Yes, if you are eating sugar while sitting around all day, it will increase your risk of developing type 2 diabetes. But someone who trains regularly is already preventing the metabolic damage that leads to type 2 diabetes. And right after a workout is when the carbohydrate goes straight to the muscles and restocks the muscle glycogen as well as the liver glycogen levels. So there is no risk in consuming fast carbohydrate after workouts. It's what your body needs.

Although the amount of fast carbohydrate you consume after a workout depends on your weight and the intensity and length of the workout, a general recommendation is to shoot for about 20 to 40 grams of fast carbs such as dextrose within 30 minutes after the workout is over. Limit the fast carbs to about 60 grams for two main reasons. The first is that for optimal absorption by the intestines, 60 to 70 grams of one type of carbohydrate is the maximum before absorption by the intestines becomes limited. If you're consuming more than this, add some fructose, such as from fruit, to your postworkout meal in addition to the dextrose or glucose. The second reason is that consuming too much fast carbohydrate can make you feel terrible after it's all been quickly taken up by the liver and muscles and your blood glucose levels drop. This is known as hypoglycemia and can make you feel dizzy, lethargic, and just lousy in general. If you find that this happens to you even with smaller amounts of fast carbohydrate, then mix your postworkout carbohydrate so that you are getting some fast and some slow carbohydrate, such as fruit, oats, whole-wheat bread, and sweet potatoes.

GOAL 8: SUPPLEMENT BEFORE AND AFTER WORKOUTS

The two most critical windows for supplying your body the nutrients it needs to grow bigger and stronger is the preworkout window and the postworkout window. Getting the right nutrients right before you work out can have a significant impact on your muscle strength, energy levels, muscle endurance, and overall intensity of your training. Plus it will prime your body for muscle growth when the workout is over.

Taking in the proper nutrients immediately after the workout will help to better replenish what was used up during the workout, aid recovery, and allow for better muscle growth and strength gains.

In addition to protein powder blend and carbohydrate before and after workouts, the three critical supplements that you should consider taking before and after workouts are BCAAs, creatine, and beta-alanine. Along with the protein and carbohydrate, these can have a dramatic impact on muscle growth and strength gains. In fact, research from Victoria University (Australia) found that when participants consumed whey protein, creatine, and glucose immediately before and after workouts for

10 weeks they had an 80 percent greater increase in muscle mass and about a 30 percent greater increase in muscle strength than participants taking the same supplements in the morning and at night (Cribb and Hayes 2006). They also lost body fat while taking the supplements pre- and postworkout, while the group taking the supplements in the morning and night lost no body fat. The pre- and postworkout supplement group also had significantly higher muscle glycogen levels, which is critical for performance and muscle growth.

branched-chain amino acids (BCAAs)—The BCAAs are the three amino acids leucine, isoleucine, and valine. These amino acids are critical to take before and after workouts because of their ability to boost energy, reduce fatigue, and instigate muscle growth.

Supplementing with BCAAs before exercise promotes muscle endurance and blunts fatigue. One reason for this is the fact that the BCAAs, unlike most other amino acids, are used directly by the muscle fibers as an energy source. This is especially true during intense exercise, such as weight training.

Another way the BCAAs keep you energized during workouts is thanks to valine. During exercise tryptophan is taken up by the brain in large amounts. Tryptophan is converted in the brain to 5-hydroxytryptamine (5-HT), or what you likely know better as serotonin. Having higher serotonin during exercise signals the brain that the body is fatigued. This leads to a reduction in muscle strength and endurance. Valine competes with tryptophan for entry into the brain and typically wins. This means that less tryptophan gets in and gets converted to serotonin, which allows your muscles to contract with more force for a longer time before getting fatigued. This also can help you to stay more alert and keep your brain sharper during the day when you are not exercising.

After workouts you want another dose of BCAAs because they are the most critical amino acids for muscle growth. Leucine is the key player here; it has one of the most critical roles in muscle growth. Leucine acts much like a key does to an ignition of a car. The car in this case is a muscle cell or fiber. The ignition turns on the process of muscle protein synthesis, which builds up the muscle protein that leads to muscle growth. In more scientific terms, leucine activates a complex called mTOR, which ramps up muscle protein synthesis

and therefore muscle growth. Those who add extra leucine to postworkout protein and carbohydrate have significantly greater muscle protein synthesis than those just getting protein and carbohydrate.

Another way that leucine acts as a potent anabolic agent is by spiking insulin levels. Much like eating high-glycemic carbs, leucine increases the release of insulin from the pancreas, which helps to drive it into the muscle cells where it can work to stimulate muscle growth. Insulin also encourages muscles' growth itself by encouraging greater muscle protein synthesis and decreasing muscle protein breakdown.

Take a 5- to 10-gram dose of BCAAs within 30 minutes before workouts and another 5 to 10 grams of BCAAs within 30 minutes after workouts. Even though whey protein, which you will also take at these points, is rich in BCAAs, taking extra BCAAs in their free form can get them to your muscles faster and ensure that you have ample BCAAs at the time they are most critical.

creatine—Both clinical data and anecdotal evidence suggest that creatine provides the best results when taken before and after workouts. The main reason to get a dose of creatine before workouts is that it provides the muscle fibers with a powerful energy source. Once inside the muscle fibers, creatine gains a high-energy phosphate to form phosphocreatine (PCr). Phosphocreatine is simply a molecule of creatine with a phosphate group attached to it. During very high-intensity exercise, such as weightlifting, creatine donates this high-energy phosphate group to the muscle to form ATP (adenosine triphosphate). This rapidly generated ATP fuels the muscle contractions during a set. The more phosphocreatine you have stored in your muscle fibers, the more reps you can get during a set. This is the main way that supplementing with creatine leads to greater gains in muscle strength and muscle hypertrophy over time. It allows you to complete more reps with a given weight. That eventually allows you to lift heavier and heavier weight. And that greater overload placed on the muscle in combination with greater work performed eventually leads to greater muscle growth. Getting a dose of creatine before workouts ensures that your levels of phosphocreatine in the muscle fibers are maximized.

Supplementing with creatine leads to significant gains in muscle strength and power as well as muscle growth. Numerous studies have reported significant improvements in one-rep max strength of people taking creatine. For example, Vandenberghe and colleagues (1997) reported that untrained participants taking creatine while following a 10-week weight training program increased their one-rep max on the squat by 25 percent more than those taking a placebo while following the same program. Another study by Noonan and colleagues (1998) found that trained collegiate football players taking creatine while following an 8-week weight training program had a 6 percent increase in their one-rep bench press strength, while those taking a placebo had no strength gains at all. A 2003 review by Rawson and Volek on creatine reported that out of 16 studies investigating the effects of creatine on one-rep max strength, the average increase in strength was about 10 percent more in those taking creatine than in those taking a placebo.

Studies also show that creatine enables people to complete more reps with a given weight. Competitive powerlifters taking creatine while preparing for a competition increased the number of reps they were able to complete with 85 percent of their one-rep max by 40 percent, while those taking a placebo had no change in the number of reps they were able to complete with the same weight (Kelly and Jenkins, 1998). Rawson and Volek (2003) determined that out of the 16 studies they reviewed, the average increase in reps performed while taking creatine was about 15 percent more than for those taking a placebo. Figure 27.2 shows the average percent increase in muscle strength

and repetitions completed when participants supplemented with creatine as compared to a placebo.

Most of the studies performed on creatine indicate that supplementing with it significantly enhances athletic ability because it produces higher muscle force and power during short bouts of exercise. The participants in these studies had mixed athletic ability and training status, from relatively untrained novices to competitive college-level athletes. Some of the exercise performances that are improved include various types of short-term and all-out cycling, sprinting, repeated jumping, swimming, soccer, kayaking, rowing, and of course weightlifting, which was discussed previously. The greatest improvements in athletic performance seem to be found during a series of repetitive high-power output exercise bouts. For example, after a short rest period (20-60 seconds) after a short sprint, speed may be increased on the second bout of sprinting. Athletic performance during these latter bouts of exercise can be increased by 5 to 20 percent with creatine over the placebo group. This means that athletes in sports such as football and soccer, in which continuous play typically lasts for only a few seconds, can expect a significant boost in performance from creatine.

Several studies show that creatine significantly boosts lean muscle mass. Kelly and Jenkins (1998), as noted earlier, found that the powerlifters taking creatine gained an average of over 6 pounds of lean body weight; some participants gained up to 11 pounds of lean body weight in less than 4 weeks, while those taking a placebo had

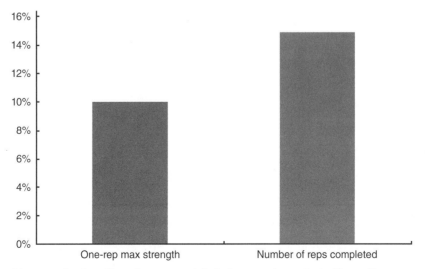

FIGURE 27.2 Percent increase in strength and reps completed when supplementing with creatine versus a placebo.

Source: E.S. Rawson and J.S. Volek, 2003, "Effects of creatine supplementation and resistance training on muscle strength and weightlifting performance," *Journal of Strength & Conditioning Research* 17(4): 822-831.

no change in body weight. Becque and colleagues (2000) reported that trained weightlifters taking creatine gained almost 5 pounds of lean body weight in 6 weeks, while those taking a placebo had no change in body weight. Since creatine supplementation likely does not increase bone mass or organ mass, the increase in lean body weight is more reasonably the result of a gain in muscle mass. In these short periods a good deal of that gain in muscle mass likely comes from water, because the muscle fibers gain a higher volume of fluid when stocked with higher levels of creatine. However, that can lead to long-term muscle growth via greater protein synthesis. Figure 27.3 shows the average increase in lean body weight (muscle mass) in pounds that participants gained while taking creatine and following a weight training program. Both studies found no change in lean body weight in those taking a placebo.

The majority of benefits from creatine involve its ability to supply fast energy during workouts. This allows you to recover faster between bouts of exercise, such as fast running or weightlifting. But today we know that creatine works through a number of mechanisms, one of which is through muscle cell volumization. This is a fancy term that means the muscle cells fill up with water. Since creatine is essentially a protein, it draws water from the blood and the space outside of the muscle cells (known as the interstitial fluid) into the muscle through the process of osmosis. This is the major reason for the rapid weight gain that is associated with creatine supplementation in the early stages of supplementation. However, this increase in cell volume causes the cell membranes to stretch, which is thought to initiate long-term increases in muscle growth and strength through greater protein synthesis—the method that muscle cells use to grow.

Another way that creatine has been found to work is by increasing the number of satellite cells in muscle fibers. Satellite cells are basically muscle stem cells, and one way that muscles grow bigger and stronger is by the addition of muscle satellite cells to existing muscle fibers. A 2006 study by Olsen and colleagues found that after 8 weeks of supplementing with creatine while following a weight training program, participants had almost 100 percent more satellite cells in their muscle fibers than those taking a placebo. As expected, the greater number of satellite cells was associated with greater muscle size. This can also lead to greater muscle strength and power.

Creatine also appears to work through increases in insulin-like growth factor-I (IGF-I). IGF-I is critical in initiating processes in muscle cells that lead to enhanced muscle growth and muscle strength. Burke (2008) reported that weight-trained participants taking creatine while following a weightlifting program for 8 weeks had significantly higher IGF-I content in their muscle fibers than those taking a placebo.

Another way that creatine appears to work is by inhibiting myostatin. Participants taking creatine while following a weightlifting program for 8 weeks had significantly lower myostatin levels than those

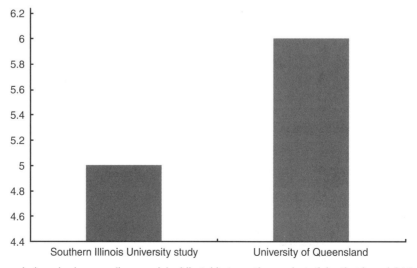

FIGURE 27.3   Increase in lean body mass (in pounds) while taking creatine and participating in weight training program.

Sources: V.G. Kelly and D.G. Jenkins, 1998, "Effect of oral creatine supplementation on near-maximal strength and repeated sets of high-intensity bench press exercise," *Journal of Strength & Conditioning Research* 12(2): 109-115, and M.D. Becque, J.D. Lochmann, and D.R. Melrose, 2000, "Effects of oral creatine supplementation on muscular strength and body composition," *Medicine & Science in Sports & Exercise* 32(3): 654-658.

taking a placebo (Saremi et al. 2010). Myostatin is a protein that limits muscle growth. The Iranian researchers concluded that since myostatin levels were lower in the participants taking creatine, one way that creatine may work to increase muscle size and strength is by reducing myostatin levels, which reduces the limitation that this protein places on muscle growth.

Although there is ample research showing that creatine is safe for almost anyone at any age to use, there are still myths regarding safety and side effects. One of the longest-standing myths is that creatine can cause muscle cramps. Numerous studies debunk this claim. Greenwood and colleagues (2003b) concluded that NCAA football players taking creatine over the course of 3 years had no increase in incidence of muscle cramps or muscle injures. In fact, another 2003 study found that NCAA football players taking creatine for one full season actually had a significant reduction in muscle cramps and muscle injuries (Greenwood et al. 2003a).

Another misconception about creatine is that it can lead to impaired liver and kidney function. Studies done in the 1990s were some of the first to show that short-term creatine supplementation does not impair kidney function in healthy adults (Poortmans et al. 1997; Poortmans and Francaux 1999). Another study (Cancela et al. 2008) has further shown that 8 weeks of creatine supplementation in football (soccer) athletes had no effect on health markers that included kidney and liver function. Longer-term studies have also been done to confirm creatine's safety. Mayhew and colleagues (2002) concluded that NCAA football players taking creatine for up to about 6 years had no long-term detrimental effects on overall health or kidney or liver functions. In another study (Kreider et al. 2003) NCAA football players taking creatine for close to 2 years exhibited no negative effects on general health or kidney and liver function. The most recent study (Lugaresi et al. 2013) involved weight-trained participants who were following a high-protein diet (0.6-1.5 grams of protein per pound of body weight) and consumed 5 grams of creatine for 1 year. Kidney function was not compromised.

Instead of being detrimental to your health, creatine actually provides numerous health benefits. Because phosphocreatine is important for energy production involved in nerve cell function, creatine has been shown to provide numerous benefits to the brain and the rest of the nervous system.

For example, research has found that creatine supplementation enhances cognitive function and memory and may help in the treatment of Parkinson's disease, Huntington's disease, and even depression. It may also protect against brain injury.

Creatine has also been found to aid cardiovascular health, such as improvement of symptoms in those with congestive heart failure, and may even lower cholesterol levels. One study (Earnest et al. 1996) discovered that male and female participants taking creatine for 8 weeks had a drop of more than 5 percent in total cholesterol and a drop in LDL cholesterol (the bad type of cholesterol) of more than 20 percent. Similarly, researchers reported that 28 days of creatine supplementation decreased total cholesterol by 10 percent in healthy young males (Arciero et al. 2001). And healthy young males taking creatine plus a multivitamin supplement significantly reduced their levels of homocysteine (an amino acid associated with heart disease), compared to those taking just the multivitamin supplement (Korzun 2004).

So be sure to get a dose of creatine before workouts to ensure that your levels of it in the muscle cells are maximized. And get another dose after workouts, when it will be preferentially taken up by the muscle cells, and replenish any that was lost during the workout. How much you take pre- and postworkout depends on the form of creatine you use. If you go with creatine monohydrate, take 3 to 5 grams before and after workouts. Although creatine monohydrate is the most studied form of creatine, creatine hydrochloride is a form of creatine that I have worked with extensively. It tends to be absorbed better than creatine monohydrate and causes less stomach distress. If using this form, take 1.5 to 2 grams before and after workouts.

beta-alanine—A nonessential amino acid that is produced naturally in the liver. You also get it in your diet from meat sources, such as beef and poultry. In the body, beta-alanine, whether from the liver or ingested from food or supplements, is taken up by the muscle fibers and combines with the amino acid histidine to form the dipeptide (two-amino-acid protein) carnosine. Carnosine provides all the benefits associated with beta-alanine, which include greater strength and power, better endurance, and even greater fat loss and muscle growth.

Carnosine works by increasing the muscle's buffering capacity of hydrogen (H+) ions, which are produced when lactic acid levels rise during intense exercises, such as weight training. This increases the muscle's ability to maintain stronger contractions for longer periods during exercise. In other words, you can lift more weight and complete more reps during the later stages of your workouts. And this ability leads to greater gains in strength and power, as well as muscle mass, while also promoting greater fat loss.

Participants taking just over 4 grams of beta-alanine per day for 30 days were able to increase the number of reps they could complete during a squat workout by almost 25 percent more than those taking a placebo (Hoffman et al. 2008). Another study found that 4 weeks of beta-alanine supplementation in amateur boxers increased their average punching power in the last 10 seconds of simulated 3-minute rounds by 2000 percent more than those taking a placebo (Donovan et al. 2012). The ability to maintain punching power late in the round is similar to the ability to maintain more strength and power later in workouts, meaning you can lift more weight for more reps. The most recent study, found that soldiers taking beta-alanine for four weeks increased jumping power and even marksmanship. This suggests not only a muscle performance benefit of beta-alanine, but also possible improved psychomotor performance (Hoffman et al. 2014).

Research also shows a great synergy of beta-alanine with creatine. One study reported that weight-trained athletes consuming 3.2 grams of beta-alanine plus 10 grams of creatine daily for 12 weeks gained significantly more muscle mass while simultaneously losing significant body fat, as compared to those taking just 10 grams of creatine alone and those taking a placebo (Hoffman et al. 2006). Both the creatine-only group and the placebo group did not lose any body fat.

The absolute lowest amount of beta-alanine consumed to provide the benefits listed previously is 1.6 grams per day. However, research on various levels of supplementation shows that around 2 grams per day or 4 grams per day each may provide even better benefits. Since the uptake of nutrients such as amino acids beta-alanine is improved around workouts, I recommend getting a dose of beta-alanine preworkout and postworkout. Blood levels of beta-alanine peak within 30 minutes of supplementing with it, and it completely leaves the circulation within 3 hours of consuming. So it makes sense to get about a 2-gram dose of beta-alanine both before workouts and then immediately after.

GOAL 9: COVER YOUR VITAMIN AND MINERAL NEEDS WITH A SUPPLEMENT

Athletes and those who train intensely lose many critical vitamins and minerals, such as B vitamins, vitamin C, chromium, selenium, zinc, magnesium, and copper. This is due to a variety of factors, such as loss of the minerals in sweat and urine, as well as increased use for energy production during the workout and recovery and protein synthesis after training.

Even if you were careful to eat a well-rounded diet, you may not be getting adequate amounts of critical micronutrients. That's because our food supply today is lower in many of these vitamins and minerals due to conventional farming practices, such as overfarming, which dwindles the nutrient density of the soil. And the grain feeding of conventional cattle and chickens also dwindles the micronutrient content of milk, beef, eggs, and chicken. Plus certain foods inhibit the absorption of some micronutrients. Refined sugar, as well as white-flour products (like white bread), can lower blood levels of minerals, such as zinc and magnesium. Foods rich in calcium (such as dairy products) inhibit absorption of both zinc and magnesium by the small intestine. Foods rich in phytates (phosphorous compounds found in whole-grain breads, cereals, and legumes) also hinder the absorption of zinc by the small intestine.

Numerous studies also show that vitamin and mineral supplements reduce the risk of certain diseases and death. The most recent was from Li and colleagues (2012). The researchers reported that in about 24,000 people, those taking vitamin and mineral supplements at the start of the study had a 42 percent reduced risk of all-cause mortality over the 11 years of the study and a 48 percent reduced risk of cancer-related death. A 2012 study by Arul and colleagues suggests that supplementing with a multivitamin could reduce the risk of colon cancer. A study reported that supplementing with multivitamins, especially those including vitamins A, C, and E, reduced the risk of colon cancer (Park et al. 2010). Another study reported that women using multivitamins had a 30 percent reduced risk of heart attack (Rautiainen et al. 2010). A 2009 study by Pocobelli and colleagues suggests that multivitamin use over 10 years reduces the risk of death from cardiovascular disease by 16 percent, while vitamin E supplementation specifically can reduce the risk by almost 30 percent. Xu and colleagues (2009) reported that women taking a multivitamin supplement have a younger biological age based on telomere length compared to those not supplementing. And a study reported that taking selenium along with a multivitamin reduced the risk of prostate cancer by 40 percent (Peters et al. 2007). A study found that in 130 adults, those taking a multivitamin and mineral supplement for 1 year had significantly less infection, such as respiratory, gastrointestinal, and urinary tract infections and influenza, and a lower rate of illness-related absenteeism, than those receiving a placebo (Barringer et al. 2003).

The bottom line is that you definitely should be using a multivitamin and mineral supplement to boost overall health, brain function, athletic performance, and even fat loss and muscle recovery and growth. Your best bet is to take your multivitamin with your first meal of the day to enhance absorption of most of the nutrients and to stock up on them for your day ahead.

Look for a multivitamin that provides as close to 100 percent as possible of the daily value (DV) of the following:

- Vitamin A (only if it is mostly beta-carotene; otherwise keep it under 4000 IU)
- Vitamins B_1 (thiamin), B_2 (riboflavin), B_3 (niacin), B_6, B_{12}, and folic acid (B_9)
- Vitamin C
- Chromium
- Copper
- Iodine (especially if you follow a low-sodium diet)
- Iron
- Manganese
- Selenium

Don't worry about the amount of calcium in your multivitamin. In fact, because calcium interferes with the absorption of other minerals such as zinc and magnesium, the less calcium the better. You should take a calcium supplement separate from when you take a multivitamin. Don't worry too much about the amount of zinc or magnesium since you should take them separately from a multivitamin anyway.

Consider getting more than the DV, or likely what's in your multivitamin, of the following vitamins and minerals:

- B vitamins: These water-soluble vitamins are typically low in those who train. They are often lost in sweat. Take a B-complex 100 that provides 100 milligrams of B_1, B_2, B_3, pantothenic acid (B_5), and B_6 and at least 100 micrograms of B_{12}, 400 micrograms of folic acid, and 300 micrograms of biotin once or twice a day.
- Vitamin C: This is also a water-soluble vitamin that can be lost in sweat. Take 250 to 500 milligrams of vitamin C once a day.
- Vitamin D: This vitamin is critical for your health, physique, and performance. It aids fat loss, testosterone levels, bone health, and mood. Take 2000 to 6000 IU of vitamin D_3 per day.
- Vitamin E: New research shows that vitamin E is critical for muscle recovery. Unless your multivitamin has at least 400 IU of E, you will want to take a vitamin E supplement providing 400 to 800 IU per day. Be sure to buy the natural forms, called d-alpha-tocopherols, which are absorbed and used better than the synthetic forms, called dl-alpha tocopherols.
- Calcium: Important for bone health, fat loss, and even testosterone levels, calcium in the amount of 1000 to 2000 milligrams per day is required. Take 500 to 600 milligrams of calcium (any more may not get absorbed properly) one or two times per day (depending on how much calcium you get from your diet) separately from other minerals and vitamins.
- Zinc and magnesium: Get 30 milligrams of zinc and 450 milligrams of magnesium 30 to 60 minutes before bedtime. It will help increase sleep quality and keep your testosterone levels and muscle strength up. An easy way to do this is to take a ZMA supplement.
- For any vitamin or mineral that does not add up to 100% DV in your multivitamin, consider taking as a separate supplement to keep your bases covered, unless you are certain to get adequate amounts of the nutrient in your daily diet.

GOAL 10: FIND WHAT WORKS FOR YOU

The first nine rules work very well for most people. However, maybe you are that one person who doesn't respond so well to a few of these goals. Maybe your schedule doesn't allow for frequent meals. Maybe you're a vegan, and dairy-based protein powders are not on your diet. Whatever it is, use these goals as a guideline, but stick only with the ones that work for you. Take these goals and adapt them to your schedule and your body, or find ones that work better for you, or create your own. You have a unique biochemistry, and not everyone reacts the same way to food or training. Be your own guinea pig. If something works for you, it doesn't matter whether or not it works for anyone else.

SAMPLE MEAL PLANS

The following meal plans are based on the guidelines discussed previously. I have provided one sample day for those who train at any of the four times of day:

1. First thing in the morning (see table 27.1)
2. At lunch time (see table 27.2)
3. Before dinner (see table 27.3)
4. After dinner later at night (see table 27.4)

These are the four most common workout windows of the day. The following meals are samples to be followed on workout days and provide roughly 3,300 calories, 290 grams of protein, 330 grams of carbohydrate, and 90 grams of fat. For a 180-pound person, that equates to about 18 calories, a little over 1.5 grams of protein, almost 2 grams of carbohydrate, and 0.5 gram of fat per pound. On rest days, skip the postworkout meal and supplements and have the preworkout meal as a snack that day. Take the suggested preworkout supplements with breakfast on rest days. That means a reduction to about 3,000 calories, 260 grams of protein, 290 grams of carbohydrate, and 85 grams of fat. For a 180-pounder, that equates to about 17 calories, a bit under 1.5 grams of protein, a bit over 1.6 grams of carbohydrate, and just under 0.5 gram of fat per pound. These sample diets will work well as a starting point for those weighing 160 to 200 pounds. If you weigh significantly less or more than this range, modify the macronutrients and calories for your body weight.

TABLE 27.1 Sample Meal Plan When Exercising First Thing in the Morning

Preworkout 1 (as soon as you wake/30-45 minutes before workout)

5-10 grams BCAAs

2-5 grams creatine (depending on form)

2-3 grams beta-alanine

20-30 grams protein from a mixed protein powder (whey/casein)

1 large apple

Postworkout (within 30 minutes after workout)

20-40 grams protein from a mixed protein powder (whey/casein)

30-40 grams fast digesting carbs (dextrose, Pixy Stix, gummy bears, white bread)

5-10 grams BCAAs

2-5 grams creatine (depending on form)

2-3 grams beta-alanine

Breakfast (30-60 minutes after postworkout meal)

20-30 grams protein of a mixed protein powder (whey/casein)

3 whole eggs, 3 egg whites, and 1 tbsp olive oil (scrambled eggs cooked in olive oil)

2 cups cooked oatmeal (1 cup dry oats before cooking) and 1 tbsp honey (mix honey in oatmeal)

Late-morning snack

1 cup low-fat cottage cheese and 1 cup sliced pineapple (mix pineapple in cottage cheese)

Lunch

6 oz. can albacore tuna

2 slices whole-wheat (or Ezekiel) bread

1 tbsp light mayonnaise

1 large piece of fruit (e.g., apple, orange, banana)

Afternoon snack

20-30 grams protein of a mixed protein powder (whey/casein)

1 tbsp peanut butter, 1 tbsp jam, 2 slices whole-wheat (or Ezekiel) bread (make peanut butter sandwich to eat with shake)

Dinner

8 oz. steak (or salmon or other fish, or chicken or other poultry, or pork)

1 medium sweet potato (or cup of brown rice or cup of beans)

2 cups mixed green salad

2 tbsp salad dressing (olive oil and vinegar)

Bedtime snack

20-30 grams protein from a mixed protein powder (whey/casein) or 1 cup cottage cheese or 1 cup Greek yogurt (with 1 teaspoon honey)

1 tbsp peanut butter (can add to shake or Greek yogurt or eat separately)

TABLE 27.2 Sample Meal Plan When Exercising at Lunchtime

Breakfast

20-30 grams protein of a mixed protein powder (whey/casein)

3 whole eggs, 3 egg whites, and 1 tbsp olive oil (scrambled eggs cooked in olive oil)

2 cups cooked oatmeal (1 cup dry oats before cooking) and 1 tbsp honey (mix honey in oatmeal)

Late-morning snack

1 cup low-fat cottage cheese and 1 cup sliced pineapple (mix pineapple in cottage cheese)

Preworkout 1 (30-45 minutes before workout)

5-10 grams BCAAs

2-5 grams creatine (depending on form)

2-3 grams beta-alanine

20-30 grams protein from a mixed protein powder (whey/casein)

1 large apple

Postworkout (within 30 minutes after workout)

20-40 grams protein from a mixed protein powder (whey/casein)

30-40 grams fast digesting carbs (dextrose, Pixy Stix, gummy bears, white bread)

5-10 grams BCAAs

2-5 grams creatine (depending on form)

2-3 grams beta-alanine

Lunch (30-60 minutes after postworkout meal)

6 oz. can albacore tuna

2 slices whole-wheat (or Ezekiel) bread

1 tbsp light mayonnaise

1 large piece of fruit (e.g., apple, orange, banana)

Afternoon snack

20-30 grams protein of a mixed protein powder (whey/casein)

1 tbsp peanut butter, 1 tbsp jam, and 2 slices whole-wheat (or Ezekiel) bread (make peanut butter sandwich to eat with shake)

Dinner

8 oz. steak (or salmon or other fish, or chicken or other poultry, or pork)

1 medium sweet potato (or cup of brown rice or cup of beans)

2 cups mixed green salad

2 tbsp salad dressing (olive oil and vinegar)

Bedtime snack

20-30 grams protein from a mixed protein powder (whey/casein) or 1 cup cottage cheese or 1 cup Greek yogurt (with 1 teaspoon honey)

1 tbsp peanut butter (can add to shake or Greek yogurt or eat separately)

TABLE 27.3 Sample Meal Plan When Exercising Before Dinner

Breakfast
20-30 grams protein of a mixed protein powder (whey/casein)
3 whole eggs, 3 egg whites, and 1 tbsp olive oil (scrambled eggs cooked in olive oil)
2 cups cooked oatmeal (1 cup dry oats before cooking) and 1 tbsp honey (mix honey in oatmeal)
Late-morning snack
1 cup low-fat cottage cheese and 1 cup sliced pineapple (mix pineapple in cottage cheese)
Lunch
6 oz. can albacore tuna
2 slices whole-wheat (or Ezekiel) bread
1 tbsp light mayonnaise
1 large piece of fruit (e.g., apple, orange, banana)
Afternoon snack
20-30 grams protein of a mixed protein powder (whey/casein)
1 tbsp peanut butter, 1 tbsp jam, and 2 slices whole-wheat (or Ezekiel) bread (make peanut butter sandwich to eat with shake)
Preworkout 1 (30-45 minutes before workout)
5-10 grams BCAAs
2-5 grams creatine (depending on form)
2-3 grams beta-alanine
20-30 grams protein from a mixed protein powder (whey/casein)
1 large apple
Postworkout (within 30 minutes after workout)
20-40 grams protein from a mixed protein powder (whey/casein)
30-40 grams fast digesting carbs (dextrose, Pixy Stix, gummy bears, white bread)
5-10 grams BCAAs
2-5 grams creatine (depending on form)
2-3 grams beta-alanine
Dinner (30-60 minutes after postworkout meal)
8 oz. steak (or salmon or other fish, or chicken or other poultry, or pork)
1 medium sweet potato (or cup of brown rice or cup of beans)
2 cups mixed green salad
2 tbsp salad dressing (olive oil and vinegar)
Bedtime snack
20-30 grams protein from a mixed protein powder (whey/casein) or 1 cup cottage cheese or 1 cup Greek yogurt (with 1 teaspoon honey)
1 tbsp peanut butter (can add to shake or Greek yogurt or eat separately)

TABLE 27.4 Sample Meal Plan When Exercising After Dinner

Breakfast
20-30 grams protein of a mixed protein powder (whey/casein)
3 whole eggs, 3 egg whites, and 1 tbsp olive oil (scrambled eggs cooked in olive oil)
2 cups cooked oatmeal (1 cup dry oats before cooking) and 1 tbsp honey (mix honey in oatmeal)
Late-morning snack
1 cup low-fat cottage cheese and 1 cup sliced pineapple (mix pineapple in cottage cheese)
Lunch
6 oz. can albacore tuna
2 slices whole-wheat (or Ezekiel) bread
1 tbsp light mayonnaise
1 large piece of fruit (e.g., apple, orange, banana)
Afternoon snack
20-30 grams protein of a mixed protein powder (whey/casein)
1 tbsp peanut butter, 1 tbsp jam, and 2 slices whole-wheat (or Ezekiel) bread (make peanut butter sandwich to eat with shake)
Dinner
8 oz. steak (or salmon or other fish, or chicken or other poultry, or pork)
1 medium sweet potato (or cup of brown rice or cup of beans)
2 cups mixed green salad
2 tbsp salad dressing (olive oil and vinegar)
Preworkout 1 (30-45 minutes before workout)
5-10 grams BCAAs
2-5 grams creatine (depending on form)
2-3 grams beta-alanine
20-30 grams protein from a mixed protein powder (whey/casein)
1 large apple
Postworkout (within 30 minutes after workout)
20-40 grams protein from a mixed protein powder (whey/casein)
30-40 grams fast digesting carbs (dextrose, Pixy Stix, gummy bears, white bread)
5-10 grams BCAAs
2-5 grams creatine (depending on form)
2-3 grams beta-alanine
Bedtime snack
20-30 grams protein from a mixed protein powder (whey/casein) or 1 cup cottage cheese or 1 cup Greek yogurt (with 1 teaspoon honey)
1 tbsp peanut butter (can add to shake or Greek yogurt or eat separately)

CHAPTER 28

Nutrition for Maximizing Fat Loss

Before you read this chapter you should read chapter 27. The guidelines discussed in chapter 27 are the same guidelines you want to follow to maximize fat loss. After all, when you talk about dropping body fat, you still want to at least maintain, if not build, lean muscle mass and muscle strength. And using the programs in chapter 13 along with the information in chapter 27 and 28, you can.

While chapter 27 broke down the nutrition guidelines into goals, chapter 28 breaks down the nutrition information to maximize fat loss into steps. That's because fat loss is a continual process, and your diet must change gradually over time. The worst thing that you can do is to immediately jump down to a very low-calorie and low-carbohydrate diet. For example, many people ask me if going on a keto diet where almost all carbohydrate is removed from the diet is a smart plan. The answer is no. Yes, it can result in very rapid fat loss at the beginning of the diet. But after a couple of months or less, when the fat loss stops and they hit a plateau, they have little wiggle room to remove more calories from their diet and continue losing body fat.

When you diet, your body responds by going into starvation mode. That basically means that your body slows down your metabolic rate, which is the number of calories you burn just sitting around. The reason for this is to conserve energy stores, namely your body fat. Your body prefers to not be lean, since body fat is stored energy that it can rely on in times of food scarcity. In developed countries, food scarcity is obviously not a real threat for most people. But your body has developed this process should there be a time when food is scarce. So once you reduce your caloric intake, your body

reacts by slowing down your metabolic rate. The greater you reduce your caloric intake, the bigger the drop in your metabolic rate and the quicker this will happen.

To prevent a massive slowing of your metabolic rate, you need to gradually reduce your caloric intake little by little. Of course, exercise will help to keep your metabolic rate higher, but it cannot prevent the gradual reduction of it as you reduce calories. So you actually want to start a diet for fat loss by eating as many calories as you can while still losing weight. This way you will have ample room to keep reducing calories as your metabolic rate drops and fat loss hits a plateau. This way you can keep losing body fat. Figure out how many calories to start your diet with by reading through step 1: analyze your diet.

STEPPING UP FAT LOSS

Following are the eight steps you want to follow to maximize fat loss while building muscle and strength or, at the very least, maintaining muscle mass.

Step 1: Analyze Your Diet

To get the best estimate of where you should start for calories, you will need to take an honest look at your current diet. I typically recommend recording everything you eat for one full week. But if that seems daunting, do at least two weekdays and one weekend day. If you have a scale, weigh food such as chicken, beef, and fish. For liquids and grains like rice and cereal, use measuring cups and measuring spoons. Or if you have a good take on how much one cup of something is, or how much 8 ounces of chicken breast is, then take your best estimate. For packaged foods, use the nutrition facts label on the box; for other foods, use a reliable source, such as USDA site. The direct link to their food database is http://ndb.nal.usda.gov/ndb/search/list.

It's important that you do not alter your typical diet when you record your food intake. One trick that we use to keep people from steering astray from a diet is to have them record everything they eat. When they have a weak moment and crave doughnuts, knowing that they have to record that in a food log helps them avoid eating the doughnuts. But during this week, do not avoid eating any of the foods that you normally do. The point is to assess your true current diet so that you know where to start your new diet. If you alter it, it can actually work against your fat-loss efforts.

Calculate the amount of calories, grams of protein, grams of carbohydrate, and grams of total fat for each food that you eat. Then add these up for all the foods that you eat each day. Once you have the total amount of calories and grams of protein, carbohydrate, and fat for each day, you need to get an average of all the days. So if you recorded 7 days of food intake, then add the calories up for all 7 days and divide this number by 7 to get the average caloric intake for the 7 days. If you did just 3 days, then obviously you would add up the total calories for the 3 days and divide by 3. Do this also for grams of protein, grams of carbohydrate, and grams of fat. But the critical factor is your average caloric intake. Take your average caloric intake and divide it by your body weight in pounds to calculate your average calories relative to your body weight. For example, if you weigh 200 pounds and you consumed an average of 4,000 calories per day, you currently consume an average of 20 calories per pound of body weight.

Step 2: Build Your Initial Diet

Using the muscle building guidelines in chapter 27, the most critical goals that you want to focus on to build your initial diet are goal 1 (focus on protein) and goal 2 (get ample fat). Start your diet by making sure that you consume 1.5 grams of protein per pound of body weight and 0.5 gram

of fat per pound. Since there are 4 calories per gram of protein, that means that you will consume 6 calories from protein per pound of body weight. Since fat has about 9 calories per gram, you will be consuming 4.5 calories from fat per pound of body weight. Adding the calories from protein and the calories from fat equates to 10.5 calories per pound of body weight. Subtract 10.5 calories from 20 calories (the number of calories per pound of body weight you currently eat), which equals 9.5 calories. This is the number of calories you can consume from carbohydrate per pound of body weight. Since there are 4 calories per gram of carbohydrate, that equals about 2.5 grams. Round down to 2 grams of carbohydrate per pound of body weight. So your new diet will consist of about 1.5 grams of protein, 2 grams of carbohydrate, 0.5 gram of fat, and 18.5 calories per pound of body weight. For the 200-pounder, that equates to 3,700 calories, 300 grams of protein, 400 grams of carbohydrate, and 100 grams of fat per day. See sample diet for a 200-pound person following these guidelines in tables 28.1, 28.2, 28.3, or 28.4 based on when you work out. Note that the sample meal plans in this chapter are very similar for reasons of illustrating how to change the diet when you move through the steps. This does not mean that you should eat the same foods every day and the same foods in each step of the diet. Quite the contrary. You want to have as much variety in your diet as possible. For food alternatives to replace the foods in the sample diets, refer to the food alternatives list in appendix B.

Follow this diet for as long as you continue losing fat. Note that you will likely gain muscle mass even though you are dropping body fat. So do not use the scale as your major indicator of fat loss. Use the mirror and waist size or the fit of the waist on your pants. An even better option is to have your body fat professionally measured by a seven-site skinfold caliper, underwater weighing, or DEXA scan. Do not use bioelectrical impedance, which calculates percent body fat on how fast it takes a current to travel through your body. That method is not accurate.

The sample meals are for workout days. On rest days, skip the postworkout meal and have the preworkout meal as a snack.

TABLE 28.1 Sample Meal Plan When Exercising First Thing in the Morning

Preworkout 1 (as soon as you wake/30-45 minutes before workout)
5-10 grams BCAAs
2-5 grams creatine (depending on form)
2-3 grams beta-alanine
20-30 grams protein from a mixed protein powder (whey/casein)
1 large apple

Postworkout (within 30 minutes after workout)
20-40 grams protein from a mixed protein powder (whey/casein)
30-40 grams fast-digesting carbohydrate (dextrose, Pixy Stix, gummy bears, white bread)
5-10 grams BCAAs
2-5 grams creatine (depending on form)
2-3 grams beta-alanine

Breakfast (30-60 minutes after postworkout meal)
20-30 grams protein of a mixed protein powder (whey/casein)
3 whole eggs, 3 egg whites, and 1 tbsp olive oil (scrambled eggs cooked in olive oil)
2 cups cooked oatmeal (1 cup dry oats before cooking) and 1 tbsp honey (mix honey in oatmeal)

Late-morning snack
1 cup low-fat cottage cheese, 1 cup sliced pineapple, and 5 Triscuit whole-wheat crackers (mix pineapple in cottage cheese and eat with crackers)

Lunch
6 oz. can albacore tuna
2 slices whole-wheat (or Ezekiel) bread
1 tbsp light mayonnaise
1 large piece of fruit (e.g., apple, orange, banana)

Afternoon snack
20-30 grams protein of a mixed protein powder (whey/casein)
1 tbsp peanut butter, 1 tbsp jam, and 2 slices whole-wheat (or Ezekiel) bread (make peanut butter sandwich to eat with shake)

Dinner
8 oz. steak (or salmon or other fish, or chicken or other poultry, or pork)
1 cup of cooked brown rice
1 cup of cooked black beans (or pinto beans)
2 cups mixed green salad
2 tbsp salad dressing (olive oil and vinegar)

Bedtime snack
20-30 grams protein from a mixed protein powder (whey/casein) or 1 cup cottage cheese or 1 cup Greek yogurt (with 1 teaspoon honey)
1 tbsp peanut butter (can add to shake or Greek yogurt or eat separately)

TABLE 28.2 Sample Meal Plan When Exercising at Lunchtime

Breakfast
20-30 grams protein of a mixed protein powder (whey/casein)
3 whole eggs, 3 egg whites, and 1 tbsp olive oil (scrambled eggs cooked in olive oil)
2 cups cooked oatmeal (1 cup dry oats before cooking) and 1 tbsp honey (mix honey in oatmeal)

Late-morning snack
1 cup low-fat cottage cheese, 1 cup sliced pineapple, and 5 Triscuit whole-wheat crackers (mix pineapple in cottage cheese and eat with crackers)

Preworkout 1 (30-45 minutes before workout)
5-10 grams BCAAs
2-5 grams creatine (depending on form)
2-3 grams beta-alanine
20-30 grams protein from a mixed protein powder (whey/casein)
1 large apple

Postworkout (within 30 minutes after workout)
20-40 grams protein from a mixed protein powder (whey/casein)
30-40 grams fast-digesting carbohydrate (dextrose, Pixy Stix, gummy bears, white bread)
5-10 grams BCAAs
2-5 grams creatine (depending on form)
2-3 grams beta-alanine

Lunch (30-60 minutes after postworkout meal)
6 oz. can albacore tuna
2 slices whole-wheat (or Ezekiel) bread
1 tbsp light mayonnaise
1 large piece of fruit (e.g., apple, orange, banana)

Afternoon snack
20-30 grams protein of a mixed protein powder (whey/casein)
1 tbsp peanut butter, 1 tbsp jam, and 2 slices whole-wheat (or Ezekiel) bread (make peanut butter sandwich to eat with shake)

Dinner
8 oz. steak (or salmon or other fish, or chicken or other poultry, or pork)
1 cup of cooked brown rice
1 cup of cooked black beans (or pinto beans)
2 cups mixed green salad
2 tbsp salad dressing (olive oil and vinegar)

Bedtime snack
20-30 grams protein from a mixed protein powder (whey/casein) or 1 cup cottage cheese or 1 cup Greek yogurt (with 1 teaspoon honey)
1 tbsp peanut butter (can add to shake or Greek yogurt or eat separately)

TABLE 28.3 Sample Meal Plan When Exercising Before Dinner

Breakfast

20-30 grams protein of a mixed protein powder (whey/casein)

3 whole eggs, 3 egg whites, and 1 tbsp olive oil (scrambled eggs cooked in olive oil)

2 cups cooked oatmeal (1 cup dry oats before cooking) and 1 tbsp honey (mix honey in oatmeal)

Late-morning snack

1 cup low-fat cottage cheese, 1 cup sliced pineapple, and 5 Triscuit whole-wheat crackers (mix pineapple in cottage cheese and eat with crackers)

Lunch

6 oz. can albacore tuna

2 slices whole-wheat (or Ezekiel) bread

1 tbsp light mayonnaise

1 large piece of fruit (e.g., apple, orange, banana)

Afternoon snack

20-30 grams protein of a mixed protein powder (whey/casein)

1 tbsp peanut butter, 1 tbsp jam, and 2 slices whole-wheat (or Ezekiel) bread (make peanut butter sandwich to eat with shake)

Preworkout 1 (30-45 minutes before workout)

5-10 grams BCAAs

2-5 grams creatine (depending on form)

2-3 grams beta-alanine

20-30 grams protein from a mixed protein powder (whey/casein)

1 large apple

Postworkout (within 30 minutes after workout)

20-40 grams protein from a mixed protein powder (whey/casein)

30-40 grams fast-digesting carbohydrate (dextrose, Pixy Stix, gummy bears, white bread)

5-10 grams BCAAs

2-5 grams creatine (depending on form)

2-3 grams beta-alanine

Dinner (30-60 minutes after postworkout meal)

8 oz. steak (or salmon or other fish, or chicken or other poultry, or pork)

1 cup of cooked brown rice

1 cup of cooked black beans (or pinto beans)

2 cups mixed green salad

2 tbsp salad dressing (olive oil and vinegar)

Bedtime snack

20-30 grams protein from a mixed protein powder (whey/casein) or 1 cup cottage cheese or 1 cup Greek yogurt (with 1 teaspoon honey)

1 tbsp peanut butter (can add to shake or Greek yogurt or eat separately)

TABLE 28.4 Sample Meal Plan When Exercising After Dinner

Breakfast

20-30 grams protein of a mixed protein powder (whey/casein)

3 whole eggs, 3 egg whites, and 1 tbsp olive oil (scrambled eggs cooked in olive oil)

2 cups cooked oatmeal (1 cup dry oats before cooking) and 1 tbsp honey (mix honey in oatmeal)

Late-morning snack

1 cup low-fat cottage cheese, 1 cup sliced pineapple, and 5 Triscuit whole-wheat crackers (mix pineapple in cottage cheese and eat with crackers)

Lunch

6 oz. can albacore tuna

2 slices whole-wheat (or Ezekiel) bread

1 tbsp light mayonnaise

1 large piece of fruit (e.g., apple, orange, banana)

Afternoon snack

20-30 grams protein of a mixed protein powder (whey/casein)

1 tbsp peanut butter, 1 tbsp jam, and 2 slices whole-wheat (or Ezekiel) bread (make peanut butter sandwich to eat with shake)

Dinner

8 oz. steak (or salmon or other fish, or chicken or other poultry, or pork)

1 cup of cooked brown rice

1 cup of cooked black beans (or pinto beans)

2 cups mixed green salad

2 tbsp salad dressing (olive oil and vinegar)

Preworkout 1 (30-45 minutes before workout)

5-10 grams BCAAs

2-5 grams creatine (depending on form)

2-3 grams beta-alanine

20-30 grams protein from a mixed protein powder (whey/casein)

1 large apple

Postworkout (within 30 minutes after workout)

20-40 grams protein from a mixed protein powder (whey/casein)

30-40 grams fast-digesting carbohydrate (dextrose, Pixy Stix, gummy bears, white bread)

5-10 grams BCAAs

2-5 grams creatine (depending on form)

2-3 grams beta-alanine

Bedtime snack

20-30 grams protein from a mixed protein powder (whey/casein) or 1 cup cottage cheese or 1 cup Greek yogurt (with 1 teaspoon honey)

1 tbsp peanut butter (can add to shake or Greek yogurt or eat separately)

Step 3: Adjust the Diet by Reducing Carbohydrate by 0.25 Gram per Pound

As mentioned previously, as you reduce calories, your body adjusts by lowering metabolic rate, and your body burns fewer calories throughout the day. The only way to combat this and continue losing body fat is to reduce your calories. Since you want to keep protein and fat where they are to maximize muscle growth and strength gains, your best bet is to whittle away at your carb intake. Each time you hit a plateau in your diet and it seems like you have not made any progress in losing fat for at least a week, it's time to reduce carbohydrate. You will reduce carbohydrate by 0.25 gram per pound of body weight each time you need to cut again. That will reduce your total caloric intake by about 1 calorie per pound of body weight. So for a 200-pound person, that equates to about a 200-calorie cut.

Because our sample 200-pounder is currently consuming 2 grams of carbohydrate per pound of body weight, his first cut will be bring him down to 1.75 grams per pound of body weight. Where you start reducing your carbohydrate depends on when you train. But regardless of when you train, you will cut postworkout carbohydrate absolutely last. For those who train first thing in the morning, start reducing carbohydrate from the end of the day and working up as you continue to drop. For those who train at night, start reducing your carbohydrate from the start of the day and work down as you continue to cut. It gets a little trickier, if you train at lunch or before dinner. This will bounce around from end to end a bit. See the sample diets for guidelines on dropping carbohydrate from your diet with each 0.25-gram-per-pound cut.

You will progressively cut carbohydrate each time fat loss hits a plateau until you are down to around just 0.25 gram of carbohydrate per pound. That is, if you ever have to get that low. Many will not have to get anywhere close to that. But it all depends on where you are starting from, how active your training is, and how your body responds to the training and diet.

The following sample meals in tables 28.5 through 28.8 are for those making their first cut in carbohydrate from 2.0 to 1.75 grams per pound of body weight (or 350 grams of carbohydrate total for the 200-pounder). This drops calories to 17 per pound of body weight or about 3,400 for the 200-pound sample person. Remember that these meal plans are based on workout days. On rest days, skip the postworkout meal and have the preworkout meal as a snack.

TABLE 28.5 Sample Meal Plan When Exercising First Thing in the Morning

Preworkout 1 (as soon as you wake/30-45 minutes before workout)
5-10 grams BCAAs
2-5 grams creatine (depending on form)
2-3 grams beta-alanine
20-30 grams protein from a mixed protein powder (whey/casein)
1 large apple
Postworkout (within 30 minutes after workout)
20-40 grams protein from a mixed protein powder (whey/casein)
30-40 grams fast-digesting carbohydrate (dextrose, Pixy Stix, gummy bears, white bread)
5-10 grams BCAAs
2-5 grams creatine (depending on form)
2-3 grams beta-alanine
Breakfast (30-60 minutes after postworkout meal)
20-30 grams protein of a mixed protein powder (whey/casein)
3 whole eggs, 3 egg whites, and 1 tbsp olive oil (scrambled eggs cooked in olive oil)
2 cups cooked oatmeal (1 cup dry oats before cooking) and 1 tbsp honey (mix honey in oatmeal)
Late-morning snack
1 cup low-fat cottage cheese, 1 cup sliced pineapple, and 5 Triscuit whole-wheat crackers (mix pineapple in cottage cheese and eat with crackers)
Lunch
6 oz. can albacore tuna
2 slices whole-wheat (or Ezekiel) bread
1 tbsp light mayonnaise
1 large piece of fruit (e.g., apple, orange, banana)
Afternoon snack
20-30 grams protein of a mixed protein powder (whey/casein)
1 tbsp peanut butter, 1 tbsp jam, and 2 slices whole-wheat (or Ezekiel) bread (make peanut butter sandwich to eat with shake)
Dinner
8 oz. steak (or salmon or other fish, or chicken or other poultry, or pork)
1 cup of cooked black beans (or pinto beans)
2 cups mixed green salad
2 tbsp salad dressing (olive oil and vinegar)
Bedtime snack
20-30 grams protein from a mixed protein powder (whey/casein) or 1 cup cottage cheese or 1 cup Greek yogurt (with 1 teaspoon honey)
1 tbsp peanut butter (can add to shake or Greek yogurt or eat separately)

TABLE 28.6 Sample Meal Plan When Exercising at Lunchtime

Breakfast

20-30 grams protein of a mixed protein powder (whey/casein)

3 whole eggs, 3 egg whites, and 1 tbsp olive oil (scrambled eggs cooked in olive oil)

1 cup cooked oatmeal (1/2 cup dry oats before cooking)

Late-morning snack

1 cup low-fat cottage cheese, 1 cup sliced pineapple, and 5 Triscuit whole-wheat crackers (mix pineapple in cottage cheese and eat with crackers)

Preworkout 1 (30-45 minutes before workout)

5-10 grams BCAAs

2-5 grams creatine (depending on form)

2-3 grams beta-alanine

20-30 grams protein from a mixed protein powder (whey/casein)

1 large apple

Postworkout (within 30 minutes after workout)

20-40 grams protein from a mixed protein powder (whey/casein)

30-40 grams fast-digesting carbohydrate (dextrose, Pixy Stix, gummy bears, white bread)

5-10 grams BCAAs

2-5 grams creatine (depending on form)

2-3 grams beta-alanine

Lunch (30-60 minutes after postworkout meal)

6 oz. can albacore tuna

2 slices whole-wheat (or Ezekiel) bread

1 tbsp light mayonnaise

1 large piece of fruit (e.g., apple, orange, banana)

Afternoon snack

20-30 grams protein of a mixed protein powder (whey/casein)

1 tbsp peanut butter, 1 tbsp jam, 2 slices whole-wheat (or Ezekiel) bread (make peanut butter sandwich to eat with shake)

Dinner

8 oz. steak (or salmon or other fish, or chicken or other poultry, or pork)

1 cup of cooked brown rice

1 cup of cooked black beans (or pinto beans)

2 cups mixed green salad

2 tbsp salad dressing (olive oil and vinegar)

Bedtime snack

20-30 grams protein from a mixed protein powder (whey/casein) or 1 cup cottage cheese or 1 cup Greek yogurt (with 1 teaspoon honey)

1 tbsp peanut butter (can add to shake or Greek yogurt or eat separately)

TABLE 28.7 Sample Meal Plan When Exercising Before Dinner

Breakfast

20-30 grams protein of a mixed protein powder (whey/casein)

3 whole eggs, 3 egg whites, and 1 tbsp olive oil (scrambled eggs cooked in olive oil)

1 cup cooked oatmeal (1/2 cup dry oats before cooking)

Late-morning snack

1 cup low-fat cottage cheese, 1 cup sliced pineapple, and 5 Triscuit whole-wheat crackers (mix pineapple in cottage cheese and eat with crackers)

Lunch

6 oz. can albacore tuna

2 slices whole-wheat (or Ezekiel) bread

1 tbsp light mayonnaise

1 large piece of fruit (e.g., apple, orange, banana)

Afternoon snack

20-30 grams protein of a mixed protein powder (whey/casein)

1 tbsp peanut butter, 1 tbsp jam, and 2 slices whole-wheat (or Ezekiel) bread (make peanut butter sandwich to eat with shake)

Preworkout 1 (30-45 minutes before workout)

5-10 grams BCAAs

2-5 grams creatine (depending on form)

2-3 grams beta-alanine

20-30 grams protein from a mixed protein powder (whey/casein)

1 large apple

Postworkout (within 30 minutes after workout)

20-40 grams protein from a mixed protein powder (whey/casein)

30-40 grams fast-digesting carbohydrate (dextrose, Pixy Stix, gummy bears, white bread)

5-10 grams BCAAs

2-5 grams creatine (depending on form)

2-3 grams beta-alanine

Dinner (30-60 minutes after postworkout meal)

8 oz. steak (or salmon or other fish, or chicken or other poultry, or pork)

1 cup of cooked brown rice

1 cup of cooked black beans (or pinto beans)

2 cups mixed green salad

2 tbsp salad dressing (olive oil and vinegar)

Bedtime snack

20-30 grams protein from a mixed protein powder (whey/casein) or 1 cup cottage cheese or 1 cup Greek yogurt (with 1 teaspoon honey)

1 tbsp peanut butter (can add to shake or Greek yogurt or eat separately)

TABLE 28.8 Sample Meal Plan When Exercising After Dinner

Breakfast

20-30 grams protein of a mixed protein powder (whey/casein)

3 whole eggs, 3 egg whites, and 1 tbsp olive oil (scrambled eggs cooked in olive oil)

1 cup cooked oatmeal (1/2 cup dry oats before cooking)

Late-morning snack

1 cup low-fat cottage cheese, 1 cup sliced pineapple, and 5 Triscuit whole-wheat crackers (mix pineapple in cottage cheese and eat with crackers)

Lunch

6 oz. can albacore tuna

2 slices whole-wheat (or Ezekiel) bread

1 tbsp light mayonnaise

1 large piece of fruit (e.g., apple, orange, banana)

Afternoon snack

20-30 grams protein of a mixed protein powder (whey/casein)

1 tbsp peanut butter, 1 tbsp jam, and 2 slices whole-wheat (or Ezekiel) bread (make peanut butter sandwich to eat with shake)

Dinner

8 oz. steak (or salmon or other fish, or chicken or other poultry, or pork)

1 cup of cooked brown rice

1 cup of cooked black beans (or pinto beans)

2 cups mixed green salad

2 tbsp salad dressing (olive oil and vinegar)

Preworkout 1 (30-45 minutes before workout)

5-10 grams BCAAs

2-5 grams creatine (depending on form)

2-3 grams beta-alanine

20-30 grams protein from a mixed protein powder (whey/casein)

1 large apple

Postworkout (within 30 minutes after workout)

20-40 grams protein from a mixed protein powder (whey/casein)

30-40 grams fast-digesting carbohydrate (dextrose, Pixy Stix, gummy bears, white bread)

5-10 grams BCAAs

2-5 grams creatine (depending on form)

2-3 grams beta-alanine

Bedtime snack

20-30 grams protein from a mixed protein powder (whey/casein) or 1 cup cottage cheese or 1 cup Greek yogurt (with 1 teaspoon honey)

1 tbsp peanut butter (can add to shake or Greek yogurt or eat separately)

You can find additional sample meals for the following cuts in carbohydrate at www.humankinetics.com/products/all-products/Jim-Stoppanis-Encyclopedia-of-Muscle--Strength-2nd-edition:

- 1.75 to 1.5 grams per pound of body weight
- 1.5 to 1.25 grams per pound of body weight
- 1.25 to 1 gram per pound of body weight
- 1 to 0.75 gram per pound of body weight
- 0.75 to 0.5 gram per pound of body weight

Step 4: Add a High-Carbohydrate Day

This step might be a favorite one for you because it gives you the opportunity to eat some of the foods you might have been craving on a low-carbohydrate diet. Once carbohydrate drops to 0.5 gram per pound of body weight, it is advisable to include a higher-carbohydrate day every week or so. This can help to keep your metabolic rate higher despite the fact that carbohydrate and caloric intake is so low. Plus, it works well as an incentive to get through the week. Knowing that you have a higher-carb day to look forward to helps you make it through the low-carb period. Most people find that they better police themselves during the low-carbohydrate days so that they can feel like they earned the high-carb day. Once you have enjoyed the higher-carb day and enjoyed some of the food you were craving, like bread and pasta, it's easier to go back to the lower-carbohydrate diet.

It doesn't matter what day of the week your high-carbohydrate day is, but you don't want to go any less frequent than about every 7 days. A weekend day works best for most people, but any day of the week will work. Protein and fat should stay about the same; however, you can drop them somewhat on your higher-carbohydrate day. But don't allow protein to drop much lower than 1 gram per pound of body weight, and don't allow fat to go any lower than 0.25 gram per pound. You should shoot for about 2 grams of carbohydrate per pound of body weight on your high-carb day. That's about 400 grams for the 200-pounder.

Your best options for high-carbohydrate foods are low-glycemic or slow-digesting carbohydrate, such as oatmeal, whole-wheat breads and pastas, and sweet potatoes. However, if you train on your high-carb day, then you should still consume high-glycemic carbohydrate immediately after the workout. While the majority of your carbohydrate should come from low-GI carbohydrate, you can enjoy some high-GI carbohydrate throughout the day. Having a boost in insulin will help to keep your metabolism higher. And this will allow you to enjoy some of the sweets you may have been craving.

When it comes to fruit, you should consume it just through the first half of the day.

Foods on the high-carb days should not also be high-fat foods like doughnuts, ice cream, or pizza. However, if you really have been craving one of these foods, then feel free to have a reasonable portion to keep cravings at bay and stay on your diet.

The following sample meals in tables 28.9 through 28.12 are for workout days. On rest days, skip the postworkout meal and have the preworkout meal as a snack.

TABLE 28.9 Sample Meal Plan When Exercising First Thing in the Morning

Preworkout 1 (as soon as you wake/30-45 minutes before workout)
5-10 grams BCAAs
2-5 grams creatine (depending on form)
2-3 grams beta-alanine
20-30 grams protein from a mixed protein powder (whey/casein)
1 large apple
Postworkout (within 30 minutes after workout)
20-40 grams protein from a mixed protein powder (whey/casein)
30-40 grams fast-digesting carbohydrate (dextrose, Pixy Stix, gummy bears, white bread)
5-10 grams BCAAs
2-5 grams creatine (depending on form)
2-3 grams beta-alanine
Breakfast (30-60 minutes after postworkout meal)
3 whole eggs, 3 egg whites, and 1 tbsp olive oil (scrambled eggs cooked in olive oil)
3 four-inch pancakes and 2 tbsp maple syrup
½ cantaloupe
Late-morning snack
20-30 grams protein of a mixed protein powder (whey/casein)
¼ whole-wheat Boboli crust, ¼ cup light mozzarella cheese, and ¼ cup marinara sauce (add sauce to crust and top with cheese; cook at 400 degrees F for 10-15 min or until cheese is browned)
Lunch
6-inch Subway turkey and ham (double meat) on 9-grain wheat bread
1 bag Baked Lays potato chips
Regular diet soda

Afternoon snack
3 sticks light string cheese
6 cups air-popped popcorn (or bag of low-fat microwave popcorn)
Dinner
6 oz. chicken breast (or fish, or lean beef or other poultry, or pork)
1 cup of cooked brown rice
1 cup of cooked black beans (or pinto beans)
1 cup chopped broccoli
Bedtime snack
1 cup reduced fat Greek yogurt, 1 tbsp honey, and 7 walnut halves (crushed) (add honey and walnuts to yogurt and eat)

TABLE 28.10 Sample Meal Plan When Exercising at Lunchtime

Breakfast
20-30 grams protein of a mixed protein powder (whey/casein)
3 whole eggs and 1 tbsp olive oil (scrambled eggs cooked in olive oil)
3 four-inch pancakes and 2 tbsp maple syrup
½ cantaloupe
Late-morning snack
20-30 grams protein of a mixed protein powder (whey/casein)
¼ whole-wheat Boboli crust, ¼ cup light mozzarella cheese, and ¼ cup marinara sauce (add sauce to crust and top with cheese; cook at 400 degrees F for 10-15 min or until cheese is browned)
Preworkout 1 (30-45 minutes before workout)
5-10 grams BCAAs
2-5 grams creatine (depending on form)
2-3 grams beta-alanine
20-30 grams protein from a mixed protein powder (whey/casein)
1 large apple
Postworkout (within 30 minutes after workout)
20-40 grams protein from a mixed protein powder (whey/casein)
30-40 grams fast-digesting carbohydrate (dextrose, Pixy Stix, gummy bears, white bread)
5-10 grams BCAAs
2-5 grams creatine (depending on form)
2-3 grams beta-alanine
Lunch (30-60 minutes after postworkout meal)
6-inch Subway turkey and ham (double meat) on 9-grain wheat bread
1 bag Baked Lays potato chips
Regular diet soda

Afternoon snack
3 sticks light string cheese
6 cups air-popped popcorn (or bag of low-fat microwave popcorn)

Dinner
6 oz. chicken breast (or fish, or lean beef or other poultry, or pork)
1 cup of cooked brown rice
1 cup of cooked black beans (or pinto beans)
1 cup chopped broccoli

Bedtime snack
1 cup reduced fat Greek yogurt, 1 tbsp honey, and 7 walnut halves (crushed) (add honey and walnuts to yogurt and eat)

TABLE 28.11 Sample Meal Plan When Exercising Before Dinner

Breakfast
20-30 grams protein of a mixed protein powder (whey/casein)
3 whole eggs and 1 tbsp olive oil (scrambled eggs cooked in olive oil)
3 four-inch pancakes and 2 tbsp maple syrup
½ cantaloupe

Late-morning snack
20-30 grams protein of a mixed protein powder (whey/casein)
¼ whole-wheat Boboli crust, ¼ cup light mozzarella cheese, and ¼ cup marinara sauce (add sauce to crust and top with cheese; cook at 400 degrees F for 10-15 min or until cheese is browned)

Lunch
6-inch Subway turkey and ham (double meat) on 9-grain wheat bread
1 bag Baked Lays potato chips
Regular diet soda

Afternoon snack
3 sticks light string cheese
6 cups air-popped popcorn (or bag of low-fat microwave popcorn)

Preworkout 1 (30-45 minutes before workout)
5-10 grams BCAAs
2-5 grams creatine (depending on form)
2-3 grams beta-alanine
20-30 grams protein from a mixed protein powder (whey/casein)
1 large apple

Postworkout (within 30 minutes after workout)
20-40 grams protein from a mixed protein powder (whey/casein)
30-40 grams fast-digesting carbohydrate (dextrose, Pixy Stix, gummy bears, white bread)

5-10 grams BCAAs
2-5 grams creatine (depending on form)
2-3 grams beta-alanine

Dinner (30-60 minutes after postworkout meal)
6 oz. chicken breast (or fish, or lean beef or other poultry, or pork)
1 cup of cooked brown rice
1 cup of cooked black beans (or pinto beans)
1 cup chopped broccoli

Bedtime snack
1 cup reduced fat Greek yogurt, 1 tbsp honey, and 7 walnut halves (crushed) (add honey and walnuts to yogurt and eat)

TABLE 28.12 Sample Meal Plan When Exercising After Dinner

Breakfast
20-30 grams protein of a mixed protein powder (whey/casein)
3 whole eggs and 1 tbsp olive oil (scrambled eggs cooked in olive oil)
3 four-inch pancakes and 2 tbsp maple syrup
½ cantaloupe

Late-morning snack
20-30 grams protein of a mixed protein powder (whey/casein)
¼ whole-wheat Boboli crust, ¼ cup light mozzarella cheese, and ¼ cup marinara sauce (add sauce to crust and top with cheese; cook at 400 degrees F for 10-15 min or until cheese is browned)

Lunch
6-inch Subway turkey and ham (double meat) on 9-grain wheat bread
1 bag Baked Lays potato chips
Regular diet soda

Afternoon snack
3 sticks light string cheese
6 cups air-popped popcorn (or bag of low-fat microwave popcorn)

Dinner
6 oz. chicken breast (or fish, or lean beef or other poultry, or pork)
1 cup of cooked brown rice
1 cup of cooked black beans (or pinto beans)
1 cup chopped broccoli

Preworkout 1 (30-45 minutes before workout)
5-10 grams BCAAs
2-5 grams creatine (depending on form)
2-3 grams beta-alanine
20-30 grams protein from a mixed protein powder (whey/casein)
1 large apple

> continued

TABLE 28.12   Sample Meal Plan When Exercising After Dinner *(continued)*

Postworkout (within 30 minutes after workout)
20-40 grams protein from a mixed protein powder (whey/casein)
30-40 grams fast-digesting carbohydrate (dextrose, Pixy Stix, gummy bears, white bread)
5-10 grams BCAAs
2-5 grams creatine (depending on form)
2-3 grams beta-alanine

Bedtime snack
1 cup reduced fat Greek yogurt, 1 tbsp honey, and 7 walnut halves (crushed) (add honey and walnuts to yogurt and eat)

Step 5: Cut Carbohydrate by 0.25 Gram One Final Time

You can slash carbohydrate once more before you hit the lowest you can go in carbohydrate. After all, you still need vegetables. And although they provide a good deal of fiber, they also provide real net carbohydrate. Some experts recommend not counting carbohydrate from vegetables as part of your daily total of carbohydrate due to the high fiber content of most vegetables. Yet the carbohydrate content of most vegetables is less than 50 percent fiber. So if you're eating a lot of vegetables, this can add up. Instead, I prefer to count even fiber as part of daily carb intake, but realizing that at the lowest point, carb intake will still be a good 30 to 60 grams depending on the diet, or roughly about 0.25 gram per pound of body weight. Small amounts of carbohydrate are also in most protein shakes. And since you need to rely on it to maximize your results in the gym, you'll need to leave room for it in your diet. The bottom line is that at the lowest point, you can never truly get to zero grams of carbohydrate.

Remember that during this phase of the diet, you should definitely include one high-carbohydrate day each week as discussed in step 4. Having this high-carb day to look forward to will make a difference in your ability to tolerate such extremes in dieting.

You can find sample meals for making the final cut in carbohydrate from 0.5 to 0.25 gram per pound of body weight (or 50 grams of carbohydrate total for the 200-pounder) at www.humankinetics.com/products/all-products/Jim-Stoppanis-Encyclopedia-of-Muscle--Strength-2nd-edition. This drops calories to about 10 per pound of body weight or about 2,000 for the 200-pound sample person. Protein and fat stay steady as they have throughout. Remember that these meal plans are based on workout days. On rest days, skip the postworkout meal and have the preworkout meal as a snack.

Step 6: Switch to Intermittent Fasting (IF)

Once you get down to 0.25 gram of carbohydrate per pound of body weight, it's next to impossible to go any lower in carbohydrate. This small amount of carbohydrate is coming from protein sources and vegetables. If you get this low in carbohydrate and hit a plateau, then there is a very good chance that it is because you are at extremely low levels of body fat but want to get even lower. For men, this would be somewhere around 5 percent; for women it is somewhere around 12 percent. To keep losing body fat, you could continue by dropping protein and fat, but that could compromise muscle mass. So an alternative to try first is intermittent fasting.

Intermittent fasting is a technique where you fast for a good portion of the day and then you have a window of time where you can eat. The type of intermittent fasting that I have found to work best for losing body fat and maintaining muscle is 16/8 intermittent fasting. That means that you fast for 16 hours and your feeding window is 8 hours. For the average person, the time of day you fast and the time of day you eat make no difference. However, those who work out should manipulate their fasting and feeding windows based on when they train.

If you train in the morning, then I suggest that you start your 8-hour feeding window with your postworkout meal. That means that you would train completely fasted and your first meal would be your postworkout shake. But since you skipped your preworkout shake, your postworkout shake should include both your pre- and postworkout shakes and supplements. For example, if you train from 7:00 to 8:30 a.m., then your feeding window starts at 8:30 a.m. with your postworkout shake and ends at 4:30 p.m. with your bedtime snack of slow-digesting protein. If you train in the morning, yet ending your feeding window in the late afternoon is too early for you, then you could postpone your postworkout shake by 2 to 3 hours. It's not ideal for maintaining muscle mass, but it certainly will not hamper fat loss. The following sample meal plans in tables 28.13 through 28.16 show you how to apply intermittent fasting for the four main training times throughout the day. And while I suggest that you schedule your fasting and eating around the time you train, you can also adjust the time you train to better match when you want to fast and eat. If you normally train in the morning but find that it's almost impossible for you to fast at night because your cravings are stronger at night, then train later in the day so that you fast in the morning and eat at night.

Intermittent fasting has become increasingly popular in the last few years. However, I have been interested in its application for fat loss for a couple of decades. The lab where I did my postdoctoral at Yale University School of Medicine did a bit of work on fasting and fat loss before 2000. Our group published several papers showing that one of the key mechanisms in fasting-induced fat loss has to do with an increase in the activity of genes that increase the number of calories the body burns (Pilegaard et al. 2003; Hildebrandt et al. 2000). More specifically, when you fast, it turns on genes that encode for certain uncoupling proteins. In simple terms, these uncoupling proteins poke holes in the mitochondria inside muscle cells. The mitochondria are where most of your energy is derived from, especially at rest. By poking holes in the mitochondria, they produce less energy. So they have to burn far more calories to produce the same amount of energy in the form of ATP.

Fasting also works through a number of mechanisms that lead to increased calorie and fat burn and enhanced fat loss. Research also suggest that fasting provides numerous health benefits, such as lower cholesterol and triglyceride levels (Mattson and Wan 2005).

Some proponents claim that IF even benefits muscle building. But this is where I disagree with their logic. There really is no research suggesting that IF benefits muscle growth over a traditional diet. In fact, from my personal experience and the data I've collected over the years, it would appear that IF would limit muscle growth as compared to following the rules covered in chapter 27 for eating to maximize muscle growth.

There is no debating the fact that intermittent fasting works well to enhance fat loss. However, it is not a method of dieting that needs to be used from the get-go. Instead, I recommend using it once

you've hit a plateau and you can no longer lower carbohydrate. Since you want to keep protein and fat as high as possible, IF allows you one more step before you need to start whittling away at those two critical macros to lower calories and continue losing body fat.

The following sample diets in tables 28.13 through 28.16 show how to apply IF based on when you train. You will still consume the same number of calories, grams of protein, carbohydrate, and fat as you did in the prior phase of the diet. You should even consume the same number of meals. Since you are cramming so many meals into an 8-hour time frame, meals will come more frequently than you were eating, maybe an hour or two apart and as soon as 30 minutes in some cases. If you find that you cannot consume this many meals, you can also combine some of them. For example, the snack before dinner is a protein shake and peanut butter. You can have this shake with dinner and enjoy the peanut butter as a dessert.

While you should do your best to consume the same amount of food as your previous diet phase, it is not the end of the world if you simply cannot. This is one of the fringe benefits of IF. You often cannot consume that much food in the 8-hour time window, which lowers calories and aids fat loss. Yet this is also one reason why you should wait until a later stage in your diet to employ IF. If you start it too soon, you may not be able to consume enough food during your feeding window, which will make it hard to drop calories in later stages as your fat loss plateaus.

Although the meals in the sample diets still list breakfast, lunch, and dinner, these meals may not necessarily be consumed at the normal time for that meal. In the sample morning workout, if you finish your workout at 8:00 a.m. and consume your postworkout meal at this time, your feeding window ends at 4:00 p.m. That means that lunch will be some time before noon and dinner would probably be before 3:00 p.m.

You should also continue to include one high-carbohydrate day each week with IF. You can either do the high-carb day as an IF day with an 8-hour feeding window or try eating at any hour of the day to see what works best for you. Some like having the ability to let the IF go for a day when getting their high-carb day. It helps them stay true to their diet during the rest of the week. If that works for you, then use it.

TABLE 28.13 Sample IF Meal Plan When Exercising First Thing in the Morning

During workout (drink during workout)

5-10 grams BCAAs

2-5 grams creatine (depending on form)

2-3 grams beta-alanine

Postworkout (within 30 minutes after workout, which starts your 8-hour eating window)

40-60 grams protein from a mixed protein powder (whey/casein)

5-10 grams BCAAs

2-5 grams creatine (depending on form)

2-3 grams beta-alanine

Breakfast (30 minutes after postworkout meal)

20-30 grams protein of a mixed protein powder (whey/casein)

3 whole eggs, 3 egg whites, and 1 tbsp olive oil (scrambled eggs cooked in olive oil)

Late-morning snack

1 cup low-fat cottage cheese

Lunch

6 oz. can albacore tuna (add tuna to salad)

2 cups mixed green salad

1 tbsp salad dressing (olive oil and vinegar)

Snack

20-30 grams protein of a mixed protein powder (whey/casein)

1 tbsp peanut butter

Dinner

8 oz. steak (or salmon or other fish, or chicken or other poultry, or pork)

2 cups mixed green salad

2 tbsp salad dressing (olive oil and vinegar)

Snack (within 8 hours from when you consumed postworkout meal)

20-30 grams protein from a mixed protein powder (whey/casein) or 1 cup cottage cheese

TABLE 28.14 Sample IF Meal Plan When Exercising at Lunchtime

Preworkout 1 (30 minutes before workout; this starts your 8-hour feeding window)

5-10 grams BCAAs

2-5 grams creatine (depending on form)

2-3 grams beta-alanine

20-30 grams protein from a mixed protein powder (whey/casein)

Postworkout (within 30 minutes after workout)

20-40 grams protein from a mixed protein powder (whey/casein)

5-10 grams BCAAs

2-5 grams creatine (depending on form)

2-3 grams beta-alanine

Breakfast (30-60 minutes after postworkout meal)

20-30 grams protein of a mixed protein powder (whey/casein)

3 whole eggs, 3 egg whites, and 1 tbsp olive oil (scrambled eggs cooked in olive oil)

Late-morning snack

1 cup low-fat cottage cheese

Lunch

6 oz. can albacore tuna (add tuna to salad)

2 cups mixed green salad

1 tbsp salad dressing (olive oil and vinegar)

Afternoon snack

20-30 grams protein of a mixed protein powder (whey/casein)

1 tbsp peanut butter

Dinner

8 oz. steak (or salmon or other fish, or chicken or other poultry, or pork)

2 cups mixed green salad

2 tbsp salad dressing (olive oil and vinegar)

Snack (within 8 hours from preworkout meal)

20-30 grams protein from a mixed protein powder (whey/casein) or 1 cup cottage cheese

TABLE 28.15 Sample IF Meal Plan When Exercising Before Dinner

Breakfast (this starts your 8-hour feeding window so have this 8 hours before you plan on having your last meal)

20-30 grams protein of a mixed protein powder (whey/casein)

3 whole eggs, 3 egg whites, and 1 tbsp olive oil (scrambled eggs cooked in olive oil)

Late-morning snack

1 cup low-fat cottage cheese

Lunch

6 oz. can albacore tuna (add tuna to salad)

2 cups mixed green salad

2 tbsp salad dressing (olive oil and vinegar)

Afternoon snack

20-30 grams protein of a mixed protein powder (whey/casein)

1 tbsp peanut butter

Preworkout 1 (30-45 minutes before workout)

5-10 grams BCAAs

2-5 grams creatine (depending on form)

2-3 grams beta-alanine

20-30 grams protein from a mixed protein powder (whey/casein)

Postworkout (within 30 minutes after workout)

20-40 grams protein from a mixed protein powder (whey/casein)

5-10 grams BCAAs

2-5 grams creatine (depending on form)

2-3 grams beta-alanine

Dinner (30-60 minutes after postworkout meal)
8 oz. steak (or salmon or other fish, or chicken or other poultry, or pork)
2 cups mixed green salad
2 tbsp salad dressing (olive oil and vinegar)
Snack (within 8 hours of breakfast)
20-30 grams protein from a mixed protein powder (whey/casein)
or 1 cup cottage cheese

TABLE 28.16 Sample IF Meal Plan When Exercising After Dinner

Breakfast (this starts your 8-hour feeding window so have this 8 hours before you plan on having your last meal)
20-30 grams protein of a mixed protein powder (whey/casein)
3 whole eggs, 3 egg whites, and 1 tbsp olive oil (scrambled eggs cooked in olive oil)
Late-morning snack
1 cup low-fat cottage cheese
Lunch
6 oz. can albacore tuna (add tuna to salad)
2 cups mixed green salad
2 tbsp salad dressing (olive oil and vinegar)
Snack
20-30 grams protein of a mixed protein powder (whey/casein)
1 tbsp peanut butter
Dinner
8 oz. steak (or salmon or other fish, or chicken or other poultry, or pork)
2 cups mixed green salad
2 tbsp salad dressing (olive oil and vinegar)
Preworkout 1 (30-45 minutes before workout)
5-10 grams BCAAs
2-5 grams creatine (depending on form)
2-3 grams beta-alanine
20-30 grams protein from a mixed protein powder (whey/casein)
Postworkout (within 30 minutes after workout)
20-40 grams protein from a mixed protein powder (whey/casein)
5-10 grams BCAAs
2-5 grams creatine (depending on form)
2-3 grams beta-alanine
Bedtime snack (within 8 hours of breakfast)
20-30 grams protein from a mixed protein powder (whey/casein) or 1 cup cottage cheese

Step 7: Lower Fat and Protein

The low-carbohydrate IF should get you as low in body fat as you ever need to go. However, every body reacts differently. So if you have hit a fat-loss plateau with low-carbohydrate IF, then you will need to adjust your diet yet again. As mentioned, once you are down to 0.25 gram of carbohydrate per pound of body weight, it's fairly impossible to go any lower in carbohydrate without removing vegetables and protein shakes, which you really do not want to do. The only thing left to do now is lower the other macronutrients—fat and protein. This will bring calories down again and allow you to burn more body fat.

So you will cut out some protein shakes, such as with breakfast, and cut out some fat from peanut butter and by reducing the amount of salad dressing you use. This will bring protein intake down to about 1.25 grams per pound of body weight and fat to about 0.25 gram per pound of body weight. And calories will now be just 9 per pound of body weight, or about 1,800 calories total for the 200-pound person.

Of course, you will also continue to employ intermittent fasting to help with fat loss because you are reducing calories through less protein and fat. Be sure to add a high-carbohydrate day, but keep it within the 8-hour feeding window with IF. See tables 28.17 through 28.20.

TABLE 28.17 Sample IF Meal Plan When Exercising First Thing in the Morning

During workout (drink during workout)
5-10 grams BCAAs
2-5 grams creatine (depending on form)
2-3 grams beta-alanine
Postworkout (within 30 minutes after workout, which starts your 8-hour eating window)
40-60 grams protein from a mixed protein powder (whey/casein)
5-10 grams BCAAs
2-5 grams creatine (depending on form)
2-3 grams beta-alanine
Breakfast (30 minutes after postworkout meal)
3 whole eggs, 3 egg whites, and 1 tbsp olive oil (scrambled eggs cooked in olive oil)
Late-morning snack
1 cup low-fat cottage cheese
Lunch
6 oz. can albacore tuna (add tuna to salad)
2 cups mixed green salad
1 tbsp salad dressing (olive oil and vinegar)

> continued

TABLE 28.17 Sample IF Meal Plan When Exercising First Thing in the Morning *(continued)*

Snack
20-30 grams protein of a mixed protein powder (whey/casein)

Dinner
8 oz. steak (or salmon or other fish, or chicken or other poultry, or pork)
2 cups mixed green salad
1 tbsp salad dressing (olive oil and vinegar)

Snack (within 8 hours from when you consumed postworkout meal)
20-30 grams protein from a mixed protein powder (whey/casein) or 1 cup cottage cheese

TABLE 28.18 Sample IF Meal Plan When Exercising at Lunchtime

Preworkout 1 (30 minutes before workout; this starts your 8-hour feeding window)
5-10 grams BCAAs
2-5 grams creatine (depending on form)
2-3 grams beta-alanine
20-30 grams protein from a mixed protein powder (whey/casein)

Postworkout (within 30 minutes after workout)
20-40 grams protein from a mixed protein powder (whey/casein)
5-10 grams BCAAs
2-5 grams creatine (depending on form)
2-3 grams beta-alanine

Breakfast (30-60 minutes after postworkout meal)
3 whole eggs, 3 egg whites, and 1 tbsp olive oil (scrambled eggs cooked in olive oil)

Late-morning snack
1 cup low-fat cottage cheese

Lunch
6 oz. can albacore tuna (add tuna to salad)
2 cups mixed green salad
1 tbsp salad dressing (olive oil and vinegar)

Afternoon snack
20-30 grams protein of a mixed protein powder (whey/casein)

Dinner
8 oz. steak (or salmon or other fish, or chicken or other poultry, or pork)
2 cups mixed green salad
1 tbsp salad dressing (olive oil and vinegar)

Snack (within 8 hours from preworkout meal)
20-30 grams protein from a mixed protein powder (whey/casein) or 1 cup cottage cheese

TABLE 28.19 Sample IF Meal Plan When Exercising Before Dinner

Breakfast (this starts your 8-hour feeding window so have this 8 hours before you plan on having your last meal)
3 whole eggs, 3 egg whites, and 1 tbsp olive oil (scrambled eggs cooked in olive oil)

Late-morning snack
1 cup low-fat cottage cheese

Lunch
6 oz. can albacore tuna (add tuna to salad)
2 cups mixed green salad
2 tbsp salad dressing (olive oil and vinegar)

Afternoon snack
20-30 grams protein of a mixed protein powder (whey/casein)

Preworkout 1 (30-45 minutes before workout)
5-10 grams BCAAs
2-5 grams creatine (depending on form)
2-3 grams beta-alanine
20-30 grams protein from a mixed protein powder (whey/casein)

Postworkout (within 30 minutes after workout)
20-40 grams protein from a mixed protein powder (whey/casein)
5-10 grams BCAAs
2-5 grams creatine (depending on form)
2-3 grams beta-alanine

Dinner (30-60 minutes after postworkout meal)
8 oz. steak (or salmon or other fish, or chicken or other poultry, or pork)
2 cups mixed green salad
1 tbsp salad dressing (olive oil and vinegar)

Snack (within 8 hours of breakfast)
20-30 grams protein from a mixed protein powder (whey/casein) or 1 cup cottage cheese

TABLE 28.20 Sample IF Meal Plan When Exercising After Dinner

Breakfast (this starts your 8-hour feeding window so have this 8 hours before you plan on having your last meal)
3 whole eggs, 3 egg whites, and 1 tbsp olive oil (scrambled eggs cooked in olive oil)

Late-morning snack
1 cup low-fat cottage cheese

Lunch
6 oz. can albacore tuna (add tuna to salad)
2 cups mixed green salad
2 tbsp salad dressing (olive oil and vinegar)

Snack
20-30 grams protein of a mixed protein powder (whey/casein)

Dinner
8 oz. steak (or salmon or other fish, or chicken or other poultry, or pork)
2 cups mixed green salad
1 tbsp salad dressing (olive oil and vinegar)

Preworkout 1 (30-45 minutes before workout)
5-10 grams BCAAs
2-5 grams creatine (depending on form)
2-3 grams beta-alanine
20-30 grams protein from a mixed protein powder (whey/casein)

Postworkout (within 30 minutes after workout)
20-40 grams protein from a mixed protein powder (whey/casein)
5-10 grams BCAAs
2-5 grams creatine (depending on form)
2-3 grams beta-alanine

Bedtime snack (within 8 hours of breakfast)
20-30 grams protein from a mixed protein powder (whey/casein) or 1 cup cottage cheese

Step 8: Drop Protein and Fat Again, If Needed

Step 7 should be the last step that anyone would need to make to reach a goal, even if it is getting to ridiculously low levels of body fat for a fitness or bodybuilding competition or photo shoot. But, as I have said earlier, every body is different, and there is always one person who is an outlier and does not respond as you would expect. So if you have hit a plateau in fat loss and have some more body fat to strip away, then you would simply continue making small reductions in your calories by dropping more fat and protein. You could cut out olive oil completely and use noncaloric cooking spray and just vinegar for salad dressing. And you could reduce your protein meals by about a quarter of the serving size. These small changes will allow you to keep calories slowly dropping while you continue losing fat.

MAINTAINING YOUR NEW LEAN BODY

A common question I get from those dieting down to low levels of body fat is how to maintain that lean body without gaining body fat while trying to build more muscle. It is quite possible to do so if you are very careful and detailed with your diet. You simply can't go back to the way you were eating before you started to get serious with your fat-loss diet. That will lead to rapid fat gain because your metabolism is a bit slower at this moment. Just like reducing carbohydrate and calories was a slow and progressive process, so should be your return to a higher-carb and higher-calorie diet. Simply put, you will reverse the steps that brought you to where you now are.

Your strategy for gaining muscle but not fat will be to slowly move to the step before your current step in the diet process. So if you left off at step 7, then you will move into step 6 of the diet. How long you stay there depends on how your body reacts. I would suggest staying with a diet step no less than two weeks before moving to the next step. Your body will need time to adjust to the higher carbohydrate and caloric intake. It will respond by increasing your metabolic rate, which will allow you to consume more carbohydrate and more calories without adding body fat or at least not adding much body fat. You will likely not be able to maintain the exact amount of body fat that you reached in your final stages of the diet while you are adding carbohydrate and calories. But if you do it slowly enough, a very minimal amount of fat will be added.

If you find that you are gaining fat readily when you move up a step, do some diet cycling. For example, if you are currently at 0.5 gram of carbohydrate per pound of body weight and find that moving up to 0.75 gram of carbohydrate per pound is putting some fat on your physique, then stick with the 0.5 gram for two days and then doing a day of 0.75 gram and then back to 0.5 gram for two days and back to 0.75 gram. Then eventually move to alternating 0.5 gram and 0.75 gram every day. Then eventually move into consuming 0.75 gram of carbohydrate every day.

The nice thing about maintaining your lean physique by slowly increasing carbohydrate and calories is that you can afford to include a real cheat day once per week. So instead of having a "clean" high-carb day once a week where fat is relatively low and you are focusing on low-fat carbohydrate like rice, oatmeal, and popcorn, and you can also include some "dirty" foods like ice cream, doughnuts, and pizza.

Metric Equivalents for Dumbbells and Weight Plates

Following are tables giving conversions for common dumbbell and weight plate increments. For weights not listed here, you can calculate conversions using this equivalent: 1 kilogram = 2.2 pounds.

TABLE A.1 Pound Increments Converted to Kilograms

DUMBBELLS		WEIGHT PLATES	
Pounds	Kilograms	Pounds	Kilograms
5	2.3	2.5	1.1
10	4.5	5	2.3
15	6.8	10	4.5
20	9	25	11.4
25	11.4	35	15.9
30	13.6	45	20.5
35	15.9		
40	18.2		
45	20.5		
50	22.7		

TABLE A.2 Kilogram Increments Converted to Pounds

DUMBBELLS		WEIGHT PLATES	
Kilograms	Pounds	Pounds	Kilograms
2.5	5.5	1.25	2.75
5	11	2.5	5.5
7.5	16.5	5	11
10	22	10	22
12.5	27.5	15	33
15	33	20	44
17.5	38.5	25	55
20	44		
22.5	49.5		
25	55		
30	66		

List of Alternative Foods

In the nutrition chapters of *Jim Stoppani's Encyclopedia of Muscle & Strength* you will notice that the sample meal plans do not offer much variety. This does not mean that you should be eating those exact foods and only those foods. When it comes to nutrition, variety is always best. Yet many people worry that eating a different type of meat for dinner or a different kind of fruit will throw off their diets. In reality, you can replace most foods with similar yet different foods without having it affect your macronutrient and calorie totals much, if at all.

The key to using these diets as templates but replacing the foods with different selections is to choose foods that are of a similar kind and size. For example, if you don't have 8 ounces of top sirloin steak, you can replace it with 8 ounces of chicken or other poultry, fish, or lean pork. If you want to replace a medium apple, you can choose a medium peach or orange or pear. One cup of chopped broccoli can be replaced with one cup of green beans or chopped zucchini or chopped asparagus.

Refer to the following list of food alternatives so that your diet doesn't become boring and lacking in nutrient diversity.

MEAT REPLACEMENTS

The following meats can be used for any meal with the sample diet. You can also replace any meats with about 2 servings of the dairy products listed later or 2 scoops of protein powder:

Chicken breast	Lean ground beef
Chicken thighs	Top sirloin steak
Chicken drumstick	Tri-tip steak
Turkey breast	Flank steak
Turkey leg	Pork tenderloin
Lean ground turkey	Bison

Venison	Shrimp
Ostrich	Crab
Lamb	Scallops (sea or freshwater)
Goat	
Salmon	Clams
Sardines	Mussels
Herring	Oysters
Trout	Lobster
Tilapia	Squid
Cod	Octopus
Halibut	Lean deli turkey breast
Sole or flounder	Lean deli chicken breast
Arctic char	Lean deli ham
	Lean deli roast beef

DAIRY REPLACEMENTS

Unless you are allergic to milk protein or are lactose intolerant, you should consider eating dairy at several meals to maximize muscle growth. Dairy provides a good blend of whey and casein protein, which have been shown to be superior for muscle growth. Each cup (8 oz.) of milk provides about 12 to 15 grams of carbohydrate in addition to 8 grams of protein. So watch your carbohydrate intake if you are lowering carbohydrate.

Greek yogurt

Cottage cheese

Low-fat string cheese

3 slices or ounces of low-fat cheese (such as American, cheddar, Swiss, feta)

1 scoop of protein powder

4-6 oz. of any of the meats listed previously

2 oz. beef jerky

EGG REPLACEMENTS

Unless you are allergic to eggs, I highly recommend that you do not replace the eggs due to the benefits they provide for muscle growth and strength. However, I understand that some people cannot stand eggs, others are allergic, and some just get sick of eating them. So if you must, feel free to replace the eggs with the following:

- 1-2 scoops egg protein
- 1-2 scoops of a milk protein blend (whey/casein)
- 1 serving of the dairy foods listed
- 6 oz. of any of the meats listed

VEGETABLE REPLACEMENTS

These vegetables can replace any vegetables listed in the sample diets.

Mixed green salad	Eggplant
Asparagus	Bok choy (chinese cabbage)
Green beans	
Broccoli	Mushrooms
Cauliflower	Spinach
Onion	Cucumber
Bell peppers	Okra
Brussels sprouts	1 cup prepared stir-fry vegetables
Zucchini	

FRUIT REPLACEMENTS

Replace any of the fruit with any of these:

Apple	1 cup raspberries
Orange	1 cup blackberries
Grapefruit	1 cup cherries
Peach	1 cup grapes
Nectarine	1 cup sliced pineapple
Banana	1 cup sliced watermelon
Pear	
Asian pear	Kiwi fruit
1 cup sliced strawberries	½ small cantaloupe
1 cup blueberries	½ small honey dew melon

CEREAL REPLACEMENTS

While oatmeal makes a great breakfast carbohydrate, you can replace it with any of the following:

- Whole-grain cold cereal (such as Cheerios, Quaker Oat Squares, Kashi)
- Granola
- Whole-wheat waffle
- Whole-wheat or buckwheat pancakes
- Any of the following breads

BREAD REPLACEMENTS

The following breads can be used wherever bread is listed.

Whole-wheat bread	Whole-wheat english muffin
Ezekiel bread	
Rye bread	Whole-wheat pita bread
Sourdough bread	
	Whole-wheat bagel
	Whole-wheat tortilla

GRAIN REPLACEMENTS

While bread and cereal are grains, I separated them according to when they are consumed. Cereals are usually eaten at breakfast or as a snack, and bread is often used at lunch to make sandwiches or as snacks. The grains here are typically eaten at dinner but can be eaten any time of day when grains (breads and cereals included) are listed.

- Brown rice
- Whole-wheat pasta (small amount of marinara sauce)
- 1 cup quinoa
- Any of the following beans listed
- Medium sweet potato

BEAN REPLACEMENTS

The following beans can be used wherever beans are listed or in place of any grains.

Black beans	Lima beans
Pinto beans	Baked beans
Kidney beans	Lentils
Navy beans	Garbanzo beans

GLOSSARY

In every discipline there is a lexicon of common terms that members understand and use. These terms include both formal nomenclature and slang terms that have been established by the community. To better understand the language used in the chapters of this book as well as in the gym, consider the following terms. This collection of terms is not exhaustive; it includes only the definitions that are not found elsewhere in the book or those that need a clearer explanation.

abduction—Movement away from the body such as what occurs when you raise your arm straight out to the side.

abs—A slang term referring to the abdominal muscles.

adduction—Movement of a limb toward the body such as what occurs when your arm is straight out to your side and you lower it down to the side of your body.

adenosine triphosphate (ATP)—The molecular "currency" that provides energy in cells for everything from protein synthesis to muscle contraction.

adipose tissue—Where fat is stored in the body.

advanced weightlifter—A person who has strength-trained steadily and systematically for at least one full year.

aerobic exercise—Prolonged (usually performed for at least 20 minutes continuously), moderate-intensity exercise that uses up oxygen at or below the level at which the cardiorespiratory system can replenish oxygen in the working muscles. Common aerobic exercise activities are walking, jogging, running, cycling, stair climbing, working out on elliptical exercise machines, rowing, swimming, dancing, and aerobic dance classes.

agonist muscle—A muscle responsible for producing a specific movement through concentric muscle action. For example, during the biceps curl exercise, the biceps muscle is the agonist muscle.

anaerobic exercise—Exercise that is higher in intensity than aerobic work. Anaerobic exercise uses up oxygen more quickly than the body can replenish it in the working muscles. Anaerobic exercise uses stored-muscle ATP, phosphocreatine, and glycogen to supply its energy needs. Common anaerobic activities are weightlifting and sprinting.

antagonist muscle—The muscle responsible for actively opposing the concentric muscle action of the agonist muscle. Although this seems counterintuitive, the opposing force is necessary for joint stability during the movement. For example, during the biceps curl exercise, the triceps muscle is the antagonist muscle.

anterior—Anatomical term referring to the front of the body.

assistance exercise—Typically single-joint exercises such as the biceps curl, triceps extension, and deltoid lateral raise. These exercises involve only a single muscle group.

ATP—See *adenosine triphosphate.*

atrophy—Wasting away of any part, organ, tissue, or cell, such as the atrophy of muscle fibers caused by inactivity.

ballistic stretch—This type of muscle stretch involves dynamic muscle action in which the muscles are stretched suddenly in a bouncing movement. A ballistic stretch for the hamstrings might involve touching your toes repeatedly in rapid succession.

basal metabolic rate—The rate at which the body burns calories while awake but at rest (usually measured in calories per day).

beginning weightlifter—A person with less than six months of strength training experience.

belt—See *weight belt.*

bis—A slang term for the biceps muscles.

BMR—See *basal metabolic rate.*

bodybuilding—A type of strength training applied in conjunction with nutritional practices to alter the shape of the body's musculature. The sport of bodybuilding is a competitive sport in amateur and professional categories for males and females.

body fat percentage—The amount of fat in your body, generally expressed as a percentage.

bulking up—To gain body size and mass, preferably muscle tissue.

burn—A slang term for the intense and painful sensation felt in a muscle that has been fatigued by high-rep sets.

cardio—See *aerobic exercise.*

chalk—Also known as magnesium carbonate, it is often used by powerlifters and Olympic lifters to keep the hands dry for a more secure grip on the weights.

cheating—The condition in which strict form is ignored in order to get a few additional reps out of a set. Cheating is not generally recommended because it can lead to injury. However, it can sometimes help a lifter push the muscles beyond muscle failure. An example of cheating would be forcibly swinging the upper body to help complete a standing biceps curl.

compound exercise—An exercise that involves more than one muscle group to perform the exercise. Therefore, movement occurs at more than one joint. For this reason, compound exercises are often called multijoint exercise. These types of exercises are the best choices for developing strength. Examples are the squat, bench press, and barbell row.

cool-down—Low-intensity exercise performed at the end of a high-intensity workout. The purpose of the cool-down is to allow the body's systems (cardiovascular, respiratory, metabolic, and so on) that were used during the workout to gradually return to resting levels.

core—The superficial and deep muscles of the abdominals and low back that stabilize the spine and help to prevent back injuries as well as enhance greater overall strength.

cross-training—Participation in two or more sports or activities that can improve performance in each and help an athlete achieve a higher level of fitness. Examples are strength training and football.

cutting—The process of dieting in an effort to shed all visible body fat to emphasize the individual muscles.

definition—Visibility of the shape and detail of individual muscles. This occurs in people with low body fat.

delayed-onset muscle soreness (DOMS)—Muscle soreness that develops a day or two after a heavy bout of exercise.

delts—A slang term referring to the deltoid muscles.

DOMS—See *delayed-onset muscle soreness.*

dorsiflexion—Moving the top of the foot upward and toward the shin.

EPOC—See *excess postexercise oxygen consumption.*

excess postexercise oxygen consumption (EPOC)—Elevated oxygen consumption above that of resting levels after exercise.

extension—The act of straightening a joint. For example, during the triceps pressdown exercise, the elbow extends. The opposite of extension is flexion.

failure—See *muscle failure.*

false grip—A type of grip in which the thumb remains against the side of the palm rather than wrapped around the bar as in a normal grip.

fast-twitch muscle fibers—Muscle fibers that contract quickly and powerfully but not with great endurance. Fast-twitch muscle fibers are best developed through strength training programs that employ heavy weight and low reps or light weight and low reps that are performed in a quick and explosive manner.

flexibility—Suppleness of joints, muscle fibers, and connective tissues. This suppleness allows a greater range of motion about the joints. Flexibility is an important component of overall fitness and is best developed through systematic stretching.

flexion—The act of bending a joint. For example, during the biceps curl exercise the elbow flexes. The opposite of flexion is extension.

form—Refers to the use of proper biomechanics during an exercise. This means that all movements are performed in such a manner that only the required muscle groups are used during the exercise and all movements are performed in a safe manner to avoid the risk of injury.

GH—See *growth hormone.*

gloves—See *weightlifting gloves.*

glutes—A slang term for the gluteal muscles.

glycogen—The form of carbohydrate stored in the body, predominantly in the muscles and liver.

growth hormone (GH)—An anabolic hormone that stimulates fat metabolism and promotes muscle hypertrophy.

hypertrophy—The scientific term denoting an increase in muscle size.

insertion—The point of attachment of a muscle most distant from the body's midline or center.

intermediate strength trainer—A person with 6 to 12 months of bodybuilding experience.

isolation exercise—An exercise that involves just one muscle group and the movement of the one joint that that muscle group crosses. These types of exercises are sometimes called single-joint exercises. Examples are the dumbbell fly, lateral raise, and leg extension.

knee wrap—A band of elastic fabric that is wound tightly around the knee to support the joint during squats and other heavy leg exercises.

knurling—A grooved or roughened area along the gripping portion of a barbell or dumbbell that lessens the tendency for the hand to slip.

lean body mass—Total body mass minus fat mass; this includes muscle, bone, organs, and water.

lifter—Slang term that refers to a person who regularly strength-trains.

macrocycle—A phase in periodization that typically involves six months to one year but may be up to four years, such as with Olympic athletes.

mass—A term used to refer to muscle size, as in muscle mass.

mesocycle—A phase in periodization usually lasting several weeks to months.

microcycle—A phase in periodization lasting a week.

multijoint exercise—See *compound exercise.*

muscle atrophy—See *atrophy.*

muscle failure—The point during an exercise at which the muscles have fully fatigued and can no longer complete an additional rep of that exercise using strict form.

muscle hypertrophy—See *hypertrophy.*

negative phase of repetition—A term used to describe the eccentric portion of a muscle contraction. Emphasizing the eccentric, or negative, portion of the rep induces greater muscle damage than that caused by the concentric portion of the rep. An example of a negative phase is the lowering of the weight down to the chest during a bench press.

Olympic weightlifting—The type of weightlifting contested at the Olympic Games every four years as well as at national and international competitions each year. Olympic lifting involves two lifts: the snatch and the clean and jerk.

origin—The point of attachment of a muscle closest to the body's midline, or center.

overhand grip—This type of grip, also known as a pronated grip, involves grabbing the bar with the palms down and the knuckles on the front or the top of the bar. An example is the grip used for the reverse barbell curl or shrug.

overreaching—Scientific term used to describe exercise training that pushes the body beyond its limits to recover and adapt. This usually involves training with too much volume, too much intensity, too much frequency, or all of these. Overreaching is the stage that occurs just before the athlete becomes overtrained. If an athlete stops overreaching in time, the athlete can avoid the deleterious effects of overtraining and actually rebound with rapid advances in strength and muscle mass.

overtraining—When an athlete overreaches for too long, he or she reaches the point of overtraining. Chronically exceeding the body's ability to recover by overreaching causes the body to stop progressing and actually lose some of the gains that were made in strength and muscle mass. Besides impairing athletic performance, overtraining can increase the risk of injury or disease. The early signs of overtraining from too much weight include increased resting heart rate, difficulty in sleeping, increased sweating, and altered emotions. The early signs of overtraining from lifting too much volume or too often include decreased resting heart rate, digestion problems, fatigue, and lower blood pressure.

passive stretching—This type of stretching involves having a partner assist in moving joints through their ranges of motion. This allows for a greater range of motion than what can be reached when stretching alone.

peak—The absolute zenith of competitive condition achieved by an athlete.

pecs—A slang term that refers to the pectoralis muscles.

periodization—The systematic manipulation of the acute variables of training over a period that may range from days to years.

phosphocreatine (PCr)—An energy-rich compound that plays a critical role in providing energy for muscle action by maintaining ATP concentration.

plantar flexion—Moving the top of the foot away from the shin, such as when pointing the toes down for heel raises.

positive phase of repetition—The concentric portion of the repetition. Examples of the positive phase include the pressing of the barbell off the chest during the bench press and the curling up of the weight during a barbell curl.

powerlifting—A form of competitive weightlifting that features three lifts: the squat, bench press, and deadlift. Powerlifting is contested both nationally and internationally in a variety of weight and age classes for both men and women.

preexhaust—The use of single-joint exercises before multijoint exercises in an effort to exhaust a particular muscle group so that it becomes the weak link in the multijoint exercise.

primary exercise—An exercise that is most specific to the goals of the lifter. These exercises must involve the muscle groups in which the person is most interested in gaining strength.

pronation—Rotating the wrist inward.

prone—Lying horizontally on the abdomen.

pump—A term commonly used by bodybuilders to refer to the swelling that muscles undergo during a workout. The pump occurs because when muscles contract repeatedly they create metabolic waste products that draw water into the muscle. The greater water volume increases the overall size of the muscle cells. This can lead to temporary increases in total muscle size of one to two inches. The pump typically lasts until the metabolic waste products have been cleared from the muscle.

quads—A slang term referring to the quadriceps muscles on the front thigh.

range of motion (ROM)—The range through which a joint can be moved, usually its range of flexion and extension. Exercises also have a specific range of motion that involves the movement from start to finish.

rep—Slang term for repetition.

repetition—Refers to a single execution of an exercise. For example, if you curl a barbell through the entire range of motion once from start to finish, you have completed one repetition (rep) of the movement.

repetition speed—The length of time it takes to complete one rep.

resistance—The amount of weight used in an exercise. Sometimes referred to as *intensity*.

resting metabolic rate (RMR)—The metabolic rate measured under conditions of rest. This is the minimal number of calories a person will need during a day to maintain body weight.

rest interval—The brief pause lasting between 30 seconds and 2 minutes, and in some cases even longer, which occurs between sets to allow the body to partially recuperate before initiating the succeeding set.

ripped—A term that means a body has clearly visible muscles and very little fat.

routine—A term that refers to an individual training program.

RMR—See *resting metabolic rate*.

set—A group of consecutive repetitions of an exercise that are performed without resting.

single-joint exercise—See *isolation exercise*.

six-pack—A slang term used to refer to defined abdominal muscles. The term is used because most people's abdominal muscles create six bulges (three per side) when they are well developed and body fat levels are low.

slow-twitch muscle fiber—A type of muscle fiber that has high endurance capacity and poor ability to generate quick, powerful contractions.

split routine—A training program in which the body is divided into segments and trained more than three times per week, as most beginners do. The most basic split routine is done four days per week. The most popular type of split routine involves dividing the body into three parts, which are worked over three consecutive days, followed by a rest day and a repeat of the routine on day five. This is called a three-on and one-off split.

spotter—A training partner or a person who gives assistance to a lifter while the lifter is performing an exercise. The purpose of the spotter is to be on hand in case the lifter fails to complete a rep. In this case, the spotter can help the lifter complete the rep, which allows the lifter to train past muscle failure as well as avoid injury on dangerous exercises such as the bench press.

stabilizer muscles—Muscles that assist in the performance of an exercise by steadying the joint or limb being moved but not increasing the force applied to move the weight.

staggered grip—A grip in which the left and right hand have opposite styles of grip. One hand uses an underhand grip while the other uses an overhand grip. This is a common grip used during the deadlift because the alternated gripping allows for stronger grip strength.

static stretch—A low-force, long-duration stretch that holds the desired muscle at the greatest possible length for 20 to 30 seconds.

sticking point—The point in an exercise where the muscle is at its weakest.

striations—Fine grooves or bands on the surface of a muscle. The grooves are caused by the molecular machinery of the muscle fibers that are visible through the skin in ripped bodybuilders.

supination—Rotating the wrist outward.

supine—Lying horizontally on the back.

synergist—A muscle that assists in the performance of an exercise by adding to the force required for executing the movement. For example, the triceps muscle is a synergist to the pectoralis muscles during the bench press exercise.

tendon—A band of dense white fibrous tissue that connects a muscle to a bone. The movement of the bone is produced by the transmission of force from the muscle through the tendon to the bone.

testosterone—The primary natural androgenic and anabolic steroid hormone produced primarily by the testes in the male. It is also produced in smaller quantities by the adrenal glands in both males and females. Testosterone is the hormone responsible for maintenance of muscle mass and strength as well as the development of secondary male sexual characteristics such as a deep voice, body and facial hair, and male pattern baldness.

training log—A log that a lifter keeps for recording workouts. The information recorded usually includes exercises performed, weight used, number of sets performed, number of reps completed per set, amount of rest taken between sets, how the lifter felt during or after exercises, and what the lifter ate before and after the workout. This information helps the lifter assess progress and stay motivated to reach goals.

training partner—A person who trains with you on the majority of your training days.

traps—A slang term for the trapezius muscles.

tris—A slang term referring to the triceps muscles.

underhand grip—The opposite of an overhand grip. The lifter should grip the barbell or dumbbell with the hands under the bar.

vascularity—The visibility of veins through the skin.

volume training—The use of a very high number sets for each bodypart.

warm-up—Before any workout it is important to gradually prepare the body through low-intensity exercise. This helps to get the heart rate elevated so that oxygen uptake and blood flow to muscle tissue are enhanced. It also increases body temperature, which enhances the mobility of joints and the contractibility of muscle fibers. Good warm-up exercises include walking on a treadmill, riding a stationary cycle, doing light calisthenics, and doing lightweight lifting slowly and rhythmically.

washboard abs—a slang term used to describe ripped abs.

weight belt—A wide belt usually made of leather or nylon that is worn tightly around the waist to help support the low back and increase abdominal pressure. This is supposed to help prevent back injury and increase strength. Today it is recommended that belts be worn only during exercise training in which near-maximal weights are being lifted.

weightlifting gloves—Gloves made of leather or synthetic materials are often worn during weightlifting to aid in the grip and prevent calluses from developing on the palms.

working set—The set performed after finishing the warm-up sets.

workout—A single training session.

wrist straps—Strips of material (often canvas, nylon, or leather) that are about 2 inches (5 centimeters) wide and 12 inches (30.5 centimeters) long with a looped end. They are wrapped around the wrist and the bar or handle that the lifter is holding onto to increase grip strength.

wrist wraps—Bands of elastic material that are tightly wrapped around the wrists to support them during heavy lifting or while performing exercises that place a high amount of stress on the wrists.

Ahtiainen, J.P., et al. 2003. Acute hormonal and neuromuscular responses and recovery to forced vs. maximum repetitions multiple resistance exercises. *International Journal of Sports Medicine* 24:410-418.

Altena, T.S., et al. 2003. Effects of continuous and intermittent exercise on postprandial lipemia. *Medicine & Science in Sports and Exercise* (5cSuppl).

Almuzaini, K.S., et al. 1998. Effects of split exercise sessions on excess postexercise oxygen consumption and resting metabolic rate. *Canadian Journal of Applied Physiology* 23(5):433-43.

Arciero, P.J., et al. 2001. Comparison of creatine ingestion and resistance training on energy expenditure and limb blood flow. *Metabolism.* 50(12):1429-1434.

Arul, A. B., et al. 2012. Multivitamin and mineral supplementation in 1,2-dimethylhydrazine induced experimental colon carcinogenesis and evaluation of free radical status, antioxidant potential, and incidence of ACF. *Canadian Journal of Physiology and Pharmacology* 90(1):45-54.

Babraj, J.A., et al. 2009. Extremely short duration high intensity interval training substantially improves insulin action in young healthy males. *BMC Endocrine Disorders* 28;9:3.

Baker, D. and Newton, R.U. 2005. Acute effect on power output of alternating an agonist and antagonist muscle exercise during complex training. *Journal of Strength and Conditioning Research* 19(1):202-205.

Barringer, T. A., et al. 2003. Effect of a multivitamin and mineral supplement on infection and quality of life: a randomized, double-blind, placebo-controlled trial. *Annals of Internal Medicine* 138(5):365-371.

Becque, M.D., et al. 2000. Effects of oral creatine supplementation on muscular strength and body composition. *Medicine & Science in Sports and Exercise* 32(3):654-658.

Blahnik, J. 2011. *Full-body flexibility.* 2nd ed. Champaign, IL: Human Kinetics.

Borg, G.A.V. 1982. Psychophysical bases of perceived exertion. *Medicine and Science in Sports and Exercise* 14:377-381.

Boirie, Y., et al. 1997. Slow and fast dietary proteins differently modulate postprandial protein accretion. *Proceedings of the National Academy of Sciences of the United States of America* 94(26):14930-14935.

Bosco, C., et al. 2000. Hormonal responses to whole-body vibration in men. *European Journal of Applied Physiology* 81:449-454.

Borshein, E. and Bahr, H. 2003. Effect of exercise intensity, duration and mode on postexercise oxygen consumption. *Sports Medicine* 33(14):1037-1060.

Bosse, J. D. and B.M. Dixon. 2012. Dietary protein to maximize resistance training: a review and examination of protein spread and change theories. *Journal of the International Society of Sports Nutrition* 9(1):42.

Boutcher, S.H., et al. 2007. The effect of high intensity intermittent exercise training on autonomic response of premenopausal women. *Medicine & Science in Sports & Exercise* 39(5 suppl):S165.

Breil, F. A., et al. 2010. Block training periodization in alpine skiing: effects of 11-day HIT on $\dot{V}O_2$max and performance. *European Journal of Applied Physiology* 109(6):1077-1086.

Burd, N.A., et al. 2010. Low-load high volume resistance exercise stimulates muscle protein synthesis more than high-load low volume resistance exercise in young men. *PLOS ONE* 5(8):e12033.

Burd, N.A., et al. 2011. Enhanced amino acid sensitivity of myofibrillar protein synthesis persists for up to 24 h after resistance exercise in young men. *Journal of Nutrition* 1;141(4):568-73.

Burke, D. G, et al. 2001. The effect of whey protein supplementation with and without creatine monohydrate combined with resistance training on lean tissue mass and muscle strength. *International Journal of Sport Nutrition and Exercise Metabolism* 11(3):349-364.

Burke, D. G. 2008. Effect of creatine supplementation and resistance-exercise training on muscle insulin-like growth factor in young adults. *International Journal of Sport Nutrition and Exercise Metabolism.* 18(4):389-98.

Cancela, P., et al. 2008. Creatine supplementation does not affect clinical health markers in football players. *British Journal of Sports Medicine* 42(9):731-5.

Candow, D. G., et al. 2006. Effect of whey and soy protein supplementation combined with resistance training in young adults. *International Journal of Sport Nutrition and Exercise Metabolism* 16(3):233-244.

Cribb, P. J., et al. 2007. Effects of whey isolate, creatine, and resistance training on muscle hypertrophy. *Medicine & Science in Sports & Exercise* 39(2):298-307.

Cribb, P. J. and Hayes, A. 2006. Effects of supplement timing and resistance exercise on skeletal muscle hypertrophy. *Medicine & Science in Sports & Exercise* 38(11):1918-25.

Daly, W., et al. 2005. Relationship between stress hormones and testosterone with prolonged endurance exercise. *European Journal of Applied Physiology* 93(4):375-80.

Davis, W.J., et al. 2008. Elimination of delayed-onset muscle soreness by pre-resistance cardioacceleration before each set. *Journal of Strength and Conditioning Research* 22(1):212-25.

Deighton, K., et al. 2012. Appetite, energy intake and resting metabolic responses to 60 min treadmill running performed in a fasted versus a postprandial state. *Appetite* 58(3):946-54.

DeLorme, T.L. 1945. Restoration of muscle power by heavy resistance exercises. *Journal of Bone and Joint Surgery American Volume* 27:645-667.

DeLorme, T.L., and A.L. Watkins. 1948. Techniques of progressive resistance exercise. *Archives of Physical Medicine* 29:263-273.

Donovan, T., et al. 2012. β-alanine improves punch force and frequency in amateur boxers during a simulated contest. *International Journal of Sport Nutrition and Exercise Metabolism* 22(5):331-7.

Drinkwater, E.J., et al. 2004. Repetition failure is a key determinant of strength development in resistance training. *Medicine and Science in Sports and Exercise* 36(5):S53.

Drinkwater, E.J., et al. 2005. Training leading to repetition failure enhances bench press strength gains in elite junior athletes. *Journal of Strength and Conditioning Research* 19(2):382-388.

Earnest, C., et al. 1996. High-performance capillary electrophoresis-pure creatine monohydrate reduces blood lipids in men and women. *Clinical Science* 91(1):113-118.

Ebben, W. P., et al. 2011. Antagonist knockout training increases force and the rate of force development. Annual Meeting of the National Strength & Conditioning Association.

Falvo, M.J., et al. 2005. Effect of loading and rest internal manipulation on mean oxygen consumption during the bench press exercise. *Journal of Strength and Conditioning Research* 19(4):e12.

Farthing, J.P., and P.D. Chilibeck. 2003. The effects of eccentric and concentric training at different velocities on muscle hypertrophy. *European Journal of Physiology* 89(6):578-586.

Fincher, G.E. 2004. The effect of high intensity resistance training on body composition among collegiate football players. *Journal of Strength and Conditioning Research* 18(4):e354.

Fish, D.E., et al. 2003. Optimal resistance training: Comparison of DeLorme with Oxford techniques. *American Journal of Physical Medicine and Rehabilitation* 82:903-909.

Fleck, S.J., and W.J. Kraemer. 2004. *Designing resistance training programs*. 3rd ed. Champaign, IL: Human Kinetics.

Fleck, S.J., and R.C. Schutt. 1985. Types of strength training. *Clinical Sports Medicine* 4:159-168.

Friedmann, B., et al. 2004. Muscular adaptations to computer-guided strength training with eccentric overload. *Acta Physiologica Scandinavica* 182(1):77-88.

Gonzalez, J.T., et al. 2013. Breakfast and exercise contingently affect postprandial metabolism and energy balance in physically active males. *British Journal of Nutrition* 23:1-12.

Gorostiaga, E.M., et al. 1991. Uniqueness of interval and continuous training at the same maintained exercise intensity. *European Journal of Applied Physiology* 63(2):101-107.

Goto, K., et al. 2004. Muscular adaptations to combinations of high- and low-intensity resistance exercises. *Journal of Strength and Conditioning Research* 18(4):730-737.

Goto. K., et al. Inserted rest enhances fat metabolism during and after prolonged exercise. Annual Meeting of the American College of Sports Medicine, 2007.

Greenwood, M., et al. 2003a. Cramping and injury incidence in collegiate football players are reduced by creatine supplementation. *Journal of Athletic Training* 38(3):216-219.

Greenwood, M., et al. 2003b. Creatine supplementation during college football training does not increase the incidence of cramping or injury. *Molecular & Cellular Biochemistry* 244(1-2):83-8.

Hamalainen EK, et al. 1983. Decrease of serum total and free testosterone during a low-fat high-fibre diet. *Journal of Steroid Biochemistry* 18(3):369-70.

Hansen, K., et al. 2005. The effects of exercise on the storage and oxidation of dietary fat. *Sports Medicine* 35:363-373.

Hatle, H., et al. 2014. Effect of 24 sessions of high-intensity aerobic interval training carried out at either high or moderate frequency, a randomized trial. *PLoS ONE* 9(2):e88375.

Hernandez, J.P., et al. 2003. Bilateral index expressions and iEMG activity in older versus young adults. Journals of Gerontology Series A: Biological Sciences and Medical Sciences 58:536-541.

Hildebrandt, A.L., and P.D. Neufer. 2000. Exercise attenuates the fasting-induce transcriptional activation of metabolic genes in skeletal muscle. *American Journal of Physiology—Endocrinology and Metabolism* 278(6):E1078-E1086.

Hoffman, J. R., et al. 2014. β-alanine supplementation improves tactical performance but not cognitive function in combat soldiers. *Journal of the International Society of Sports Nutrition* 10;11(1):15.

Hoffman J. R., et al. 2008. Short-duration beta-alanine supplementation increases training volume and reduces subjective feelings of fatigue in college football players. *Nutrition Research* 28(1):31-5.

Hoffman J. R., et al. 2006. Effect of creatine and beta-alanine supplementation on performance and endocrine responses in strength/power athletes. *International Journal of Sport Nutrition and Exercise Metabolism* 16(4):430-46.

Hoshino, D., et al. 2013. High-intensity interval training increases intrinsic rates of mitochondrial fatty acid oxidation in rat red and white skeletal muscle. *Applied Physiology, Nutrition, and Metabolism* 38(3):326-33.

Issurin, V.B., and G. Tenenbaum. 1999. Acute and residual effects of vibratory stimulation on explosive strength in elite and amateur athletes. *Journal of Sports Science* 17(3):177-182.

Izquierdo, M., et al. 2004. Maximal strength and power, muscle mass, endurance and serum hormones in weightlifters and road cyclists. *Journal of Sports Science* 22(5):465-78.

Kaminsky, L.A., et al. 1990. Effect of split exercise sessions on excess post-exercise oxygen consumption. *British Journal of Sports Medicine* 24(2):95-8.

Kanda, A., et al. 2013. Post-exercise whey protein hydrolysate supplementation induces a greater increase in muscle protein synthesis than its constituent amino acid content. *British Journal of Nutrition* 110(6):981-7.

Kelleher, A., et al. 2010. The metabolic costs of reciprocal supersets vs. traditional resistance exercise in young recreationally active adults. *Journal of Strength and Conditioning Research* 24(4):1043-1051.

Kelly, V. G., and D. G. Jenkins. 1998. Effect of oral creatine supplementation on near-maximal strength and repeated sets of high-intensity bench press exercise. *Journal of Strength & Conditioning Research* 12(2):109-115.

Kerksick, CM, et al. 2006. The effect of protein and amino acid supplementation in performance and training adaptations during ten weeks of resistance training. *Journal of Strength and Conditioning Research* 20(3):643–653.

King, J.W. 2001. *A comparison of the effects of interval training vs. continuous training on weight loss and body composition in obese pre-menopausal women* (thesis). East Tennessee State University.

Knuttgen, H.G., and W.J. Kraemer. 1987. Terminology and measurement in exercise performance. *Journal of Applied Sport Science Research* 1:1010.

Kraemer, W.J. 2003. Strength training basics: Designing workouts to meet patients' goals. *Physician and Sportsmedicine* 31(8).

Kraemer, W.J., et al. 2006.The effects of amino acid supplementation on hormonal responses to resistance training overreaching. *Metabolism* 55(3):282-291.

Kraemer, W.J., et al. 2003. Physiological changes with periodized resistance training in women tennis players. *Medicine and Science in Sports Exercise* 35(1):157-68.

Kraemer, W.J., et al. 2002. American College of Sports Medicine position stand: Progression models in resistance training for healthy adults. *Medicine and Science in Sports and Exercise* 34(2):364-380.

Kraemer, W.J., et al. 2000. Influence of resistance training volume and periodization on physiological and performance adaptations in collegiate women tennis players. *American Journal of Sports Medicine* 28(5):626-633.

Kraemer, W.J., et al. 1996. Strength and power training: Physiological mechanisms of adaptation. In *Exercise and Sport Sciences Reviews*, ed. J.O. Holoszy, 363-398. Baltimore: Williams & Wilkins.

Kreider, R. B., et al. 2003. Long-term creatine supplementation does not significantly affect clinical markers of health in athletes. *Molecular and Cellular Biochemistry* 244(1-2):95-104.

Leosdottir, M., et al. 2005. Dietary fat intake and early mortality patterns - data from The Malmo Diet and Cancer Study. *Journal of Internal Medicine* 258(2):153-65.

Li, K., et al. 2012. Vitamin/mineral supplementation and cancer, cardiovascular, and all-cause mortality in a German prospective cohort (EPIC-Heidelberg). *European Journal of Nutrition* 51(4):407-13.

Lugaresi, R., et al. 2013. Does long-term creatine supplementation impair kidney function in resistance-trained individuals consuming a high-protein diet? *Journal of the International Society of Sports Nutrition* 10(1):26.

Macpherson, R.E.K., et al. 2011. Run sprint interval training improves aerobic performance but not maximal cardiac output. *Medicine and Science in Sports and Exercise* 43(1):115-122.

Marx, J.O., et al. 2001. Low-volume circuit versus high-volume periodized resistance training in women. *Medicine and Science in Sports Exercise* 33(4):635-643.

Mattson, M. P. and Wan, R. 2005. Beneficial effects of intermittent fasting and caloric restriction on the cardiovascular and cerebrovascular systems. *Journal of Nutritional Biochemistry* 16(3):129-37.

Mayhew, D. L., et al. 2002. Effects of long-term creatine supplementation on liver and kidney functions in American college football players. *International Journal of Sport Nutrition and Exercise Metabolism*. 12(4):453-60.

Mazzetti, S., et al. 2007. Effect of explosive versus slow contractions and exercise intensity on energy expenditure. *Medicine & Science in Sports & Exercise* 39(8):1291-1301.

Meuret, J.R., et al. 2007. A comparison of the effects of continuous aerobic, intermittent aerobic, and resistance exercise on resting metabolic rate at 12 and 21 hours post-exercise. *Medicine & Science in Sports & Exercise* 39(5 suppl):S247.

Mirela, V., et al. 2009. Continuous versus intermittent aerobic exercise intermittent in the treatment of obesity. 6th European Sports Medicine Congress.

Mitchell, C.J., et al. 2012. Resistance exercise load does not determine training-mediated hypertrophic gains in young men. *Journal of Applied Physiology* 113(1):71-7.

Moore, D. R., et al. 2012. Daytime pattern of post-exercise protein intake affects whole-body protein turnover in resistance-trained males. *Nutrition & Metabolism (Lond)* 9(1):91.

Noonan, D., et al. 1998. Effects of varying dosages of oral creatine relative to fat free body mass on strength and body composition. *Journal of Strength & Conditioning Research* 12(2):104-108.

Nosaka, K. and Newton, M. Repeated eccentric exercise bouts do not exacerbate muscle damage and repair. *Journal of Strength & Conditioning Research* 16(1):117–122, 2002.

Olsen, S., et al. 2006. Creatine supplementation augments the increase in satellite cell and myonuclei number in human skeletal muscle induced by strength training. *Journal of Physiology.* 573(Pt 2):525-34.

O'Shea, P. 1966. Effects of selected weight training programs on the development of strength and muscle hypertrophy. *Research Quarterly* 37:95-102.

Paoli, A., et al. 2009. The effect of stance width on the electromyographical acitivity of eight superficial thigh muscles during back squat with different bar loads. biomechanical comparison of back and front squats in healthy trained individuals. *Journal of Strength & Conditioning Research* 23(1):246-250.

Park, Y. et al. 2010. Intakes of vitamins A, C, and E and use of multiple vitamin supplements and risk of colon cancer: a pooled analysis of prospective cohort studies. *Cancer Causes Control* 21(11):1745-57.

Paton, C.D., et al. 2009. Effects of low- vs. high-cadence interval training on cycling performance. *Journal of Strength and Conditioning Research* 23(6):1758–1763.

Pearson, D., A. Faigenbaum, M. Conley, and W.J. Kraemer. 2000. The National Strength and Conditioning Association's basic guidelines for the resistance training of athletes. *Strength and Conditioning Journal* 22(4):14-27.

Peters, U., et al. 2007. Serum selenium and risk of prostate cancer-anested case-control study. *The American Journal of Clinical Nutrition* 85(1):209-217.

Pilegaard, H., et al. 2003. Effect of short-term fasting and refeeding on transcriptional regulation of metabolic genes in human skeletal muscle. *Diabetes* 52:657-662.

Pocobelli, G., et al. 2009. Use of supplements of multivitamins, vitamin C, and vitamin E in relation to mortality. *American Journal of Epidemiology* 170(4):472-83.

Poortmans, J. R., and M. Francaux. 1999. Long-term oral creatine supplementation does not impair renal function in healthy athletes. *Medicine and Science in Sports and Exercise* 31:1108-1110.

Poortmans, J. R., et al. 1997. Effect of short-term creatine supplementation on renal responses in men. *European Journal of Applied Physiology* 76:566-567.

Pullinen, T., et al. 2002. Hormonal responses to a resistance exercise performed under the influence of delayed-onset muscle soreness. *Journal of Strength & Conditioning Research* 16(3):383–389.

Racil, G., et al. 2013. Effects of high vs. moderate exercise intensity during interval training on lipids and adiponectin levels in obese young females. *European Journal of Applied Physiology* 113(10):2531-40. doi: 10.1007/s00421-013-2689-5. Epub 2013 Jul 4.

Ratamess, N.A., et al. 2003. The effects of amino acid supplementation on muscular performance during resistance training overreaching. *Journal of Strength and Conditioning Research* 17(2):250-258.

Ratamess, N.A., et al. 2007. The effect of rest interval length on metabolic responses to the bench press exercise. *European Journal of Applied Physiology* 100(1):1-17.

Rautiainen, S., et al. 2010. Multivitamin use and the risk of myocardial infarction: a population-based cohort of Swedish women. *American Journal of Clinical Nutrition* 92(5):1251-6.

Rawson, E. S. and Volek, J. S. 2003. Effects of creatine supplementation and resistance training on muscle strength and weightlifting performance. *Journal of Strength & Conditioning Research* 17(4):822-31.

Reed M.J., et al. 1987. Dietary lipids: an additional regulator of plasma levels of sex hormone binding globulin. *Journal of Clinical Endocrinology & Metabolism* 64(5):1083-85.

Reidy, P.T. et al. 2014. Soy-dairy protein blend and whey protein ingestion after resistance exercise increases amino acid transport and transporter expression in human skeletal muscle. *Journal of Applied Physiology* 116(11):1353-64.

Reidy, P. T., et al. 2013. Protein blend ingestion following resistance exercise promotes human muscle protein synthesis. *Journal of Nutrition* 143(4):410-416.

Rhea, M.R., and B.L. Alderman. 2004. A meta-analysis of periodized versus nonperiodized strength and power training programs. *Research Quarterly for Exercise and Sport* 75(4):413-422.

Rhea, M.R., et al. 2002. A comparison of linear and daily undulating periodized programs with equated volume and intensity for strength. *Journal of Strength and Conditioning Research* 16(2):250-255.

Rhea, M.R., et al. 2003. A comparison of linear and daily undulating periodized programs with equated volume and intensity for local muscular endurance. *Journal of Strength and Conditioning Research* 17(1):82-87.

Robbins, D. W., et al. 2010. The effect of an upper-body agonist-antagonist resistance training protocol on volume load and efficiency. *Journal of Strength and Conditioning Research* 24(10):2632-40.

Robertson, R.J. 2004. *Perceived exertion for practitioners*. Champaign, IL: Human Kinetics.

Robertson, R.J., et al. 2003. Concurrent validation of the OMNI perceived exertion scale for resistance exercise. *Medicine and Science in Sports and Exercise* 35(2):333-341.

Saremi, A., et al. 2010. Effects of oral creatine and resistance training on serum myostatin and GASP-1. *Molecular and Cellular Endocrinology* 317(1-2):25-30.

Sartor, F., et al. 2010. High-intensity exercise and carbohydrate-reduced energy-restricted diet in obese individuals. *European Journal of Applied Physiology* 110(5):893-903.

Scalzo, R.L. et al. 2014. Greater muscle protein synthesis and mitochondrial biogenesis in males compared with females during sprint interval training. *FASEB Journal.* 28(6):2705-2714.

Selye, H.A. 1936. Syndrome produced by diverse nocuous agents. *Nature* 138:32.

Sijie, T., et al. 2012. High intensity interval exercise training in overweight young women. *Journal of Sports Medicine and Physical Fitness* 52(3):255-62.

Smith, G.I., et al. 2011. Omega-3 polyunsaturated fatty acids augment the muscle protein anabolic response to hyperinsulinaemia-hyperaminoacidaemia in healthy young and middle-aged men and women. *Clinical Science* 121(6):267-278.

Smith, A.E., et al. 2009. Effects of β-alanine supplementation and high-intensity interval training on endurance performance and body composition in men: A double-blind trial. *Journal of the International Society of Sports Nutrition* 6:5.

Soop, M., et al. 2012. Coingestion of whey protein and casein in a mixed meal: demonstration of a more sustained anabolic effect of casein. *American Journal of Physiology—Endocrinology and Metabolism* 303(1):E152-62.

Souza-Junior, T.P., et al. 2011. Strength and hypertrophy responses to constant and decreasing rest intervals in trained men using creatine supplementation. *Journal of the International Society of Sports Nutrition 8:17.*

Springer, B.L., and P.M. Clarkson. 2003. Two cases of exertional rhabdomyolysis precipitated by personal trainers. *Medicine and Science in Sports and Exercise* 35(9):1499-1502.

Stone, W.J., and S.P. Coulter. 1994. Strength/endurance effects from three resistance training protocols with women. *Journal of Strength and Conditioning Research* 8:134-139.

Stone, M.H., et al. 1996. Training to muscle failure: Is it necessary? *Strength and Conditioning Journal* 10(1):44-48.

Tabata, I. et al. 1996. Effects of moderate-intensity endurance and high-intensity intermittent training on anaerobic capacity and $\dot{V}O_2$max. *Medicine and Science in Sports and Exercise* 28(10):1327-30.

Tabata, I., et al. 1997. Metabolic profile of high intensity intermittent exercises. *Medicine and Science in Sports and Exercise.* 29(3):390-5.

Talanian, J.L. et al. 2010. Exercise training increases sarcolemmal and mitochondrial fatty acid transport proteins in human skeletal muscle. *American Journal of Physiology—Endocrinology and Metabolism* 299(2):E180-8.

Talanian, J.L. et al. 2007. Two weeks of high-intensity aerobic interval training increases the capacity for fat oxidation during exercise in women. *Journal of Applied Physiology* 102(4):1439-1447.

Tanisho, K., and K. Hirakawa. 2009. Training effects of endurance capacity in maximal intermittent exercise: Comparison between continuous and interval training. *Journal of Strength and Conditioning Research* 23(8):2405-2410.

Taylor, K., et al. Warm-up affects diurnal variation in power output. *International Journal of Sports Medicine* 32(3):185-189, 2011.

Tjonna, A.E., et al. 2007. Superior cardiovascular effect of interval training versus moderate exercise in patients with metabolic syndrome. *Medicine & Science in Sports & Exercise* 39(5 suppl):S112.

Tower, D.E., et al. 2005. National Strength and Conditioning Associations Annual Meeting, Las Vegas.

Trapp, E.G. 2008. The effects of high-intensity intermittent exercise training on fat loss and fasting insulin levels of young women. *International Journal of Obesity* 32(4):684-91.

Trapp, E. G. and Boutcher, S. 2007. Metabolic response of trained and untrained women during high-intensity intermittent cycle exercise. *American Journal of Physiology—Regulatory, Integrative, and Comparative Physiology* 293(6):R2370-5.

Tremblay, A., et al. 1994. Impact of exercise intensity on body fatness and skeletal muscle metabolism. *Metabolism.* 43(7):814-8.

Treuth, M.S. et al. 1996. Effects of exercise intensity on 24-h energy expenditure and substrate oxidation. *Medicine & Science in Sports & Exercise* 28(9):1138-1143.

Vandenberghe, K., et al. 1997. Long-term creatine intake is beneficial to muscle performance during resistance training. *Journal of Applied Physiology.* 83:2055-2063.

Weiss, L.W., et al. 1999. Differential functional adaptations to short-term low-, moderate- and high-repetition weight training. *Journal of Strength and Conditioning Research* 13:236-241.

Willis, F.B., et al. 2009. Frequency of exercise for body fat loss: A controlled, cohort study. *Journal of Strength and Conditioning Research* 23(8):2377-2380.

Willoughby, D.S. 1993. The effect of meso-cycle-length weight training programs involving periodization and partially equated volumes on upper and lower body strength. *Journal of Strength and Conditioning Research* 7:2-8.

Witard, O. C., et al. 2011. Effect of increased dietary protein on tolerance to intensified training. *Medicine & Science in Sports & Exercise* 43(4):598-607.

Yarrow, J. F., et al., "Neuroendocrine responses to an acute bout of eccentric-enhanced resistance exercise," *Medicine & Science in Sports & Exercise*, 39(6):941-47, 2007.

Ziemann, E. et al. 2011. Aerobic and anaerobic changes with high-intensity interval training in active college-aged men. *Journal of Strength and Conditioning Research* 25(4):1104-12.

INDEX

Note: The italicized *f* and *t* following page numbers refer to figures and tables, respectively.

Jim Stoppani, PhD, received his doctorate in exercise physiology with a minor in biochemistry from the University of Connecticut. After graduation, he served as a postdoctoral research fellow in the prestigious John B. Pierce Laboratory and department of cellular and molecular physiology at Yale University School of Medicine, where he investigated the effects of exercise and diet on gene regulation in muscle tissue. For his ground-breaking research he was awarded the Gatorade Beginning Investigator in Exercise Science Award in 2002 by the American Physiological Society. From 2002 to 2013 Stoppani was senior science editor for *Muscle & Fitness*, *Muscle & Fitness Hers,* and *Flex* magazines. He is currently the owner of JYM Supplement Science and jimstoppani.com.

Stoppani has written thousands of articles on exercise, nutrition, and health. He is coauthor of the *New York Times* best-seller *LL Cool J's Platinum 360 Diet and Lifestyle* (Rodale, 2010) as well as *Stronger Arms & Upper Body* (Human Kinetics, 2009) and *PrayFit* (Regal, 2010). He is also coauthor of the chapter "Nutritional Needs of Strength/Power Athletes" in the textbook *Essentials of Sports Nutrition and Supplements* (Humana Press, 2008). Dr. Stoppani is the creator of the popular training and nutrition programs Shortcut to Size and Shortcut to Shred, as seen on bodybuilding.com. Dr. Stoppani has been the personal nutrition and health consultant for numerous celebrity clients such as LL Cool J, Dr. Dre, Mario Lopez, and Chris Pine.

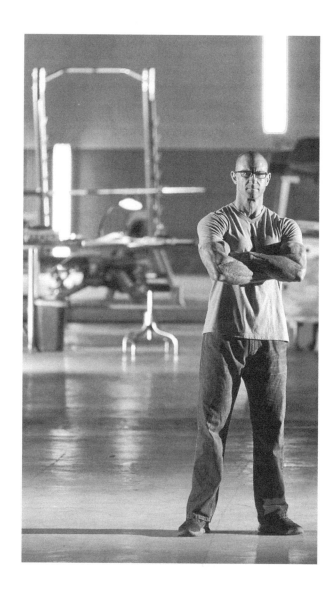